Emerging Trends in IoT and Computing Technologies

About the Conference

A 'Second International Conference of Emerging Trends in IoT and Computing Technologies' (ICEICT 2023) is an inventive event organized with motive to make available an open international forum for the researches, academicians, technocrats, scientist engineers, industrialist and students around the globe to exchange their innovations and share the research outcomes which may lead the young researchers, academicians and industrialist to contribute to the global society.

The conference was inaugurated with auspicious Saraswati vandana, garlanding and lamp lighting of Maa Saraswati. The inaugural function was attended by Chief Guest Prof. (Dr.) J. P. Pandey - Hon'ble Vice Chancellor AKTU, Guest of Honour Dr. Dharmendra Singh Yadav - Sr. Director (IT), Scientist-F, National Informatics Centre (NIC), New Delhi, India, Prof. (Dr.) Yogendra Narain Singh - Director, REC, Pratapgarh, Prof. (Dr.) Rajeev Srivastava - IIT BHU, Dr. Satish Kumar Singh -IIIT, Allahabad, Prof.(Dr.) Gaurav Bansal - University of Wisconsin-Green Bay USA, Dr. Veronika Berdnikova -University of Dodoma, Tanzania, Prof. (Dr.) Celestine Lwendi - University of Bolton, UK, Prof. (Dr.) Victor Chang - Aston University, Birmingham, United Kingdom, Dr. Siddharth Chaurasia - Head AI, AI Cloud- Life Science and Health Care business, Tata Consultancy Services, Mr. Dipan Sahu - Assistant Innovation Director MoE, Innovation Cell, Dr. Seethalekshmi K. - Dean PG & R, AKTU, Institute of Engineering and Technology, Lucknow (U.P.), India, Prof (Dr.) Xin-She Yang - Middlesex University, London, United Kingdom, Dr. Anup Shukla - IIT, Jammu, Prof (Dr.) Farhan Sabir Ujager - De Monfort University, United Kingdom, Prof. (Dr.) Rishi Asthana- Director GITM, Dr. Devendra Agarwal - Dean Academic GITM, Dr Anita Pal – Head of Department CSE and all heads from different departments of GITM with faculty members.

The inaugural ceremony was preceded with the felicitation of honourable dignitaries. The Convener of ICEICT-2023, Dr. Anita Pal began the session by delivering introductory speech about the conference. The session was preceded with inspirational words by Chief Patron and inviting Chief guest Er. Mahesh Agarwal - Chairman, Goel Group of Institutions who insisted that constant updation of technical knowledge in new research areas is necessary for the academic growth of oneself. After that the souvenir of the conference ICEICT-2023 was released. The inaugural session was continued with valuable words by all present dignitaries and concluded by vote of thanks by Prof. (Dr.) Devendra Agarwal - Dean Academic GITM, who expressed his gratitude to everyone for being part of this grand intellectual gathering.

The conference closed with the valedictory session. The valedictory session start by sharing the valuable words from our chief guests Dr. Siddharth Chaurasia - Head AI, AI Cloud- Life Science and Health Care business, Tata Consultancy Services, Mr. Dipan Sahu - Assistant Innovation Director MoE, Innovation Cell, Dr. Seethalekshmi K. - Dean PG & R, AKTU, Institute of Engineering and Technology, Lucknow (U.P.), India. After that the glimpsing of ICEICT-2023 souvenir was released. The session was followed by keynote talks Prof. (Dr.) Xin-She Yang - Middlesex University, London and Dr. Anup Shukla - IIT, Jammu. The summary of two days conference and vote of thanks was presented by the Prof. (Dr.) Devendra Agarwal - Professor & Dean, GITM.

Emerging Trends in IoT and Computing Technologies

Proceedings of Second International Conference on
Emerging Trends in IoT and Computing Technologies – 2023 (ICEICT-2023),
Goel Institute of Technology & Management Lucknow, India

Edtitors

Suman Lata Tripathi

Lovely Professional University,
Jalandhar, India

Devendra Agarwal

Goel Institute of Technology & Management
Lucknow, India

Anita Pal

Goel Institute of Technology & Management
Lucknow, India

Yusuf Perwej

Goel Institute of Technology & Management
Lucknow, India

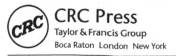

CRC Press

Taylor & Francis Group
Boca Raton London New York

CRC Press is an imprint of the
Taylor & Francis Group, an **informa** business

First edition published 2025
by CRC Press
4 Park Square, Milton Park, Abingdon, Oxon, OX14 4RN

and by CRC Press
2385 NW Executive Center Drive, Suite 320, Boca Raton FL 33431

British Library Cataloguing-in-Publication Data
A catalogue record for this book is available from the British Library

ISBN: 978-1-032-87924-6 (pbk)
ISBN: 978-1-003-53542-3 (ebk)

DOI: 10.1201/9781003535423

Typeset in Times LT Std
by Aditiinfosystems

Contents

List of Figures

Emerging Trends in IoT and Computing Technologies – Suman Lata Tripathi et al. (eds)
© 2024 Taylor & Francis Group, London, ISBN 978-1-032-87924-6

Emerging Trends in IoT and Computing Technologies – Suman Lata Tripathi et al. (eds)
© 2024 Taylor & Francis Group, London, ISBN 978-1-032-87924-6

List of Tables

Emerging Trends in IoT and Computing Technologies – Suman Lata Tripathi et al. (eds)
© 2024 Taylor & Francis Group, London, ISBN 978-1-032-87924-6

Introduction

Second International Conference on Emerging Trends in IOT and Computing Technologies (ICEICT – 2023) is organised with a vision to address the various issues to promote the creation of intelligent solution for the future. It is expected that researchers will bring new prospects for collaboration across disciplines and gain ideas facilitating novel concepts. Second International Conference of Emerging Trends in IoT and Computer Technologies (ICEICT-2023) is an inventive event organised in Goel Institute of Technology and Management, Lucknow, India, with motive to make available an open International forum for the researches, academicians, technocrats, scientist, engineers, industrialist and students around the globe to exchange their innovations and share the research outcomes which may lead the young researchers, academicians and industrialist to contribute to the global society. The conference ICEICT- 2023 is being organised at Goel Institute of Technology and Management, Lucknow, Uttar Pradesh, during 12-13 January 2024. It will feature world-class keynote speakers, special sessions, along with the regular/oral paper presentations. The conference welcomes paper submissions from researcher, practitioners, academicians and students will cover numerous tracks in the field of Computer Science and Engineering and associated research areas.

Programme Committee

Emerging Trends in IoT and Computing Technologies – Suman Lata Tripathi et al. (eds)
© 2024 Taylor & Francis Group, London, ISBN 978-1-032-87924-6

Organizing Committee of Second ICEICT-2023

Chief Patron

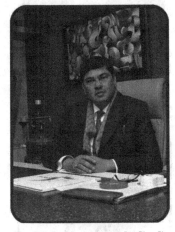

Er. Mahesh Agarwal (Goel)

Chairman, Goel Group of Institutions

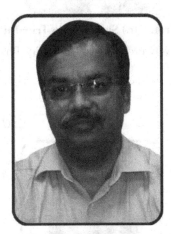

Prof. (Dr.) J.P. Pandey

Vice Chancellor, Dr. A P J Abdul Kalam Technical University

Patron

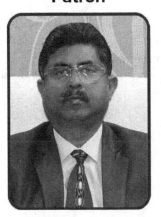

Dr. Rishi Asthana

Director, Goel Institute of Technology & Management, Lucknow, India

Chief-Editors of ICEICT-2023

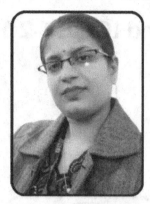

Prof. (Dr.) Suman Lata Tripathi

Professor, Lovely Professional University, Phagwar, India

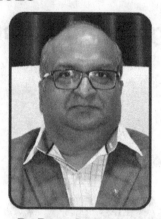

Dr. Devendra Agarwal

Professor & Dean, Goel Institute of Technology & Management, Lucknow, India

Editors of ICEICT-2023

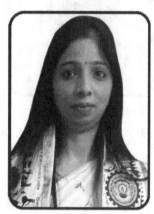

Dr. Anita Pal

HOD CSE, Goel Institute of Technology & Management, Lucknow, India

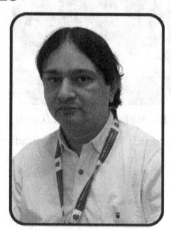

Dr. Yusuf Parwej

Professor CSE, Goel Institute of Technology & Management, Lucknow, India

Guest of Honour of ICEICT-2023

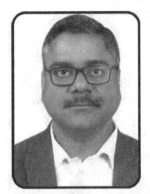

Prof. (Dr.) Rajeev Srivastava

IIT- Banaras Hindu University, Varanasi, India

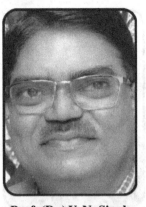

Prof. (Dr.) Y. N. Singh

Rajkiya Engineering College, Pratapgarh, India

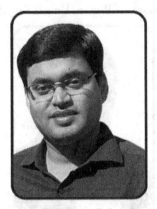

Mr. Dipan Sahu

Assistant Innovation Director, MoE, Innovation Cell, New Delhi, India

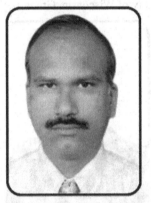

Dr. Dharmendra Singh Yadav

Sr. Director (IT), Scientist-F, The National Informatics Centre, New Delhi, India

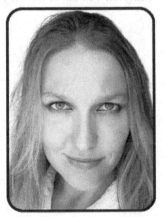

Dr. Veronika Berdnikova

University of Dodoma, Tanzania

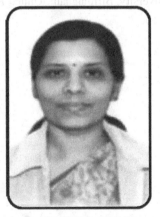

Dr. Seethalekshmi K

Dean PG & R, Dr A P J AKTU, India

Keynote Speaker of ICEICT-2023

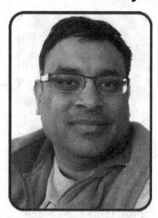

Prof. (Dr.) Gaurav Bansal

University of Wisconsin, Green Bay, USA

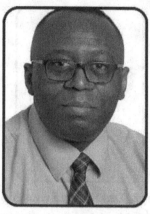

Prof. (Dr.) Celestine Iwendi

University of Bolton, United Kingdom

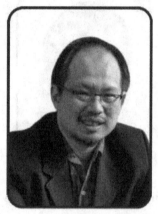

Prof. (Dr.) Victor Chang

Aston University, Birmingham, United Kingdom

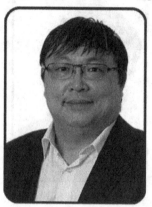

Prof. (Dr.) Xin-she Yang

Middlesex University, London, United Kingdom

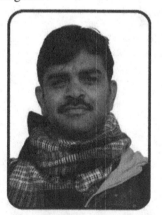

Dr. Anup Shukla

Indian Institute of Technology, Jammu, India

Session Chairs of ICEICT-2023

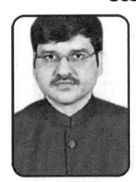

Dr. Arun Kumar Singh

Rajkiya Engineering College, Kannauj, India

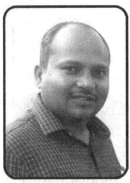

Dr. Vipin Chandra Pal

National Institute of Technology, Silchar, India

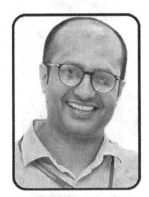

Dr. Aleem Ali

Chandigarh University, India

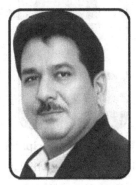

Dr. Ihtiram Raza Khan

Jamia Hamdard University, New Delhi, India

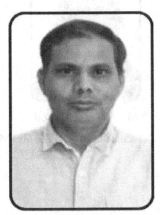

Dr. Natthan Singh

Institute of Engineering & Technology, Lucknow, India

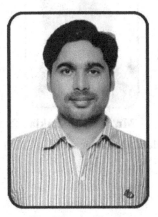

Dr. Bharat Singh

National Institute of Technology, Ranchi, India

Steering Committee of ICEICT-2023

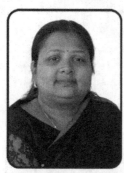

Dr. Jyoti Agarwal

HoD, Department of Management, GITM

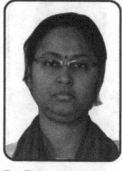

Dr. Priyanka Jaiswal

HoD, Department of EEE, GITM

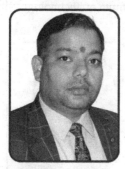

Mr. Shiv Kumar Tripathi

HoD, Department of ME, GITM

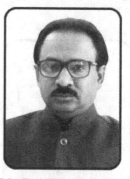

Mr. Raj Kumar Gupta

HoD, Department of CE, GITM

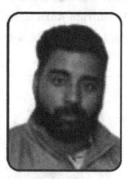

Mr. Shivam Shukla

HoD, Department of IT, GITM

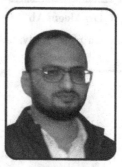

Mr. Ahsan Masood

HoD, Department of BTE, GITM

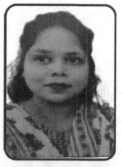

Dr. Nikhat Akhtar

Associate Professor CSE, GITM

Coordinators of ICEICT-2023

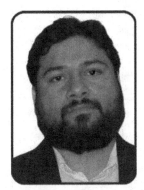

Dr. Piyush Pal

Associate Professor, ME, GITM

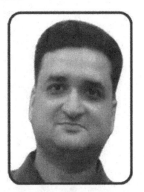

Mr. Peeyush Kumar Pathak

Asstt. Professor, CSE, GITM

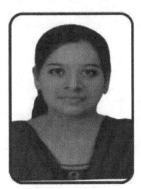

Ms. Namita Srivastava

Asstt. Professor CSE, GITM

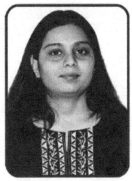

Ms. Prachi Yadav

Asstt. Professor CSE, GITM

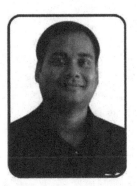

Mr. Dileep Kumar Gupta

Asstt. Professor CSE, GITM

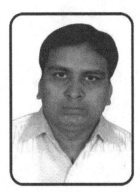

Mr. Kumar Bibhuti Bhusan Singh

Asstt. Professor CSE, GITM

Emerging Trends in IoT and Computing Technologies – Suman Lata Tripathi et al. (eds)
© 2024 Taylor & Francis Group, London, ISBN 978-1-032-87924-6

Sentiment Analysis Based on NLP Using Machine Learning Techniques

Jaishree Jain[1], Shashank Sahu[2]

Ajay Kumar Garg Engineering College,
Department of Computer Science & Engineering, Ghaziabad, India

Neeta Sahu[3]

Ajay Kumar Garg Institute of Management, Ghaziabad, India

Abstract: The most popular platform for sharing people's opinions on many subjects is social media. Machine learning is used in sentiment analysis, and without any human intervention, the machine will provide an accurate sentiment of the populace. Text can be classified as good, negative, or neutral via sentiment analysis. Therefore, any business, foundation, or movie critic is free to solicit public opinion and act accordingly. The growth of social networking has made the Internet a promising platform for online learning, idea exchange, and opinion voicing. A significant amount of sentiment data may be found on social media in the form of tweets, blogs, status updates, postings, etc. SVM, Random Forest, and Naive Bayes are just a few of the machine learning methods covered in this article for sentiment analysis. Experimental analyses demonstrate the effectiveness and superior accuracy and speed of the suggested machine learning classifiers.

Keywords: Machine learning, Sentimental analysis, SVM, Naïve Bayes, Social media

1. Introduction

Machines learn to analyze human emotion autonomously, without human input or intervention. Social media is a commonplace aspect of modern life. Expedia Canada demonstrates how widely and well sentiment analysis is used. Canadians utilize sentiment analysis to their advantage when they notice that their audience dislikes the music that is being played on their television station. Expedia is able to take advantage of a critical comment rather than ignore it by airing fresh, soulful music on their channel.

Sentimental analysis involves computing whether the writers' opinions or attitudes are good, negative, or neutral. Sentiment analysis is another name for data mining. Determining the sentimental analysis is crucial in many domains, including business, politics, and public affairs. In the context of business, it is highly helpful to comprehend the feelings of the client in order to grow the business. In politics, next: It can even be used to forecast the outcome of an election. There are two different classification methods: lexicon-based classification and machine learning classification. Since most politicians, well-known people and even average people routinely tweet about their feelings; emotional analysis using machine learning classifiers is used in this study.

1.1 Analysis of Sentiment Levels

(a) *Document level:* The entire document is subjected to document level analysis. An individual topic-focused paper is included in this level of classification. Customers have the idea that it is impossible to compare two themes or two papers at the document level.

[1]jaishree3112@gmail.com, [2]sahushashank75@gmail.com, [3]nsahu@akgim.edu.in

DOI: 10.1201/9781003535423-1

(b) *Sentence level:* Sentence level is strongly related to subjectivity classification. Sentence level sentiment analysis uses all of the classifier from document level sentiment analysis.

(c) *Aspect level:* Let's use the phrase "My car has good handling but it is a little heavy" as an example. In this instance, the opinion of the weight of the car is contrary to that regarding the handling of the car. The competitive statement is a result of a sentiment analysis at the aspect level.

(d) *Phrase level:* These both have advantages and disadvantages since advantages are found in places where the exact opinion of the subject is present. However, there is a contextual polarity issue that puts results at risk of being inaccurate.

(e) *Level of Feature:* Product characteristics are distinguishing features. Document feature level sentiment analysis is the study of these features to detect feelings.

1.2 Sentiment Analysis in Practice

(a) *Monitoring market research:* To determine what new products have entered the market and what consumers demand. You can adjust your business plan in light of that analysis.

(b) *To see the competition:* To see what your competitors are launching or which product they put into the market. To study the competitor's strategy according to people's opinion.

(c) *Product Analysis:* To learn what people think of the product after it has been released or to see reactions you have never seen before. You may quickly assess a product review by searching the term for a certain characteristic of the product.

(d) *Social media monitoring:* You can simply track people's sentiment on different points of view by using sentiment analysis and a keyword search.

(e) *Customer comments:* The most crucial aspect of any market or organization is customer feedback. A corporation can quickly see user reviews of a product by applying sentiment analysis, and based on those reviews, make modifications to the product.

1.3 Advantages of Sentiment Analysis

(a) Less expensive than assistance for customer insight.

(b) It is the quickest method of gathering customer insight data.

(c) Making use of sentiment analysis will make it simple to implement client suggestions.

(d) Finding a company's or organization's strengths or shortcomings will get much simpler.

(e) Consumer feedback will be more reliable.

2. Background

2.1 Sentimental Examination

These days, social media is among the best channels for communication. Nowadays, a company or organisation must be able to understand the feelings of its customers (Govindarajan) [1]. Sentiment analysis, also referred to as opinion mining, is a technique for evaluating the degree of positivity or negativity in an author's or user's viewpoint on a given subject. Sentiment analysis is the practice of utilizing natural processing techniques to extract relevant features and semantics from text in order to ascertain the writer's attitude, which can be either positive, negative, or neutral (Aggarwal et al.) [2]. Since sentiment analysis classifies opinionated writings as either positive or negative based on polarity—it can also be neutral—the dataset's class range is not limited to only positive or negative, either wonderful or terrible, or agreed upon or disagreed upon. According to Aggarwal et al., you can rate it from strongly disagree, disagree, agree, or strongly agree on a scale of 1 to 5 [3]. Singh et al., for instance, used sentiment analysis to analyze reviews of US and European vacation spots, whose ratings varied from 1 to 5 [4]. In order to create a lexicon corresponding sentiment values (Pak et al.) the three more that follows [5]. The Yelp dataset was subjected to machine learning techniques in (Ingle et al.) [6]. It comprises service provider ratings on a 1 to 5 scale. The following sections outline the three steps of sentiment analysis classification.

2.2 Sentiment Analysis Levels

Twitter is one well-known social media site that gets a sizable number of tweets each day. This data can be used for government, social, industrial, and economic techniques by arranging and assessing the tweets according to our demands (Rodreguj et al.)

[7]. The study (Sahayak) covered a model for sentiment extraction from Twitter, a popular microblogging site where users express their opinions about everything [8]. The sentiment is identified at the document level and is present across the whole document or record. Documentation is needed to extract overall emotion from lengthy texts with noise and repetitive local patterns Kamal et al [9]. Reflecting the composition of documents by considering the most difficult component of document-level sentiment classification considering the relationships between words and sentences in addition to the general context of the semantic information (Mukhtar et al.) [10]. It requires a more thorough comprehension of the complex structural makeup of dependent words and emotions (Nasim et al.) [11].Sentiment analysis determines opinion at the aspect level about a particular characteristic or aspect. For instance, this device has a fast CPU speed in spite of its expensive price. Here, there are two factors or viewpoints: cost and speed. Speed is an explicit component because it is stated in the statement, but cost is an implicit factor. A technique for determining how frequently an aspect co-occurs with feature indicator was proposed by (Hammad et al.) by leveraging the connection between opinionated words and explicit aspects [12].

As was previously indicated, academics employ terminology that differs in a few areas quite regularly. Polarity plays a more significant role in emotion recognition than sentiment analysis when it comes to identifying the emotional, psychological, or mood state. Sentiment analysis is more subjective, but emotion identification is more precise and objective.

2.3 Recognizing Emotions

These feelings affect how people make decisions and improve our ability to communicate with others. Emotion identification from text is challenging, but some bodily behaviors like heart rate, hand trembling, perspiration, and vocal pitch can also reveal a emotional state of an individual (Ahmad et al.) [13]. Additionally, complicating the task of identifying emotions from text are the many uncertainties and frequently introduced new terms. Furthermore, according to Senevirathne et al., emotion recognition tends to go beyond only recognising the three basic psychological states (happy, sad, and furious), often reaching a 6- or 8-scale [14].Sentiment analysis has only been the subject of two deep learning-based studies, and both of them only examined document-level sentiment analysis for the binary case. Tusar et al. used just three different kinds of deep learning models in their research [15]. This study goes much further into the use of more recent, cutting-edge models,

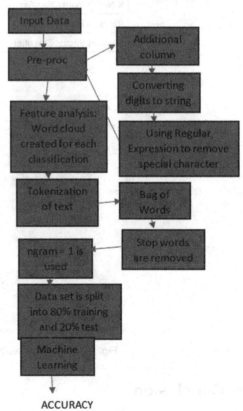

such as capsule networks and hierarchical attention hybrid neural networks in addition to more traditional sequence models such as Bi-LSTM, LSTM, and RNN (Brummerloh et al.) [16]. Using sentiment analysis, we categorise the images according to appropriate posture. Customer satisfaction is currently one of the top goals for corporate growth. Companies are devoting substantial financial and human resources to a range of strategies aimed at understanding and meeting the needs of their customers. Presumably, the text on the page where the picture appears either agrees or disagrees (positive emotion) with a particular position on a contentious issue.

3. Proposed Work

Sentiment analysis is a natural language processing (NLP) technique used to find out the sentiment information expressed in text. It determines sentiment or emotional tone conveyed by sentences for understanding the attitudes or emotions of the speaker.

It uses natural language processing concepts. A twitter dataset has been taken from Kaggle. It consists of four columns: id, information, type and text. The column 'type' has four classifications as mentioned above. It will be used as predicted value. The proposed model uses various machine learning algorithms classifiers. Figure 1.1 shows the architecture of proposed model:

(a) *Input Data:* Total number of rows in the dataset is 74682. Column id has tweet 'id'. Column 'information' provides the brand information for which tweet is there. Column 'type' provides the information sensitivity type like positive, negation etc. And column 'text' consists of tweets.

Fig. 1.1 Proposed architecture

(b) *Pre-Processing:* As dataset consists of four columns, an additional column is created named 'lower'. This column is needed to pre-process the data of the column 'text' into string format and remove the special characters from the text. This pre-processing is needed for machine learning algorithm to learn the data accurately.

(c) *Feature analysis:* For feature analysis of the data, word cloud is created for each sensitive classification. As mentioned, there are four sentiments are considered in the model, which are positive, negative, irrelevant and neutral. The four word clouds have been created using word cloud python library. Feature analysis shows that there more tweets for neutral, then tweets are related to negative classification.

(d) *Tokenization:* Tokenization is used for dataset to find out unique identification symbols that presents in the text. There are more than 30 thousand unique words in the dataset. Bag of words is constructed using ngram = 1.

(e) *Splitting the dataset:* Data set have been divided into training and testing data, in which 80% of training data and 20% test data is considered.

4. Results and Analysis

The experiments are performed in an Intel i5 processor with 8GB RAM and windows 11 operating system. Goggle Colab is used for executing the machine learning algorithms. The result of model shows that Logistics Regression has 83.34% accuracy, Decision Tree Classifier has 82.25%, K Neighbors Classifier has 85.76% accuracy, Random Forest Classifier has 90.98% and Support Vector Classifier has 84.01%. The highest accuracy is achieved by Random Forest Classifier.

Table 1.1 Accuracy of various machine learning algorithms

Machine Learning Classifiers	Accuracy
Logistic Regression	83.34
Decision Tree Classifier	82.25
K Neighbours Classifier	85.76
Random Forest Classifier	90.98
Support Vector Classifier	84.01

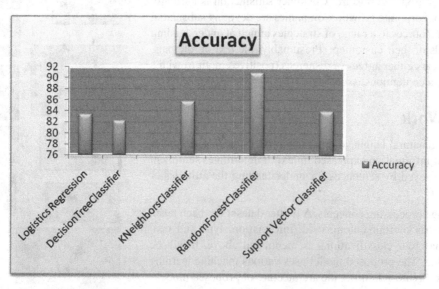

Fig. 1.2 Result of sentiment analysis of twitter tweets using various classifiers

5. Conclusion

The ability to extract emotion using sentiment analysis has become essential for many companies and even individuals. A relatively new but rapidly expanding aspect of decision-making is sentiment analysis. Since people have started sharing their opinions online, there is a greater need than ever for opinionated online content analysis for a range of useful applications. The literature has a vast amount of research on text sentiment detection. Still, these current attitudes may use a great deal of improvement. The Random Forest Classifier outperforms the other machine learning algorithms in terms of accuracy, according to the experiment analysis.

REFERENCES

1. Govindarajan, M. (2013). Sentiment analysis of movie reviews using hybrid method of naive bayes and genetic algorithm. International Journal of Advanced Computer Research, 3(4), 139.
2. Agarwal, A., Xie, B., Vovsha, I., Rambow, O., & Passonneau, R. J. (2011, June). Sentiment analysis of twitter data. In Proceedings of the workshop on language in social media (LSM 2011) (pp. 30–38).
3. Agarwal, A., & Sabharwal, J. (2012, December). End-to-end sentiment analysis of twitter data. In Proceedings of the Workshop on Information Extraction and Entity Analytics on Social Media Data (pp. 39–44).
4. Singh, V. K., Piryani, R., Uddin, A., &Waila, P. (2013, March). Sentiment analysis of movie reviews: A new feature-based heuristic for aspect-level sentiment classification. In 2013 International mutli-conference on automation, computing, communication, control and compressed sensing (imac4s) (pp. 712–717). IEEE.
5. Pak, A., &Paroubek, P. (2010, May). Twitter as a corpus for sentiment analysis and opinion mining. In LREc (Vol. 10, No. 2010, pp. 1320–1326).
6. Ingle, A., Kante, A., Samak, S., & Kumari, A. (2015). Sentiment analysis of twitter data using hadoop. International Journal of Engineering Research and General Science, 3(6), 144–147.
7. Rodrigues, A. P., Rao, A., & Chiplunkar, N. N. (2017, December). Sentiment analysis of real time Twitter data using big data approach. In 2017 2nd International conference on computational systems and information technology for sustainable solution (CSITSS) (pp. 1–6). IEEE.
8. Sahayak, V., Shete, V., & Pathan, A. (2015). Sentiment analysis on twitter data. International Journal of Innovative Research in Advanced Engineering (IJIRAE), 2(1), 178–183.
9. Kamal, A., &Abulaish, M. (2013, August). Statistical features identification for sentiment analysis using machine learning techniques. In 2013 International Symposium on Computational and Business Intelligence (pp. 178–181). IEEE.
10. Mukhtar, N., & Khan, M. A. (2018). Urdu sentiment analysis using supervised machine learning approach. International Journal of Pattern Recognition and Artificial Intelligence, 32(02), 1851001.
11. Nasim, Z., Rajput, Q., & Haider, S. (2017, July). Sentiment analysis of student feedback using machine learning and lexicon based approaches. In 2017 international conference on research and innovation in information systems (ICRIIS) (pp. 1–6). IEEE.
12. Hammad, M., & Al-Awadi, M. (2016). Sentiment analysis for arabic reviews in social networks using machine learning. In Information Technology: New Generations: 13th International Conference on Information Technology (pp. 131–139). Springer International Publishing.
13. Ahmad, M., Aftab, S., & Ali, I. (2017). Sentiment analysis of tweets using svm. Int. J. Comput. Appl, 177(5), 25–29.
14. Senevirathne, L., Demotte, P., Karunanayake, B., Munasinghe, U., & Ranathunga, S. (2020). Sentiment analysis for sinhala language using deep learning techniques. arXiv preprint arXiv:2011.07280.
15. Tusar, M. T. H. K., & Islam, M. T. (2021, September). A comparative study of sentiment analysis using NLP and different machine learning techniques on US airline Twitter data. In 2021 International Conference on Electronics, Communications and Information Technology (ICECIT) (pp. 1–4). IEEE.
16. Brummerloh, T., Carnot, M. L., Lange, S., &Pfänder, G. (2022). Boromir at Touché 2022: Combining natural language processing and machine learning techniques for image retrieval for arguments. Working Notes Papers of the CLEF.

Emerging Trends in IoT and Computing Technologies – Suman Lata Tripathi et al. (eds)
© 2024 Taylor & Francis Group, London, ISBN 978-1-032-87924-6

Detection of Counterfeit Currency

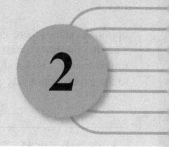

Angotu saida[1]

Department of ECE KG Reddy College of Engineering & Technology, Hyderabad, India

Mirza Sajid Ali Baig[2]

Department of ECE Vidya Joythi Institute of Technology Aziznagar, Hyderabad, India

Ch. Sreedhar[3]

Department of ECE AVN Institute of Engineering and Technology Ranga reddy, Hyderabad, India

Madugula Ramesh[4]

Department of ECE AVN Institute of Engineering and Technology Ranga reddy, Hyderabad, India

Rikkala Spoorti[5]

Department of ECE KG Reddy College of Engineering and Technology, Hyderabad, India

Kuruvenla Kaveri[6]

Department of ECE KG Reddy College of Engineering & Technology, Hyderabad, India

Abstract: Regarding counterfeit currency, we've got a new trick up our sleeves: UV light and clever computers. Here's the deal: real money often has hidden marks that only appear under UV light. But fakes need help to copy them. So, we use special UV LED lights to make these secret marks pop out. When we shine the light on money, it's like revealing a hidden message. But that's not all. We take pictures of the money under this light. Then, intelligent computer programs kick in. They're like super detectives with an eye for detail. They analyze the pictures and look for authentic money patterns that fakes can't replicate. It's like catching a fake red-handed. Why is this cool? Because it's faster and better than old methods, it's like having a quick and reliable way to tell real money from fakes, especially in busy places like stores. Ultimately, using UV light and intelligent computers is a genius move to fight fake money. By showing us hidden patterns and letting computers think, we're one step ahead of those trying to mess with our money. And as this idea grows, it could be a game-changer for keeping our cash safe.

Keywords: Counterfeit currency, UV LED, Image processing, Deep learning, Security features

1. Introduction

Financial systems worldwide continue to face a severe threat from counterfeit money, necessitating the development of effective and trustworthy detection techniques. The suggested UV LED system has use cases in the banking, retail, and law enforcement industries, among other sectors. Banks can improve their currency verification systems and ensure the quick identification of fake banknotes while conducting cash-handling activities by integrating UV LED technology into the detection process.

[1]angotusaida2@gmail.com, [2]mirjasir@gmail.com, [3]sridhar.ch@avniet.ac.in, [4]madugularamesh5@gmail.com, [5]spoorthi1061@gmail.com, [6]kaverikurvindla9030@gmail.com

DOI: 10.1201/9781003535423-2

Similarly, retail establishments can swiftly reduce the risk of accepting counterfeit money by using UV LED-equipped devices at point-of-sale terminals to authenticate banknotes. By examining the UV-induced features on seized currency, helping to find counterfeiters, and interfering with their activities, law enforcement organizations can also use this technology to support investigations.

2. Problem Statement

Fake currency in India was detected in 6.9% of reserve banks and 93.1% of other banks. Most people need help identifying counterfeit currency notes [2]. This phoney currency is 500, 2000 notes. The culprit places the fake notes between bunches of many actual notes. In this busy world, people cannot check each note. People cannot give it to the bank for replacement, too. In such situations, we reluctantly accept the loss. Most of the time, people doing small business will encounter this problem because they need help to afford machines that detect fake notes due to high costs.

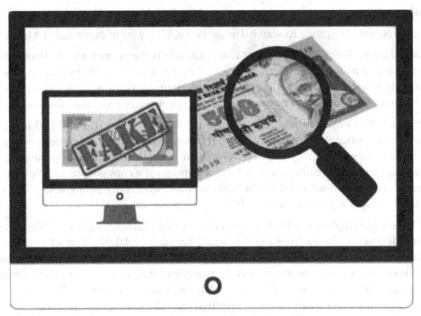

Fig. 2.1 Fake note identification [3]

2.1 Problem Scoping

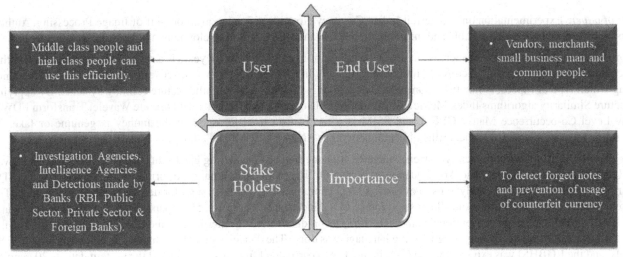

Fig. 2.2 Problem scoping

3. Literature Survey

Title of the paper: Fake money identification system for Bharath notes using picture refining methods. Author: Dr. D. Regan, SK Saajid Rehman, N Hari Babu, T Naveen Kumar, T Subhash, P Sai. Published in: Journal of Emerging Technologies and Innovative Research (JETIR), Year of publish: April 2019. The usage and distribution of counterfeit cash poses serious risks to a country's capacity to maintain its economic stability. With the help of digital image processing algorithms, counterfeit money use is now being reduced digitally. The printing of fake currency is done with the highest level of accuracy possible. Therefore, it is challenging to identify phony currency through basic visual inspection, and here is where the application of digital image processing techniques becomes crucial. Both the chemical characteristics of the cash and its physical appearance can be used as potential detection methods. The methodology used in this study is based on how the Indian money actually looks. For example, intaglio printing (RBI logo), discriminating proof imprint and security thread, which are recognized as security highlights of Indian currency, have been exposed using image processing algorithms [4].

Title of the paper: A study on Indian fake currency detection. Author: Devid Kumar, Surendra Singh Chauhan.

Published in: International Journal of Creative Research Thoughts (IJCRT), Year of publishes: 3 March 2020.

The identification of counterfeit currency is a significant issue that affects the economies of almost every country, including India. One of the important concerns being examined in today's world is the use of phony money. Due to the forgers' use of significantly ground-breaking innovation, they are becoming increasingly difficult to track down. One of the most effective methods to stop forging is to use fake location programming, which is both effectively available and skilled [5].

Title of paper: A Review of Fake Currency Recognition Methods, Author: Sruthy R, Published in: IRJET, Year of publish: July 2022. The world economy is susceptible to money fraud. It is now typical due to advancements in printing and scanning technology. The detection of counterfeit money is a severe problem for both individuals and businesses. For counterfeiters, producing fake banknotes that can hardly be distinguished from real money is a constant process. Several conventional methods and techniques based on colors, widths, and serial numbers are available to identify phony notes. This essay explores various image processing techniques for spotting fraudulent cash [6].

Title of the paper: Real Time counterfeit money identification using Deep Learning, Author: V. Vijayaraghavan, M. Laavanya, published in: International Journal of Engineering and Advanced Technology IJEAT, Year of publish: December 2019. The scanning and printing industries' significant technology evolution contributed to the counterfeiting issues accelerated growth. Therefore, counterfeit money has an impact on the society economy and further down the value of currency, because of this finding counterfeit money is highest importance. The most of the previous technology rely on hardware image processing technical methods. These techniques approaches are less effective and take more effort to detect fake money. The suggested utilizing deep convolutional artificial technology to detect counterfeit cash in order to resolve the foregoing issue, through analysis of the money photos, our approach detects counterfeit money. The web is prepared to recognize deceptive currencies in concurrent. The suggested method takes effectively and in less time identifies forgeries of the 2000, 500, 200, and 50 currencies [7].

Title of paper: Experimentation on counterfeit Indian Currency Note identification avail oneself of Image Processing, Author: Miss. I. Irulappasamy Santhiya Published in: International Journal of Scientific Development and Research.

Year of publish: March 2021. The increase in everyday transactions in India last few years is a reflection of several factors that have contributed to the growth of currency transactions in daily life. This article how to discover the counterfeit Indian money along which type of rupees, is functioned and elucidated along with by considering the picture refining systems. By applying Structure Similarity algorithms Index Metric SSIM, Adaptive histogram equalization, Fast Discrete Wavelet Transform FDWT, Gray Level Co-occurrence Matrix GLCM and SSIM is a mechanism used to ascertain the money is genuine or fake. To determine the note's currency value, artificial neural networks (ANNs), GLCM, and additional FDWT are used [8].

Title of paper: A Counterfeit Fiduciary Currency identification method by considering UV Light based on LVQ, Author: Dewan to Harjun Wibowo, Sri Hartati, and Aris Budanov, published in: International Journal on Informatics for Development (IJID), Year of publishes: 2012. This study aims to evaluate a LVQ neural network-based system for detecting fake paper money. The system's input image is an ultraviolet-fluorescent image of a dancer made out of Rs. 50 in paper money. Data about fiduciary currency has extracted from conventional banks. The LVQ technique is used to determine or the Fiduciary Currency test is not original. Using a visual the coding, programming language was done. The dancer tested object had features measuring 114×90 pixels, and the RGBHSI was extracted as the LVQ input. The experimental findings indicate that the system detects 20 genuine test case data with a 100% accuracy rate and 22 simulated test case data with a 96% accuracy rate. The brightness of the picture message was changed to produce the simulated case data. Ten actual paper bills and ten counterfeit bills are included in the real test case data. 11 genuine paper bills and 11 fake bills are included in the simulated case data. The method works well with the following settings: Learning Rate = 0.01 and Max Posh = 10 [9].

Title of paper: UV counterfeit currency detector. Author: Mark Dobbs, Jeffrey Kelsoe, Dwight Haas. Published in: United States Patent Dobbs et al, Year of publish: May 11, 2010. An ultraviolet (UV) detector that uses UV light and white light back lighting to detect and confirm the authenticity of papers that are placed within, in addition to detector housing, the UV detector has a viewing room with an observing mirror installed inside for examining papers. For adding papers into the viewing room next to the viewing glass, the identifier housing also has a document insertion slot. The detector housing also has an LED container that can carry more LEDS. This spring of UV light illuminates the observing chamber, viewing mirror, and documents, allowing for the identification of UV-activated characteristics on the data. The identifier housing also has translucent and an LED component inside it that emits diffuse visible white light that can be used to detect watermarks on papers [10].

4. Methodology

Key characteristics of UV LEDs include:

Wavelength Range:

Between visible light and X-rays, there is a wavelength spectrum called UV light. UV LEDs have the ability to emit light in variety of UV wavelength ranges, which are commonly diverge into UVA (315–400 nm), UVB (280–315 nm) & UVC (100–280 nm). These price points each have various applications and impacts on materials. EFFICIENCY and Longevity, Compact Size, Specificity, Safety Considerations and Cost

Faking invisible dyes on fake currency notes: It's difficult to simulate invisible colors on false cash notes. Genuine money notes frequently have invisible security dyes applied to them to prevent counterfeiting. Although some dyes are undetectable under regular daylight, they can be found utilizing specialized tools or methods. It is difficult to fake invisible dyes for the following reasons. Specialized materials, Manufacturing processes, Authentication methods, Evolving security measures, Ultraviolet (UV) light, Fluorescence, UV and currency Detection

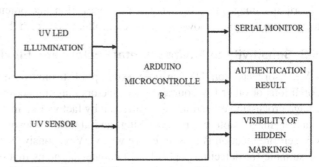

Fig. 2.3 Counterfeit currency detection using IoT technique

How fluorescence works: The process of fluorescence involves several steps, Absorption: UV photons are absorbed by fluorescent molecules in the ink, causing them to move from a lower energy state to an excited state. Excitation state: The molecules have extra energy in the excited state. The molecules swiftly release a photon of visible light as they revert to their lower energy ground state in order to remove the extra energy.

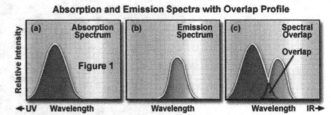

Fig. 2.4 Absorption and emission spectra with overlap profile [13].

Serial monitor: For real-time and dynamic interaction with Arduino projects, the serial monitor is a crucial tool. The serial monitor offers a view into the internal workings of the Arduino board and considerably facilitates the development process, whether testing code, debugging, or monitoring sensor readings.

Hardware and software components: Arduino UNO, UV LED, DC Power supply, Jumper wires (Male to male and Male to female wires), Bread board, 470 Ohms resistor, Software: Arduino IDE v 1 works, Python

5. Result and Discussion

Comparative analysis between UV sensor detection and image processing detection in the context of counterfeit note detection can help us understand their strengths, limitations and suitability for different scenarios. Here is a comparison between UV sensor detection and image processing detection.

5.1 Principle of Operation and Detection Accuracy

UV sensor detection: UV sensors measure the intensity of ultraviolet light, which can be used as a feature to differentiate between genuine and counterfeit currency notes. UV security features, such as fluorescent inks or threads, are often present in natural notes and emit distinctive UV patterns. Image processing detection: Image processing techniques involve analysing the visual features and patterns present in images of currency notes. These features can include watermarks, security threats, micro printing or specific patterns unique to genuine notes. UV sensors can accurately measure the UV index or the presence of UV-responsive security features. However, more than UV detection is required to detect all types of counterfeit notes, especially those without UV features or more sophisticated counterfeits. Image processing detection: A wider variety of fake notes can be found using image processing techniques since they can analyze a variety of visual attributes. However, the accuracy of image processing detection pivots on the quality of the images and the complexity of the counterfeit notes. The sophistication of image processing algorithms employed.

5.2 Complexity of Implementation

UV Sensor Detection: Implementing UV sensor detection with Arduino or similar platforms is relatively straightforward. It involves connecting the UV sensor to the Arduino board, reading the UV index, or analysing the UV-responsive features. Image Processing Detection: Image processing detection can be more complex and resource-intensive. It requires computer vision algorithms, image pre-processing, feature extraction, and potentially machine learning techniques. This typically involves using a computer or a more powerful microcontroller to perform the necessary image-processing tasks.

5.3 Sensitivity to Environmental Factors and Flexibility and Adaptability

UV Sensor Detection: UV sensors are susceptible to environmental factors affecting UV light intensity, such as ambient lighting conditions or other UV sources. These factors may impact the accuracy of UV-based detection. Image Processing Detection: Image processing detection can be affected by factors like image quality, lighting conditions, noise, and complex backgrounds. Careful image capture, pre-processing, and algorithm design are necessary to mitigate these factors. UV Sensor Detection: UV sensor detection is most effective when UV-responsive security features are present on genuine currency notes. It may not be suitable for detecting sophisticated counterfeit notes that do not rely on UV features. Image Processing Detection: Image processing detection can be more versatile and adaptable. It allows for analysing multiple visual features and can be updated or modified to accommodate new counterfeit techniques or security features.

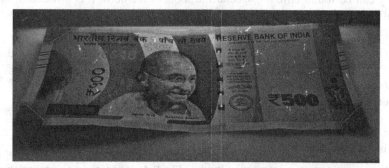

Fig. 2.5 Indication of hidden marks on genuine currency notes under UV rays

In summary, UV sensor detection is straightforward and can provide accurate results when UV features are present on genuine currency notes, as shown in Fig. 2.5. Image processing detection offers more versatility, enabling analysis of various visual features, but requires more computational resources and expertise. Combining UV sensor detection and image processing techniques can enhance counterfeit note detection systems' detection accuracy and robustness.

6. Conclusion

The project effectively demonstrates using a UV LED and image processing with Arduino to construct a counterfeit currency detecting system. The device provides a reliable method for identifying false banknotes by integrating UV LED illumination, image capture, and image processing algorithms. The technology solves a significant real-world issue by offering an automatic and accurate way of spotting fake money. Its applications cover many industries, including banks, retail outlets, and money exchange facilities, where identifying counterfeit currency is essential. The system can illuminate banknotes using UV LED technology with ultraviolet light, revealing secret UV-reactive security features that distinguish authentic banknotes from fake ones. The control system is an Arduino board, which makes it easier to coordinate UV LED illumination, image capturing, and processing algorithms. Overall, the counterfeit currency detection system is a valuable weapon in the struggle against fake money, bolstering the existing security precautions and lowering financial risks. It offers a practical and effective solution that aids in preserving the reliability of economic systems and safeguards businesses from the negative consequences of fake money. The number of fake notes on the society is emerging quickly daily. Various processes are currently being utilized to assess whether a note is original or fraudulent money. This study suggests using convolutional neural networks to identify counterfeit Indian cash. CNN employed four predefined networks, namely Alex Net, Resnet50, Darknet53, and Google Net, to confirm the accuracy of the dataset it produced. The findings demonstrated that each of the four preconfigured networks excels at one criterion while compromising on the others. Future dataset verification will employ a revolutionary CNN architecture to address this issue and produce superior results by considering all characteristics.

REFERENCES

1. https://i0.wp.com/ommcomnews.com/wp-content/uploads/2023/09/Fake Note.jpg?fit=750%2C430&ssl=1
2. Satokar, Harshal. Project Report On. Diss. Rashtrasant Tukadoji Maharaj Nagpur University. Kumar, T. Naveen, et al. "Fake Currency Recognition System for Indian Notes Using Image Processing Techniques." Journal of Emerging Technologies and Innovative Research 6.4 (2019): 30–35.
3. https://www.google.com/imgres?imgurl=https%3A%2F%2Fwww.pantechsolutions.net%2Fwp content%2Fuploads%2F2021%2F09%2Ffakecurrencydetectionusingimageprocessing_1.jpg&tbnid=-_pwRlPmLe70tM&vet=1&imgrefurl=https%3A%2F%2Fwww.pantechsolutions.net%2Ffake currency-detection-using-image-processing&docid=fa8I6sLdncArWM&w=1000&h=1000&source=sh%2Fx%2Fim%2Fm4%2F2#vhid=-_pwRlPmLe70tM&vssid=l
4. Kumar, T. Naveen, et al. "Fake Currency Recognition System for Indian Notes Using Image Processing Techniques." Journal of Emerging Technologies and Innovative Research 6.4 (2019): 30–35.
5. Kumar, Devid, and Surendra Singh Chauhan. "A study on Indian fake currency detection." IJCRT 8.3 (2020).
6. Rajee, Alimul. "Fake Currency Detection."
7. Laavanya, M., and V. Vijayaraghavan. "Real time fake currency note detection using deep learning." Int. J. Eng. Adv. Technol. (IJEAT) 9 (2019).
8. Irulappasamy, Santhiya. "Research on Fake Indian Currency Note Detection using Image Processing." IJSDR 6.3 (2021).
9. Harjunowibowo, Dewanto, Sri Hartati, and Aris Budianto. "A counterfeit paper currency recognition system using LVQ based on UV light." IJID (International Journal on Informatics for Development) 1.2 (2012): 9–13.
10. Dobbs, Mark, Jeffrey Kelsoe, and Dwight Haas. "UV counterfeit currency detector." U.S. Patent No. 7,715,613. 11 May 2010.
11. https://www.wyckomaruv.com/UVTechnology.html
12. https://wtamu.edu/~cbaird/sq/2015/05/15/what-makes-a-fluorescent-highlighter-marker-so-bright/
13. https://www.olympus-lifescience.com/en/microscope-resource/primer/lightandcolor/fluoroexcitation/

Emerging Trends in IoT and Computing Technologies – Suman Lata Tripathi et al. (eds)
© 2024 Taylor & Francis Group, London, ISBN 978-1-032-87924-6

AI based Post Disaster Recce Bot using FPGA Controller

3

D. Preethi[1], N. Navya Sai Sailesh[2], T. Karthik[3], K. Bhanu Prakash[4]
Vel Tech Rangarajan Dr. Sagunthala R&D Institute of Science and Technology,
Dept. Electronics & Communication Engineering, Chennai, India

Abstract: In the aftermath of natural or man-made disasters, rapid and efficient rescue operations are critical to saving lives and minimizing the impact on affected communities. This abstract presents a novel approach to AI based post-disaster recovery operations through the utilization of a specialized autonomous vehicle, empowered by a Field Programmable Gate Array [FPGA] controller. The proposed Recovery bot is designed to navigate and operate in challenging and hazardous environments, such as collapsed buildings, debris covered areas, and unstable terrains. The FPGA [PYNQ Z2] based controller plays a pivotal role in enhancing the robot's capabilities by enabling real-time processing of sensor data, efficient decision making and versatile control strategies. The FPGA [PYNQ Z2] based Recovery bot consists of a ov7670 camera sensor operated at a voltage of 3.3v and the resolution is 640x480 VGA which is responsible for capturing the images of the affected person in the Disaster stricken area, and it also consists of MQ2 gas sensor responsible for detecting flammable gas leakage which causes fire accidents, and the output of the gas sensor is connected to input of ADC of PYNQ Z2 FPGA Controller. Now the collected data will be processed, and the data is transferred to the rescue team. In order to mobilize the bot to the target location, shortest path algorithm such as A-star algorithm is administered. To differentiate between the victim and the obstacle/non-victim debris, CNN algorithm is used for the precise decision of the bot. To transfer the data which is collected, we are using a HC-05 Bluetooth module which communicates with FPGA using serial UART protocol. With the help of the data which is collected and transmitted by the Recovery bot, the rescue teams can provide their services to the affected people quickly.

Keywords: Recovery bot, PYNQ Z2 FPGA controller, CNN algorithm, Shortest path algorithm

1. Introduction

An important and cutting-edge technical tool called the Post-Disaster Recovery Bot was created to facilitate and speed up the recovery process following natural or man-made disasters. Infrastructure, communities, and ways of life can all be severely damaged by catastrophes like earthquakes, storms, floods, and wildfires. The restoration of normalcy and assistance for impacted people and communities require a planned and effective strategy during the recovery phase that follows[1]. Modern artificial intelligence and chatbot technologies are used by the Post-Disaster Recovery Bot to give disaster survivors, aid providers, and recovery teams support and information in real time. This AI-powered bot assists people in navigating the complexities of recovery operations by acting as a primary source of knowledge, direction, and assistance. The Post-Disaster Recovery Bot's salient attributes are as follows:

---
[1]prettz_d@yahoo.in, [2]vtu17150@veltech.edu.in, [3]vtu15377@veltech.edu.in, [4]vtu15359@veltech.edu.in

DOI: 10.1201/9781003535423-3

Dissemination of Information: The bot shares current details regarding the emergency services, evacuation routes, shelter places, medical facilities, and other vital resources that are available in the impacted area.

Personalized Support: Through user interaction, the bot may identify user needs and make personalized suggestions for recovery resources like financial aid, medical care, psychological support, and housing support.

Resource Coordination: By establishing connections with pertinent relief organizations and governmental organizations, the bot can assist in coordinating the allocation and distribution of resources including food, water, medical supplies, and other necessities.

Navigational Support: The bot can give displaced people maps and directions to make it easier for them to find temporary housing, healthcare services, and other locations important to the rehabilitation process.

Emotional Support: Understanding the psychological toll that disasters exact, the bot can provide emotional support by connecting users to counselling services, mental health resources, and coping mechanisms.

Progress Monitoring: The bot can help authorities and recovery teams monitor the status of their activities, spot problem regions, and allocate resources more efficiently.

Communication in many languages: The bot's ability to converse ensures that it can connect with a variety of afflicted people and offer inclusive support.

Data gathering: By examining the interactions and questions it receives, the bot can give disaster response teams insightful information that will help them decide what to do and how to improve their plans.

2. Literature Review

Robin R. Murphy, Raymond S. T. Lee proposed a paper titled, 'Rescue Robots for Complex Environments' that discusses the challenges and advancements in the field of disaster rescue robots, including the use of drones, ground robots, and underwater robots. Nikolaos Tsiogkas, Nikolaos Mavridis published a paper titled, 'A Review of Disaster Robotics: Concepts and Applications', which provides an overview of disaster robotics, including classifications, challenges, and potential applications in various disaster scenarios. T. Balch, R. C. Arkin, J. A. Redi introduced the RoboCup Rescue Simulation Platform, an influential research platform for testing and developing disaster rescue robot algorithms titled 'The RoboCup Rescue Simulation Platform'. 'Human-Robot Interaction in USAR: Lessons Learned from Field Exercises with Rescue-Robots' proposed by Robin R. Murphy, Brian J. Gerkey was published in Journal of Field Robotics, which discusses the challenges of human-robot interaction in urban search and rescue (USAR) environments, based on field exercises and lessons learned. Bradley Hayes, Robin R. Murphy has studied upon, 'Challenges in Deploying Robots in Post-Disaster Environments: Results from Deployments in a Simulated Suburban Environment' that presents findings from robot deployments in a simulated suburban disaster environment and discusses the challenges faced by rescue robots.

The paper titled, 'Disaster Robotics' authored by Satoshi Tadokoro, Masaki Ogino, provides insights into the development of disaster rescue robots and their role in disaster management. Erion Plaku, Stefano Carpin in their article titled, 'A Review of Robots for Search and Rescue in Urban Environments' has covered the use of robots for urban search and rescue missions, highlighting various robotic systems and their capabilities. Using Convolutional Neural Networks (CNNs) in disaster rescue robots is an active area of research, especially for tasks like object recognition, navigation, and decision-making in complex environments. Below are some research papers that discuss the application of CNNs in disaster rescue robots:

Kaiming He, Xiangyu Zhang, Shaoqing Ren, et al. has presented the focuses on disaster robots, this paper introduces the ResNet architecture, which has been widely used for deep learning-based tasks, including object recognition in disaster scenarios in their article titled, 'Deep Residual Learning for Image Recognition'. Todd Hester, Peter Stone has published their article, 'Object Recognition for Disaster Response Robots Using Convolutional Neural Networks' to explore the use of CNNs for object recognition in the context of disaster response robots. It discusses the challenges and solutions in training CNNs for real-world disaster scenarios. Mark Pfeiffer, Maren Bennewitz, Wolfram Burgard has published an article titled, 'CNN-Based Object Detection and Navigation for Autonomous Search and Rescue Robots' in which a CNN-based approach for object detection and navigation in search and rescue scenarios are discussed. It focuses on using deep learning to enhance the robot's perception and decision-making capabilities.

These research papers cover a range of topics related to disaster rescue robots, from their design and capabilities to human-robot interaction and real-world deployments.

3. Architectural Model of the Robot

A 'Recce bot', short for reconnaissance robot, is a type of robot designed for various reconnaissance and surveillance tasks. These robots can be implemented using a combination of hardware and software components to achieve their objectives effectively[4]. Here's an overview of how such a robot is implemented.

The FPGA based system is a promising approach for developing post-disaster rescue robots. The FPGA's high performance, reconfigurability, low power consumption, and small size make it an ideal platform for implementing the complex algorithms and logic required for these robots[5]. The system has the potential to save lives and reduce property damage in the aftermath of a disaster. The architectural diagram of a post- disaster rescue robot using an FPGA shown in Fig. 3.1 typically consists of the following components:

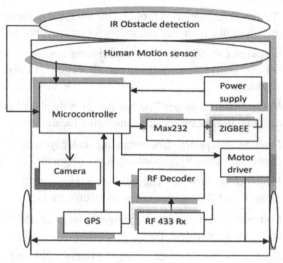

Sensors: The sensors are responsible for gathering information about the environment around the robot. This information can include temperature, pressure, humidity, gas concentration, obstacle detection, and victim detection.

Fig. 3.1 Block diagram of post disaster recce bot

FPGA: The FPGA is the central processing unit of the robot. It is responsible for processing the sensor data, generating control signals for the actuators, and implementing the robot's logic.

Actuators: The actuators are responsible for moving the robot. This can include motors, wheels, tracks, arms, and grippers.

Power supply: The power supply provides electrical power to the robot's components. The power supply can also be replaced by a battery, a fuel cell, or a solar panel.

Communication module: The communication module allows the robot to communicate with the operator. This can be done through a wired or wireless connection. The operator can use the communication module to send commands to the robot, to receive status updates from the robot, and to view images from the robot's camera.

The architectural diagram of the proposed system is designed to be modular and scalable. This means that the system can be easily adapted to different disaster scenarios. For example, the system can be equipped with different sensors, actuators, and communication modules depending on the specific needs of the mission.

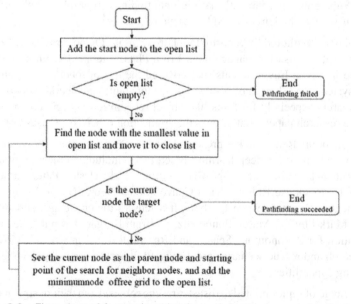

Fig. 3.2 Flow chart of A-star algorithm for path finding in post disaster bot

4. Software/Algorithmic Model of the Robot

FPGA are known for their low latency and high-throughput capabilities, making them suitable for robotics applications where quick responses are essential. Path Planning and Navigation in FPGA based rescue robots often incorporate advanced path planning and navigation algorithms.

4.1 A * algorithm for path finding

Algorithms help the robot navigate through complex and dynamic disaster environments to reach victims or perform specific tasks for effective and shortest path navigation of the robot. There is less computational complexity. The following steps provide the pseudocode description of the A* algorithm, a well-liked pathfinding method that finds the shortest path from a start node to a goal node in a graph or grid by combining the features of Dijkstra's algorithm and a heuristic function:

```
function AStar(initial, target):
open_Path := {initial}        // nodes to be evaluated
 closed_Path := {}            // nodes already evaluated
previous := {}           // For each node, the previous node that most efficiently reached it
gScore[initial] := 0         // Cost from start node to start node is 0
fScore[initial] := heuristic(initial, target) // Estimated total cost
present := node with lowest fScore in openSet if current equals goal:
return reconstructPath(past, present)  // Found a path, return it remove current from open_Path
    for each neighbor in getNeighbors(presentt)
    if robot in closed-Path:
    continue    // Ignore if exists
    estimated tentative_g_Score := g_Score[current] + distance(current, neighbor)
    if neighbor not in open_Path: add neighbor to open_Path
    else if tentative_g_Score >= g_Score[neighbor]:
    continue    // If better results are achieved
```

The algorithm proceeds by iteratively evaluating nodes with the lowest fScore value and updating the costs and paths as it goes. Once the goal node is reached, it reconstructs the path by backtracking through the came from map.

4.2 CNN Algorithm for Object Recognition

In computer vision, Convolutional Neural Networks (CNNs) are a class of deep learning models that are frequently utilised for object recognition tasks. They have transformed the area and serve as the basis for a number of applications, including as segmentation, object identification, and image classification. An overview of the CNN object recognition algorithm is provided below:

Gather a labelled dataset comprising pictures of items and the labels that go with them (e.g., rocks, debris, humans, etc.). Preprocess the photos by normalising the pixel values (usually in the range [0, 1] or [-1, 1]) and shrinking them to a uniform size (e.g., 224x224 pixels). Make training, validation, and test sets out of the dataset. The CNN algorithm's pseudocode representation is given below:

```
# Define hyperparameters
training_rate = 0.01
num_iterations = 10
cluster_size = 32
# Initialize weights and biases randomly
initialize_weights_and_bias()
# Main training loop
For iteration in range(num_epochs):
    for cluster to get_mini_batches(training_data, cluster_size):
# Forward pass
conv_output = convolution_layer(batch)
flattened_output = flatten(conv_output)
fully_connected_output = fully_connected_layer(flattened_output)
```

```
estimated_labels = soft_max(fully_connected_output)
 # Compute loss
loss = calculate_loss(estimated_labels, cluster_labels)
# Backpropagation
gradient = compute_gradient
update_weights_and_bias(gradient, training_rate)
# Print the loss for this epoch
print("Epoch {}: Loss = {}".format(epoch, loss))
# After training, use the model for predictions
for image in test_data:
conv_output = convolution_layer(image)
flattened_output = flatten(conv_output)
fully_connected_output= fully_connected_layer(flattened_output)
predicted_label = argmax(softmax(fully_connected_output))
print("Predicted label:", predicted_label)
```

5. Experimentation and Results

The AI-based Post Disaster Recovery Bot is equipped with various sensors to perceive its environment. These sensors collect data, which is then processed by the FPGA controller. The FPGA controller is programmed with AI algorithms (e.g., machine learning models) that analyze this data to make decisions. The AI algorithm such as CNN can perform tasks such as identifying survivors in disaster-stricken areas, mapping out safe paths for rescue operations, or determining the stability of damaged structures. The FPGA controller then sends commands to the actuator.

The process of capturing visual data through cameras, sensors, or other imaging devices are enhanced by techniques to improve the quality of images by adjusting contrast, brightness, and reducing noise. Applying filters or convolution operations to modify images for specific purposes, such as edge detection or smoothing.

A critical component of the UI is the display of live video feeds from the robot's on board cameras Operators rely on these feeds to navigate the robot and gather visual information from its surroundings to carry out actions based on the AI's decisions through A* algorithm. Throughout this process, the AI model continually adapts to new data and changing conditions, improving its performance over time. The prototype model in Fig. 3.3 and 3.4, serves as a demonstration of how this system would work in practice, allowing developers and stakeholders to test and refine the technology before moving on to full-scale production. It is a preliminary version of a robot designed to assist in disaster recovery efforts.

Utilizing the strength of PYNQ-Z2 FPGA controllers, the Post-Disaster Recce Bot is a unique robotic system created to help in disaster-stricken areas. With cutting-edge electronics and sensors, this sophisticated robot can navigate around disaster areas, evaluate damage, and gather crucial data for first responders and relief organizations.

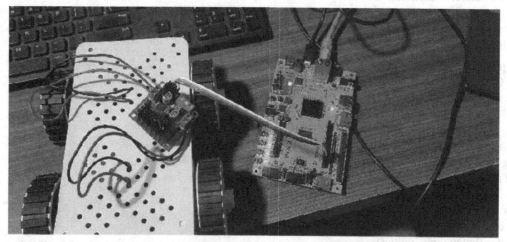

Fig. 3.3 Prototype model of post disaster recce bot using PYNQ Z2 FPGA controller

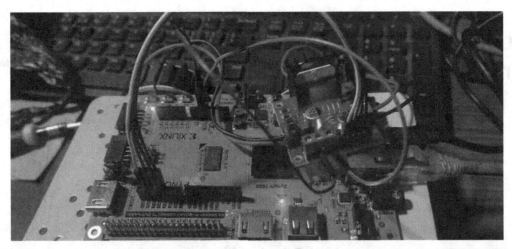

Fig. 3.4 Experimentation set up completed of post disaster recce bot using PYNQ Z2 FPGA controller

6. Conclusion

In conclusion, the PYNQ-Z2 FPGA controller-powered Post-Disaster Recce Bot offers a revolutionary approach to disaster response and recovery. The cutting-edge technology and human compassion that come together in this creative robotic system are intended to lessen the catastrophic effects of disasters on communities and people. This bot is essential in disaster-stricken areas thanks to its cutting-edge sensors, autonomous navigation abilities, and real-time communication facilities. It provides first responders with essential assistance, assisting them in their goal to save lives and protect communities. The bot contributes to more informed decision-making by quickly and safely gathering crucial data on the disaster's aftermath, thereby shortening reaction times and lowering risks.

References

1. Robin R. Murphy, Raymond S. T. Lee, "Rescue Robots for Complex Environments", Introduction to Autonomous Robots, 2019
2. J Trevelyan, WR Hamel, SC kang "Robotics in Hazardous Applications", Springer Handbook of Robotics, 2016
3. T. Balch, R. C. Arkin, J. A. Redi, "The RoboCup Rescue Simulation Platform", 2010
4. Robin R. Murphy, Brian J. Gerkey, "Human-Robot Interaction in USAR: Lessons Learned from Field Exercises with Rescue-Robots", Transactions on Systems, Man, and Cybernetics, vol 34, 2004
5. Bradley Hayes, Robin R. Murphy "Challenges in Deploying Robots in Post-Disaster Environments: Results from Deployments in a Simulated Suburban Environment", IEEE Open Journal of the Communications Society, vol 3, pp 1177-1205, 2022.

Emerging Trends in IoT and Computing Technologies – Suman Lata Tripathi et al. (eds)
© 2024 Taylor & Francis Group, London, ISBN 978-1-032-87924-6

Deep Learning-Based Image Segmentation for Early Detection of Lung Tumors

Happila T[1],
Assistant Professor, Karpagam College Engineering,
Electronic and Communication Engineering, Coimbatore, India

Rajendran A[2],
Professor, Karpagam College Engineering,
Electronic and Communication Engineering, Coimbatore, India

Kalaivanan D[3], Nithish Selva M[4], Dharshang[5], Kawashkar V[6]
Student, Karpagam College Engineering, Electronic and Communication Engineering, Coimbatore, India

Abstract: A patient's prognosis and response to treatment are greatly improved by early diagnosis of lung tumors. Lung tumors are frequently diagnosed and monitored using computed tomography (CT) scans, however segmenting these tumors with accuracy is challenging. A novel deep learning-based technique for image segmentation that enables the early identification of lung cancers in CT scan images is presented in this work. Convolutional neural networks (CNNs) are used in our suggested strategy to automatically and precisely define lung tumor locations inside CT data. To improve the quality of the raw CT scan pictures, we use image normalization and noise reduction techniques during the preprocessing stage. To extract useful spatial and contextual information from the photos, the feature extraction stage uses a sophisticated CNN architecture. On a sizable dataset of annotated CT scans, we hone a pre-trained model to segregate lung tumors. In the post-processing stage, the segmentation findings are improved by lowering false positives and ensuring smooth and exact tumor boundaries. We used a sizable dataset of CT scan images, including lung cancers in both the early and advanced stages, to test our method. Our findings show that the suggested strategy is effective in achieving high segmentation accuracy and resilience. The capacity of our approach to precisely identify tumor boundaries can assist radiologists and clinicians in making knowledgeable decisions about patient care. Early diagnosis of lung tumors is essential for early action. The deep learning-based image segmentation technique described in this study offers the potential Possibility of using CT scan images for early lung tumor identification, in light of the above. Our approach may speed up and improve the accuracy of lung cancer detection, which will eventually lead to better patient outcomes. This is accomplished by automating the segmentation process and offering precise tumor delineation.

Keywords: (CNN) Convolutional neural network, (CT) Computed tomography

1. Introduction

In large part because of late-stage diagnosis that has few treatment options, One of the leading causes of cancer-related deaths worldwide is lung cancer. It is essential to find lung tumors early in order to increase patient survival rates and treatment

[1]Happila.t@kce.ac.in, [2]rajendranav@gmail.com, [3]201121@kce.ac.in, [4]201136@kce.ac.in, [5]201113@kce.ac.in, [6]211504@kce.ac.in

DOI: 10.1201/9781003535423-4

effectiveness. Due to its ability to provide precise anatomical data, computed tomography (CT) scans are essential for the diagnosis and monitoring of lung cancer. However, manually identifying and segmenting lung tumors in CT scans takes time, is prone to error due to inter-observer variability, and is laborious. Using deep learning-based picture segmentation, This study suggests a novel approach for the early identification of lung cancers from CT scans. Our suggested approach overcomes the aforementioned difficulties by utilizing the strength of convolutional neural networks (CNNs) to automatically and precisely define lung tumor regions. Our research is driven by the possibility of transforming lung cancer diagnostics. We can give clinicians a dependable, effective, and impartial tool to recognize tumors in their early stages using deep learning. Early detection enables quick treatment, potentially lowering lung cancer's morbidity and fatality rates. This work proposes a novel method for using CT images to detect lung tumors early. including image pre-processing, feature extraction with a tailored CNN architecture, and post-processing to enhance segmentation outcomes. We also provide thorough analyses of several CT scan datasets, illustrating the sturdiness and precision of our technique. In the end, we believe that our research will aid in the early detection of lung tumors, hence improving patient outcomes and lowering lung cancer-related mortality.

2. Literature Review

Choosing the appropriate deep learning architectures, such as Transformer models, Recurrent Neural Networks (RNNs), or Convolutional Neural Networks (CNNs), for a given healthcare task.[6]: extracting relevant information from CT scan images and smoking-related data that can be utilized to forecast the development of lung cancer.[13] The selected deep learning model is given the pre-processed lung images, and its parameters are iteratively changed to optimize task performance.[2] choosing a machine learning technique, such as Support Vector Machines (SVM), Random Forest, or Gradient Boosting, that is appropriate for the identification and classification of lung cancer. Support Vector Machines (SVM), Random Forest, or Gradient Boosting are utilized with the Multinomial Bayesian method for the

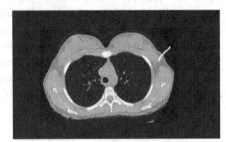

Fig. 4.1 CT scan lung image

diagnosis and classification of lung cancer [1].[16] removing noise, cleaning, and preparing the image data to ensure consistency before using it to train the Deep CNN model.[18]. using deep learning models that have already been trained, such as CNNs for pictures, to extract important information from the medical images. These complex features hold important patterns and information regarding the incidence of cancer.[8].

3. Architecture of Deep Learning

The layers of interconnected neurons that make up the deep learning architecture comprise input, hidden, and output layers. Recurrent neural networks for sequences, Transformers for language processing, Convolutional neural networks for images, and Feedforward neural networks for general tasks are examples of common forms. Architectures like Autoencoders, and ResNets tackle certain difficulties. Because these networks learn from data and adjust their parameters during training, they are useful instruments for a wide range of machine learning applications.

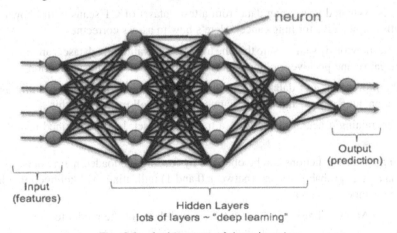

Fig. 4.2 Architecture of deep learning

4. Methodology

The data gathering and preprocessing phase of the convolutional neural network (CNN) approach involves curating and preparing a labeled dataset, which frequently entails scaling, normalization, and data augmentation. Next, a suitable CNN architecture is chosen, which can be anything from more established models like LeNet to cutting-edge designs like ResNet or VGG. To hasten convergence, the model is initialized with either pre-trained weights from a big dataset or random weights. Input data is processed through the convolutional and pooling layers of the network during training to extract hierarchical features. A suitable loss function is selected based on the kind of problem because activation

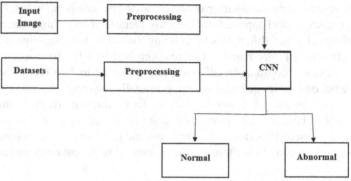

Fig. 4.3 Block diagram of CNN

functions like ReLU introduce non-linearity. The model can iteratively change its weights by using optimization algorithms like Stochastic Gradient Descent (SGD) or Adam since back propagation estimates the gradients of the loss. Overfitting is avoided by using regularisation techniques like dropout and weight decay. While training is carried out on the training dataset for a predetermined number of epochs, performance is monitored on a validation set. The learning rate, batch size, and network-specific parameters are optimized by hyperparameter tweaking after the model has been evaluated using the relevant metrics on a separate test dataset. The trained CNN is then installed in the target application and is continuously maintained.

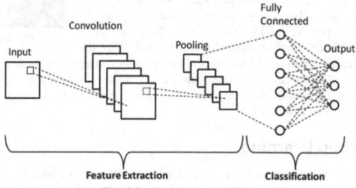

Fig. 4.4 Architecture of CNN

5. Estimation of Accuracy in Lung Cancer Detection

The model's performance is evaluated using scan data from a test dataset of CT scans with known ground truth labels, i.e., whether each scan is positive or negative for lung cancer. Here's how to assess correctness:

Make the test dataset: As was previously said, ensure that the training and validation datasets are not the same as the test dataset. CT scans that are both --negative and positive for lung cancer must be included in this collection.

Pre-process Test Data: Pre-process the test dataset using the same procedures as during training and validation. Rescaling, normalization, noise reduction, lung region, and nodule segmentation are all included in this.

Load Trained Model: After training a neural network on a training dataset, load the trained neural network model that was created.

Utilise Test Data to Run Inference: Predictions can be obtained by feeding the loaded neural network model the preprocessed CT images from the test dataset. A probability score (between 0 and 1) indicating the likelihood that lung cancer was detected in each CT scan should be the model's output.

The Classification Threshold: Apply a threshold to the output probabilities of the model to turn them into binary predictions. For instance, categorize it as lung cancer present if the chance is greater than or equal to 0.5; otherwise, classify it as lung cancer absent.

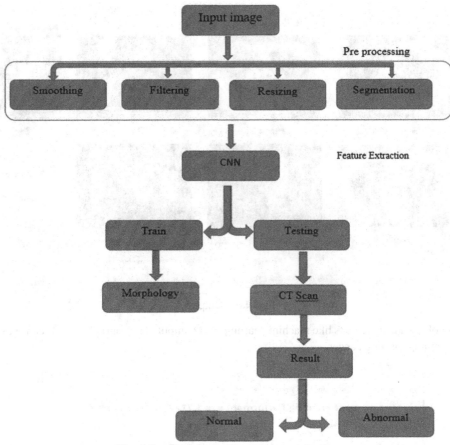

Fig. 4.5   Flowchart of lung tumor detection

6. Training

A back-propagation approach is used in order to train the Deep CNN to identify lung tumours on a CT scan with a size of 5*20*20. It happens in two stages. Corrected linear units and numerous volumetric convolution make up a CNN's first stage. To extract useful information, layers of (ReLU) and maximum pooling volumetric characteristics from the input data. The following stage is the classifier. It conducts a thorough examination of the brain's neural network by trailing many FC and threshold layers with a Soft Max layer in between. The CT didn't get scaled in any way.to preserve the original values of the dataset, photos of the As many jpeg images as you can. Training is when the randomly selected volumes from the CT scans of the and are normalised using an estimation of the training set's what is often distributed in the voxel values in the dataset.

Calculate Accuracy: Evaluate the model's binary predictions in comparison to the test dataset's actual labels (ground truth). The percentage of correctly categorized samples in the test dataset is what is referred to as accuracy. Accuracy is calculated as follows:

$$\text{Accuracy} = \frac{\text{Current Data}}{\text{Total Data}} \times 100$$

For instance, the accuracy would be as follows if your model accurately classified 90 of the 100 CT scans in the test dataset: 90% accuracy is the same as 90% of the total.

Please be aware that there are many different evaluation measures that are utilized in machine learning. Accuracy may not always be the most informative metric, depending on the issue and the class distribution.. In particular, for imbalanced datasets where the proportion of positive and negative samples differs noticeably, it is crucial to consider additional metrics like precision, recall, F1-score, and area under the receiver operating characteristic curve (AUC-ROC) in order to obtain a deeper understanding of the model's performance.

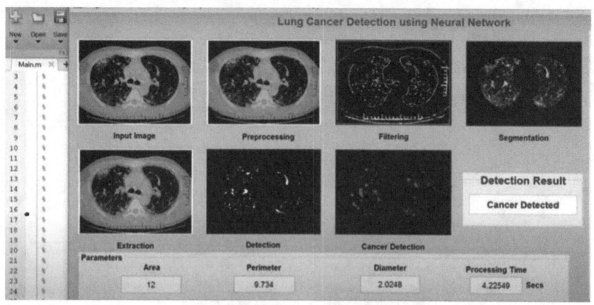

Fig. 4.6 Output

Medical imaging technology advancements like machine learning and computed tomography (CT) scans have greatly enhanced early diagnosis and treatment of lung cancer.

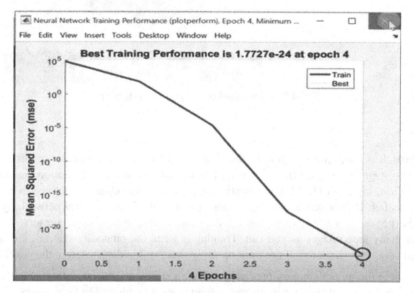

Fig. 4.7 Graph for best training performance

One sort of deep learning model that excels at extracting certain patterns and features from lung images to assist in identifying potential malignancies is Convolutional NeuralNetworks(CNNs).

7. Conclusion

By improving the speed and accuracy of diagnosis, these technologies may enable earlier interventions and better patient outcomes. While AI-driven tools are effective assistance, it is crucial to keep in mind that they should be used in conjunction with the knowledge of healthcare experts who make the final diagnostic choices. Collaboration between technological advancements and medical knowledge is still essential in the fight against lung cancer. AI-driven technologies, such as cutting-edge deep learning models and multimodal data integration, hold the key to the identification of lung cancer in the future, offering more precise, early-stage diagnosis and customized treatment strategies.

REFERENCES

1. lung cancer detection and classification using deep learning, Ruchita Tekade, prof. Dr. K. Rajeswari, IEEE-2018
2. Susmita Das, Lung Cancer Detection using Deep Learning Network: A Comparative Analysis, 2020-ICRCICN.
3. Radhika P R, Rakhi..S.Nair, A Comparative Study of Lung Cancer Detection using Machine Learning Algorithms, 2018-IEEE.
4. Syed Saba Raoof, M a.Jabbar, Syed Aley Fathima, Lung Cancer Prediction using Machine Learning: A Comprehensive Approach,2020-ICIMIA.
5. Amjad Rehman, Muhammad Kashif, Ibrahim Abunadi, Noor Ayesha, Lung Cancer Detection and Classification from Chest CT Scans Using Machine Learning Learning Techniques,2021-CAIDA.
6. Wasudeo Rahane,Himali Dalvi,Yamini Magar, Anjali Kalane, Lung Cancer Detection Using Image Processing and Machine Learning HealthCare,2018-IEEE.
7. K. Karthick,S.Rajkumar, N.Selvanatham,U.K.Balaji Saravanan,M.Murali, B.Dhiyanesh, Analysis Of Lung Cancer Detection Based On The Machine Learning Algorithm an IOT,2021-IEEE.
8. F.Taher, N.Prakash, A.Shaffie, A.Soliman, A.El-Baz, An overview of lung cancer Classification Algorithms and their Performances, IAENG-2021.
9. Puneet, Anamika Chauhan, Detection of Lung cancer using Machine Learning Techniques based on Routine Blood Indices, IEEE-2020.
10. wood Abdul, An Automatic Lung Cancer Detection and Classification (ALCDC) System Using Convolutional Neural Network, IEEE-2020.
11. Freddie Bray, Jacques Ferlay, Isabelle Soerjomataram, Rebecca L.Siegel, Lindsey, Global cancer Statistics 2018, CLIN-2018.
12. Geoffrey Hinton, Deep Learning-A technology With the potential to Transform Health Care, American Medical Association-2018.
13. Vineet K Raghul, Wei Zhao, Jiatao Pu, Joseph Leader, renewed Wang, James Herman, Jian-Min yuan, Panayiotis, Feasibility of lung Cancer Prediction from low dose CT scan and Smoking factors using Causal models, THORAXjinl-2018.
14. Mearj Begum Shaikh Ismail, Lung Cancer Detection and Classification using machine Learning Algorithm, Turkish Journal of Computer and Mathematics education-2021.
15. Ms.Bhagyashree, Akshay Panchal, Dilip Chavan, Lung Cancer Detection Using Deep Learning, ICAST-2019.
16. Mr.Sandeep A.Dwivedi, R.P.borse, Anil m.Yametkar, Lung Cancer Detection and Classification by using machine learning & multinomial Bayesian, IOSR-JECE-2016.
17. Pragya Chaturvedi,Prediction and Classification of lung cancer using machine learing Techniques,IOPC-2021.
18. Mehedi Masud, Niloy Sikder, Abdullah-Al nahid, Anupam Kumar Bairagi, A Machine learning Approach to Diagnosing Lung and Colon cancer using a Deep learning-based Classification framework,sensors-2021.
19. S.Sasikala,m. Bharathi, B.R.Sowmiya, Lu g cancer detection and classification using Deep CNN, IJITEE-2018.

Emerging Trends in IoT and Computing Technologies – Suman Lata Tripathi et al. (eds)
© 2024 Taylor & Francis Group, London, ISBN 978-1-032-87924-6

Analysis of Brain Disorder Based on MRI Using Artificial Intelligence

5

Sadaf Qasim[1], Nandita Pradhan[2]
United University, Electronics and Communication Engineering, Prayagraj, India

Abstract: The new development yield new technology which is neuroimaging that has significantly marked its presence for diagnosing schizophrenia ever since it is originated, and varieties of modalities have been introduce. There are different technologies that are used in this invention of neuroimaging. For demonstrating the connection between audible hallucinations and absolute gyrus loss in volume, which is the form of structural neuroimaging, a negative symptom of schizophrenia turns up which show loss of volume in prefrontal lobe. A default model was assigning to a part of brain function where functional neuroimaging diagnose disseminate functional abnormalities track down at various areas of brain in patient of schizophrenia. In this paper, we have observed varieties of modalities influences on different subclasses of schizophrenia and tried on looking to the imaging and its findings. Clinical image technique is employed for schizophrenia that helps in excluding the structural form of lesions who can be responsible to generation of symptom that imitate the same condition as that of patients of schizophrenia. Although, the findings here may purely be dependent on neurologic behavior of positive and negative, as per data, demonstrated by patients.

Keywords: Brain disorder, Psychosis, Schizophrenia (SZ), MRI4, DTI, PET, Psychiatry, Neuroimaging

1. Introduction

Through this analysis, it has been integrated the range of modalities that include CT scan, MRI, MRS, and PET in the various literature of schizophrenia patients. With the employment of TMS therapy, which is transcranial magnetic stimulation, the investigation on dataset of different schizophrenia patient's finding and its substitute can easily be define [1]. Thus, in this paper it will give the result that has advanced imaging outcome which is the repercussion of two class of schizophrenia patients, unattended and attended patient. All the survey and reviewing of the article was done as per the guideline followed by PRISMA. Schizophrenia is considered the most challenging psychiatric disorder to define [8]. It is characterized by illusion, hallucinations, and disturbances in belief during crucial phase, and suspension of social, unconcern, slothful, and motivational deficiency in the atrocious phase. Additionally, it is interconnected with various cognitive impairments that are not exclusively related to psychosis, suggesting result in a range of neuropsychiatric disorders. The exact cause of schizophrenia remains undetermined.

1.1 Structural Brain Disorder: Schizophrenia

Initially, the fact that believe interconnection with mental disorder and brain structural view, sociodemographic state of art, or mental health [2]. However, some scientists have assumed that brain structural view, i.e. size can be associated with postpartum impediment or neuropsychiatric deformity, or it can be both, though it is still debatable and vague (see Table 5.1). For investigation of any specific area or any portion of the it, entire volume of brain was evaluated to supervised that. For example,

[1]sadaf.riya@gmail.com, [2]nanditapradhan123@yahoo.com

DOI: 10.1201/9781003535423-5

to investigate a small portion of hippocampi that are recognize in any field in connection with the other, it will be crucial to discover whether specific portion is responsible for small size of brain or incommensurate that specific hippocampi, irrespective of brain structural size. Ther are may techniques to estimate the brain dimension such as we can compute the neurocranium or cranial cavity with Gray, white and cerebrospinal fluid [3]. The ventricle expansion was estimated by expulsion of ventricles autopsy of brain.

Table 5.1 Clinical remark

Clinically Remark	Symptom
One month period	Hallucinations, disorganized speech, disorganized behavior, elusions, decreased motivation, less expressive
Since onset of the distress	Work, mutual relations, or self-care
At least 6 months	Professional functioning absence
Total duration	Continuous indication of the disturbance
Autism history	Evaluation of cognition, depression, and mania symptom

1.2 Vaticination

This brain disease, schizophrenia can be medicated however cannot be cure rather symptom can be attended. A group of patients suffering from schizophrenia have recuperated completely. Study have reported that the schizophrenia patient has acknowledge a growth in their treatment and treated back to pharmaceutical with productively and progressively thereby leading a life, healthy and normally [4]. This brain disorder is not mortal, but their behaviour sometimes can be unfavourable for both sufferers and gathering around. Almost 12% of patients suffering from schizophrenia leads to take their life and commit suicide [9]. They also suffer some heart related issues. Horrible history of their family ancestor, or some unattended patient from their known ones, longer issue of psychosis can be an outcome of worst scenario. Therefore, some risk factors are associated with diseases can be seen in Table 5.2.

Table 5.2 Risk factor

Factor	Issues
Genetic risk	Parent or some relative
Environmental	Exposure to nitrogen dioxide, sulphur dioxide, winter birth, entertaining drugs etc
Constitute risk	Nutrition deficiency, herpes virus type 2, influenza etc.
Birth factors	Preeclampsia, maternal diabetes, twin gestation, C-Section delivery etc.

2. Imaging Techniques

2.1 Importance Characteristics

The primary function of imaging is to preclude structural contusion of brain which is the main source and indication that imitate the effect of schizophrenia, psychiatric clutter. With an example, it can be illustrated that any effect on frontal lobe is a cause of mental illness which result in hallucinations is a case of meningioma which mislead to the diagnosis of schizophrenia [5]. However, these imaging techniques such as MRI and CT scan gives a vague illustration of diagnosing schizophrenia, but with the help of several laceration can prove to be an effective way of investigating patient with this symptom.

2.2 Computed Tomography (CT scan)

Traditional way of imaging any patient is done with the help of severe psychotic section generally done staring with head section in Emergency Subdivision [6]. This should be understood that CT scan shows no indorsement of schizophrenia. However, this may be the primary investigation of any lesions in brain that may imitate the sign of schizophrenia. CT Scan are used to examine the different lobes of brains such as frontal, temporal, cold-blooded vertebrate heads, and thalmencephalon of brain of patient suffering from schizophrenia.

2.3 Magnetic Resonance Imaging (MRI)

For this paper, Structural MRI (sMRI) has provided non-invasive technique for the conceptual, evaluation and identification in biological variation created by brain disorder. Measurements for substantial size, of image that include gray area as well as white region and the width detection can be done for investigation purpose [7]. Because of exceptional resolution of MRI, several disabilities of schizophrenia patient which may include increment in CSF fluid or decrement in white or gray area, can easily be seen with these techniques (see Fig. 5.1).

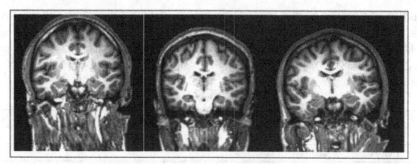

Fig. 5.1 This shows the image of patient suffering from schizophrenia (three attendee). It can be seen that T1-weighted images give high resolution to ascertain for defined gray area and CSF thus illustrating that schizophrenia patient led to volume decrement in Gray area and large CSF region. Cortical area will be supreme for quantitively analysis on group and for voxel-based analysis. In contrast, all the three contexts give the findings that there is volume variation between right hippocampal and left hippocampal whereas no such indication can be seen in remaining subset at this group. Hence, visual scrutiny is not appreciated at individual stage.

2.4 Functional MRI

This technique involves an imaging method which validate the assessment of brain contractility non-surgically at the tissues arena and is known as Arterial spin labelling (ASL). The main function of ASL is to sweep out the extracellular agent which form contrasting effect rather than convergence magnetically flow of blood. It uses radiofrequency to form autogenous dissemination traits. It investigates the cerebral flow of blood. The main function of fMRI (resting state, rs-fMRI) is considerably occupied quantitively investigation of patients suffering schizophrenia (refer Table 5.3). However, besides the factor of patient mentioned above, that are uncontrollable, encourages to make use of epidemic several specific dissimilarities, then this rs-fMRI can cross examine neurological investigation in the brain (see Fig. 5.2). With the use of fMRI (resting state), numbers of brains connection and modal have brought up in light which includes default, central, salience network, auditory, sensing and visualization modal etc.

Table 5.3 Study of MRI for change in Volume in Schizophrenia

References	Specimen	N	ROIs	Carry over interval	Findings
Chakos et al. (1994)	First episode SZ Controls Schizophrenia	20 8 11	caudate	17 months	Caudate volume with increment Volume corresponding with dose; inversely correspond with age
Chakos et al. (1995)	SZ	15	caudate	1.5 year	caudate volumes reduce
Corson et al. (1999b)	Chronic SZ Psychosis NOS Controls	19 2 4	caudate, lenticular nucleus	2 years	size of caudate is increase atypical size decrease
Degreef et al. (1991)	First episode SZ Controls	12 8	cortical ventricular	1–2 years	rate change shows no difference
DeLisi et al. (1995)	First episode SZ Controls	20 4	cerebral temporal corpus	5 years	left ventricle has rate change with greater in SZ
DeLisi et al. (1997)	First episode SZ Controls	50 25	medial lobe lateral, corpus, Sylvian	≥ 4 years	Rate change increases in SZ: left and right hemispheres,
Gur et al. (1998b)	SZ patients Controls	42 17	whole brain CSF, frontal lobes	2–3.5 years	Rate change: increased of frontal lobe in SZ. reduced in vol. temporal lobe
Jacobson et al. (1998)	Childhood SZ Controls	10 16	cerebral volume superior, amygdala hippocampus	2 years	Rate change in volume of entire cerebral and temporal lobe increased SZ
Keshavan et al. (1998b)	First episode psychosis Controls	16 16	superior temporal gyrus cerebellum	2 years	temporal gyrus of supreme vol. is inversely corresponded to psychosis time. Rate change increased in SZ with gyrus
rate change is change in volume with fast response rate in SZ patient than healthy group					

2.5 Diffusion Tensor Imaging (DTI)

Another Imaging Modality that come under the category of MRI is, Diffusion tensor imaging. These techniques provide a strong support in diagnosis of brain disorder as it has the assess of rectitude in finding the cerebral white matter fibre sweep. In an environment consisting of fluid, molecules of water typically exhibit random motion in all directions, referred to as Brownian motion. This phenomenon is described as isotropic diffusion of molecules. When a cell tissue acts as a barrier, molecules of water exhibit a particular direction of diffusion. This principle is known as anisotropic diffusion and serves as the foundation for diffusion tensor imaging.

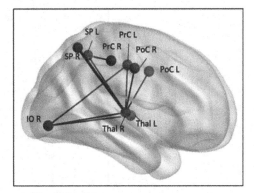

Fig. 5.2 Abnormal synchrony region

The procedure for demonstrating the white area expanse within brain carried out in a livingly, has made surface with the help of Diffusion tensor imaging (DTI) for providing the outcome in health and illness. A comprehensive study conducted by the ENIGMA group revealed extensive abnormalities in white matter micropattern among individuals with severe schizophrenia. Later, these DTI abnormalities were found to be prevalent among individuals diagnosed with alpha patient of schizophrenia. The DTI findings may vary among patients who respond to treatment and those who do not. This relates to the connection between the productiveness of antipsychotic biologic treatment and their attraction to dopa stat sensory receptors, especially in the striatum where production is increased in schizophrenia [9]. Figure 5.3 illustrates that individuals experiencing their first episode in SZ that exhibit reduction in fractional heterogeneity in white matter throughout the entire brain when compared to command [7]. This decline in fractional heterogeneity is associated with a decrease in cognitive relation among these patients. In individuals experiencing their first episode of SZ patients, abnormalities in DTI and fMRI were detected primarily in the thalamus. These findings align with previous volumetric and functional MRI studies that also provide evidence for the theory of dysfunction in the thalamocortical connection (Fig. 5.4).

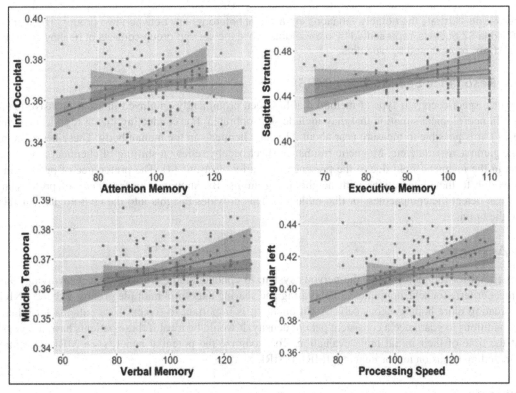

Fig. 5.3 The graph illustrates the relationship between fractional heterogeneity in different brain portion (Y) and execution in examining the cognitive (X). The red spots represent individuals with alpha SZ (n = 55), while the blue spots represent healthy controls matched for age and sex. The dark area constitutes the 92% fiducial interval for the linear regression line.

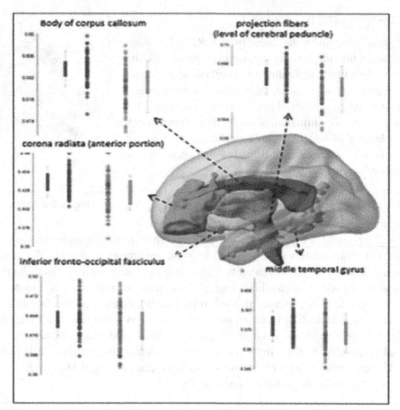

Fig. 5.4   The box-plots illustrate the notable variations in fractional heterogeneity between two groups. The first group consists of 58 alpha SZ patients, represented by orange dots, while the second group consists of healthy controls matched for age and sex, represented by blue dots.

2.6 Magnetic Resonance Spectroscopy (MRS)

Magnetic resonance spectroscopy is type of method that has been prominently employed in a non-invasive manner to assess brain anabolism in neurological situation that may include schizophrenia. For conducting this at high level of magnetic field strengths (like 7T), it is possible to measure near about 22 neurochemicals in the human body. These neurochemicals involve transmitters like gamma, aspartate etc. Magnetic resonance spectroscopy relies on shifting of chemical circumstances, which is the alteration in the magnetic field due to the presence of nearby electrons [4]. The preference of protons in complicated molecules varies due to their interactions with neighbouring atoms. By knowing the frequency of protons in a particular molecule, MRI can detect the compactness of that molecule. This provides insights into the neurological characteristics of a specific area of the brain.

3. Future Aspect

It would be beneficial for the radiology of the nervous system to conduct studies on large panel involving individuals who have recently meet criteria for schizophrenia. Collaborating and sharing data from multiple groups, like the ENIGMA project, would help in creating more homogeneous cells. Additionally, it is important to screen these patients for other medical and psychological conditions to guarantee a consistent patient density. It would be ideal if these patients have not yet started taking medications at the time of their initial brain evaluation. To maximize the potential benefits, an MRI convention should be implemented, including diffusion tensor imaging, fMRI, rsMRI, MRS.

4. Conclusion

MRI findings and potential avenues for future research are summarized here. With the advancement, our knowledge about the pathology concern with neural like that of schizophrenia has significantly developed. The use of MRI has provided confirmation of brain irregularities associated with this condition. These discoveries have expanded the range of investigations in both clinical and fundamental scientific studies, prompting a significant emphasis on understanding the neuroanatomy underlying these disorders. MRI findings in schizophrenia patient consist of several areas of the brain being affected. These areas include:

1. Enlargement of the ventricles

2. Engagement of the medial temporal lobe, specifically the amygdala, hippocampus gyrus

3. Engagement of the superior temporal gyrus (STG)

4. Engagement of the parietal lobe, especially the inferior parietal lobule, which is further divided into the angular and SMG.

5. Engagement of cortical brain regions such as the cerebellum, corpus thalamus etc.

REFERENCES

1. Adler LE, Olincy A, Waldo M, et al. Schizophrenia, sensory gating, and nicotinic receptors. Schizophora. Bull 998; 24:189–202. [PubMed: 9613620]

2. Andreasen NC, Ehrhardt JC, Swayze VW II, et al. Magnetic resonance imaging of the brain in schizophrenia. The pathophysiologic significance of structural abnormalities. Arch. Gen. Psychiatry 1990; 47:35–44. [PubMed: 2294854]

3. Becker T, Elmer K, Schneider F, et al. Confirmation of reduced temporal limbic structure volume on magnetic resonance imaging in male patients with schizophrenia. Psychiatry Res 1996; 67:135–143.[published erratum appears in Psychiatry Res 1997 May 16;74(2):1278]. [PubMed: 8876013]

4. Brown R, Colter N, Corsellis JA, et al. Postmortem evidence of structural brain changes in schizophrenia Differences in brain weight, temporal horn area, and parahippocampal gyrus compared with affective disorder. Arch. Gen. Psychiatry 1986;43:36–42.

5. Cumming, P., Abi-Dargham, A., and Gründer, G. (2021). Molecular imaging of schizophrenia: Neurochemical findings in a heterogeneous and evolving disorder. Behav. Brain Res.

6. Falkenberg, L. E., Westerhausen, R., Johnsen, E., Kroken, R., Løberg, E. M., Beresniewicz, J., et al. (2020). Hallucinating schizophrenia patients have longer left arcuate fasciculus fiber tracks: A DTI tractography study. Psychiatry Res. Neuroimaging 302:111088. doi: 10.1016/j.pscychresns.2020.111088

7. Garrity, A. G., Pearlson, G. D., McKiernan, K., Lloyd, D., Kiehl, K. A., and Calhoun, V. D. (2007). Aberrant "default mode" functional connectivity in schizophrenia. Am. J. Psychiatry 164, 450–457. doi: 10.1176/ajp.2007.164.3.450

8. Häfner, H.,Maurer, K., Löffler, W., Fätkenheuer, B., an der Heiden, W., Riecher-Rössler, A., et al. (1994). The epidemiology of early schizophrenia: Influence of ageand gender on onset and early course. Br. J. Psychiatry 164, 29–38. doi: 10.1192/S0007125000292714

9. Lee, M. H., Smyser, C. D., and Shimony, J. S. (2013). Resting-state fMRI: A review of methods and clinical applications. Am. J. Neuroradiol. 34, 1866–1872. doi: 10.3174/ajnr.A3263

Emerging Trends in IoT and Computing Technologies – Suman Lata Tripathi et al. (eds)
© 2024 Taylor & Francis Group, London, ISBN 978-1-032-87924-6

Lung Nodule Detection of CT Image Using Size and Shape-Based Features

6

Happila T[1]

Assistant Professor, Karpagam College Engineering,
Electronic and Communication Engineering, Coimbatore, India

**Rajendran A[2], Aravind S[3], Logesh V N[4],
Rishikeshan A K[5], Sivajithesh S[6]**

Professor, Karpagam College Engineering,
Electronic and Communication Engineering, Coimbatore, India

Abstract: A prominent contributor to cancer-related death worldwide, lung cancer highlights the urgent need for early identification and care. For the detection of lung nodules, which are frequently early signs of cancer, Computed Tomography (CT) imaging has become an essential technique. The use of size- and shape-based characteristics is highlighted in this survey's thorough analysis of lung nodule identification methods in CT scans. The size and shape characteristics of lung nodules are pivotal indicators for assessing their potential malignancy. Extracting these features from CT images has become increasingly important in automating and improving the precision of nodule detection. This survey explores the evolution of image processing and machine learning methodologies in this domain, providing insights into their strengths and limitations

Keywords: CT imaging, Size-based features, Shape-based features, Lung nodules

1. Introduction

It is crucial to detect tiny, irregular lung nodules on CT scans because they might be indicative of lung cancer, the leading cause of cancer-related mortality. Reliable technology is required to ensure timely detection and treatment. The two most common ways for this are deep learning and feature engineering. Lung cancer is one of the most frequent and deadliest kinds of cancer, and its continuous global influence underscores the crucial necessity of early detection and diagnosis. Because computed tomography (CT) imaging can detect even the tiniest irregularities in lung tissue, it is shown to be a very effective method for identifying and characterizing lung nodules. Lung nodules are often located in the lung parenchyma and might look as small, round, or oval lesions. They can be malignant or benign growths. Not only does early management become possible with a precise and timely diagnosis of these nodules, but patient outcomes are also markedly enhanced. In recent times, machine learning algorithms and advanced image processing techniques have been developed for use in medical imaging. An accurate and prompt identification of these nodules not only allows for early care, but also improves patient outcomes significantly.

---
[1]happila@gmail.com, [2]rajendranav@gmail.com, [3]201305@kce.ac.in, [4]201324@kce.ac.in, [5]201342@kce.ac.in, [6]201349@kce.ac.in

DOI: 10.1201/9781003535423-6

2. Proposed Methodology

CNN architectures and CNN's function as a classifier for lung CT scan image categorization are examined in the test data set as part of the suggested system's approach. This study proposes and tests the image Net-VGG-f feature-based CNN model, one of the numerous CNN architectures that have been researched. The model has been trained using a particular dataset. A reduction in the number of layers in a modified and simpler version of Image Net VGG-f CNN has been suggested. With externally extracted features provided as an input, the convolution layer—which is responsible for extracting features from the input image—is eliminated in the proposed CNN design. Hence, this design consists of one max-pooling layer, one ReLU layer, and one layer of categorization after a thick layer.

3. Literature Review

The study of this work deals with completely automated approach for lung CT image-based nodule identification. The grayscale CT image histogram is produced in order to automatically separate the lung location from the foundation. Morphological operators are used for result refinement. The

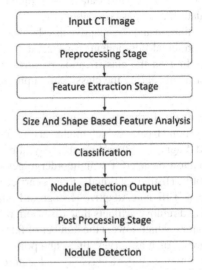

Fig. 6.1 Work flow of proposed methodology

parenchyma is then opened to reveal the interior structures. It is suggested to use a threshold-based method to distinguish the potential nodules from other structures, such as blood vessels and bronchioles. Support vector machines are used to classify the nodule feature vectors, which are created by extracting various statistical and shape-based features from the nodule. On a sizable CT dataset of the lungs obtained from the (LIDC), the suggested approach is assessed. Comparing the suggested approach to similar existing methods, it produced good results; its efficacy is demonstrated by its 93.75% sensitivity rate [1].

Here in this study the work deals with detecting nodules and making further decisions based on visual examination, medical professionals and radiological specialists utilize HRCT images. Consequently, techniques for computer-aided (CADe) have been created to accurately detect and segment nodules. In order to enhance lung nodule segmentation, an adaptive morphological filter was designed for this research project, introducing the adaptive morphology-based segmentation method (AMST). The flexible morphological filter increases the accuracy of decreasing FPs from the CT slices while simultaneously identifying potential nodule locations using adaptive structuring element (ASE). After that, the identified nodule candidate areas are processed to extract features. This work employed a SVM identification, utilizing morphological, texture, and intensity-based variables. Using the (LIDC/IDRI) dataset and obtained from a consultant radiologist, the suggested framework's performance has been assessed through the application of a 10-fold cross-validation approach [2].

The further study deals with review on this field with an update on the artworks' current condition and their development toward lung nodule detection. The published papers from 2009 to April 2018 were considered in this review study. This study provides a detailed description of several nodule identification techniques. Deep learning (DL)-based techniques have been widely used for nodule identification and characterization, it has been noted recently. CNN-based deep learning techniques have so been highlighted, with many CNN-based networks being described [3].

In order to automatically recognize and categorize, this work builds (CAD) system that can concurrently detect and classify (GGO), part-solid, and solid nodules. Ten characteristics in total were chosen for training and testing of artificial neural networks (ANNs) based on the morphological and local imaging aspects of pulmonary nodules. This was done to make sure the system could identify and categorize pulmonary nodules. Next, of every lung nodule slice was measured. The Euclidean distance method was used to determine the response (RECIST) value, and the area computation was based on the count of pixels in the maximal cross-sectional area. Utilizing the marching nodule volume with 3D reconstruction and Riemann integral formula with cube algorithm the system's sensitivity was 93.13% and 92.70%, respectively. The suggested system processes a single picture in only 0.1 seconds and can recognize GGO, part-solid, and solid nodules. Physical samples for this investigation were simulated lung nodule morphology using a clay model. Three CTs were performed on each physical sample. The volume estimated from this investigation differed, on average, by 0.37% from the actual volume. The system's detection and classification findings improved the clinical identification of absent nodules. When a patient has a second CT scan, provide information about their development rate and volume doubling time, which can improve diagnostic and treatment outcomes [4].

The study deals with proposed work where the aim is to distinguish between benign and malignant nodules. A portion of the publicly accessible dataset—the picture collection from the Lung picture Database Consortium (LIDC-IDRI)—is used to evaluate the suggested methodology. Noise reduction and filtering is done in the stage of preparation. In addition, semantic segmentation and the adaptive thresholding approach (OTSU) are employed to precisely identify lung nodules that are harmful. The principal components analysis approach has been used to extract information from 13 nodules overall. Furthermore, depending on the classification performance, four ideal characteristics are chosen. Nine distinct classifiers are used in the experiments during the classification phase. The suggested solution uses a logit boost classifier and delivers 99.23% accuracy [5].

As a result, Errors can occur while visually examining CT scans because it is difficult to differentiate lung nodules from background tissues, which might vary across observers. In order to help radiologists accurately identify lung nodules, computer-aided diagnosis is therefore critically important. Here in this system deep learning is used to automatically detect lung cancer from a low dosage CT scan in order to get around this problem. In addition, the proposed image pre-processing using Efficient Adaptive Histogram Equalization is carried out. Early detection of lung cancer is crucial for improving the survival rate of cancer patients. Efficient Adaptive Histogram Equalization –Region Of Interest [EAHE-ROI] is extracted in order to improve the CT scan and remove artifacts that arise from noise and image variations. The ROI is extracted from CT scans using morphological operators, which lowers the number of false positives. The geometric features are selected because they extract more geometric elements, such as curves, lines, and points of cancer nodules. The Non-Gaussian Convolutional Neural Networks [NG-CNN] architecture includes a classifier and feature extractor, which are applied on training, validation, and test datasets. The suggested methodology provides better-classified outcomes and effective cancer detection by surpassing the other competing methods and yields an AUC of 0.896 and test accuracy of 94.97% [6].

4. Performance Justification

To promote the use of size and shape-based characteristics for CT scan-based lung nodule detection, many critical criteria must be considered. Performance justification is based on demonstrating their advantage over competing procedures and how successfully they identify lung nodules. Important item store members are:

Clinical Significance: It is important to identify and characterize lung nodules as soon as possible since they may be early signs of lung cancer. Features that are based on size and shape make it possible to measure important metrics including volume, surface area, and irregularity, which helps with thorough nodule assessment.

Non-intrusive Approach: Early detection without intrusive treatments is ensured using CT imaging, a widely acknowledged non-invasive technology for screening for lung nodules. Preserving patient comfort and safety can be achieved by utilizing current CT scans for features based on size and shape.

Quantitative Information: By measuring nodule volume and diameter, size-related features provide quantitative information that makes it easier to identify malignant nodules and track nodule growth. Geometric insights are given by shape-based factors, like sphericity and irregularity indices, to distinguish between benign and cancerous cases.

Objectivity and Reproducibility: Subjectivity in interpretation is reduced by standardized algorithms for size- and shape-based feature calculation. By reducing radiologists' variation in nodule evaluations, this method improves diagnosis accuracy.

Early Detectionand Risk Assessment: Size-based feature scan assist categorize nodules, with bigger nodules being associated with a higher risk of malignancy. Shape-based features can be used to distinguish between benign and malignant nodules.

Feature Complementarily: Combining size and shape-based characteristics with other image-based data (for example, texture and density) can offer a more thorough characterization of lung nodules, improving the detection system's overall performance.

Research Validation: Previous research and studies have shown that size and shape-basedcriteriaareusefulindetectingandclassi fyinglungnodules, justifying their usage.

Machine Learning Applications: Size-and shape-based metrics may be easily used as input features in machine learning algorithms for automated lung nodule recognition and classification, allowing for data-driven decision support.

Integration with Clinical Workflow: Lung nodule identification systems that use size and shape-based characteristics can be incorporated into clinical processes, assisting radiologists in their everyday practice and increasing diagnostic accuracy.

In conclusion, size- and shape-based parameters provide significant benefits when used to identify lung nodules in CT scans. They provide quantitative, objective, and clinically relevant information that can aid in early detection, risk assessment, and decision support for healthcare professionals. Their effectiveness is supported by clinical relevance, research validation, and their compatibility with machine learning approaches.

5. Estimation of Accuracy in Lung Cancer Detection

Using a test dataset of CT scans with known ground truth labels—specifically, whether each scan is positive or negative for lung cancer—scan data is used to assess the model's performance. Here is how to determine accuracy:

Table 6.1   Epoch Vs accuracy

S. N.	Epoch	Accuracy (%)
1	0-2	40
2	0-4	55
3	0-6	62
4	0-8	75
5	0-10	89

1. *Create the test dataset:* As was discussed earlier, make sure that the test dataset is distinct from the training and validation datasets. This dataset needs to be made up of both lung cancer-positive and --negative CT images.

2. *Preprocess Test Data:* Preprocess the test dataset using the same procedures as during training and validation. Rescaling, normalization, noise reduction, lung region, and nodule segmentation are all included in this.

3. *Load Trained Model:* After training a neural network on a training dataset, load the trained neural network model that was created.

4. *Utilize Test Data to Run Inference:* Predictions can be obtained by feeding the loaded neural network model the pre-processed CT images from the test dataset. A probability score (between 0 and 1) indicating the likelihood that lung cancer was detected in each CT scan should be the model's output.

5. *The Classification Threshold:* Apply a threshold to the output probabilities of the model to turn them into binary predictions. For instance, categorize it as lung cancer present if the chance is greater than or equal to 0.5; otherwise, classify it as lung cancer absent.

Calculate Accuracy: Evaluate the model's binary predictions in comparison to the test dataset's actual labels (ground truth). The percentage of correctly categorized samples in the test dataset is what is referred to as accuracy.

$$\text{Accuracy} = (TP+TN)/(TP+TN+FP+FN)$$

Where TP is true positive which refers to correctly identified lung nodule, TN is true negative which refers to incorrectly identified lung nodule. FP is false positive which refers to correctly identified non nodules. FN is False negative which refers to incorrectly identified non nodules.

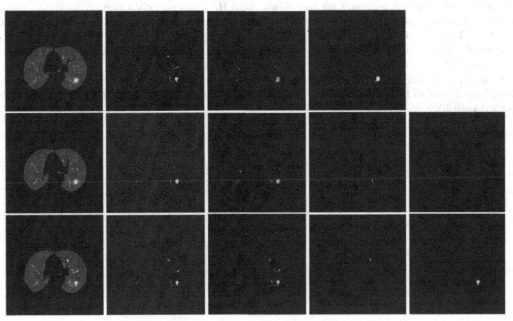

Fig. 6.2   Image segmentation for feature extraction

6. Limitation of Proposed Methodology

Table 6.2 Comments on limitation

S. N.	Limitation	Comment on limitation
1	Variability in Nodule Characteristics	Irregular or subtle nodules can be particularly challenging to detect.
2	False Positives	Lung nodules come in various shapes, sizes, and densities. Size and shape-based features might not capture the entire spectrum of nodule characteristics, making it challenging to detect certain types of nodules accurately.
3	Segmentation Errors	Precise segmentation of lung nodules from CT images can be error-prone, especially in cases of poorly defined or overlapping nodules.

7. Conclusion

In conclusion, the research on "Lung Nodule Detection Using CT Image Using Size and Shape-Based Features" has yielded significant insights and contributions to the field of medical imaging and early lung cancer diagnosis. This work has improved the precision and efficacy of nodule identification and categorization in CT scans by utilizing the capabilities of computer-aided detection systems. In order to characterize lung nodules, our technique included extracting characteristics based on form and size. These features not only aided in accurately distinguishing between benign and malignant nodules but also provided a deeper understanding of their morphological characteristics

REFERENCES

1. Noor Khehrah, Muhammad Shahid Farid, Saira Bilal, Muhammad Hassan Khan. Lung Nodule Detection in CT Images using Statistical and Shape-Based Features. Journal of Imaging (2020).
2. Amitava Halder, Saptarshi Chatterjee, Debangshu Dey, Surajit Kole, Sugata Munshi. An adaptive morphology based segmentation technique for lung nodule detection in thoracic CT image. Computer Methods and Programs in Biomedicine (2020)
3. Amitava Halder, Debangshu Dey, Anup K. Sadhu. Lung Nodule Detection from Feature Engineering to Deep Learning in Thoracic CT Images: a Comprehensive Review. Journal of digital imaging (2020).
4. Chung-Feng Jeffrey Kuo, Jagadish Barman, Chia Wen Hsieh, Hsian-He Hsu. Fast fully automatic detection, classification and 3D reconstruction of pulmonary nodules in CT images by local image feature analysis, Biomedical Signal Processing and Control (2021)
5. Talha Meraj, Hafiz Tayyab Rauf, Saliha Zahoor, Arslan Hassan, M. Ikram Ullah Lali, Liaqat Ali, Syed Ahmad Chan Bukhari, Umar Shoaib. Lung nodules detection using semantic segmentation and classification with optimal features. Hybridization of neural computing with nature-inspired algorithms (2020).
6. Johnsirani Venkatesan, Nikitha, Nam, Choon Sung, Ryeol Shin, Dong, Lung Nodule Classification on CT Images Using Deep Convolutional Neural Network Based on Geometric Feature Extraction. Journal of Medical Imaging and Health Informatics, Volume 10, Number 9, August 2020, pp. 2042-2052(11)

Emerging Trends in IoT and Computing Technologies – Suman Lata Tripathi et al. (eds)
© 2024 Taylor & Francis Group, London, ISBN 978-1-032-87924-6

A Smart Home Assessment of Security and Comfort for Elderly People: A Review

7

Shweta Tiwari[1]

Chandigarh University, CSE, Mohali, India

Puneet Kumar Yadav[2]

Alliance University, CSE, Bangalore, India

Animesh Srivastava[3]

Graphic Era Hill University, CSE, Dehradun, India

Parul Parihar[4]

Chandigarh University, CSE Mohali, India

Abstract: Home automation is already a widespread feature of Internet of Things services and products, and it offers a number of guarantees to enhance consumer welfare, lifestyle, and health. Due to the varied, vast, and complex nature of IoT, intelligent homes have several safety concerns regarding its functionality and perceived value for people. But high-quality smart home security support is also a major factor in the sector's rapid expansion. Most of the time, intrusions from the outside that result in malfunctions or equipment damage do not lead to security issues in smart homes. Privacy leakage is the greatest security threat to the smart home, at least from the standpoint of apps. Strengthening privacy security from the perspectives of networks, systems, and data processing is the primary objective of current research. The need for technology-related services will surely increase because of the urgent demands of the aging population. When used appropriately, technological advances will not only enhance the quality of life of seniors but also make it simpler for caregivers to provide the care that these senior citizens need. Without a doubt, these older folks need care and aid with their daily tasks.

Keywords: Smart homes, Elderly person, Healthcare, Internet of things, Security

1. Introduction

Smart home technology, also referred to as home automation, encourages homeowners to monitor their properties, typically using a mobile application, and also offers security, affordability, comfort, and energy efficiency. A smart home is essentially a setup that allows you to keep tabs on it via a mobile app on your laptop or smartphone. Home appliances like smart doors, ventilation, air conditioning, and lighting may all be monitored by it. In order to remotely monitor devices, Bluetooth or Wi-Fi is employed. Automated home system control, including adaptive heating, ventilation, and lighting, is a key component of the smart house movement. Even if businesses try to develop specific items like smart lights and thermostats, efforts have been made to understand the full spectrum of household solutions [1]. The system's parts are configured to talk to one another through a central hub, which the user can control and administer using mobile or web applications.

[1]shweta.tiwari2006@gmail.com, [2]punityadav9151@gmail.com, [3]er.animesh10@gmail.com, [4]parulparihar9@gmail.com

DOI: 10.1201/9781003535423-7

1.1 Categories of SmartHome Devices

Despite the fact that they frequently come under one of those headings: recreation, supervision and security, house upkeep, lighting, health and fitness, or fuel & resource management, the market for smart homes appears to be home to a sizable number of IoT devices and applications [2].

1.2 Significant Innovations: SPA

Voice technology is now used in a variety of computing applications as a result of recent rapid change or development. The creation of intelligent dwelling personal assistants (SPA), like Amazon Echo, Google Home, among other brands and others, is one of voice technology's most important advances. Two broad categories can be used to categorized connected home systems: systems with remote or local control.

Present-day cloud-based Samsung Sensible Items, Amazon AWS, Smart home systems include many other Internet of Things (also known as IoT) gadgets. An example of the way a home gadget can increase sensitivity while transmitting every piece of information over the clouds or through a central hub. Dozens of sensors that measure things are crowded into the smart house, as well as additional proof like smart gadgets that will be used for individualization, autonomous services, and improving both the functionality and quality of the residents [3].

The smart home is one of the most recent developments in user-controlled technology. They give senior citizens more independence and convenience than typical residences can. The primary goals of the functions are to increase the convenience and standard of existence in the house. Connected, remote-controllable equipment also makes it feasible to achieve additional goals like increased security and energy efficiency. Different smart home policies for senior care were prioritized at various stages of development. Different countries see smart houses for senior care as policy or technological innovations rather than popular items. These unique qualities of smart homes for elder care not only spur quick expansion but also create a variety of challenges to that growth, such as a lack of demand and an uncoordinated growth [4].

The paper is organized as follows: In the second section specification of Smart Home specialized for elders has been discussed. The security of data and the possible challenges are presented with relevant details. Following the second section we drafted the literature survey from the past few years. In the same section a few recent models of smart homes are mentioned, followed by the methodology used for the present research development.

2. Smart Home for Elders

In addition to other evidence, such as intelligent gadgets that will be used for customization, autonomous services, and improving the usability and reliability of elderly citizens, the smart house is crammed with numerous sensors that measure various aspects. The various elements which are important and should be highlighted while designing the smart home for elderly are mentioned in Table 7.1. This table defines the relationship between the concern element, the services offered by those elements and important aspects addressed.

The 'Internet of Things' idea has advanced beyond science fiction and is already a part of our everyday life now objective is to make it beneficial for elderly person. The usage of tools and programs designed to support gadgets and systems for smart homes is among the most prevalent manifestations of IoT in action. Based on a number of concepts and requirements, many equipment manufacturers offer a wide range of equipment that is integrated into a home environment. The unprecedentedly quick growth in the number of connected devices opens up new entry points for criminals and makes it easier than ever to gather and eventually share more of our information [5].

2.1 Protection Criteria

When working with protection in IOTs, the processes to evaluate the operation of a number of protected systems include the following crucial safety criteria. The Privacy issue of the user of Smart Home appears as the main challenge. This will affect the integrity of user's data while using a variety of sensors. Table 7.2 describes certain protection criteria that should be taken care of while selecting the sensor and the mode of transmission of the sensory information.

Table 7.2 Smart home criteria for security specification

S. No	Criteria	Description
1.	Availability	Stopping unauthorized users or programs from interfering with authorized users' utilization of the network resources is its main goal.
2.	Authenticity	In order to ensure that the system acknowledges this user comes first, it is necessary to retain the genuine self of the system's consumer or organization and link the current self to the system-embedded self.
3.	Authorization	Regarding access control in general, information security in specific, and data security in particular, The process for establishing access credentials and resource permissions is known as authorization.
4.	Confidentiality	This has to do with limiting the distribution of data to illegal users, organizations, and gadgets.
5.	Integrity	It has to do with stopping unauthorized individuals or things from altering or fabricating data sent over a network.

2.2 Challenges

Since smart homes contain several users and numerous device networks, they present special security, safety, and usability problems. This affects the cognitive experiences of the vast majority of home inhabitants. Modern smart home hardware typically disregards fundamental access controls and other methods to make the device obvious and available to all apps, making it inadequate for many applications [6]. Since older persons frequently lack computer literacy, it's probable that they found it challenging to adjust to life in a smart home.

The majority of Smart Home Technologies (SHTs) are being built with the elderly in mind, and it is most likely that they will have the highest demand for services related to smart home technology. Seniors 60 and older strongly prefer to remain in their homes for as long as is practicable when given the choice between staying there or relocating into an institutional facility. SHT enhances quality of life, reduces healthcare costs, and enables senior adults to live more sustainably and independently at home. These elderly people may show signs of functional and cognitive deficits, chronic illnesses, a breakdown in social networks, and a lack of physical exercise [7].

The goal of SHTs is to facilitate and support a comfortable, self-sufficient, and healthy way of life at home. The ability of a smart home to automatically manage amenities and appliances both inside and outside the building is its most fundamental technological characteristic. Figure 7.1 defines the possible no of devices connected within the smart home and the no of entities through which the sensory data can be shared. Thanks to the development of networks at home and the widespread usage of high-speed Internet, users may easily control or monitor devices in their residences from outside. modern innovations like the online world connected devices and artificial intelligence, which allow communication and data collection between smart objects and people as well as the analysis of habitation patterns, giving up the idea of a home network that merely manages the linked devices was realistic. [8].This has led to the development of technology that could offer inhabitants individualized services by foreseeing their needs and desires. Modern sensing technologies can now help individuals without requiring physical control of the apparatus, including motion sensors and video cameras.

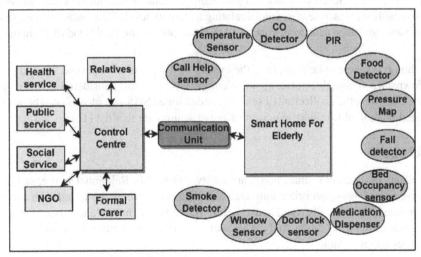

Fig. 7.1 Variety of technology in a smart home

3. Literature Review

Understanding senior users' actions and attitudes in the UAE and the factors influencing technology acceptance, Arar et al. set out to explore interests and expectations for home automation technologies. The approach involved surveying and interviewing 110 persons between the ages of 40 and 60. IBM SPSS Statistics the following statistical analyses were performed using data from 105 of the 105 legitimate survey responses: frequency, mean, cross-analysis, unbiased sample t-test, a single-direction variance assessment, and multiple regression. The two most important variables are age and liking for computer technology. The fear of technology among older users in the UAE had an impact on the uptake of smart home technologies [9].

Almutairi et al. gave a thorough recent update on the innovations, methods, and practical applications for old behavior detection in smart homes, smart medical centers, smart medical establishments, and smart retirement communities for the elderly. [10]. The research article demonstrates that the convolutional neural net architecture and its variations are the deep learning technique that has garnered the most attention from scientists.

To live independently and save money on healthcare, many older people choose to live alone in single-resident homes. Therefore, prolonging the time that elderly people may live independently requires early dementia detection. Tan-Hsu et al. offer a unique front-door events model using accessible data sets (n = 14) collected from 14 testing environments using anonymized wireless binary sensors. [exit, entry, guest, others, and brief-return-and-exit (BRE)] categorization approach (passive infrared sensors and magnetic sensors). When four things happen in a row (exit-entry-exit-entry) occur inside specific time windows, BRE events—some of which may be forgotten events occurring [11].

The opinions of older persons who have utilized smart home monitoring technology personally and those who haven't are contrasted by Ghorayeb et al. Four focus groups were conducted, with six elderly residents of the area and seven members of a massive multidisciplinary research partnership building a sensing platform for home health and lifestyle. With use and time by those who had already used the item, its acceptance grew [12]. Participants who showed little interest in smart homes concentrated on how exposed a household would be as a result of this technology and how noticeable and obtrusive it was.

The emergence of wearable technology has made fall detection technologies for smart home care conceivable., smartphones, the Internet of Things (IoT), artificial intelligence (AI), and other technologies. The most effective deep convolutional neural network for elderly fall detection (IMEFD-OD) the CNN is utilized to develop an IoT-enabled elder collapse detection strategy for smart home care. (IMEFD-OD) the CNN is used by Vaiyapuri et al. [13] The IMEFD-OD the CNN model enables the identification of falls that occur in smart homes by utilizing innovative deep learning (DL) techniques and smartphones.

The study by Debjyoti et al. established and empirically tested a theoretical framework for identifying the essential aspects that may affect elder customers' adoption of healthcare-related smart home services 254 seniors from four Asian countries who were all 55 or older participated in an online survey as a consequence. Using structural equation modelling with partial least squares, the effects of eight hypothesized predictive components were examined [14].

Using passive infrared (PIR) motion sensors and data processing, an inconspicuous dementia prediction method is provided by Kim et al. for tracking the exercise levels of senior citizens residing alone or with another individual in a variety of housing types. [15]. Their proposed method extracts feature values relating to activity levels from basic infrared sensors that are passively placed in each room space and uses deep neural networks, or DNNs, to predict the likelihood of Alzheimer's in a home utilizing sensor technology.

A comprehensive smart home system can help improve the quality of life for elderly people. Hee Jo et al. evaluate the SHS's possible benefits and downsides. Through interviews were conducted based on considered comfort, perceived ease of use, accepted privacy, and perceived benefit, a collection of sensors needed for an SHS was identified. The wireless sensor equipment set was subsequently tested on nine older adults in a South Korean senior care facility. [16].

4. Technology Used

The most crucial components of a senior's smart home are safety and health. Relational living, spatial awareness, a feeling of place, and the extensive use of age-appropriate language and imagery serve as the foundation for this framework, which is founded on four interrelated, theoretically validated criteria. We consider these standards essential for achieving marital wellbeing. To fulfil the goals of this Evaluation study. This section outlines the methods for looking at how older people use smart home devices. Various stages include.

1. *Making Plan:* We ensured that the technical and strategic strategies were developed would ensure that the approach was implemented carefully and under strict control.
2. *Developing Research:* The researchers are inspired by the significant accomplishments made in the field of smart home technologies.
3. *The Act of Searching:* Several electronic resources were taken into consideration and explored to find relevant papers on the application of smart home technology for the elderly. The relevant URLs and the databases that were searched are listed in the table. The manual search method to find publications in conference proceedings and journals, respectively, was used to pull every article from a database on the internet.
4. *Standards For Including and Discarding:* To be considered for this analysis, a study had to meet a number of criteria; if not, it was excluded. The Article must have the published piece of writing must be in English that can be understood. Each article must cover a senior-friendly smart home. Each article must provide either evidence from a real study addressing the research issue or a plan for incorporating technologies for elderly people's homes that are smart.
5. *Data Collection:* The writers came to a consensus and discussed a scenario where issues with an article were brought up throughout the review process. The authors conducted a more thorough study of the data they had gleaned from each piece, paying special attention to data on older people's use of smart home technologies as well as crucial data on ongoing smart house projects.
6. *Data Analysis:* Choose the Columns item using the MS Word Extended toolbar, and then from the selection palette, choose the appropriate number of columns. Utilized the data further in accordance with the problem's domain.

5. Discussion

The current presumptions that support aging-in-place, such as the value of independence, are sometimes entangled with ideas of power as well as static, as opposed to flexible, concepts of "home" and "place." The various representations of "older people" and aging can also support certain development or policy directions. Many IoT devices become easy targets due to a lack of security features, sometimes even without the victim's understanding that they have been infected. In this study, we attempted to provide a risk assessment for an IoT-based smart connected home environment. Emphasis is placed mostly on emphasizing concerns connected to privacy and security that are spread throughout key areas like human-related, the network, computer software, hardware, and information.

6. Conclusion

Building and promoting wellbeing has been highlighted by our framework, along with the importance of adopting an ontological perspective that values relational living over independent living, paying more awareness to disparities and inequalities, maintaining a "sense of home" while living in HSH, and, most importantly, the use of more suitable and positive language. Headings, often known as headings, are structuring elements that direct someone to read through the document. Constituent headers and text heads are the two categories. Component headers distinguish the various parts of the article and are not arranged in any topological order.

REFERENCES

1. Abdur, M., Habib, S., Ali, M., & Ullah, S.(2017). Security Issues in the Internet of Things (IoT):A   Comprehensive Study. International Journal of Advanced
2. Alam, T., A. Salem, A., O. Alsharif, A., & M.Alhejaili, A. (2020). Smart home automation towards the developmentof smart cities. Computer Science and Information Technologies, 1(1), 17–25. https://doi.org/10.11591/csit.vlil.p17-25
3. Ali, B., & Awad, A. I. (2018). Cyber and physical security vulnerability assessment for IoT-based smart homes. Sensors (Switzerland), 18(3), 1–17.
4. Zhang, Q., Li, M. & Wu, Y. Smart home for elderly care: development and challenges in China. BMC Geriatr 20, 318 (2020). https://doi.org/10.1186/s12877-020-01737-y
5. Davis, B. D., Mason, J. C., & Anwar, M. (2020). Vulnerability Studies and Security Postures of IoT Devices:A Smart Home Case Study. IEEE Internet of Things Journal, 4662(c), 1–1.
6. Desai, D., & Upadhyay, H. (2014). Security and Privacy Consideration for Internet of Things in Smart Home Environments. International Journal of Engineering Research and Development, 10(11), 73–83.

7. Arar, M., Jung, C., Awad, J. and Chohan, A.H., 2021. Analysis of Smart Home Technology Acceptance and Preference for Elderly in Dubai, UAE. Designs 2021, 5, 70.

8. Jararweh, Y.; Otoum, S.; Al Ridhawi, I. Trustworthy and sustainable smart city services at the edge. Sustain. Cities Soc. 2020,62, 102394.

9. Arar, Mohammad, Chuloh Jung, Jihad Awad, and Afaq Hyder Chohan. 2021. "Analysis of Smart Home Technology Acceptance and Preference for Elderly in Dubai, UAE" Designs 5, no.4:70https://doi.org/10.3390/designs5040070

10. M. Almutairi, L. A. Gabralla, S. Abubakar and H. Chiroma, "Detecting Elderly Behaviors Based on Deep Learning for Healthcare: Recent Advances, Methods, Real-World Applications and Challenges," in IEEE Access, vol. 10, pp.69802-69821,2022, doi: 10.1109/ACCESS.2022.3186701.

11. T. -H. Tan, M. Gochoo, F. -R. Jean, S. -C. Huang and S. -Y. Kuo, "Front-Door Event Classification Algorithm for Elderly People Living Alone in Smart House Using Wireless Binary Sensors," in IEEE Access, vol. 5, pp. 10734-10743, 2017, doi: 10.1109/ACCESS.2017.2711495.

12. "Older adults' perspectives of smart home technology: Are we developing the technology that older people want?" International Journal of Human-Computer Studies 147, (2021): 102571. Accessed February 3, 2023. https://doi.org/10.1016/j.ijhcs.2020.102571.

13. T. Vaiyapuri, E. L. Lydia, M. Y. Sikkandar, V. G. Díaz, I. V. Pustokhina and D. A. Pustokhin, "Internet of Things and Deep Learning Enabled Elderly Fall Detection Model for Smart Homecare," in IEEE Access, vol. 9, pp. 113879-113888, 2021, doi: 10.1109/ACCESS.2021.3094243.

14. D. Pal, S. Funilkul, N. Charoenkitkarn and P. Kanthamanon, "Internet-of-Things and Smart Homes for Elderly Healthcare: An End User Perspective," in IEEE Access, vol. 6, pp. 10483-10496, 2018, doi: 10.1109/ACCESS.2018.2808472.

15. J. Kim, S. Cheon and J. Lim, "IoT-Based Unobtrusive Physical Activity Monitoring System for Predicting Dementia," in IEEE Access, vol. 10, pp. 26078-26089, 2022, doi: 10.1109/ACCESS.2022.3156607.

16. Jo, Tae Hee, Jae Hoon Ma, and Seung Hyun Cha. 2021. "Elderly Perception on the Internet of Things-Based Integrated Smart-Home System" Sensors 21, no. 4: 1284. https://doi.org/10.3390/s21041284

Emerging Trends in IoT and Computing Technologies – Suman Lata Tripathi et al. (eds)
© 2024 Taylor & Francis Group, London, ISBN 978-1-032-87924-6

Predictive Analytics for Better Crop Management and Production using Machine Learning

8

Qaim Mehdi Rizvi[1], Er. Sarika Singh[2],
Shri Ramswaroop Memorial College of Engineering & Management, Lucknow

Atul Kumar[3]
Maharana Pratap Engineering College, Kanpur

Abstract: Predictive analytics and machine learning have appeared as powerful tools, capitalizing on the wealth of agricultural data to inform data-driven decisions for farmers and agribusinesses. Traditional crop management relied on historical practices, often limited by their inability to leverage modern data sources such as climate data, soil characteristics, and real-time sensor data. In contrast, predictive analytics, underpinned by machine learning algorithms, taps into this data to offer accurate forecasts and actionable insights. Ensuring food security and sustainable agriculture relies significantly on the effective management and production of crops. This paper presents a comprehensive overview of the utilization of predictive analytics and machine learning in the context of crop management and production, focusing on their applications, challenges, and potential benefits. It emphasizes the necessity for interdisciplinary collaboration between scientists, agriculturalists, technology developers, and policymakers to overcome barriers and foster the widespread adoption of predictive analytics in agriculture.

Keywords: Agriculture, Data science, Machine learning, Predictive analysis, Artificial intelligence, Predictive analytics, Agricultural data, Data-driven decisions, Soil characteristics, Real-time sensor data and accurate forecasts

1. Introduction

Agriculture plays a critical role in feeding the growing global population, and efficient crop management and production are essential for confirming food protection and ecological agricultural systems. Traditionally, crop management decisions have been based on historical knowledge, experience, and local practices. However, these approaches cannot often leverage the wealth of data available today, including climate data, soil characteristics, crop genetics, and real-time sensor data. Predictive analytics, powered by machine learning algorithms, can leverage this data to make accurate predictions and generate actionable recommendations for crop management. For instance, a study by Liu et al. [1] demonstrated the effectiveness of machine learning algorithms in predicting the yield of maize crops based on weather and soil data. Similarly, a study by Mondal et al. [2] used data from remote sensing and machine learning techniques to identify the early onset of wheat rust disease.

The principal purpose of this research paper is to explore the applications, challenges, and potential benefits of utilizing predictive analytics and machine learning in crop management and production. We will delve into the various components of predictive analytics, including data collection, pre-processing, feature selection, model training, and evaluation. By analyzing data from sensors, satellite imagery, and other sources, machine learning models can identify patterns and indicators of pest

[1]sirqaim@gmail.com, [2]sarikasingh2494@gmail.com, [3]atulverma16@gmail.com

DOI: 10.1201/9781003535423-8

and disease outbreaks, enabling timely interventions and targeted treatments [3]. Machine Learning algorithms can generate reliable predictions that aid in strategic planning [4] and can analyze soil moisture levels, weather forecasts, and crop growth patterns to determine optimal irrigation schedules and fertilizer application rates [5][6][7].

Accurate yield predictions can help farmers plan their operations, optimize resource allocation, and make informed harvesting, storage, and marketing decisions [8]. Machine learning algorithms can generate reliable predictions that aid in strategic planning by considering historical yield data along with factors such as weather patterns, soil conditions, and pest/disease prevalence [9].

Another important application is the detection and management of pests and diseases. Early identification of pests and diseases is crucial for preventing widespread damage to crops [10]. Through the examination of data obtained from sensors, satellite imagery, and various other resources, machine-learning models can identify patterns and indicators of pest and disease outbreaks, enabling timely interventions and targeted treatments [11][12].

In addition, predictive analytics can optimize irrigation and fertilization practices, helping to conserve water resources and minimize environmental impact. Using machine learning models, it is possible to assess soil moisture levels, analyze weather forecasts, and study crop growth patterns for the purpose of identifying the most effective irrigation schedules and fertilizer application rates. Despite the immense potential of predictive analytics and machine learning in crop management, several challenges need to be addressed [13]. By leveraging large datasets and advanced algorithms, farmers can prepare data-driven findings, enhance resource sharing, and moderate risks correlated with climate flexibility and pests/diseases [14][15].

2. Methodology

Data Collection

Gather diverse and comprehensive data from several resources such as historical records, remote sensing, soil sensors, weather stations, and crop-specific databases. Here we collected more than 20 crops and for each crop, we collected a minimum of 100 individual data. The given Table 8.1 contains all the average data of the following crops:

Table 8.1   All the crops having their average data value

Soil ph-Level	Rainfall	Temperature	Crop Name
5.9297	112.6548	22.6309	APPLE
5.9766	175.6866	27.4099	COCONUT
6.7903	158.0663	25.5405	COFFEE
6.0259	69.6118	23.8496	GRAPES
5.7666	94.7045	31.2088	MANGO
6.3588	24.6900	28.6631	MUSKMELON
7.0170	110.4750	22.7657	ORANGE
6.7414	142.6278	33.7239	PAPAYA
6.4292	107.5284	21.8378	POMEGRANATE
6.4255	236.1811	23.6893	RICE

Data Pre-processing

Clean the collected data by removing duplicates, handling missing values, and correcting inconsistencies. Normalize or standardize the data to ensure compatibility and facilitate model training. Perform feature engineering to transform and extract meaningful features from the raw data, considering domain knowledge and expert insights. However, this data is refined so that we have no requirement to clean the data but as it is a part of our process if we find any of the information is missing or it has dramatic changes, we will put their NULL value. Now we process all the data by neutralizing their data value using the following formula:

Neutralize Value = (Avg. value − Real value)/Std. Deviation of all value

By neutralizing all the values in Table 8.2 we have all the neutralized values which can be seen in the following data:

Table 8.2 All the crops have their standardized data value

Soil ph-Level	Rainfall	Temperature	Crop Name
-0.9985	-0.1800	-0.8722	APPLE
-0.8860	0.8936	0.3184	COCONUT
1.0651	0.5935	-0.1473	COFFEE
-0.7678	-0.9132	-0.5686	GRAPES
-1.3895	-0.4858	1.2648	MANGO
0.0305	-1.6784	0.6306	MUSKMELON
1.6087	-0.2171	-0.8386	ORANGE
0.9479	0.3305	1.8914	PAPAYA
0.1993	-0.2673	-1.0698	POMEGRANATE
0.1904	1.9241	-0.6085	RICE

Feature Selection

Apply strategies for feature selection to choose the most pertinent and educational elements for the predictive models. Principal Component Analysis (PCA) and Correlation-Based Feature Selection (CFS) are the two distinct feature selection techniques used by the authors.

PCA is a method for reducing a dataset's dimensionality while preserving as much of the original data as feasible [16]. In this paper, the authors use PCA to identify the most important variables that contribute to crop yield. These components are then used as the input variables for the predictive models. CFS is another technique used for feature selection, which involves identifying the variables that are highly correlated with the target variable (crop yield).

In the above figures (Fig. 8.1 and Fig. 8.2) you can easily find the graph variations that is their data value that has to be varied so that the standardized data will be more important and effectively participate in predictive analysis.

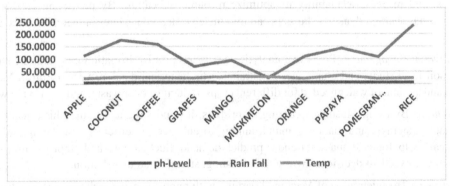

Fig. 8.1 Figure shows the crops and their average data value

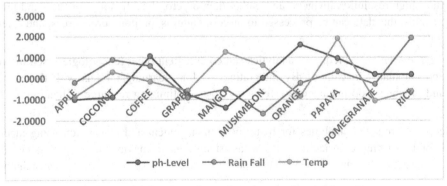

Fig. 8.2 All the crops have their standardized data value

Model Selection and Training:

Select suitable machine learning algorithms according to the objectives and characteristics of the crop management issue. Explore algorithms like decision trees, random forests, support vector machines, neural networks, or ensemble models. Divide the pre-processed data into training and validation sets for the training and evaluation of the model, respectively [17, 18].

Model Evaluation:

Utilize evaluation metrics such as accuracy, precision, recall, F1 score, and area under the curve (AUC) to gauge the performance of the trained models. Employ cross-validation to validate the model's generalization capability and address concerns such as overfitting or underfitting [19].

Continuous Monitoring and Improvement:

Continuously monitor the performance of the deployed predictive analytics system, gathering feedback and updating the models if necessary [20, 21]. Incorporate new data and insights into the models periodically to enhance their accuracy and relevance.

By following this methodology, predictive analytics can be effectively applied to enhance crop management practices and optimize production processes using machine learning techniques.

3. Future Scope

The future scope of predictive analytics for better crop management and production using machine learning is quite promising. Here are some potential developments and opportunities in this field:

Improved crop yield prediction: By employing Machine Learning algorithms, extensive datasets surrounding past weather patterns, land conditions, crop varieties, and farming practices can be analyzed. This enables accurate predictions about future crop yields, providing valuable information for farmers to optimize planting strategies, manage resources efficiently, and make well-informed decisions regarding harvesting and storage.

Optimal resource allocation: Machine Learning algorithms could analyze facts and figures on soil composition, meteorological conditions, crop types, and resource availability to optimize resource allocation. By predicting crop water requirements, fertilizer needs, and optimal planting densities, farmers can minimize waste, reduce environmental impact, and maximize crop productivity.

Smart irrigation and water management: Predictive analytics can help optimize irrigation programs by studying factors like weather predictions, soil level study, and crop water constraints. The historical data are very useful in Machine Learning to suggest the ideal time and amount of water needed for different crops, reducing water waste, and improving water use efficiency.

Supply chain optimization: By using Machine Learning algorithms, it is possible to examine historical data related to crop production, transportation, storage, and market demand, aiming to enhance the efficiency of the agricultural supply chain. Predictive analytics can help forecast market trends, predict demand fluctuations, and improve inventory management, permitting farmers to make excellent decisions involving harvesting, storage, and distribution.

Remote sensing and drones: The integration of Machine Learning with remote sensing technologies and drones offers valuable insights into crop management. Nowadays we have many advanced drones that are equipped with various agricultural sensors and cameras, can capture high-resolution imagery, and gather data on crop health, soil moisture, and temperature. Utilizing machine learning algorithms, this data can be processed to discern patterns, pinpoint crop stress, and offer recommendations for targeted interventions.

Integration with precision agriculture: Predictive analytics can complement other technologies used in precision agriculture, such as GPS, GIS, and automated machinery. By integrating machine learning models with these technologies, farmers can achieve precise and efficient crop management, reducing costs, optimizing resource utilization, and improving overall productivity.

Overall, the future scope of predictive analytics for better crop management and production using machine learning holds tremendous potential for transforming agriculture. It can assist farmers in making better judgments, optimizing resource allocation, reducing the impact on the environment, and improving overall crop productivity and sustainability.

4. Conclusion

In conclusion, the integration of predictive analytics and machine learning techniques in crop management and production holds great promise for transforming agriculture into a more efficient, sustainable, and productive industry. By leveraging the power of data-driven decision-making, farmers and agribusinesses can optimize crop management practices, increase productivity, and mitigate risks associated with climate variability, pests, and diseases.

Throughout this paper, we have surveyed the various purposes, challenges, and potential assistance of utilizing predictive analytics in crop management using machine learning algorithms. One of the key applications identified is yield prediction, where accurate predictions can assist farmers in planning their operations, optimizing resource allocation, and making informed decisions regarding harvesting, storage, and marketing. Machine learning algorithms can generate reliable predictions that aid in strategic planning by considering historical yield data along with factors such as weather relationships, land conditions, and pest/disease prevalence. By merging predictive analytics and machine learning also provides prospects for precision agriculture and site-specific management. Through the utilization of geospatial data, farmers can execute variable rate application of inputs, customizing interventions based on the specific requirements of different zones within their fields. This focused strategy reduces input waste and enhances the overall efficiency of crop management. Despite the considerable potential of predictive analytics in crop management, several challenges must be tackled for successful implementation. The availability and quality of data emerge as one of the primary challenges. The process of collecting and integrating data from various sources can be intricate, and ensuring data accuracy, reliability, and standardization is pivotal for deriving meaningful insights. Collaboration among farmers, researchers, and technology providers becomes essential to establish data-sharing frameworks and develop standardized protocols for data collection.

Providing farmers with transparent and interpretable models is essential to build trust and confidence in technology. Developing explainable AI techniques and visualizations can help farmers understand the reasoning behind the predictions and make informed decisions based on them. Overfitting, a common challenge in machine learning, must be addressed to ensure the generalization and robustness of the predictive models. Applying proper model validation techniques, such as cross-validation, and optimizing hyperparameters are crucial steps in preventing overfitting and achieving reliable predictions. Additionally, model performance should be continuously monitored and updated to incorporate new data and adapt to changing conditions.

REFERENCES

1. Liu, Z., Zhu, Q., Zhao, J., & Chen, X., Yield Prediction of Maize Crops Based on Machine Learning Algorithms. Remote Sensing, 13(4), 740, 2021.
2. Mondal, P., Kumar, U., & Jat, M. L., Early Detection of Wheat Rust Disease Using Machine Learning and Remote Sensing. Computers and Electronics in Agriculture, 185, 106006, 2021.
3. Wan, J., Zeng, W., Pan, H., Qian, L., Gong, J., & Ding, S., Deep Learning for Image-Based Weed Detection in Turf Grass. Frontiers in Plant Science, 10, 1172, 2019.
4. Priyadharshini, Aayush Kumar, Swapneel Chakraborty and Omen Rajendra, "Intelligent Crop Recommendation System using Machine Learning", Proceedings of the Fifth International Conference on Computing Methodologies and Communication (ICCMC 2021) IEEE Xplore Part Number: CFP21K25-ART.
5. Nishit Jain, Amit Kumar, Sahil Garud, Vishal Pradhan and Prajakta Kulkarni, "Crop Selection Method Based Various Environmental Factors Using Machine Learning", International Research Journal of Engineering and Technology (IRJET), vol. 04, no. 02, Feb 2017.
6. Devdatta A. Bondre and Santosh Mahagaonkar, "Prediction of Crop Yield and Fertilizer Recommendation using Machine Learning Algorithms", vol. 4, no. 5, pp. 371–376, Sept 2019.
7. Lobell, D. B., & Asseng, S., Predicting the effects of climate change on crop yields: Progress and challenges. Annual Review of Plant Biology, 68, 669–688, 2017.
8. Huang, M., Li, J., Zhang, H., Wang, P., & Gao, X., A Survey of Machine Learning Models in Renewable Energy Predictions. Appl. Sci. 2020, 10, 5975; doi:10.3390/app10175975.
9. Jiao, R.; Huang, X.; Ma, X.; Han, L.; Tian, W., A Model Combining Stacked Auto Encoder and Back Propagation Algorithm for Short-Term Wind Power Forecasting. IEEE Access 2018, 6, 17851–17858.
10. Huang, C.J.; Kuo, P.H. A Short-Term Wind Speed Forecasting Model by Using Artificial Neural Networks with Stochastic Optimization for Renewable Energy Systems. Energies 2018, 11, 2777.
11. Lobell, D. B., & Asseng, S., Predicting the Effects of Climate Change on Crop Yields: Progress and Challenges. Annual Review of Plant Biology, 68, 669–688, 2017.
12. Piryonesi, S. M., & Bakhshipour, A., A Review of Machine Learning Approaches for Yield Prediction in Precision Agriculture. Computers and Electronics in Agriculture, 184, 106040, 2021.

13. Acharya, A., Shree, C., & Agrawal, A., Agricultural Productivity Improvement using Data Mining Techniques. Indian Journal of Agricultural Research, 49(4), 334–343, 2016.
14. Fuentes, A., Yoon, S., Kim, S., & Park, D. S., A Review of Image Processing Techniques for Plant Disease Detection Using Digital Images. Multimedia Tools and Applications, 75(20), 12499-12520, 2016. https://doi.org/10.1007/s11042-015-2971-8
15. Mohanty, S. P., Hughes, D. P., & Salathé, M., Using Deep Learning for Image-Based Plant Disease Detection. Frontiers in Plant Science, 7, 1419, 2016. https://doi.org/10.3389/fpls.2016.01419
16. Kamilaris, A., Prenafeta-Boldú, F. X., & Sudhakar, P., Deep Learning in Agriculture: A Survey. Computers and Electronics in Agriculture, 147, 70-90, 2018. https://doi.org/10.1016/j.compag.2018.02.016
17. Sladojevic, S., Arsenovic, M., Anderla, A., Culibrk, D., & Stefanovic, D., Deep Neural Networks Based Recognition of Plant Diseases by Leaf Image Classification. Computational Intelligence and Neuroscience, 2016, 3289801. https://doi.org/10.1155/2016/3289801
18. Singh, A., Ganapathysubramanian, B., Sarkar, S., & Singh, A. K., Machine Learning for High-Throughput Stress Phenotyping in Plants. Trends in Plant Science, 21(2), 110–124, 2016.
19. Huan Liu and Lei Yu, "Toward integrating feature selection algorithms for classification and clustering", IEEE Transactions on Knowledge and Data Engineering, vol. 17, no. 4, pp. 491–502, 2005.
20. Baris Senliol et al., "Fast Correlation Based Filter (FCBF) with a different search strategy", Computer and Information Sciences 2008. ISCIS'08. 23rd International Symposium on, 2008.
21. Hanchuan Peng, Fuhui Long and Chris Ding, "Feature selection based on mutual information criteria of max-dependency max-relevance and min-redundancy", IEEE Transactions on pattern analysis and machine intelligence, vol. 27, no. 8, pp. 1226–1238, 2005.

Emerging Trends in IoT and Computing Technologies – Suman Lata Tripathi et al. (eds)
© 2024 Taylor & Francis Group, London, ISBN 978-1-032-87924-6

Challenges and Benefits in Future Direction of Internet of Things

9

Pooja Kumari Singh[1]

School of IT, FIMT, GGSIP University, New Delhi, India

Akash Sanghi[2]

CSE Department, Invertis University, Bareilly, Uttar Pradesh, India

Gaurav Agarwal[3]

CSE Department, Invertis University, Bareilly, Uttar Pradesh, India

Mohammed Shakeel[4]

FOCA, Invertis University, Bareilly, Uttar Pradesh, India

Yashi Bajpai[5]

CSE Department, Invertis University, Bareilly, Uttar Pradesh, India

Abstract: IoT The (Internet of Things) represents a transformative force in our digital world, promising a future where everyday objects and devices are interconnected to enhance efficiency, convenience, and productivity. This abstract explores the challenges and benefits that lie ahead in the future direction of IoT. Challenges in IoT's future direction encompass issues like security, interoperability, data management, scalability, energy efficiency, and cost concerns. These barriers must be addressed to unlock IoT's full potential. On the flip side, the benefits of IoT are abundant. It offers real-time data analysis, improved decision-making, automation of tasks, and enhanced user experiences across various fields, including healthcare, smart cities, agriculture, and industry. Comparing IoT with traditional networks emphasizes the unique scale and data diversity of IoT, while Quality of Service (QoS) considerations underscore the importance of factors like reliability, latency, and security in IoT deployments. Key enabling technologies, like virtualization, sensor networks, RFID (radio frequency identification), and communication protocol strategies, are crucial for building robust and scalable IoT ecosystems. In the evolving landscape of IoT, the focus on addressing these challenges while harnessing the associated benefits is pivotal. The future direction of IoT promises a world of innovation, efficiency, and connectivity, but it requires a thoughtful approach to overcome obstacles and seize opportunities for a more connected and intelligent future.

Keywords: IoT, Quality of service (QOS), Virtualization, Wireless sensor network, RFID, Communication protocol

1. Introduction

IoT is an innovative technological idea that has revolutionised our interactions with the physical world then collect and exchange data. It represents a system of devices connecting to each other and objects, which are equipped with software, sensors, and other embedded technologies that allow them to gather, communicate, and act upon data. These gadgets might be anything from regular household items like thermostats and refrigerators to industrial machines, vehicles, and even wearable technology. The

[1]pooja5singh23@gmail.com, [2]sanghiakash@gmail.com, [3]gaurav.a1@invertis.org, [4]shakeel@invertis.org, [5]yashibajpai877@gmail.com

DOI: 10.1201/9781003535423-9

fundamental idea behind IoT is to create a seamless and interconnected ecosystem where physical objects can communicate and engage in conversation with one another and with humans through the internet. This interaction and data exchange occur in real-time, offering numerous possibilities and applications across various industries and in our daily lives.

IoT has the potential to revolutionize industries such as healthcare, agriculture, transportation, manufacturing, and smart cities by increasing effectiveness, cutting expenses, and refining the decision-making process. For instance, IoT devices in the healthcare industry can track patients' vital indicators remotely, while in agriculture, sensors can optimize irrigation and crop management. In transportation, connected vehicles can improve road safety, and in smart cities, IoT can optimize energy usage and enhance urban planning. However, IoT also raises important concerns related to privacy, security, and data management, as the massive amounts of data generated and shared through IoT devices need robust protection and regulation. Figure 9.1 shows the flow control from sensor to actuator in IoT.

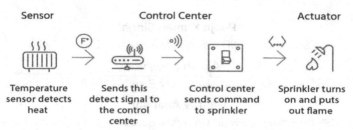

Fig. 9.1 Sensor to actuator flow

1.1 Various Segments of Internet of Things

The cloud acts as the central hub where data from myriad IoT devices is stored, managed, and processed, offering the scalability required for handling substantial data volumes. In the application layer, software and applications empower users and devices to interact with and manage IoT devices, whether through smartphones, web interfaces, or other connected devices. Security is a paramount concern in the IoT landscape, encompassing aspects like secure device authentication, data encryption, and protection against cyber threats. The underlying network infrastructure, comprising routers, gateways, and switches, is pivotal in routing data between IoT devices and the cloud, ensuring reliable and secure data transmission [5]. To facilitate seamless communication and interoperability, IoT relies on various standards and protocols such as MQTT, CoAP, and HTTP. Efficient management and monitoring tools are crucial for provisioning, troubleshooting, and optimizing IoT devices and data streams. Lastly, ensuring compliance with data protection regulations and privacy policies, it is essential to address the ethical and legal aspects of IoT data collection and usage. In unison, these components form the backbone of IoT, enabling the creation of connected and intelligent systems that enhance various aspects of our lives.

2. Use of IoT in Diverse Fields

The uses of the IoT (Internet of Things) are vast then diverse, spanning across numerous industries and enhancing our daily lives. Smart homes, for instance, leverage IoT to create a connected environment, featuring devices like smart thermostats, security cameras and lighting systems. These devices can be controlled remotely through smartphones, fostering energy efficiency and bolstering security measures. In the realm of healthcare, IoT devices play a pivotal role in monitoring vital signs of patients, making sure that medication is taken as prescribed, and transmitting information for healthcare providers for isolated patient observing. This enables early intervention and improved patient outcomes. In agriculture, precision farming is powered by IoT, as it keeps an eye on crop health, weather trends, and soil characteristics. This abundance of information enables farmers to make wise decisions, regarding irrigation, fertilization, and pest control, ultimately primary to increased crop yields and environmentally friendly farming methods. The industrial sector witnesses the rise of Industrial IoT (IIoT), which enhances efficiency and reduces downtime by monitoring the condition of machines and predicting maintenance requirements. It also streamlines supply chain operations and bolsters quality control measures. Transportation and logistics benefit from IoT technologies for vehicle and cargo tracking, route optimization, and efficient fleet management, particularly within the realm of autonomous and connected vehicles. Smart cities are making strides towards improved efficiency and sustainability by integrating IoT technologies. This includes smart traffic management, optimized waste management, intelligent street lighting, and air quality monitoring. Energy management, also employs IoT devices to monitor and control electricity, gas, and water consumption, contributing to resource conservation [3].

Retail establishments leverage IoT for inventory management, customer analytics, and personalized marketing. Innovations such as smart shelves and beacons enhance the shopping experience. Environmental monitoring sees IoT sensors deployed to track air and water quality, monitor forest fires, and gather climate change data, all of which play a crucial role in early warning systems and ecological preservation. The modernization of electrical grids is made possible by IoT in the form of smart grids, enabling real-time monitoring and control of power distribution, enhancing efficiency, and accommodating renewable energy sources [4]. Wearable technology, including smartwatches and fitness trackers, captures data on physical activity, health metrics, and biometrics, promoting healthier lifestyles. IoT's reach extends to security and surveillance, where IoT security cameras, access control systems, and sensors offer real-time monitoring and alerting capabilities. Asset tracking is another application, managing and tracking assets like vehicles, containers, and equipment in sectors such as logistics, construction, and manufacturing. The IoT technology cab be of utmost importance in a pandemic setting. IoT networking components enable remote operation of any device. [7]. Additionally, Internet of Things has found use in aiding individuals with disabilities through the implementation of smart devices, including voice-controlled home automation systems and smart prosthetics. Agricultural drones equipped with IoT technology are instrumental in surveying large agricultural areas, capturing data on crop health, irrigation needs, and pest infestations. In supply chain management, IoT streamlines operations by tracking products and assets, managing inventory, and optimizing logistics [6].

3. Internet of Things (History)

The history of the IoT has its roots in the late 20th century when the concept of connecting physical objects to the internet emerged. Notably, in 1982, computer science students at Carnegie Mellon University devised an early experiment by creating the first internet-connected appliance—a Coca-Cola machine capable of reporting its inventory and the temperature of newly loaded drinks. This experiment laid the foundational concept for IoT. The word "Internet of Things" was officially invented in 1999 by British technology pioneer Kevin Ashton, who utilised it to explain a system where things might be uniquely identified and tracked through radio-frequency identification (RFID) technology. The early 2000s marked a significant development with the adoption of RFID and sensor technologies, enabling objects to be tagged and collect data that could be shared over the internet. Mid-2000s saw the rise of wireless sensor networks, which gained prominence for various applications, such as environmental monitoring and industrial automation. By late 2000s, IoT began to make its impact in the industrial sector, often referred to as the Industrial Internet of Things (IIoT). This phase involved connecting machinery and equipment to enhance maintenance, monitoring, and operational efficiency.

In the 2010s, consumer IoT took centre stage as smart speakers, security cameras, and thermostats are examples of smart home technology. were introduced, designed to enhance convenience and energy efficiency. IoT platforms and ecosystems also emerged, providing tools and frameworks for developing, managing, and scaling IoT applications, facilitating easier integration of devices and data. Advancements in connectivity, particularly with the development and deployment of Low-power, wide-area network (LPWAN) technology and 5G networks, have significantly improved the capabilities of IoT devices for data transmission. As we entered the 2020s, IoT continued to expand its reach into various industries, including healthcare, agriculture, transportation, smart cities, and more. Use cases multiplied, encompassing remote patient monitoring, precision agriculture, autonomous vehicles, and urban management. Notably, the COVID-19 pandemic in the 2020s highlighted the vital role of IoT in addressing unprecedented challenges. It was instrumental in contact tracing, monitoring quarantine compliance, and efficiently managing healthcare resources. The evolution of IoT over the years underscores its growing significance in shaping our connected and data-driven world [2].

4. Key Barriers of Using IoT

The adoption of the IoT brings with it a set of significant challenges and barriers that must be addressed for its widespread success. One of the foremost concerns is security and privacy. IoT gadgets are susceptible to hacking and cyberattacks that may jeopardise user privacy and expose sensitive data. Robust security measures, including encryption, authentication, and regular updates, are imperative. Interoperability poses another hurdle as the lack of standardized communication protocols and data formats can impede seamless interaction between different IoT devices and platforms. Achieving interoperability is essential for the smooth functioning within the Internet of Things ecosystem. With IoT devices generating substantial volumes of data, efficient data management and storage have become a pressing challenge. This necessitates scalable cloud infrastructure and edge computing solutions to handle the data influx effectively. Scalability is crucial given that the quantity of IoT devices keeps growing surge. Ensuring that IoT networks can accommodate a vast array of devices while upholding performance and reliability is central to its success. Energy efficiency is crucial, particularly for battery-powered IoT devices, and optimizing energy consumption, extending battery life, and minimizing environmental impact is an ongoing concern. Implementing IoT systems can be costly, posing a barrier to smaller businesses and organizations. Therefore, reducing the cost of IoT components and services is pivotal in making IoT more accessible. The absence of widely accepted industry standards and regulatory frameworks creates uncertainty and hinders IoT adoption. Developing common standards for security, data privacy, and device communication is crucial to resolve this issue. Integrating IoT solutions into existing systems and processes is complex and time-consuming.

Regulatory and legal challenges, including data protection regulations like GDPR in Europe, place stringent requirements on data collection and handling. Ensuring compliance and navigating the legal landscape can be complex. Ethical and social concerns surrounding surveillance, data ownership, and potential job displacement due to automation raise important ethical questions that must be addressed as IoT proliferates. Ensuring high reliability and availability in mission-critical IoT applications, such as healthcare and industrial automation, is a substantial challenge. Downtime can have severe consequences, making this a critical aspect of IoT deployment. Sustainability in the design and use of IoT technologies is an important consideration for mitigating these effects. Lastly, human resistance to adopting IoT solutions due to concerns about data privacy and reluctance to embrace change can lead to a slow adoption rate among consumers and businesses. Addressing these barriers and challenges is vital to realizing the full potential of IoT while ensuring its responsible and secure use across various industries [3,4].

5. Difference between use of IoT and Traditional Network

IoT systems aren't the same as traditional networks. They are designed to connect and interconnect a vast number of devices, sensors, and objects, permitting them to gather and share information over the internet. It focuses on enabling machines and devices to communicate and perform tasks without human intervention. IoT networks are capable of supporting a significantly larger number of devices, often in the billions. These gadgets might be anything from basic sensors to intricate equipment. IoT networks handle a diverse range of data types, including sensor data, telemetry, and real-time data. This data can be generated from a range of sources, such as environmental sensors, industrial machines, and wearable procedures. IoT networks often involve intermittent, small data transmissions from sensors and devices which makes them having periodic and bursty traffic patterns. IoT applications may tolerate some degree of latency, as real-time requirements can vary depending on the use case. Some IoT devices can operate with short delays in data transmission IoT devices often need robust security measures due to the large number of devices and potential vulnerabilities. Ensuring secure device authentication and data encryption is a critical consideration. IoT networks often employ various network architectures, including mesh and star topologies, and edge computing to accommodate scalability and meet the specific needs of different IoT application.

On the other hand, traditional networks primarily serve human communication, connecting computers, servers, and devices that people use for data exchange and communication. Traditional networks, while also supporting many devices, are generally designed for fewer devices compared to IoT networks. Traditional networks primarily handle data generated by humans, including text, images, videos, and voice communications. Traditional networks typically deal with continuous data streams, voice calls, video streaming, and other data that may require consistent and high bandwidth. Traditional networks, especially for low latency is necessary for applications like online gaming and video conferencing. to ensure smooth user experiences. Security in traditional networks typically involves user authentication and data protection, but the scale and diversity of devices in IoT networks demand additional security measures. Traditional networks typically use a centralized architecture, such as client-server or peer-to-peer, but they may not need the same level of device scalability as IoT networks [1].

6. Key Characteristics of IoT

Impact of Internet of Things can be confirmed by the key characteristics of it. Various key aspects of IoT are discussed below.

6.1 Quality of Service for Internet of Thing

Quality of Service (QoS) is a paramount consideration in the realm of the IoT. It shows a pivotal part in ensuring that IoT applications and services meet predefined performance and reliability standards. QoS for IoT is multifaceted, encompassing several critical factors. Reliability and availability are fundamental, with IoT networks expected to deliver data and services consistently without disruptions [1]. Furthermore, latency requirements can vary based on the application, with some necessitating low latency for real-time operations, while others may tolerate slightly higher latency. Throughput, scalability, and security are also vital components of IoT QoS. The ability to transmit and receive data efficiently, scale to accommodate a growing number of devices and protect data from cyber threats are key aspects to maintain a high quality of service in the IoT ecosystem. Interoperability, adaptability, and adherence to regulatory standards round out the multifaceted considerations in the pursuit of delivering reliable and efficient IoT services.

6.2 Virtualization in Internet of Thing

Virtualization has a major part in the context of the IoT by enhancing flexibility, scalability, efficiency in IoT deployments. IoT virtualization involves creating virtual instances of physical devices or resources, allowing for the efficient use of hardware and software components. These virtualized entities can be managed, monitored, and controlled remotely, making IoT systems more adaptable and responsive to changing demands. This technology is particularly useful in scenarios where resource allocation and scaling need to be dynamic, such as in industrial IoT (IIoT) and smart cities. IoT virtualization enables the sharing of resources, enhances security by isolating critical components, and simplifies software management and updates. It also streamlines IoT device provisioning and management, making it easier to add or remove devices as needed. Virtualization is a key enabler for the scalability, cost-effectiveness, and agility of IoT deployments in diverse applications [1].

6.3 Wireless Sensor Network in Internet of Thing

The Internet of Things (IoT) is based mostly on wireless sensor networks (WSNs), serving as the sensory nervous system of this interconnected ecosystem. Wireless Sensor Networks consist of numerous tiny, power-efficient sensors equipped with data collection and communication capabilities. These sensors monitor various environmental factors, such as mobility, light, humidity, and temperature, and transmit the collected data wirelessly to a central hub or cloud-based platform. In the context of IoT, WSNs enable real-time data collection and remote monitoring, making them invaluable in applications like environmental sensing, industrial automation, agriculture, and smart cities. WSNs contribute to efficient data gathering and decision-making, offering insights that drive automation, energy savings, and improved resource management. They are essential in creating a responsive and intelligent IoT environment, as they provide the data needed for informed actions and decision-making [7].

6.4 Radio Frequency Identification in Internet of Thing

RFID technology shows a pivotal role in the IoT ecosystem by enabling the unique identification and tracking of items and resources. RFID tags come in two varieties: passive, which runs on the reader's signal, and active, which runs on its own power source, are attached to physical items, allowing them to be wirelessly scanned and identified by RFID readers or sensors. In the context of IoT, RFID enhances visibility and control over assets and products throughout their lifecycle. It is widely employed in supply chain management, logistics, inventory tracking, and retail for real-time asset tracking and inventory control. RFID technology ensures seamless, accurate data collection and helps optimize various processes, enhancing efficiency and reducing human errors. By providing the ability to collect and share real-time data on the location and status of objects, RFID contributes significantly to the automation and intelligence of IoT applications [1].

6.5 Strategy of Communication Protocols of Using Internet of Thing

Choosing the right communication protocols is a critical aspect of implementing IoT, as it profoundly influences how IoT devices and systems communicate and share data. The strategy for communication protocols in IoT is multifaceted, with several key considerations. First and foremost is scalability and interoperability, ensuring that devices from various manufacturers can communicate seamlessly, fostering scalability and compatibility. Latency and real-time requirements are essential, with applications like autonomous vehicles requiring low-latency communication, while environmental monitoring may tolerate higher latency. Data size and bandwidth considerations come into play, as some applications demand high data rates (e.g., video surveillance), while others, like temperature sensors, require minimal data transmission. Most of the IoT devices are battery-powered, thus energy efficiency is paramount. Low-power communication protocols help conserve energy and extend battery life. Security is a non-negotiable factor, with communication protocols requiring robust mechanisms such as data encryption and authentication to safeguard data and privacy. Reliability and redundancy are crucial, particularly in critical sectors like healthcare and industrial automation, where uninterrupted data transmission is essential. Cost considerations also play a significant role, especially for small and medium-sized businesses. Selecting cost-effective communication protocols for hardware, software, and infrastructure is vital. Several common communication protocols are used in IoT, including MQTT, CoAP, HTTP, and LPWAN technologies like LoRaWAN and NB-IoT. The strategy for choosing communication protocols must weigh these considerations carefully to ensure that IoT systems meet their objectives effectively and efficiently [4].

7. Future of IoT

The future of the Internet of Things (IoT) is poised for tremendous growth and transformation, but it is not without its challenges and opportunities. IoT, which began as a visionary concept, has rapidly evolved to become an integral part of our digital landscape, shaping how we interact with the world around us. The historical journey of IoT, from its early experimental stages to its current widespread applications across various fields, showcases the remarkable progress it has made. IoT has found its way into diverse domains, including smart homes, healthcare, agriculture, and industrial automation, enhancing convenience, efficiency, and productivity. Yet, the path forward is not without its obstacles. Key barriers such as security, interoperability, scalability, and energy efficiency needs to be taken care of to guarantee the responsible and secure expansion of IoT. These challenges are crucial in navigating the complex landscape of IoT versus traditional networks and in maintaining the desired Quality of Service (QoS), with an emphasis on reliability, latency, and security. Moreover, IoT's future direction relies on key enabling technologies, including virtualization, wireless sensor networks, radio frequency identification (RFID), and communication protocol strategies. These technologies are pivotal in building the foundation for efficient, scalable, and secure IoT ecosystems [4]. The future of IoT holds the promise of a more connected and intelligent world, where data-driven insights and automation empower us to make better decisions, improve our daily lives, and optimize industrial processes. Embracing these challenges while harnessing the benefits is essential for realizing the full potential of IoT and ensuring its responsible and innovative development. The future of IoT is a journey of both technical and strategic evolution that will continue to shape our digital future in profound ways.

REFERENCES

1. Zainab H. Al, Hesham A. Ali, Mahmoud M. Badawy, "Internet of Things (IoT): Definitions, Challenges and Recent Research Directions", International Journal of Computer Applications (0975 – 8887), Vol. 128, No. 1, October 2015.
2. Vivian Ukamaka Ihekoronye, Cosmas Ifeanyi Nwakanma, Goodness Oluchi Anyanwu, Dong-Seong Kim, Jae-Min Lee, "Benefits, Challenges and Practical Concerns of IoT for Smart Manufacturing", 2021 International Conference on Information and Communication Technology Convergence (ICTC), IEEE, DOI: 10.1109/ICTC52510.2021.9620771.
3. Nahida Sultana, Marzia Tamanna, "Exploring the benefits and challenges of Internet of Things (IoT) during Covid-19: a case study of Bangladesh" Discover Internet of Things (2021) 1–20, https://doi.org/10.1007/s43926-021-00020-9.
4. Hamed Taherdoost, "Security and Internet of Things: Benefits, Challenges, and Future Perspectives", Electronics 2023, 12, 1901. https:// doi.org/10.3390/electronics12081901.
5. Brous, P., Janssen, M, "Effects of The Internet of Things (IoT): A Systematic Review of The Benefits and Risks", The 2015 International Conference on Electronic Business, Taipei, December 6–10, 2015.
6. Kehinde Lawal, Hamed Nabizadeh Rafsanjani, "Trends, benefits, risks, and challenges of IoT implementation in residential and commercial buildings", Energy and Built Environment (2021), Doi: 10.1016/j.enbenv.2021.01.009, February, 2021.
7. Ankit Saxena, Akash Sanghi, Swapnesh Taterh, Neeraj Bhargava, "Role of IoT in the Prevention of COVID-19", https://onlinelibrary.wiley.com/doi/abs/10.1002/9781119836667.ch9.

Emerging Trends in IoT and Computing Technologies – Suman Lata Tripathi et al. (eds)
© 2024 Taylor & Francis Group, London, ISBN 978-1-032-87924-6

Implementation of Brute Force Attack

10

Priyanshu Sharma[1], Sarvesh Tanwar[2]
Amity Institute of Information Technology, Amity University, Noida

Vinay Kukreja[3]
Chitkara University Institute of Engineering and Technology, Chitkara University, Punjab, India

Abstract: Brute force attacks are aggressive methods employed by malicious actors to gain unauthorized access to computer systems, networks, or encrypted data. This research paper aims to provide a detailed analysis of brute force attacks, exploring their various types and demonstrating their implementation using the Python programming language. The paper delves into the underlying principles behind brute force attacks, examines the potential risks associated with them, and presents a step-by-step Python-based implementation of such attacks. It examines the significance of password complexity and strength in resisting such attacks and explores different brute force algorithms. The algorithms discussed include exhaustive search, dictionary attacks, and hybrid approaches that combine various techniques.

Keywords: Brute force attack, Python, Cryptographic attack, Exhaustive search, Dictionary attacks, Hybrid approaches

1. Introduction

Brute force attacks pose a significant threat to the security of computer systems, networks, and encrypted data. These attacks involve systematically trying every possible combination of passwords or encryption keys until the correct one is discovered, granting unauthorized access to the target [1]. The objective of this research work is to provide a comprehensive exploration of brute force attacks and demonstrate their implementation using the Python programming language. Python is a popular and versatile language known for its simplicity, readability, and extensive library support, making it an ideal choice for developing tools and scripts related to cybersecurity.

The paper will delve into the fundamental principles of brute force attacks, examining their various types and the vulnerabilities they exploit. It will explore the importance of password complexity and strength, as well as the algorithms used in brute force attacks, such as exhaustive search, dictionary attacks, and hybrid approaches. One of the key contributions of this work is the practical demonstration of implementing brute force attacks using Python. By providing step-by-step guidance and code examples, this paper aims to equip readers with the knowledge and skills to understand and develop their own Python-based brute force attack scripts [2] [5].

1.1 Methodology

Preparing the Environment: This section outlines the methodology for setting up the necessary environment to carry out the experiment effectively.

---

[1]priyanshu.sharma4@s.amity.edu, [2]s.tanwar1521@gmail.com, [3]vinay.kukreja@chitkara.edu.in

DOI: 10.1201/9781003535423-10

Research Objectives and Scope: Clearly define the objectives and scope of the research study. Identify the specific aspects of brute force attacks that will be investigated, such as types of attacks, target systems, or authentication mechanisms.

Research Ethics and Legal Considerations: Familiarize yourself with ethical guidelines and legal considerations related to conducting experiments on brute force attacks. Ensure that you comply with all applicable laws and regulations, obtain necessary permissions, and protect the privacy and security of any systems or data involved in the study [7].

Identify the Target System: Select a target system or web application for the experiment. It can be a local environment, a virtual machine, or a designated testing environment. Ensure that you have proper authorization to perform the experiment on the chosen system [11].

Set Up the Target System: Install and configure the target system according to the requirements of the research study. This may involve installing the necessary operating system, web server, and database software. Configure any authentication mechanisms or security settings that are relevant to the experiment.

Install Python and Required Libraries: Install the Python programming language on the target system. Choose the appropriate version of Python based on the compatibility requirements. Install the necessary libraries, such as 'requests' and 'BeautifulSoup', for implementing the brute force attack script [3].

Set Up a Testing Environment: Create a testing environment separate from production systems to ensure the safety and integrity of the target system. This can be a virtual machine, a containerized environment, or a separate network segment dedicated to testing purposes.

Prepare Test Data and Credentials: Generate or obtain a set of test data and credentials for the experiment. This includes usernames, passwords, and any other relevant information required for the brute force attack.

Configure Logging and Monitoring: Set up logging and monitoring mechanisms to capture relevant data during the experiment. This includes tracking login attempts, recording response times, and monitoring network traffic to analyze the behavior of the brute force attack [6].

Test System Connectivity: Ensure that the target system and the system executing the brute force attack script can communicate properly. Test network connectivity, verify firewall settings, and check any other network configurations required for the experiment.

2. Implementation

The popular computer language Python is praised for its clarity, readability, and adaptability. Python provides powerful tools and libraries that enable attackers to implement and execute brute force attacks efficiently [4][12]. In this section, we introduce Python and explore its features and capabilities in the context of brute force attacks.

2.1 Python Libraries Used

RANDOM MODULE

The random module in Python is a powerful tool that provides various functions for working with random numbers and elements. It is part of the Python Standard Library, which means it comes pre-installed with Python and can be used in any Python program without requiring any additional installation.

TQDM MODULE

The tqdm module is a Python library that provides a fast, extensible progress bar for loops and other iterable objects. The name "tqdm" stands for "taqaddum," which means "progress" in Arabic. It offers a simple and convenient way to visualize the progress of a task, making it easier to estimate the completion time and keep track of long-running processes [3].

3. Results and Discussions

3.1 Results

Brute force attacks are a method used by hackers to crack passwords or encryption by systematically trying all possible combinations until the correct one is found. The attacker starts by selecting a target, such as a user account or encrypted file, that they want to gain unauthorized access to. The attacker then employs an automated tool or script that generates and tests an exhaustive list of possible passwords or encryption keys The tool systematically tries each combination, starting from simple and commonly used passwords, and progressing to more complex and unique ones.

Case 1: Low Difficulty Password

Attempting to generate password

```
C:\Users\Sumit\PycharmProjects\pythonProject4\venv\Scripts\python.exe C:\Users\Sumit\PycharmProjects\pythonProject4\main.py
Attempting to brute force cvionm
60%|          | 14213802/23762752 [00:03<00:02, 4530965.39it/s]
```

Fig. 10.1 Password generation

Password Cracked

```
C:\Users\Sumit\PycharmProjects\pythonProject4\venv\Scripts\python.exe C:\Users\Sumit\PycharmProjects\pythonProject4\main.py
Attempting to brute force cvionm
33509670it [00:07, 4708588.84it/s]
Bruteforced password ('c', 'v', 'i', 'o', 'n', 'm') in 7 seconds

Process finished with exit code 0
```

Fig. 10.2 Password cracked

Case 2: Moderate Difficulty Password

Attempting to crack password

```
C:\Users\Sumit\PycharmProjects\pythonProject4\venv\Scripts\python.exe C:\Users\Sumit\PycharmProjects\pythonProject4\main.py
Attempting to brute force kzxelx
57%|          | 68135499/118813760 [00:26<00:14, 3460650.39it/s]
```

Fig. 10.3 Moderate difficulty password

Password cracked

```
C:\Users\Sumit\PycharmProjects\pythonProject4\venv\Scripts\python.exe C:\Users\Sumit\PycharmProjects\pythonProject4\main.py
Attempting to brute force kzxelx
130645421it [00:58, 2245619.49it/s]
Bruteforced password ('k', 'z', 'x', 'e', 'l', 'x') in 59 seconds

Process finished with exit code 0
```

Fig. 10.4 Password cracked

Case 3: High Difficulty Password

Attempting to crack password

```
C:\Users\Sumit\PycharmProjects\pythonProject4\venv\Scripts\python.exe C:\Users\Sumit\PycharmProjects\pythonProject4\main.py
Attempting to brute force qdhtro
8%|          | 15526039/190102016 [00:03<00:34, 5127133.87it/s]
```

Fig. 10.5 High difficulty password

Password cracked

```
C:\Users\Sumit\PycharmProjects\pythonProject4\venv\Scripts\python.exe C:\Users\Sumit\PycharmProjects\pythonProject4\main.py
Attempting to brute force qdhtro
191609276it [01:33, 2059154.29it/s]
Bruteforced password ('q', 'd', 'h', 't', 'r', 'o') in 93 seconds

Process finished with exit code 0
```

Fig. 10.6 Password cracked

Table 10.1 is showing analysis of brute-force attack.

Table 10.1 Analysis of Brute-Force Attack

S. No.	Password generated	Difficulty	No. of Iterations	Time taken
Case 1	cvionm	Low	33509670	7 seconds
Case 2	kzxelx	Moderate	130645421	59 seconds
Case 3	qdhtro	High	191609276	93 seconds

3.2 Discussions

The execution of this program takes place in the following steps:

- Declare a starting time using the time module.
- Define a variable and store all the lower-case ASCII characters in it obtained from the String module.
- Use the Random module to generate a string from the characters present in the above defined variable.
- Define a function that calculates the approximate time needed to try out all outcomes.
- Compare each newly generated string with the previously obtained sequence until a match is found.
- Display the final password and the time taken to crack it.

Here is a general explanation of the typical output you might expect when executing a brute force attack program:

Starting Message: The program might display an initial message indicating that the brute force attack is starting. This message could include information about the target system or the parameters being used for the attack.

Progress Updates: During the execution of the brute force attack, the program may provide periodic updates on its progress. These updates can include the number of attempts made, the current password or key being tested, or the percentage of completion.

Successful Password/Key Found: If the brute force attack is successful and the correct password or encryption key is found, the program will output a message indicating the success. This message might include the discovered password or key, and possibly additional information such as the time taken or the number of attempts made [8].

Failure: If the brute force attack is unsuccessful, the program may provide a final message stating that no valid password or key was found. This could happen when the program exhausts all possible combinations without finding the correct one.

Error Messages: Depending on the implementation and specific circumstances, the program may output error messages if there are issues during the execution of the brute force attack. These errors can occur due to network connectivity problems, system limitations, or incorrect configuration of the program.

4. Conclusion and Future Work

4.1 Conclusion

This research paper explored the implementation of brute force attacks using the Python programming language. The objective was to understand the principles, techniques, and implications of such attacks and to identify countermeasures for mitigating the risks associated with them. Through the development and implementation of Python scripts, we examined the vulnerabilities exploited by brute force attacks, such as weak passwords, lack of account lockouts, and ineffective rate limiting mechanisms. The research also emphasized the importance of password complexity and encryption techniques in bolstering security measures. Ethical considerations and legal implications were highlighted throughout the research, emphasizing the need for proper authorization and responsible disclosure. The paper discussed the potential consequences of brute force attacks, including unauthorized access, data breaches, and legal ramifications. Furthermore, various countermeasures and mitigation strategies were explored, such as implementing intrusion detection systems, utilizing account lockouts and rate limiting mechanisms, deploying CAPTCHA or token-based authentication, and enforcing strong password policies. In conclusion, the implementation of brute force attacks using Python provided valuable insights into the vulnerabilities and risks associated with weak authentication mechanisms. By understanding the principles of brute force attacks and implementing effective countermeasures, organizations can better protect their systems and applications from unauthorized access attempts [9].

4.2 Future Work

The future of brute-force programs depends on several factors, including technological advancements, computational power, and the evolution of security measures. Here are a few perspectives on the future of brute-force programs: Increased Computational Power: As computing technology advances, the computational power available to individuals and organizations continues to grow. This can enable more efficient and faster brute-force attacks, allowing attackers to test larger keyspaces and passwords in less time.

Improved Security Measures: As the threat of brute-force attacks persists, security measures and protocols are continually evolving to withstand such attacks. This includes the use of stronger encryption algorithms, longer and more complex passwords, multi-factor authentication, and rate limiting mechanisms.

Machine Learning and AI: Machine learning and artificial intelligence (AI) techniques can be applied to both offensive and defensive purposes in brute-force attacks. Attackers may use AI to optimize attack strategies and improve the efficiency of brute-force programs. On the other hand, defenders can leverage AI algorithms for anomaly detection, pattern recognition, and behavior analysis to identify and prevent brute-force attacks. Overall, while the future of brute-force programs may benefit from advancements in computational power, it is important to recognize that security measures are also advancing to mitigate such attacks. The ongoing race between attackers and defenders will likely drive the development of more secure encryption algorithms, advanced authentication mechanisms, and innovative approaches to protect sensitive information from brute-force attacks [10].

REFERENCES

1. Hacking: The Art of Exploitation by Jon Erickson (2008)
2. The Web Application Hacker's Handbook: Finding and Exploiting Security Flaws by Dafydd Stuttard and Marcus Pinto (2011)
3. Python Requests Library Documentation: https://docs.python-requests.org/en/latest/
4. Botelho, B. A. P., Nakamura, E. T., & Uto, N. (2012, December). Implementation of tools for brute forcing touch inputted passwords. In *2012 International Conference for Internet Technology and Secured Transactions* (pp. 807-808). IEEE.
5. Tyagi, R., & Rehman, U. R. (2021). Securing Web Application Against Brute Force Attack Using Continuous Authentication.
6. Tanwar, S., Paul, T., Singh, K., Joshi, M., & Rana, A. (2020, June). Classification and imapct of cyber threats in India: a review. In 2020 8th International Conference on Reliability, Infocom Technologies and Optimization (Trends and Future Directions)(ICRITO) (pp. 129-135). IEEE.
7. The Legal and Ethical Implications of Hacking, Kaspersky, https://www.kaspersky.com/resource-center/threats/legal-ethical-implications-of-hacking
8. Ethical Hacking: Overview, Benefits, and Legal Implications, Infosec, https://www.infosecinstitute.com/knowledge/ethical-hacking-overview-benefits-legal-implications/
9. Grover, V. (2020, March). An Efficient Brute Force Attack Handling Techniques for Server Virtualization. In *Proceedings of the International Conference on Innovative Computing & Communications (ICICC)*.
10. Stiawan, D., Idris, M., Malik, R. F., Nurmaini, S., Alsharif, N., & Budiarto, R. (2019). Investigating brute force attack patterns in IoT network. *Journal of Electrical and Computer Engineering, 2019*.
11. Wichmann, P., Marx, M., Federrath, H., & Fischer, M. (2021, August). Detection of brute-force attacks in end-to-end encrypted network traffic. In *Proceedings of the 16th International Conference on Availability, Reliability and Security* (pp. 1-9).
12. Tanwar, S., Gupta, N., Iwendi, C., Kumar, K., & Alenezi, M. (2022). Next generation IoT and blockchain integration. Journal of Sensors, 2022.

Emerging Trends in IoT and Computing Technologies – Suman Lata Tripathi et al. (eds)
© 2024 Taylor & Francis Group, London, ISBN 978-1-032-87924-6

Steganography through Python: Concealing Secrets in the Least Significant Bit

Cheshta Dass[1], Sarvesh Tanwar[2]
Amity Institute of Information Technology, Amity University, Noida

Vinay Kukreja[3]
Chitkara University Institute of Engineering and Technology,Chitkara University, Punjab, India

Abstract: Steganography is the art of concealing priviledged information within an innocuous cover medium, such as an image, audio, video, or text. With the advancement of digital technology, steganography has become a popular technique for secure communication and data protection. This research paper provides an overview of steganography. The study of secret communication is known as steganography. Steganography often deals with techniques for concealing the existence of conveyed data so that it can be kept private. It keeps communication between two parties secret. In picture steganography, secret communication is achieved by adding data to the cover image and producing another image knows as a stego-image. We examine the many security and data-hiding methods used to perform steganography in this work, including Least Significant Bit (LSB), ISB, and others. The article addresses common steganography tools and software as well as how to construct steganography using Python programming. It also explores several types of steganography, such as spatial and frequency domain techniques.

Keywords: Steganography, Image steganography, Stego-image, Data protection, Least significant bit, Python programming, Digital communication

1. Introduction

In today's times, any region that is developing has to have good communication. Everyone desires the privacy and security of their personal data. Even the technologies like phone and internet are not entirely secure. There are two methods that could be utilized to quietly spread the information: "cryptography" and "steganography". The message is changed in cryptography using an encryption key that is known only by the sender and the receiver. Without the encryption key, no one can access the communication [1]. However, the transmission of an encrypted communication may immediately prompt an attacker to suspect anything, and so he can forcibly intercept the message. The shortcomings of cryptography systems have led to the development of steganography techniques. The practice of concealing your communication by means of steganography is both an art and a science. This is how steganography masks data so that no one can identify it. Steganography uses the term "embedding" to refer to the process of hiding informational content within any kind of content, such as images, sounds, and videos. To strengthen the confidentiality of data exchange, these strategies may be coupled. Ancient Greece and Rome were among the first civilizations to employ this method, and it has since evolved along with modern technology. Due of its uses in digital watermarking and copyright protection, steganography has grown in popularity recently.

[1]cheshta.dass@s.amity.edu, [2]s.tanwar1521@gmail.com, [3]vinay.kukreja@chitkara.edu.in

DOI: 10.1201/9781003535423-11

1.2 Objectives

The principal objective of this research paper is to present an implementation of image steganography using the Python programming language. By leveraging the capabilities of Python, we aim to develop a practical and efficient approach to hiding information within digital images [2]. The specific objectives include:

(a) Exploring and understanding the fundamentals of image steganography.

(b) Investigating existing techniques and algorithms used in image steganography.

(c) Implementing a steganography method that can embed secret data into image pixels.

(d) Demonstrating the effectiveness and efficiency of the implemented approach through experimental results.

2. Literature Review

2.1 Overview of Image Steganography

A kind of steganography called picture steganography focuses on hiding sensitive information in digital photos. It leverages the characteristics of image files, such as the large amount of data they can store and their visual complexity, to embed hidden messages without raising suspicion. Various techniques have been developed to achieve imperceptible and secure embedding, including LSB substitution, spatial domain techniques, and transform domain techniques.

2.2 Existing Techniques and Algorithms

Various techniques, including LSB replacement, pixel differencing, histogram shifting, and random mapping, have been explored in image steganography [3]. Transform domain methods like DWT and DCT are also gaining attention for their robustness against attacks, enhancing security and minimizing visual distortion.

2.3 Comparison of Different Approaches

Research on image steganography techniques examines factors like embedding capacity, imperceptibility, security, and resistance to attacks. Some methods with high embedding capacity may cause visual artifacts, limiting covert communication suitability. Conversely, techniques prioritizing imperceptibility might have lower embedding capacity. Balancing these factors is crucial for successful implementations.

3. Problem Statement

A crucial method for safe and covert communication is image steganography, where secret information is concealed within digital images. While numerous methods and algorithms have been proposed for image steganography, there is a need for a practical and efficient implementation using the Python programming language.

The key challenges that need to be addressed in this problem statement include:

- *Designing an efficient embedding process:* Developing an embedding technique that ensures imperceptibility of the hidden message while maximizing the embedding capacity within the image pixels.

- *Ensuring secure data hiding:* Implementing encryption algorithms to protect the confidentiality of the hidden message and ensuring that the embedded information remains secure against unauthorized access.

- *Preserving image quality:* Minimizing any visual distortions introduced during the embedding process to maintain the visual integrity of the steganographic image and avoid raising suspicion.

- *Providing flexibility and ease of use:* Creating a user-friendly implementation that allows users to easily specify the input image, secret message, and optional parameters, while providing clear documentation and instructions for the implementation.

3.1 Methodology

Image Pre-processing:

Image preparation is done prior to embedding in order to assure compatibility and boost the effectiveness of the steganographic process. In this step, the incoming image is converted to a suitable format, like RGB or grayscale, and any necessary resizing or normalizing is carried out to guarantee uniformity between images.

Embedding Process:

In order to preserve visual integrity, the secret data must be hidden within the image's pixels throughout the embedding process.

LSB Substitution Technique: Consecutive covert message components are inserted into pixel LSBs using LSB replacement. The message is broken into smaller parts, and the LSBs of image pixels are swapped with matching message bits. A specific order, like left-to-right and top-to-bottom, ensures precise extraction during decoding.

Encryption and Data Compression (Optional): Before embedding, encrypting with methods like Advanced Encryption Standard (AES) enhances message confidentiality. Data compression techniques such as Huffman coding or Run-Length Encoding (RLE) reduce the secret message size, boosting embedding capacity and minimizing impact on image quality [4].

Extraction Process:

The extraction procedure entails taking the steganographic image's concealed message out. This process is performed by reverse engineering the embedding process and extracting the embedded bits from the LSBs of the image pixels. The extraction process should be designed to ensure accurate retrieval of the secret message while minimizing any distortion to the original image.

LSB Extraction Technique: The LSB extraction technique is employed to extract the hidden message from the steganographic image. This technique involves sequentially extracting the LSBs of the selected image pixels and concatenating them to reconstruct the embedded message. By reversing the process used during embedding it is possible to obtain the first covert message.

Decryption and Data Decompression (Optional): If encryption and data compression were applied during the embedding process, decryption and data decompression are performed during the extraction process. The encrypted secret message is decrypted using the corresponding decryption algorithm, and the compressed message is decompressed to its original form [8] [12]. This ensures the integrity and readability of the extracted secret information.

4. Implementation

There are many tools and software programs available for steganography, both for embedding and extracting hidden information from digital media. Here are some of the most popular tools and software programs for steganography:

- *OpenStego:* An open-source steganography tool that supports image, audio, and text-based steganography.
- *Steghide:* A command-line tool for steganography that supports image, audio, and text-based steganography
- *SteganPEG:* A steganography tool for JPEG images that uses the least significant bit (LSB) method to embed hidden information.
- *S-Tools:* A steganography tool for Windows that supports image and audio-based steganography.
- *QuickStego:* A simple steganography tool for Windows that supports image-based steganography.
- *CryptaPix:* An image viewer that also supports image-based steganography.

4.1 Algorithms for Image Steganography using Python:

LSB Substitution Technique:

One of the most often used algorithms for image steganography is the Least Significant Bit substitution technique. It involves adding the hidden message bits in place of the image's least significant pixel values [5]. The algorithm follows these steps:

a. Transform the secret message into binary form.
b. Iterate through the pixels of the cover image.
c. The pixel value is retrieved, and the LSBs are modified with the secret message bits.
d. Update the modified pixel value in the steganographic image.
e. Continue until all of the hidden message bits have been implanted.

Spatial Domain Techniques:

Spatial domain techniques exploit the spatial characteristics of images for steganography. These techniques involve directly modifying the pixel values or relationships between neighboring pixels.

Transform Domain Techniques:

In order to encode hidden information, transform domain techniques use mathematical transformations like the discrete cosine transform (DCT) or discrete wavelet transform (DWT). These methods use the representation of images in the frequency domain to conceal the hidden message. Examples of common transform domain techniques are: *Transform Coefficient Modification* and *Quantization Index Modulation.*

Error Diffusion Techniques:

Error diffusion techniques distribute the error generated during the embedding process across neighboring pixels, ensuring a better balance between image quality and imperceptibility. The most popular error diffusion algorithm used in steganography is the Floyd-Steinberg algorithm [7].

4.2 Using Library/Module in Python

Python has a sizable standard library of modules that offer many different functionalities. For instance, the 'os' module offers methods for dealing with the operating system, the 'math' module offers mathematical functions like sin and cos, and the 'random' module offers functions for generating random numbers.

Moreover, there are many third-party modules available that can be installed via the Python Package Index (PyPI) using package managers like pip [6][10]. These modules can provide additional functionalities not available in the standard library, such as web frameworks, data analysis tools, machine learning libraries, and more

To use a library or module in Python, you first need to install it. In your terminal or command prompt, use the following command to install a package using pip:

pip install package_name

Using the 'import' line, you can import a package into your Python code once it has been installed.

4.3 Python Libraries Used

The following Python libraries were imported to be used in the code for the implementation:-

- Stegano – The functions provided by this module only hide the messages without encryption using the LSB technique. The LSB module within this library will be utilized for this purpose.
- PIL (Python Imaging Library) – It supports multiple file formats and has a robust internal representation. The main picture library is designed to provide easy access to data stored in a few basic pixel formats. It should act as a solid foundation for a powerful image processing tool.
- Tkinter – Python offers various GUI development options, with Tkinter being the most popular. As a standard Python interface for the Tk GUI toolkit, Tkinter simplifies and streamlines the process of creating GUI applications, making it the quickest and easiest method [11].
- OS – The 'os' module in Python is a built-in tool for interacting with the operating system. It enables tasks like managing directories, files, processes, environment variables, and more. With 'os,' you can perform actions such as creating, deleting, renaming, and listing directories/files, manipulating paths, spawning/killing processes, retrieving process information, executing shell commands, and changing permissions.

Overall, the 'os' module is a powerful and versatile module that makes it easy to work with the operating system in Python.

5. Results

Unlocking hidden files and data, behold the fascinating outcomes of Python-powered steganography. For image steganography, the data set consists of a collection of digital images i.e. it can include images of various formats such as jpeg, png, bmp. Or gif. Let's take a look at the results:-

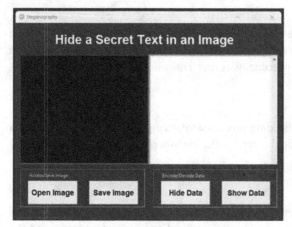

Fig. 11.1 Hiding of text in an image

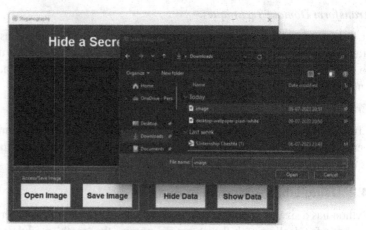

Fig. 11.2 Selecting image to open

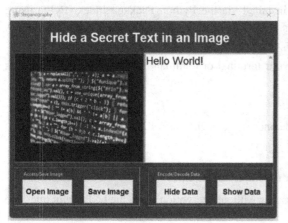

Fig. 11.3 Entering the text to be hidden, click hide data and save data

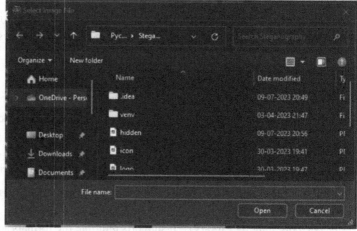

Fig. 11.4 Image saved as hidden.jpg

After implementing image steganography using Python and conducting experiments, it is essential to analyze the results obtained. This analysis aims to evaluate the effectiveness and efficiency of the implemented technique. It involves assessing various aspects, such as embedding capacity, imperceptibility, security, and robustness against different attacks. Additionally, performance metrics, including execution time and computational resources, can be considered for evaluation. The analysis of results helps to understand the strengths and weaknesses of the implemented image steganography technique.

6. Conclusion

The proposed framework for steganography using neural networks presents a promising approach that integrates privacy preservation and communication security [9]. The framework leverages neural networks for encryption and decryption, along with steganography

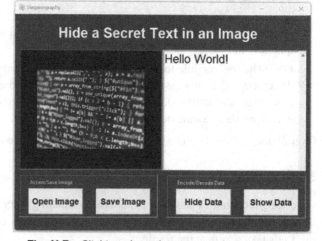

Fig. 11.5 Clicking show data to reveal text message

techniques, to hide messages within cover images in a secure and concealed manner. Encoding, transmission, and decoding—the framework's three key phases—all work together to guarantee that the concealed message is kept private and is only accessible by the intended receiver. To increase the encryption process's safety, the neural network-based encryption algorithm creates distinct encryption keys for each message. The cover image's encrypted message was concealed using a steganographic technique, which adds another level of deception. The transmission of the cover image through a secure communication channel helps prevent unauthorized access to the hidden message, maintaining the confidentiality of the communication. The decoding stage allows the receiver to derive the encrypted message from the cover image and decrypt it using the neural network-based decryption algorithm with the encryption key received from the sender.

REFERENCES

1. Fridrich, J., Goljan, M., & Du, R. (2001). Reliable detection of LSB steganography in color and grayscale images. Proceedings of the International Conference on Information Technology: Coding and Computing (ITCC 2001), 3, 320-324.

2. Provos, N., & Honeyman, P. (2003). Hide and seek: An introduction to steganography. IEEE Security & Privacy, 1(3), 32-44.

3. Riaz, N., & Hussain, I. (2018). A survey of steganography techniques in spatial and frequency domain. Journal of Information Security and Applications, 37, 1-15.

4. Al-Fatlawi, H. M., & Esmail, A. S. (2020). Comparative study of image steganography algorithms. Journal of Information Security, 11(3), 119-131.

5. Li, B., Yang, J., Wang, K., & Li, J. (2019). A comprehensive survey of image steganography: Techniques, evaluations, and trends. IEEE Access, 7, 155490-155514.

6. Westfeld, A., & Pfitzmann, A. (2000). Attacks on steganographic systems. Proceedings of the International Workshop on Information Hiding (IH 2000), 61-76.

7. Wang, R. Z., Lin, C. F., & Chang, C. C. (2003). Steganography in digital media: Principles, algorithms, and applications. CRC Press.

8. Singh, A., Kaur, K., & Gupta, V. (2018). Image steganography techniques: A review. International Journal of Advanced Research in Computer Science, 9(4), 379-384.

9. Cox, I., Miller, M., Bloom, J., & Fridrich, J. (2007). Digital watermarking and steganography. Morgan Kaufmann.

10. Chen, B., & Wornell, G. W. (2001). Quantization index modulation: A class of provably good methods for digital watermarking and information embedding. IEEE Transactions on Information Theory, 47(4), 1423-1443.

11. Morkel, T., Eloff, J. H., & Olivier, M. S. (2005, June). An overview of image steganography. In ISSA (Vol. 1, No. 2, pp. 1-11).

12. Johnson, N. F., & Jajodia, S. (1998). Exploring steganography: Seeing the unseen. Computer, 31(2), 26-34.

Emerging Trends in IoT and Computing Technologies – Suman Lata Tripathi et al. (eds)
© 2024 Taylor & Francis Group, London, ISBN 978-1-032-87924-6

A Comparative Study of the Cellular Automata Based Digital Image Watermarking Techniques in Spatial Domain

12

Iram Khurshid Bhat[1], Fasel Qadir[2]

University of Kashmir North Campus, P.G. Department of Computer Sciences,
Delina Baramulla Jammu & Kashmir, 193103, India

Abstract: The exploration of watermarking methods has attracted considerable interest within the realm of digital media security and the safeguarding of copyright. Watermarking, a technique that involves embedding subtle yet durable information, referred to as a watermark, into digital media formats like images, audio files, and videos, serves multiple purposes. These purposes encompass the enforcement of copyright, the authentication of content, and the verification of ownership. A significant set of systems with dynamic behavior and discrete nature in terms of both space and time domains are cellular automata (CA). The evolution of the CA generations relies on the transition function, which dictates the update of each cell's state within the specified cellular space. The CA's fundamental properties make it exceptionally useful in numerous applications like large-scale modeling and simulations that can benefit from the CA's parallelism property. This research presents a comprehensive examination of the fundamental elements associated with CA-based digital image watermarking methods. It provides valuable perspectives on the constantly evolving domain of digital security and the strategies implemented to protect the rights and concerns of both content creators and consumers.

Keywords: Watermarking, Cellular automata, Security, Authentication, Verification

1. Introduction

These days DIP applications are all around such as Bar-code scan and pay, camera beauty effect, face or smile detection, hand gesture detection, motion detection, background blurring, image deblurring, biometric authentication, Google Lens, Waymo LLC, face recognition, and much more. Besides, it is now simpler for people to retrieve and distribute digital images online because of the exponential growth of the internet and the easy accessibility of digital media. This has, however, also facilitated people to exploit and disseminate digital images in an unauthorized way, which has given rise to problems like the breach of copyright and piracy. To tackle these issues, the implementation of digital image watermarking offers a mechanism to track the origin or owner of digital images and spot unauthorized use or modification. Digital watermarking has been used to safeguard content creators' rights to intellectual property and ensure that their work is utilized legally and responsibly. Additionally, it can be utilized to enforce the conditions of use for digital data, digital content authenticity validation, temper detection, monitoring, fingerprinting, and integrity protection [1]. Watermarking is frequently integrated with digital rights management systems to regulate the distribution and consumption of digital media, including movies and music.

Digital image watermarking is a DIP technique using which the invisible or visible watermark information is inserted into the digital host image in a manner that there occurs no perceptual difference and it becomes challenging for the unauthorized folk to delete or modify the embedded watermark. It is an impactful tool for image identification, image authentication, preserving image copyright, enforcing terms of use set by the owner for images, and restraining piracy. Information in the form of a

---
[1]bhat.eram29@gmail.com, [2]fasel.scholars@gmail.com

DOI: 10.1201/9781003535423-12

logo, text string, image, signature or stamp, and status details such as "For Review" or "Draft" can be used as a watermark. Watermarking can be categorized as visible or invisible depending on how noticeable the watermark is to the human eye. In the context of visible watermarking, the embedded watermark is clearly noticeable to the viewer and it is made to be challenging to remove the embedded data without lowering the host image's quality. The visible approach to watermarking is usually employed for purposes like branding, advertising, and copyright infringement protection. While in invisible watermarking techniques, the embedded watermark is not noticeable to the human eye at all however it is detectable by specialized software tools. The invisible approach to watermarking is usually employed for purposes like authentication and security.

In this work, some of the cellular automata-based spatial domain methodologies for digital image watermarking will be examined. The methodologies will be examined regarding the aspects of imperceptibility, embedding capacity, robustness, and the trade-offs between them. We will discuss the techniques, challenges, and factors to be taken into account while implementing the watermarking system. We will also look at the potential uses and future developments of digital image watermarking.

2. Related Work

The transform domain and the spatial domain are the two primary domains in digital image watermarking, in which watermarking techniques can be implemented. In spatial domain approaches [2][3], the numerical values representing pixels of the host image are directly altered. Although the implementation of these methods is usually uncomplicated and rapid, they might not be robust enough to withstand various image processing operations. The least significant bit (LSB) insertion [4][5][6], intermediate significant bit (ISB) insertion [7][8], local binary pattern [9][10][11], patchwork [12], spread spectrum, and histogram modification [13][14] are different methods of watermarking in the spatial domain. *Table 12.1* summarizes the advantages and limitations of the contemporary watermarking approaches and the techniques used by them.

Table 12.1 Summary of most relevant and recent techniques for digital image watermarking

Study	Techniques Used	Advantages	Limitations
Shehab et al. [4]	The Least Significant Bit Substitution, Arnold Transform, and Singular Value Decomposition	Surpasses the current methods in terms of precision of locating tempered areas and the PSNR value of the self-recovered images.	Filtering, rotation, scaling, and cropping-like geometric attacks can easily destroy the watermark data.
Parah et al. [5]	The Least Significant Bit Substitution, Bilinear Interpolation Technique, and Magic Triangle.	The approach is secure, imperceptible, and has high data embedding capacity.	Dimensions of the resultant image do not remain the same as the original host image due to interpolation and the approach cannot withstand most of the geometric attacks.
Deeba et al. [6]	The Least Significant Bit and Artificial Neural Networks.	It is efficient and yields good PSNR values.	Complex and not tested for any kind of attack.
Zeki et al. [7]	The Intermediate Significant Bit Substitution and Neural Network.	Optimal pixel value derivation makes the approach highly imperceptible.	Less robustness.
Verma and Dutta [8]	Intermediate Significant Bits, And Block Entropy.	Higher imperceptibility.	Shows less resistance against geometrical attacks like cropping, rotation, and scaling.
Tuncer and Kaya [9]	Center Symmetric Local Binary Patterns, AES, Integer Wavelet Transform, And Logistic Map.	High visual quality, secure, and semi-fragile. Also has high data embedding capacity.	Geometric attacks and image processing robustness are required.
Pal et al. [10]	The Local Binary Pattern.	Higher embedding capacity with a high level of perceptibility. Can be used to detect tempered regions and copy-move forgery.	The LBP can be similar across different image blocks, which can cause false detection during the watermark extraction process.
Pal et al. [11]	The Local Binary Pattern and Hamming Code.	Can be used for image integrity verification and authentication. The approach caused less distortion and achieved great image quality for the high payload.	Unless the tempering is localized to a single area of the watermarked image, it won't be possible to recover the tempered image.
Li et al. [12]	The Patchwork, Logistic Map, and Discrete Cosine Transform.	Able to withstand combination attacks, Gaussian noise, rotation, JPEG compression, and filtering	More susceptible to vulnerability from cropping attacks.
Ou et al. [13]	Optional Prediction-Error Histogram Modification.	Tested on both military and standard images, it resulted in less distortion and achieved great image quality for the high payload.	Inability to withstand frequent attacks like lossy compression, cropping, and rotation.
Liu et al. [14]	The Shifting of Histogram of N-Bit Planes (Nbps).	Higher perceptibility and higher embedding capacity.	Lack of robustness.

3. Characteristics of the Digital Image Watermarking System

For a watermarking system to be efficient the characteristics it should possess are robustness, imperceptibility, high embedding capacity, security, and low computational complexity.

3.1 Robustness

A digital image watermarking system is said to be robust if it can resist and survive multiple types of attacks or DIP operations like rotating, filtering, resizing, cropping, color adjustments, and compression which purposely or accidentally attempt to alter, destroy, degrade or completely remove the embedded watermark information.

3.2 Imperceptibility

It is a significant characteristic of an image watermarking system that represents the level to which the human eye is unable to perceive or notice the embedded watermark information. The quality and the perceived aesthetics of an image should not be significantly impacted after the watermark embedment process.

3.3 Capacity

The capacity characteristic of an image watermarking system is the measure of the amount of data that can be embedded as a watermark into a host image. The upper limit for the size of the watermark is contingent upon the capabilities and capacity inherent in the employed watermarking technique.

3.4 Security

It is a significant characteristic of an image watermarking system that refers to all the measures taken or mechanisms involved, which without the right key or permission makes it challenging for anyone to delete or alter the embedded watermark information.

3.5 Computational complexity

The last characteristic is the computational complexity of the image watermarking system which refers to quantifying the number of resources like processing power, processing time, and space required to embed as well as extract the watermark data. The effectiveness and practicality of a watermarking algorithm can be significantly influenced by how computationally complex it is.

It is critical to note that robustness, imperceptibility, and capacity are frequently traded off in the design of a watermarking system.

4. Cellular Automata (CA)

In a bid to study artificial life and self-reproduction, mathematicians John von Neumann and Stanislaw Ulam pioneered the introduction of CA during the latter part of the 1940s [15]. Neumann developed a theoretical model that was biologically motivated and used a set of predefined rules in order to be able to replicate itself [16] [17]. CA systems serve as dynamic mathematical models employed for the simulation of intricate systems. These models have discrete space and time domains and show complex behavior from simple update rules. A cellular automaton is formally defined as a quadruple $= (Z^D, N, S, f)$ where:

- Z^D represents a lattice of homogeneous cells of D-dimensions called cellular space.
- $N = (n^*_1, n^*_2, n^*_3 \ldots n^*_m)$ consists of m different elements of Z^D and is called the neighborhood vector that links every cell with its neighbors. Typically, a cell's neighbors are the close cells that surround it.
- S represents the finite set of possible states.
- $f: S^m \rightarrow S$ is referred to as the local automaton rule, in accordance with which the status of each cell undergoes synchronous updates at discrete time steps. The new cell state is determined by $f = (S_1, S_2, S_3 \ldots S_m)$ where $S_1, S_2, S_3 \ldots S_m$ are the current states of all the cells within the neighborhood, and 'm' represents the neighborhood size.

The configuration of the D-dimensional CA can be described as the state of the entire cellular space at any given point in time. It is a function $c: Z^D \rightarrow S$ [18] that maps all the cells in the cellular space (Z^D) with their states from the state set (S) and set S^{ZD} contains all possible configurations. A distinct means of recognizing a cellular automaton involves the examination of its global transition function denoted by $e = G(c)$ where $G: S^{ZD} \rightarrow S^{ZD}$. There exists a strong correlation between the dimension of the CA and the CA cell neighborhood. A cellular automaton is the most prominent technique to design the dynamics of numerous processes because of its ability to generate dynamic complex patterns from simple local update rules.

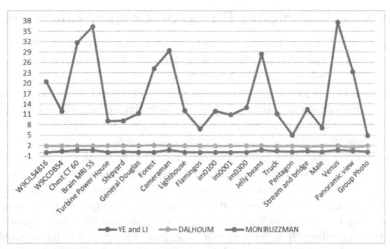

Fig. 12.1 Root Mean-squared error (RMSE) obtained by different watermarking techniques under examination for different test images

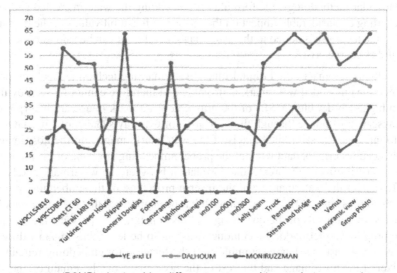

Fig. 12.2 Peak signal-to-noise ratio (PSNR) obtained by different watermarking techniques under examination for different test images

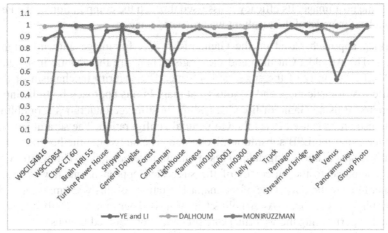

Fig. 12.3 Structural similarity (SSIM) index obtained by different watermarking techniques under examination for different test images

5. Image Watermarking Techniques Based on Cellular Automata

A novel chaotic cellular automata-based digital image scrambling and watermarking approach has been designed by Ye and Li [19]. In this work, two algorithms have been presented, one to scramble the digital image using different chaotic rules of cellular automata, and the second to embed a watermark into the scrambled host image. To analyze the behavior of certain referenced rule number cellular automata their fractal box dimensions are computed. Then the evolution patterns are observed at different iteration times and the cellular automata rules that become chaotic are selected for scrambling digital images. The set of cellular automata rules that were analyzed in this study include rules 261100, 8189, 4093, 816, 35853, and 534 and it was observed that rule numbers 35853, 819, and 534 show chaotic behavior. The chaotic cellular automata rules that were chosen in this approach for scrambling original images are rule 224 (The Game of Life), rule 816, and rule 35852. The initial random matrix A0, the chosen chaotic cellular automata rule, and the number of generations to be generated from the keys of this approach. The non-blind digital image watermarking algorithm presented in this work is based on the image scrambling scheme. Using the cellular automata-based image scrambling technique the host image is scrambled first and then the pixel values representing the watermark are incorporated into the scrambled representation of the host image. To recover the original image the scrambling algorithm's inverse procedure was applied to the scrambled image. According to the implementation of the presented work, it was observed that its scrambling technique performed well but the incorporation formula for watermarking had a notable influence on both the quality and the visual aesthetics perceived in the host image post-embedding. In this particular methodology, the formula for embedding the watermark pixels operates on the gray values of the host image pixels, exerting a considerable impact on the most significant bit values of the host image pixels. As a result, the watermark data appears like the noise is added to the host image therefore it can be said that the scheme drastically fails to incorporate the imperceptibility characteristic.

A blind two-dimensional cellular automata-based digital image watermarking technique has been proposed by Adwan et al. [20]. In the proposed method the embedded watermark is invisible and therefore cannot be seen by the viewer. In this spatial domain technique, the two highest-order bits (MSB) of the grayscale watermark image are incorporated into the two lowest-order bits (LSB) of the grayscale host image through the utilization of Conway's Game of Life (GOL).The chaotic properties of 2D CA are employed to integrate the scrambled pixels of the watermark image into the host image and therefore make it impossible to read the embedded watermark data without the proper embedding key. One of the main advantages of employing the 2D Game of Life CA is that it effectively breaks the correlation between the watermark pixels and thereby augmenting the algorithm's security. To extract the watermark data, the inverse procedure of the embedding process is performed on the watermarked image using the same Game of Life generations. It has been observed that the watermark bits are easily detectable as they are embedded into the first n pixels of the host image in this context, 'n' represents the overall count of pixels of the watermark image thus the proposed watermarking technique turns out to be less robust against different geometrical attacks like cropping. Nevertheless, watermark pixels are scrambled but the location for embedding remains permanent that is from the first pixel to the nth pixel of the host image and the rest of the host image pixels remain on the shelf which becomes the major disadvantage of the proposed approach. Cropping or modifying only the first n LSB bits of the watermarked image can completely remove or alter the watermark image. The proposed scheme focuses on scrambling the watermark pixels rather than distributing them throughout the host image. Its efficacy is assessed through the computation of the Peak Signal-to-Noise Ratio (PSNR) between the original host image and the resultant watermarked image.

A highly secure watermarking approach based on the Game-of-life CA for image authentication has been suggested by Moniruzzaman et al. in [21]. The Arnold's Cat map and the Logistic map are the chaotic maps employed in the suggested approach to intensify the level of security of the suggested scheme. The security mechanism of the suggested approach is provided by the Game-of-life CA, logistic map, and Arnold's Cat map. In this approach both the input images are scrambled, the binary watermark is scrambled using Game-of-life CA, and the host image undergoes scrambling through the utilization of Arnold's Cat map. The logistic map is used to set the CA's initial configuration. The scrambled watermark data is inserted into the scrambled host image using the LSB substitution technique. The suggested method makes use of numerous chaotic maps, creating a substantial key space, thus being able to resist unauthorized changes. Three different watermarking methods that are chaos-based were compared to the outcomes of the suggested approach and it was observed that the suggested scheme outperforms the other three techniques. One of the major limitations of this watermarking technique is that it employs Arnold's Cat map for scrambling host images. As Arnold's Cat Map is determined only for the squared plots therefore the proposed scheme is restricted to performing the watermarking procedure on squared images only.

6. Experimental Setup

In the pursuit of facilitating a fair and comprehensive comparison, a series of carefully considered modifications to the above-discussed three prominent cellular automata-based image watermarking techniques were undertaken. These alterations were meticulously designed to standardize the input conditions across all three methods, a critical step to ensure the validity of the comparative analysis. For each technique, we strategically adjusted key parameters to ensure a uniform input, thereby eliminating any confounding variables that could affect the comparative analysis. These modifications ranged from fine-tuning the embedding and extraction algorithms to adapting the watermark embedding capacity. The overarching goal was to establish an equitable testing environment where the only variables under consideration were the unique characteristics of each technique. This process involved a systematic and well-documented approach, ensuring that the resulting modifications were not only technically sound but also transparent and reproducible. Moreover, it allowed for a nuanced understanding of how these modifications impacted the performance of each watermarking technique, shedding light on their strengths and limitations in a standardized context. The watermarking methods under evaluation were tested on different grayscale host images. The two most significant bits per pixel of the grayscale watermark image were embedded into the grayscale host image. The dimensions of the grayscale watermark image were 128X64.

7. Comparative Analysis

The comprehensive analysis of the different watermarking methods under evaluation is presented in *Table 12.2*. The performance of these methods was evaluated on various test images of different dimensions. Based on the comparative evaluation Ye and Li's [19] watermarking technique demonstrates performance that has been characterized as sub-optimal. It consistently yields higher MSE and RMSE values, indicating a relatively higher level of distortion introduced to the watermarked images. The PSNR values are relatively lower, suggesting a reduced capacity to preserve image quality. Furthermore, the SSIM values are

Table 12.2 Comprehensive imperceptibility analysis of various test images, assessing image quality and impact of the different watermarking methods under evaluation

Host Image Grayscale (8 bits/pixel)	Host Image Size (pixels)	YE and LI [19]				ADWAN [20]				MONIRUZZMAN [21]			
		MSE	RMSE	PSNR	SSIM	MSE	RMSE	PSNR	SSIM	MSE	RMSE	PSNR	SSIM
W9CIL54816	524x581	418.3748	20.4542	21.9151	0.8796	3.4951	1.8695	42.6962	0.9879	N/A	N/A	N/A	N/A
W9CCDB54	512x512	141.9224	11.9131	26.6103	0.9414	3.5038	1.8718	42.6854	0.9974	0.1065	0.3264	57.8561	0.9998
Chest CT 60	256x256	1008.489	31.7567	18.0941	0.6612	3.4553	1.8588	42.7460	0.9886	0.4167	0.6456	51.9321	0.9975
Brain MRI 55	256x256	1321.865	36.3575	16.9189	0.6654	3.5439	1.8825	42.6360	0.9683	0.4535	0.6734	51.5653	0.9969
Turbine Power House	576x718	81.4850	9.0269	29.0200	0.9484	3.5431	1.8823	42.6370	0.9910	N/A	N/A	N/A	N/A
Shipyard	1024x1024	82.3662	9.0756	28.9733	0.9646	3.4589	1.8598	42.7414	0.9863	0.0270	0.1644	63.8128	0.9997
General Douglas	576x712	126.4171	11.2435	27.1127	0.9361	3.5261	1.8778	42.6579	0.9899	N/A	N/A	N/A	N/A
Forest	447x301	585.9550	24.2065	20.4522	0.8133	4.2363	2.0582	41.8610	0.9919	N/A	N/A	N/A	N/A
Cameraman	256x256	865.0880	29.4124	18.7602	0.6505	3.4359	1.8536	42.7703	0.9872	0.4228	0.6502	51.8699	0.9967
Lighthouse	480x640	143.2877	11.9703	26.5687	0.9186	3.4674	1.8621	42.7308	0.9884	N/A	N/A	N/A	N/A
Flamingos	1296x972	45.3042	6.7308	31.5694	0.9788	3.5002	1.8709	42.6899	0.9920	N/A	N/A	N/A	N/A
im0100	700x605	142.0792	11.9197	26.6055	0.9165	3.4819	1.8660	42.7126	0.9815	N/A	N/A	N/A	N/A
im0001	700x605	116.7653	10.8058	27.4577	0.9203	3.5229	1.8769	42.6618	0.9808	N/A	N/A	N/A	N/A
im0300	700x605	165.5180	12.8654	25.9424	0.9307	3.5117	1.8740	42.6756	0.9795	N/A	N/A	N/A	N/A
Jelly beans	256x256	807.4062	28.4149	19.0599	0.6258	3.4273	1.8513	42.7813	0.9884	0.4323	0.6575	51.7727	0.9956
Truck	512x512	123.5240	11.1141	27.2133	0.9025	3.1032	1.7616	43.2127	0.9928	0.1098	0.3314	57.7247	0.9993
Pentagon	1024x1024	24.4735	4.9471	34.2438	0.9845	3.3315	1.8252	42.9044	0.9936	0.0281	0.1678	63.6373	0.9999
Stream and bridge	512x512	154.5128	12.4303	26.2412	0.9341	2.3214	1.5236	44.4734	0.9997	0.0948	0.3079	58.3621	0.9997
Male	1024x1024	49.4194	7.0299	31.1918	0.9724	3.3181	1.8216	42.9220	0.9857	0.0273	0.1652	63.7709	0.9998
Venus	256x256	1418.043	37.6569	16.6139	0.5307	3.5109	1.8737	42.6767	0.9267	0.4609	0.6789	51.4945	0.9917
Panoramic view	512x512	543.8697	23.3210	20.7759	0.8449	1.9811	1.4075	45.1617	0.9827	0.1719	0.4146	55.7774	0.9971
Group Photo	1024x1024	23.5546	4.8533	34.4101	0.9848	3.4784	1.8651	42.7170	0.9893	0.0269	0.1640	63.8354	0.9998

notably lower compared to the other techniques, indicating a potential decrease in structural similarity between the original and watermarked images.

The Adwan et al. [20] watermarking technique continues to display commendable results, particularly in contrast to Ye and Li. It consistently maintains low MSE and RMSE values, indicating minimal error introduced to the watermarked images. The high PSNR values demonstrate its proficiency in maintaining image quality. This specifies that Adwan et al. [20] effectively embed watermarks while preserving image quality.

The Moniruzzaman et al. in [21] watermarking technique presents competitive imperceptibility results. It consistently delivers low MSE and RMSE values, suggesting minimal distortion in the watermarked images. High PSNR values reveal its effectiveness in maintaining image quality. The SSIM values reflect a strong ability to maintain structural similarity. The performance evaluation metric scores display variation with squared test images yielding exceptionally best scores, while others are marked as N/A. This variability suggests that Moniruzzaman's performance is influenced by the image dimension characteristic.

8. Conclusion and Future Work

In conclusion, the comparative analysis of three given watermarking techniques offers valuable insights into the applications of CA in image security and copyright protection. Ye and Li, while displaying poor performance in the analysis, appear to struggle in minimizing distortion and preserving image quality, especially when contrasted with Adwan et al. and Moniruzzaman et al. Adwan et al. continue to be a robust watermarking technique that effectively preserves image quality while introducing minimal distortion. Its performance remains consistent, making it a reliable choice in various applications. Moniruzzaman et al., while exhibiting variability in certain cases, maintain competitive imperceptibility characteristics and can be a valuable option with further fine-tuning and testing.

Future study in digital image watermarking using CA is expected to go in a number of constructive ways. The development of powerful and more secure watermarking methods that can resist increasingly complex attacks and manipulation attempts is one area of emphasis. Another topic of focus is the combination of CA, artificial intelligence, and machine learning to enable the development of adaptive and customized watermarks and automate the watermarking process that strictly considers all the associated moral and legal issues. Aside from digital rights management and copyright control, there is also a significant focus on the use of the watermarking technique for a number of other purposes, including image authentication and content-based image retrieval.

REFERENCES

1. A. Kumar, "A review on implementation of digital image watermarking techniques using lsb and dwt," Information and Communication Technology for Sustainable Development: Proceedings of ICT4SD 2018, pp. 595–602, 2020.
2. Q. Su, Z. Yuan, and D. Liu, "An approximate schur decomposition-based spatial domain color image watermarking method," IEEE Access, vol. 7, pp. 4358–4370, 2018.
3. J. Abraham and V. Paul, "An imperceptible spatial domain color image watermarking scheme," Journal of King Saud University-Computer and Information Sciences, vol. 31, no. 1, pp. 125–133, 2019.
4. A. Shehab, M. Elhoseny, K. Muhammad, A. K. Sangaiah, P. Yang, H. Huang, and G. Hou, "Secure and robust fragile watermarking scheme for medical images," IEEE access, vol. 6, pp. 10269–10278, 2018.
5. S. A. Parah, A. Bashir, M. Manzoor, A. Gulzar, M. Firdous, N. A. Loan, and J. A. Sheikh, "Secure and reversible data hiding scheme for healthcare system using magic rectangle and a new interpolation technique," in Healthcare Data Analytics and Management, pp. 267–309, Elsevier, 2019
6. F. Deeba, S. Kun, F. A. Dharejo, and H. Memon, "Digital image watermarking based on ann and least significant bit," Information Security Journal: A Global Perspective, vol. 29, no. 1, pp. 30–39, 2020.
7. A. Zeki, A. Abubakar, and H. Chiroma, "An intermediate significant bit (isb) watermarking technique using neural networks," SpringerPlus, vol. 5, pp. 1–25, 2016.
8. K. Verma and A. Dutta, "Intermediate significant bit-based approach to image watermarking using block entropy," in 2017 2nd International Conference on Telecommunication and Networks (TEL-NET), pp. 1–6, IEEE, 2017.
9. T. Tuncer and M. Kaya, "A novel image watermarking method based on center symmetric local binary pattern with minimum distortion," Optik, vol. 185, pp. 972–984, 2019.
10. P. Pal, B. Jana, and J. Bhaumik, "Watermarking scheme using local binary pattern for image authentication and tamper detection through dual image," Security and Privacy, vol. 2, no. 2, p. e59, 2019.
11. P. Pal, B. Jana, and J. Bhaumik, "An image authentication and tampered detection scheme exploiting local binary pattern along with hamming error correcting code," Wireless Personal Communications, vol. 121, no. 1, pp. 939–961, 2021.

12. Y. Li, J. Li, C. Shao, U. A. Bhatti, and J. Ma, "Robust multi-watermarking algorithm for medical images using patchwork-dct," in International Conference on Artificial Intelligence and Security, pp. 386–399, Springer, 2022.

13. B. Ou, Y. Zhao, and R. Ni, "Reversible watermarking using optional prediction error histogram modification," Neurocomputing, vol. 93, pp. 67–76, 2012.

14. L. Liu, C.-C. Chang, and A. Wang, "Reversible data hiding scheme based on histogram shifting of n-bit planes," Multimedia Tools and Applications, vol. 75, pp. 11311–11326, 2016.

15. A. W. Burks, "Essays on cellular automata," (No Title), 1970.

16. J. Von Neumann, A. W. Burks, et al., "Theory of self-reproducing automata," IEEE Transactions on Neural Networks, vol. 5, no. 1, pp. 3–14, 1966.

17. A. R. Smith III, "Real-time language recognition by one-dimensional cellular automata," Journal of Computer and System Sciences, vol. 6, no. 3, pp. 233–253, 1972.

18. J. Kari, "Basic concepts of cellular automata." Handbook of natural computing, vol. 1, pp. 3–24, 2012.

19. R. Ye and H. Li, "A novel image scrambling and watermarking scheme based on cellular automata," in 2008 International Symposium on Electronic Commerce and Security, pp. 938–941, IEEE, 2008.

20. O. Adwan, A. A. Awwad, A. Sleit, and A. L. A. Alhoum, "A novel watermarking scheme based on two dimensional cellular automata," in Proceedings of the International Conference on Computers and Computing, World Scientific and Engineering Academy and Society (WSEAS). Canary Islands, Spain, pp. 88–94, 2011.

21. M. Moniruzzaman, M. A. K. Hawlader, and M. F. Hossain, "Watermarking scheme based on game of life cellular automaton," in 2014 International Conference on Informatics, Electronics & Vision (ICIEV), pp. 1–6, IEEE, 2014.

Emerging Trends in IoT and Computing Technologies – Suman Lata Tripathi et al. (eds)
© 2024 Taylor & Francis Group, London, ISBN 978-1-032-87924-6

A Review Paper on Toxic Comment Classifier

13

Disha Sengupta[1], Zaid Rupani[2], Rajvi Jagani[3], Kashish Nahar[4]

Dr. D. Y. Patil Institute of Technology, Department of Artificial Intelligence & Data Science,
Pimpri, Pune, India

Abstract: The rapid growth of digital platforms, especially YouTube, has given rise to a surge in user-generated content. However, this abundance of content brings with it challenges, including the generation of toxic and harmful comments. Comments have turned into a significant piece of our everyday life and on social media platform they play a huge role. But what if someone misuses this freedom and comments start becoming abusive, harsh or disrespectful, making a few users uncomfortable? In this paper, we address the specificities of YouTube comments, considering the platform's unique linguistic characteristics, user engagement patterns, and the contextual intricacies of video-based discussions. A dataset comprising YouTube comments is curated and annotated for model training and evaluation. Leveraging the transformative power of BERT which is a Bidirectional Encoder Representations from Transformers, one of the deep learning model, we achieve significant advancements in accurately analyzing toxic comments. Our aim is to contribute to content moderation efforts, ultimately empowering content creators, users, and platform administrators to mitigate toxic behaviour and promote meaningful online interactions actively.

Keywords: YouTube comments, Hate analysis, BERT, Deep learning

1. Introduction

In the digital age, user-generated content on online platforms has grown exponentially, allowing individuals from around the world to engage, share, and connect over a myriad of topics and interests. Among the various platforms that have emerged as hubs for content sharing, YouTube has firmly established itself as a global community, with billions of users consuming and creating videos daily. As indicated by Alexa, the web traffic checking administration claimed by Amazon, YouTube is the second most famous site internationally with north of 300 hours of recordings transferred consistently and 5 billion recordings watched each and every day [4]. With the rise of user-generated content, however, comes the challenge of moderating the vast quantity of comments posted beneath these videos. Toxic and offensive comments can tarnish the user experience and have a detrimental impact on the well-being of content creators and their audiences. Negative social media interactions have also been shown in numerous studies to exacerbate melancholy, low self-esteem, and even suicide thoughts [2]. This is where the critical need for an efficient toxic comment classifier arises.

According to a Pew Research Centre study, 40% of adult Internet users have directly experienced harassment and 73% have witnessed it occur [17]. According to a different survey, 19% of teenagers said that unpleasant or embarrassing things had been said or posted about them on social networking sites.

[1]disha.24sharma@gmail.com, [2]zaidrupani.zr42@gmail.com, [3]rajvijagani@gmail.com, [4]kashishnhr5@gmail.com

DOI: 10.1201/9781003535423-13

Moderating these comments manually can be a daunting task, especially on platforms like YouTube, where thousands of comments can be posted in just a few minutes. For example, 87.3% of the films that were gathered were classified as news and politics on YouTube. Analysis reveals that the highest percentage of toxic comments are found in news articles about religion and violence/crime, accounting for 24.8% and 25.9% of all comments left on videos on these subjects, respectively. In contrast, the lowest percentage of toxic comments is found in news articles about the economy, accounting for 17.4% of all comments [14]. This is where automated toxic comment classifiers can play a pivotal role in maintaining a healthy online environment. With the aid of the YouTube API, we aim to harness the wealth of comments generated on the platform and provide users with tools to effectively manage these comments.

This research paper delves into the development and implementation of a toxic comment classifier, specifically tailored for YouTube video comments. With a primary focus on BERT (Bidirectional Encoder Representations from Transformers) models, we want to harness the power of cutting-edge natural language processing (NLP) models to efficiently identify and classify comments into two main groups: harmful and non-toxic. Our primary objective is to create a robust and adaptable system that can be integrated seamlessly with YouTube. Users will have the capability to access categorized comments, and, most importantly, have the means to flag and remove toxic comments to foster a more positive and inclusive online environment.

Our project's website, which is connected to the YouTube API, offers users a user-friendly interface where they can view and interact with comments. We have categorized comments into three main sections: toxic, non-toxic, and neutral. This categorization simplifies the experience for users, enabling them to quickly identify and focus on the comments that matter most to them. Furthermore, users have the authority to mark comments as toxic, thus aiding in the refinement of the classifier. Additionally, they can delete toxic comments, giving them greater control over their online space.

The development of a toxic comment classifier for YouTube comments, integrated into a website and powered by BERT, holds significant promise. This research serves a dual purpose: to contribute to the improvement of online communities by reducing toxicity and to showcase the potential of cutting-edge NLP models for content moderation and user engagement

2. Literature Survey

Various researches has taken place and all of them have different approaches to tackle a big problem which involves cyber bullying. It is not easy to classify comments and it requires a well-developed and trained model to classify comments in an efficient way.

In [2], the researchers implemented deep learning networks trained and optimised to take advantage of all that the current Elastic Cloud Computing (EC^2) infrastructure has to offer, supporting the deployment paradigm of the MXNet framework. In order to maximise the potential of numerous GPUs, they implemented LSTM/RNN (Long-short term memory/Recurrent neural networks), which were optimised with MXNet.742 toxic comments (true positive) out of 1,543 (roughly 50%) toxic comments were classified accurately. Naive Bayes was also used as benchmark, which ended up giving biased results, it is therefore inferred using Support Vector Machines (SVM) or other deep learning techniques would give more accurate results.

The authors in [4], used non-negative matrix factorisation techniques, also using Perspective AI to each comment a toxicity score, which was subsequently utilised to build a model for commenter toxicity score prediction..This method has two drawbacks: first, new users won't have a toxicity score at first, and second, the commenter-video toxicity matrix may become rather sparse with data volume grows, increasing the reconstruction error. The authors of [5] decided to take upon an approach in using Convolution Neural Network instead of the traditional bag of words approach for text classification as use of CNN is more efficient and effective.

Lexical Syntactical Feature architecture is used in [7], the authors aim to detect toxic comments and content and identify probable toxic and threatening users to the community in social media. The authors taken in account, the user's writing style, structure inorder to predict how likely a user is going to be offensive or toxic. It accomplishes 98.24% precision and 94.34% recall in sentence offensive detection and 77.9% precision and 77.8% recall in user offensive detection. However, LSF can digest sentences at a rate of about 10 msec, indicating that it might be used in social media in an efficient manner. [7].

In [3], the authors used standard Machine Learning techniques to classify comments on a Swedish YouTube channel; its findings were that 0.643% of the total comments analyzed were toxic.

3. Methodology

3.1 Data Collection and Visualization of Training Data

YouTube is a website where users may upload and share videos. When YouTube was launched in 2005, its users could only upload videos to share with others. Mr. Jawed Karim uploaded the first video, which was about visiting the zoo, and it received 2.7 million views. [8].

Youtube comments on popular channels are a task,there are more than 1000 comments on popular channels and the toxicity cannot be measured. To measure the level of toxicity of the comments on a particular channel,we need access to the comments and the data related to it. YouTube offers an application programming interface (API) for retrieving user and video-related data, including user profiles, videos, comment threads, and more. [20]It is called as Youtube API.

The YouTube API, officially known as the YouTube Data API, is a collection of Google-provided application programming interfaces (APIs) that enable users to access a range of features and information on the well-known streaming service Youtube. By making authenticated requests to the API, developers can create applications that allows them to fetch video metadata, manage comments, upload videos, search for specific content, and access analytics data. This helps us gain access and fetch comments from videos. These capabilities have made it a cornerstone for building applications like video downloaders, content curation platforms, and analytics tools, offering new ways to interact with and leverage YouTube's extensive content library. Using the Google APIs ,the user is asked to login to one's youtube channel making use of Google OAuth 2.O to gain access to the channel. The C#, Python, and R programming languages are accessible for the Google APIs, which are free Google APIs used for gathering comments. Python is a tool we use at business. Google APIs will retrieve the information from Youtube.com following login. The file will be saved in CSV format by the APIs following the collection of comments. The file can be saved in CSV, JSON, or simply text format. Our dataset of comments is saved in CSV format. [19]

This is the collection of data which is going to be actually used in our application. A different dataset is used for testing and training the model.

The act of teaching a model to make predictions or choices by subjecting it to a dataset of inputs and their intended or accurate outputs is known as "training" in machine learning. In the process of training, the model discovers the underlying correlations and patterns in the data, which enables it to forecast previously unseen data.

Eight categories are used to group the comments. 1) id, 2) comment_text, and 3) poisonous 4) highly toxic 5) vulgar; 6) menacing; 7) derogatory; 8) hate of individuality. The model learns from this data after preprocessing and cleaning in order to predict the category on unseen data.

The process of representing data graphically or pictorially to make it easier for others to grasp is known as data visualisation. It is a crucial tool for communication and data analysis since it simplifies the understanding and interpretation of complex data.

Inorder to visualize all the toxic comments or words used in the dataset,we can use wordcloud to visualize it. AA word cloud is a common visual representation of text data in which words are arranged in an eye-catching and visually appealing manner. The size of the words indicates how frequently they occur and how significant they are in a phrase.

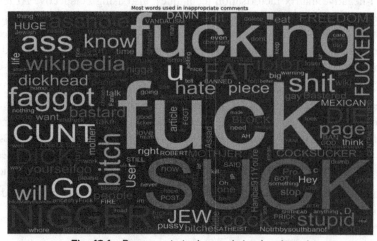

Fig. 13.1   Represents toxic words in cloudword

Visualizations is an important part,it helps understanding the data better,usually the data is not clean, before training the data in order to give accurate results we perform preprocessing. Visualisations helps find outliers, in the above wordcloud we can observe "go" is not actually toxic and visualization helps fix errors like this inorder to correctly predict on unseen data, in our case the comments received from Youtube Data API.

3.2 Data Pre-Processing

The efficiency of tasks like information retrieval, sentiment analysis, and classification is greatly influenced by pre-processing. This paper delves into a comprehensive analysis of key data pre-processing techniques, with a focus on tokenization, stemming, stopword removal, and punctuation removal.

Tokenization: The process of breaking up text into smaller pieces, usually words or subwords, is known as tokenization. This method divides textual material into tokens so that additional analysis can be done. Any word, number, or other sign that captures all the pertinent details about the data without compromising its security can be used as a token.

Stemming: brings words down to their most basic or root form. This helps to condense vocabulary and capture the essence of words. However, it can lead to imprecise results due to over-simplification. Modern NLP models sometimes favour lemmatization, which preserves linguistic accuracy.

Number Removal: Removing numbers from text data is valuable in many NLP tasks, as numbers often carry limited semantic meaning. However, in applications like sentiment analysis, retaining numbers might be essential for contextual understanding.

Punctuation Removal: Stripping text of punctuation marks can improve tokenization and text analysis. It must be eliminated in order to enhance machine learning algorithms' learning process because it causes issues throughout the learning process. Yet, context matters, and in tasks like social media analysis, some punctuation may carry valuable sentiment or meaning.

Stopword Removal: Stopwords are common words (e.g., "the," "and," "in") that may not considerably advance the text's meaning. Removing them can reduce data dimensionality and enhance processing speed. However, their removal should be task-specific, as they might contain valuable information in certain contexts.

3.3 About BERT

BERT, which stands for "Bidirectional Encoder Representations from Transformers," is a paradigm for natural language processing (NLP) that Google created in 2018. One kind of transformer model, called BERT, is a major development in natural language processing. Its capacity to grasp linguistic nuances and context has had a significant influence on a range of NLP jobs.

In practical terms, BERT is a pre-trained language model, which indicates that a substantial amount of text material from the internet is used for its first training. BERT has a thorough comprehension of general language patterns thanks to this pretraining. With comparatively little task-specific data, it can then be optimised for certain NLP tasks, such as question answering, sentiment analysis, or the classification of poisonous comments. BERT's versatility and power in NLP stem from its capacity to construct contextual word embeddings and its adaptability, which allow it to operate at the cutting edge of various language-related tasks.

3.4 Why BERT

Bidirectional Understanding: Traditional language models like LSTMs and earlier transformer models (e.g., GPT-1) read text in a unidirectional manner, which means they process words sequentially from left to right or vice versa. BERT, on the other hand, uses a bidirectional approach. It has a stronger comprehension of the context and word relationships when it learns to predict missing words in a phrase from both sides.

Contextual Word Embeddings: BERT generates contextual word embeddings. In other words, it produces word representations that vary according to the context of the word's appearance. This enables BERT to capture the meaning of a word differently in different contexts.

Pre-trained Model: BERT is pre-trained using a substantial body of textual data, which means it learns from a massive amount of text from the internet. This pretraining enables BERT to capture a broad range of language patterns, making it versatile and adaptable to various NLP tasks.

Contextual Understanding: Toxic comments often rely on subtle language, sarcasm, or contextual cues. BERT's contextual embeddings allow it to understand these nuances and identify toxicity more effectively than models with static word embeddings.

State-of-the-Art Performance: BERT routinely outperforms earlier models in a variety of NLP tasks, such as the classification of harmful comments. Its ability to capture context and nuances in text helps it achieve high accuracy in identifying toxic comments.

3.5 Comparison

Keyword-Based Classifier: Generally speaking, there have been three chronological phases in the development of online hate detection: (1) basic classifiers based on lexicons or keywords, (2) classifiers that use distributed semantics, and (3) deep learning classifiers that use sophisticated linguistic features. For instance, given a list of profane terms, one should be able to accurately identify 40% of the words as such and 52% of them as hateful or not. The researchers employed 1078 hate words from Hatebase,1, a database of nasty words, and specific hate targets (such as Black people, Mexican people, and stupid people) to prevent false positives, such as: "I really hate owing people favours" [9]. The linguistic diversity of the texts in which the sarcasm and other types of humour were not recognised is one of the limits of employing the Keyword based Classifier, despite its use in earlier studies. Moreover, as new lingo and slang emerge on social media swiftly, the dictionaries of derogatory terms and insults need to be updated frequently.

The Naive Bayes methodology is a statistical method for teaching machines to learn. The Bayes theorem, $P(A|B) = P(B|A) P(A) / P(B)$, forms its foundation. These are some of the most basic models of Bayesian networks. Next, based on the percentage of hazardous messages in the training data set, the probability that a message is toxic, or P(hazardous), was determined. Based on the naive simplification of the Bayes Theorem, the likelihood that the new message's content is discovered in the toxic word pool is required; the probability of the message content, P(message content), does not need to be calculated. Because of the naive assumption, the probability that the new message will be harmful is calculated based on whether the word appears in the pool of poisonous words or not. Similarly, it is possible to determine the probability that the new communication won't be harmful, and the likelihood ratio will determine how the new message is categorised [2]. The linguistic features of the sentence are unknown since the message content is not taken into account. Understanding the irony and sarcasm in the sentence—where the meaning of a straightforward sentence varies depending on the context—is the primary drawback of the naive Bayes approach.

By comparing the BERT model with different approaches, it gives an immense value to the contextual understanding of sentences and increases the accuracy by using different libraries. As a pretrained model, it creates the vector according to the features of the particular word and recognizing the contextual situation makes it more unique and intellectual to use it for toxicity classification.

4. Conclusion

In this research, we delved into the critical domain of toxic comment classification, with a particular focus on the dynamic and ever-evolving platform of YouTube. Our study has shed light on the toxicities and nuances that characterize comments within the YouTube ecosystem. One of the highlights of our research was the adoption of the BERT (Bidirectional Encoder Representations from Transformers) model, which stands as a cornerstone in the realm of natural language processing. BERT's bidirectional context understanding, coupled with pre-training on vast corpora of text data, making it a robust choice for toxic comment classification on YouTube.

In conclusion, our research signifies a significant stride towards an enhanced understanding of toxic comment classification on YouTube. As YouTube continues to evolve, our findings underscore the importance of advanced NLP models and tailored approaches in the relentless pursuit of enhancing online conversations and promoting a more positive, inclusive, and respectful online ecosystem.

REFERENCES

1. Salminen, J., Hopf, M., Chowdhury, S.A., Jung, S.G., Almerekhi, H. and Jansen, B.J., 2020. Developing an online hate classifier for multiple social media platforms.Human-centric Computing and Information Sciences, 10, pp.1-34.
2. Zaheri, S., Leath, J. and Stroud, D., 2020. Toxic comment classification. SMU Data Science Review, 3(1), p.13.
3. Dehkhoda, S. and Gunica, J.A., 2023. Analyzing Toxicity in YouTube Comments with the Help of Machine Learning.
4. Obadimu, A., Mead, E. and Agarwal, N., 2019. Identifying latent toxic features on YouTube using non-negative matrix factorization.In The Ninth International Conference on Social Media Technologies, Communication, and Informatics, IEEE.

5. Georgakopoulos, S.V., Tasoulis, S.K., Vrahatis, A.G. and Plagianakos, V.P., 2018, July. Convolutional neural networks for toxic comment classification. In Proceedings of the 10th hellenic conference on artificial intelligence (pp. 1-6).

6. Poojitha, K., Charish, A.S., Reddy, M. and Ayyasamy, S., 2023. Classification of social media Toxic comments using Machine learning models.arXiv preprint arXiv:2304.06934.

7. Obadimu, A., Mead, E., Hussain, M.N. and Agarwal, N., 2019. Identifying toxicity within youtube video comment. In Social, Cultural, and BehavioralModeling: 12th International Conference, SBP-BRiMS 2019, Washington, DC, USA, July 9–12, 2019, Proceedings 12 (pp. 214-223). Springer International Publishing.

8. Zhao, Z., Zhang, Z. and Hopfgartner, F., 2021, April. A comparative study of using pre-trained language models for toxic comment classification. In Companion Proceedings of the Web Conference 2021 (pp. 500-507).

9. Salminen, J., Hopf, M., Chowdhury, S.A., Jung, S.G., Almerekhi, H. and Jansen, B.J., 2020. Developing an online hate classifier for multiple social media platforms. Human-centric Computing and Information Sciences, 10, pp.1-34.

10. d'Sa, A.G., Illina, I. and Fohr, D., 2019. Towards non-toxic landscapes: Automatic toxic comment detection using DNN. arXiv preprint arXiv:1911.08395.

11. Kajla, H., Hooda, J. and Saini, G., 2020, May. Classification of online toxic comments using machine learning algorithms.In 2020 4th international conference on intelligent computing and control systems (ICICCS) (pp. 1119-1123).IEEE.

12. Murali, S.R., Rangreji, S., Vinay, S. and Srinivasa, G., 2020, October. Automated NER, sentiment analysis and toxic comment classification for a goal-oriented chatbot.In 2020 Fourth International Conference On Intelligent Computing in Data Sciences (ICDS) (pp. 1-7).IEEE.

13. Rupapara, V., Rustam, F., Shahzad, H.F., Mehmood, A., Ashraf, I. and Choi, G.S., 2021. Impact of SMOTE on imbalanced text features for toxic comments classification using RVVC model. IEEE Access, 9, pp.78621-78634.

14. Alshamrani, S., Abuhamad, M., Abusnaina, A. and Mohaisen, D., 2020, October. Investigating Online Toxicity in Users Interactions with the Mainstream Media Channels on YouTube.In CIKM (Workshops).

15. Schultes, P., Dorner, V. and Lehner, F., 2013. Leave a comment! An in-depth analysis of user comments on YouTube.

16. Chakravarthi, B.R., 2022. Hope speech detection in YouTube comments. Social Network Analysis and Mining, 12(1), p.75.

17. M. Duggan, "Online harassment," Pew Res. Center, Washington, DC, USA, Tech. Rep., 2014.[Online]. Available: https://www.pewresearch.org/internet/wp-content/uploads/sites/9/2017/07/PI_2017.07.11_OnlineHarassment_FINAL.pdf

18. Mikolov, T., Sutskever, I., Chen, K., Corrado, G.S. and Dean, J., 2013. Distributed representations of words and phrases and their compositionality.Advances in neural information processing systems, 26.

19. Nawaz, S., Rizwan, M. and Rafiq, M., 2019. Recommendation of effectiveness of YouTube video contents by qualitative sentiment analysis of its comments and replies. Pakistan Journal of Science, 71(4), p.91.

20. Khan, A.U.R., Khan, M. and Khan, M.B., 2016. Naïve Multi-label classification of YouTube comments using comparative

Emerging Trends in IoT and Computing Technologies – Suman Lata Tripathi et al. (eds)
© 2024 Taylor & Francis Group, London, ISBN 978-1-032-87924-6

Visual Content to Spoken Word Transformation for Visually Impaired People

14

Rajendran A[1], Dhanush C[2],
Hari Krishna S[3], Mohamed Abul Hasil S[4], Mohanaprasath M[5]
Karpagam College of Engineering,
Dept. Electronics and Communication Engineering, Coimbatore, India

Abstract: Blindness is becoming more and more common in this generation, as seeing and hearing are the main factors for proper communication in day-to-day life. Visually impaired people face many problems during their daily life as they struggle for interaction between people. A device which helps to read books without seeing and also helps the person to recognize the face of the other person. This method used to convert the image into text using Tesseract OCR and the text into image using e- Speak engine. When the visually impaired people need help the text-image to speech comes into place and replace any person without any struggle. In addition, we used Haar Cascade Classifier to detect the face and store the image from the facial recognition. It recognizes the faces and inform the people who uses it about them by informing their name. It will be a change of life for the visually impaired people who sought to life a normal life.

Keywords: Tesseract (OCR), TTS engine, Haar cascade classifier

1. Introduction

There are 2.2 billion blind people in the world now, out of a total population of 8 billion people. 295 million people in this group have visual impairments of various degrees, and 37 million people are totally blind. Readiness of routine activities like menu cards, signboard interpretation, and book reading can be quite difficult for people who are visually impaired. The multimedia technology space has expanded dramatically as a result, and images are now an essential component of multimedia material that includes text, people, and face features. By combining OpenCV functionalities with image processing techniques, the suggested solution makes use of Open Computer Vision (OpenCV) for word recognition. Under the guise of assessing the quality of the recognized text, the OCR engine skillfully discerns subtleties such as font types, italicized text, and clustered characters. Then the e-speak algorithm is used to turn the text that was identified into speech. A Haar cascade classifier is used for face identification, and OpenCV library functionalities are also utilized for facial recognition in addition to text recognition. Not only does this invention help the blind, but it also benefits others who are farsighted and have trouble reading print materials.

2. Literature Review

Shraddha Hingankar, Prachi Tardekar, Prof. Santoshi Pote, [1] The proposed system captures images from documents or books using a Raspberry Pi 3 camera. Image pre-processing removes noise by applying appropriate thresholds, correcting skew angles, sharpening, thresholding, and segmentation. Geetha M.N.*, Sheethal H.V., Sindhu S., Ayesha Siddiqa J. and Chandan H.C. [2] Visually impaired individuals require Braille systems for reading and writing, and face challenges to use modern

[1]rajendran.a@kce.ac.in, [2]dhanushcool2003@gmail.com, [3]harikrishvcp2002@gmail.com, [4]abulhasil234@gmail.com, [5]mohanaprasath2808@gmail.com

DOI: 10.1201/9781003535423-14

gadgets such as smartphones or computers. S Sarkar, G Pansare, B Patel, A Gupta, A Chauhan, R Yadav and N Battula [3] This algorithm uses a camera module to capture text and convert it into binary representation, converting it into gray-scale images. The Optical Character Recognition Algorithm extracts and recognizes individual characters from the grayscale image.

The technique developed by Ram Nivas Duraisamy and Sathya Manoharan uses Tesseract, Festival, and Raspberry Pi to turn input visuals into speech. To capture and understand text, they use free and open-source Computer Vision libraries. Prof. Vidhyashree. C, Supriya. A. M, Supriya. H, Vedala Dinesh, Kavya. R [11] The proposed method involves the machine learning algorithm for text-to-speech which can be used by visually impaired people and also the normal people who wants to read the book loudly at any rate of speed and pitch.

Sabin Khader, Meerakrishna M R, Reshma Roy, Willson Joseph C [12] The proposed model involves the detection of obstacles while a blind person walks outside, it detects the obstacles and capture the image and send the information as a speech format for the knowledge of the person using it. Nisha P, Dr J Vijayakumar [13] The project aims to help them to detect the bus name, boards, bus stops, shops etc. using capturing image, text localization and text to audio conversion. The technologies used are using OCR, speak algorithm and the text are recognized by the API and using Python and Java Programming. Tushar Khete, Aditya Bakshi [14] In this project there are different technologies used which are OCR, g-TTS (google Text-to-Speech) and python and terminal for the integration of the interface with the project. This convert the processed image into text which will be converted using python library in the command line Interface tool and the audio is heard by the people who uses it.

3. Proposed Method

The proposed technique helps the visually impaired individuals to do the things that a normal person do such as reading books or anything that are need to be remembered and recognize the face of other people. It is done using the images of the text and faces taken. The system converts the recognized document to voice output using an eSpeak algorithm, ensuring mobility.

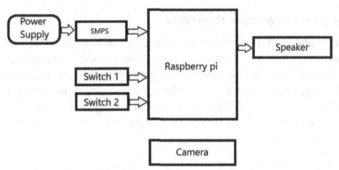

Fig. 14.1 Block diagram

The recommended technique offers both face and text recognition capabilities. It allows vision challenged people to take photographs in text recognition mode so they can read product labels, documents, and printed text. A number of processing processes are applied to these collected images, such as converting them to grayscale and performing dilation and erosion techniques to remove noise. The Tesseract OCR is then fed the binarized image as a result for text recognition. The eSpeak method is then used to convert the identified text into an audible format. Headphones plugged into a Raspberry Pi's audio port get the audio output.

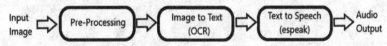

Fig. 14.2 Image to speech conversion process

Face detection, feature extraction, and face recognition are the three steps in the face recognition process. The first face detection process uses the Haar cascade classifier. Each item in the database, which is created to hold details on recognized people, consists of a pair of input photographs and labels. After that, the face recognition software locates the identified face and makes an effort to match it with pictures that are kept in the database. Through this procedure, the visual data from face recognition is transformed into a text format and saved as a text file. The text is then recognized using Optical Character Recognition (OCR) technology and e-speak algorithm will convert it into audible output. People who are blind or visually challenged may benefit from this audio output since it enables them to "read" content with their ears. It's crucial to remember that vivid, detailed images outperform darker, less detailed ones in terms of recognition system performance. For best recognition, text in a.txt file format with black font on a white backdrop is recommended for OCR.

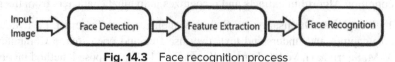

Fig. 14.3 Face recognition process

4. Software Implementation

4.1 Process of Recognizing Text From Image by using Tesseract OCR Tool

The suggested project makes use of Google's open-source Tesseract OCR technology to extract text from photos. This engine first binaries the image it has collected before performing text detection on it. Connected component analysis is the first step in the OCR process, when components are saved for further reverse text recognition. This is a methodical process that can recognize and translate writing that has been inverted, as well as recognize black text on a white backdrop. The machine then classifies the pixels in the foreground as either blobs or possible characters. After that, these characters are arranged into text lines and evaluated based on whether or not they have a proportionate or fixed pitch text layout. Character spacing is used to further break the lines into words, and any fixed pitch information is quickly separated into individual character cells.

4.2 Transformation of Text into Speech by the use of e-Speak Engine

It requires engines such as e-Speak, are used for this purpose. Using a "formant synthesis" technique, the open-source speech synthesizer E-Speak provides numerous languages in small packages. Among its main advantages is a clear and quick speech output. A command-line utility called E-Speak makes it possible to alter voice characteristics.

4.3 Face Recognition using Haar Cascade Classifier

For the purpose of image capturing and facial recognition we use the OpenCV, required OS and the python library numpy and image modules are used when we detect the face. To store the images, we can use the numpy modules and so when we want to convert the image into text it is obtained from numpy module. It starts to scan from the left top of the image to the right bottom of the image to cover the whole image and convert it to text. There are three steps involved in the process of face recognition. For the initial process there will be a face detection when we provide the image to the classifier it detects the face in the image and try to process it to the OCR as then it is converted into text file and using espeak engine we can convert the text file into audible speech.

5. Results

5.1 Software Output

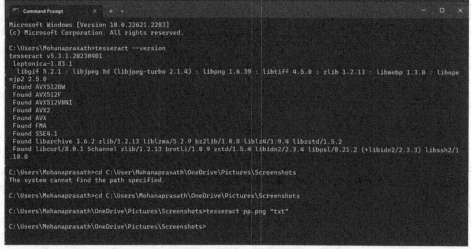

Fig. 14.4 Tesseract OCR

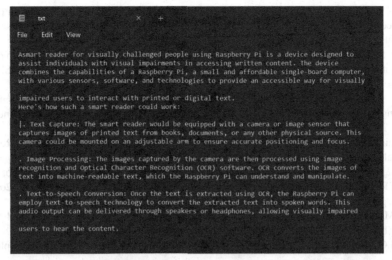

Fig. 14.5 Text output from Tesseract OCR

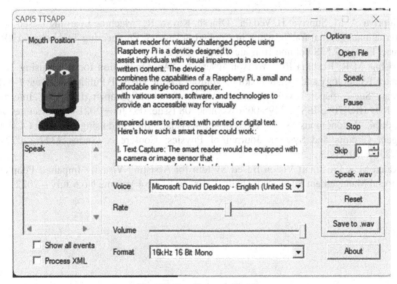

Fig. 14.6 Espeak Engine

6. Conclusion

Using Raspberry Pi technology, a small and portable reading aid for those with vision problems is created. This cutting-edge tool recognizes face features and text in photos. It uses a wired camera for quick image processing and a rechargeable battery for portability. A GPS system is integrated for position and orientation help, and object detection capabilities may be added to improve the user experience. Moreover, the availability of Wi-Fi connectivity may replace the requirement for conventional connections. This adaptable gadget is a lifesaver for those who are visually impaired, and it may be used in any setting where voice help is needed.

REFERENCES

1. Shraddha Hingankar1, Prachi Tardekar2, Prof. Santoshi Pote3," A Smart Reader for Visually Impaired Individuals", International Research Journal of Engineering and Technology (IRJET) e-ISSN: 2395- 0056 Volume: 07 Issue: 07 | July 2020 www.irjet.net p-ISSN: 2395-0072.
2. Geetha M.N.*, Sheethal H.V., Sindhu S., Ayesha Siddiqa J. and Chandan H.C.,"Survey on Smart Reader for Blind and Visually Impaired (BVI)", Indian Journal of Science and Technology, Vol 12(48), DOI: 10.17485/ijst/2019/v12i48/149408, December 2019.

3. S Sarkar, G Pansare, B Patel, A Gupta, A Chauhan, R Yadav and N Battula, "Smart Reader for Visually Impaired Using Raspberry Pi", International Conference on Innovations in Mechanical Sciences (ICIMS'21) IOP Conf. Series: Materials Science and Engineering 1132 (2021) 012032 IOP Publishing doi:10.1088/1757- 899X/1132/1/012032.

4. Ram Nivas Duraisamy, Sathya Manoharan "A Smart Reader for Visually Impaired People (Standard Image Vs Real Time Image: A Comparative Study)", International Journal of Latest Engineering and Management Research (IJLEMR) ISSN: 2455-4847 www.ijlemr.com || Volume 03 - Issue 10 || October 2018 || PP. 39-46.

5. Norharyati binti Harum, Nurul Azma Zakaria, Nurul A. Emran, Zakiah Ayop4, Syarulnaziah Anawar, "Smart Book Reader for Visual Impairment Person using IoT Device", (IJACSA) International Journal of Advanced Computer Science and Applications, Vol. 10, No. 2, 2019.

6. Muhammad Farid Zamir, Khan Bahadar Khan1, Shafquat Ahmmad Khan, and Eid Rehman, "Smart Reader for Visually Impaired People Based on Optical Character Recognition" Chapter · May 2020 DOI: 10.1007/978- 981-15-5232-8_8.

7. K. Barathkumar, S. Balaji, K. N. Desikan, S. Padhmanabha Iyappan, "Raspberry Pi based Smart Reader for Visually Impaired People", International Journal of Research in Engineering, Science and Management Volume-2, Issue-2, February-2019 www.ijresm.com | ISSN (Online): 2581-5792.

8. L Latha, V Geethani, M Divyadharshini, P Thangam, "A Smart Reader for Blind People", International Journal of Engineering and Advanced Technology (IJEAT) ISSN: 2249-8958 (Online), Volume-8 Issue-6S3, September 2019.

9. Rajkumar N, Anand M.G, Barathiraja N,"Portable Camera Based Product Label Reading for Blind People." IJETT, Vol. 10 Number 11 –Apr 2014.

10. Wilson, P. I., Fernandez, J., "Facial feature detection using haar classifiers", in journal of Computing sciences in Colleges (2006), pp.127-133.

11. Prof. Vidhyashree. C, Supriya. A. M, Supriya. H, Vedala Dinesh, Kavya. R, "Machine Learning Based Text to Speech Converter for Visually Impaired", International Journal for Research in Applied Science & Engineering Technology (IJRASET) ISSN: 2321-9653; IC Value: 45.98; SJ Impact Factor: 7.538 Volume 10 Issue VII July 2022.

12. Sabin Khader, Meerakrishna M R, Reshma Roy, Willson Joseph C, "An Application for Blind using Text to Speech Conversion", Advancement of Computer Technology and its Applications Volume 3 Issue 1 HBRP Publication Page 1-6 2020.

13. Nisha P, Dr.J.Vijayakumar, "Survey paper: Text To Speech conversion for visually impaired peoples", International Research Journal of Engineering and Technology (IRJET) e-ISSN: 2395-0056 Volume: 08 Issue: 06 | June 2021 www.irjet.net p-ISSN: 2395-0072.

14. Tushar Khete, Aditya Bakshi, "Autonomous Assistance System for Visually Impaired using Tesseract OCR & gTTS", 4th International Conference on Intelligent Circuits and Systems Journal of Physics: Conference Series 2327 (2022) 012065 IOP Publishing doi:10.1088/1742-6596/2327/1/012065.

15. Aysha Nafla P, SruthiRajan M K "A Smart Vision Based System for Assisting Visually Impaired People", International Journal of Engineering Technology and Management Sciences Website: ijetms.in Issue: 4 Volume No.6 July – 2022.

Emerging Trends in IoT and Computing Technologies – Suman Lata Tripathi et al. (eds)
© 2024 Taylor & Francis Group, London, ISBN 978-1-032-87924-6

Cybersecurity Issues and Challenges in Industry 4.0

15

B. Varshaa[1], V. Jothi Francina[2], C. Nithisha[3]
Sona College of Technology, MBA, Salem. India

Abstract: Industry4.0, which is defined by the integration of creative technologies like robotics, big data, cloud computing, Internet of Things (IoT), cyber-physical systems (CPS), cognitive computing, and artificial intelligence (AI), has been ushered in by the convergence of information technology (IT) and operational technology (OT).While Industry 4.0 promises increased productivity and efficiency, it also poses significant cybersecurity challenges, particularly in managing and securing the vast amounts of data generated by IoT devices. This article explores the key challenges and proposes a top-down approach to enhance cybersecurity in Industry 4.0.

Keywords: Internet of thing (IOT), Operational technology (OT), Cyber-physical system (CPS), Malware intrusions, Modifications in firmware, Adoption, Challenges

1. Introduction

The arrival of Industry4.0, the fourth artificial revolution, is described by the infusion of advanced technologies like cloud computing, IoT, and robotics into traditional manufacturing processes. This digital transformation has brought unparalleled opportunities but also introduced new cybersecurity threats. As industries become hyper-connected, they are more susceptible to cyberattacks. Industry 4.0's integration of cutting-edge technologies, IoT devices, and networked systems has opened the door to potentially devastating cyber threats. This article delves into the challenges posed by Industry 4.0, especially in the realm of cybersecurity.

1.1 Internet of Things (IoT)

IoT, the network of interconnected devices capable of exchanging data, collects information from physical objects and uses big data for more efficient data processing and storage. The synergy between IoT and big data enhances data collection and analysis, ultimately improving production.

1.2 Malware Intrusions

Traditional cybersecurity measures like firewalls and antivirus software are lacking to guard robotization systems from malware attempts, bushwhackers can play weakness to hazard automation and product systems, dismembering the all-work wheel. Advanced cybersecurity means, like as ubiquitous Internet tail System Integrity Monitoring, offer helped security by detecting unauthorized changes to critical network ingredients essential for operation robotization.

---

[1]Varshusuba2610@gmail.com, [2]jothifranica@sonamgmt.org, [3]cnithisha23@gmail.com

DOI: 10.1201/9781003535423-15

1.2 Modifications in Firmware

Hackers have become adept at creating alternate firmware versions that can be injected into Industrial Internet of Things (IIoT) systems to exploit security weaknesses or disrupt the entire network. To counter this threat, modern IT teams must rigorously inspect firmware and ensure driver updates before network deployment. Implementing a user-centric access control system and disabling USB ports on critical systems can further mitigate firmware-related security issues.

2. Review of Literature

I have discovered multiple reliable sources that offer valuable insights on the subject at hand. IGI Global provides a thorough examination of cybersecurity issues and challenges within the context of Industry 4.0. They delve into the ever-evolving threat landscape and discuss effective strategies to mitigate risks. In a research paper available on Diva-portal, the significance of cybersecurity in Industry 4.0 is highlighted, emphasizing the crucial need for robust protective mechanisms. CYBALT presents a white paper that specifically addresses the real-world cybersecurity challenges faced by Industry 4.0, offering practical guidance to enhance cyber resilience. Balbix brings forth a discussion on cybersecurity in the era of Industry 4.0, stressing the importance of a proactive approach to ensure strong protection against cyber threats. Lastly, ResearchGate presents a state-of-the-art review that focuses on the cybersecurity challenges present in Industry 4.0, providing a comprehensive analysis of the current landscape along with potential solutions.

3. Espousing a Top- Level Approach for Upgraded Cybersecurity In Industry 4.0

In an era where hundreds of devices and systems are interconnected, conventional cybersecurity approaches are insufficient. A multi-layered approach that establishes a framework for digital transformation and adopts a energetic top-down perspective is needed.

4. The Succeeding Steps can be Enforced

Begin with Strategic Planning

Constitute digital changeover systems powered by IoT technology from the top position, supported by strategic planning. crucial opinions should be formed catching programs, strategies, guidelines, and decrees for the undivided network and company.

Focus on Data Security

Shift the focus to data processing layers to secure critical business data. Develop a comprehensive data security strategy that accommodates future growth and evolving threats.

Design Technology Infrastructure

Design technology structures and systems with functionality and security requirements in mind. Careful selection of vendors is crucial to address potential third-party vulnerabilities.

Emphasize Network Design

With the reference framework in place, security engineers can design networks based on layered conditions, ensuring that no security is compromised in order to satisfy all business requirements.

5. Cybersecurity Challenges In Industry 4.0

The manufacturing industry, the second-most targeted sector, faces unique cybersecurity challenges due to its increased attack surface in the age of Industry 4.0. Challenges include:

- Each linked trick denotes an implicit issue.
- Manufacturing networks, similar as Industrial Control Systems (ICS), have express weakness.
- Industry4.0 connects preliminarily insulated systems, expanding the attempt exterior.
- Upgrades are frequently installed incrementally due to system difficulty.

- Manufacturing has topmost regulatory compliance norms than other sectors.
- Visibility across systems and insulated surroundings is limited.

In this dynamic landscape, organizations must cover a wide spectrum of technology and prepare for evolving cyber threats.

6. Conclusion

Industry 4.0, marked by the integration of cyber-physical systems and advanced technologies, is poised for rapid growth. However, it also faces cybersecurity challenges that demand continuous improvement. This article has reviewed the cybersecurity threats associated with Industry 4.0 and proposed potential solutions. With the right strategies and proactive measures, the manufacturing sector can navigate the complexities of Industry 4.0 and protect its operations from cyber threats. As the industry evolves, it is crucial to stay ahead in the cybersecurity game and explore innovative solutions, such as blockchain, to bolster security.

REFERENCE

1. https://www.igi-global.com/chapter/cybersecurity-issues-and-challenges-in-industry-40/255359
2. https://www.diva-portal.org/smash/record.jsf?pid=diva2%3A1590006&dswid=3044
3. https://pdfs.semanticscholar.org/6117/4ecce41d8cd86f88a804868d57f4634fd4f8.pdf?_gl=1*193m7ka*_ga*MTE5ODU5NjY0MS4x-NjY1ODQ0MjA1*_ga_H7P4ZT52H5*MTY5ODA3MDY5MS4xLjEuMTY5ODA3MDczMy4xOC4wLjA.
4. https://www.dqindia.com/industrial-revolution-4-0-cyber-security-challenges-solutions/
5. https://www.nist.gov/blogs/manufacturing-innovation-blog/cybersecurity-and-industry-40-what-you-need-know
6. https://www.sciencedirect.com/science/article/pii/S2351978917306820
7. https://www.cybalt.com/docs/default-source/white_papers/cybalt-white-paper---industry-4.0-cyber-security-challenges---how-real-it-is.pdf
8. https://www.balbix.com/insights/cybersecurity-in-the-age-of-industry-4-0/
9. https://turcomat.org/index.php/turkbilmat/article/view/4946
10. https://www.researchgate.net/publication/362884521_Cybersecurity_challenges_in_Industry_40_A_state_of_the_art_review#:~:text=Cybersecurity%20is%20an%20important%20topic,well%20as%20their%20potential%20solutions.

Emerging Trends in IoT and Computing Technologies – Suman Lata Tripathi et al. (eds)
© 2024 Taylor & Francis Group, London, ISBN 978-1-032-87924-6

Deep Learning based Framework for Smart Fruit Grading System Using Raspberry Pi

16

**M. Meenalochani[1], R. Sriranjani[2],
N. Hemavathi[3], A. Gladsun Jerom[4], A. Prince Britto[5]**
SASTRA Deemed to be University, Dept. of CSE, Thanjavur, Tamilnadu, India

Abstract: Identification of freshness of a fruit is essential in the food industry as it ensures that the fruit is safe for consumption. Also, manual grading of fruits is a tedious process as it lacks consistency in classification and prone to human errors. Hence, an attempt is made to develop a standalone embedded system which is based on the principles of Deep Learning and IoT. The system detects the freshness of fruits based on visual perception n developed using Raspberry Pi. This system uses a camera to capture the images of the fruits and machine learning algorithm to determine whether the fruit is fresh or rotten. Fresh and rotten fruit images were used to train the algorithm, and a set of test images was used to test the accuracy of the model. This system enables us to distinguish fresh fruit from rotten fruit and can be used in many places such as supermarkets, greengrocers and agricultural area. Thus, it allows only fresh fruit to be sold and eaten and has the potential to improve the food industry's quality control process and reduce food waste.

Keywords: Deep learning, Inception model, Fruit grading, Raspberry Pi, Standalone embedded system

1. Introduction

Fruits are inevitable for a healthy diet as it contains fiber, vitamins and plant polyphenols, rich in antioxidant and anti-inflammatory properties. Fruits can also lower blood pressure and reduce the occurrence of stroke and pacify digestive issues [1]. Quality of fruits are also vital in maintaining the consumer health and safety. Microorganisms can infect the fruits which on consumption can lead to harmful health issues in humans. Conventional manual grading results in variations as each individual can have different interpretations on criteria for quality check. Also, manual grading cannot be used for high volume-based processing and thus it reduces the throughput of operation [2]. Thus, automated and semi-automated fruit grading systems can be utilized to overcome the challenges faced by traditional methods.

Recently, Deep Learning approaches have improved the state of the art in various emerging fields [4]. Automated fruit grading using machine learning approaches are gaining importance to evaluate the quality of food products without much human intervention. A picture dataset comprising three different fruit samples to differentiate fresh and rotten samples is proposed [5].Convolutional Neural Networks using Histograms, grey level co-occurrence matrices, a variety of features were used for the development of the framework. A machine vision framework for robot to harvest the dates based on convolutional neural networks based on transfer learning and fine tuning on pre-trained models is suggested [6].

A dataset consisting of around 8000 images under different date types exhibiting various stages of maturity is created. Accuracies achieved by the model are 99.01%, 97.25%, and 98.59% under the type, maturity, and harvesting decision classification tasks, respectively. A method to classify fruits by combining two features extracted from Statistical color features and Gray Level

[1]meenalochani@cse.sastra.edu, [2]mathusri@eee.sastra.edu, [3]hemavathi@eie.sastra.edu, [4]jeromgladsun@gmail.com, [5]princebritto1202@gmail.com

DOI: 10.1201/9781003535423-16

Co-occurrence Matrix and into a single feature descriptor is presented [7]. Based on these features, a classification model using SVM is created to find the fruit in the dataset. A machine vision system developed using images of kiwifruit obtained from an orchard at different timing is proposed [8].

Several architectures which are the variants of existing DL algorithms were proposed in recent years. Around 2400 images were fed to a R-CNN classifier developed using VGG16 and trained. The proposed model had an average precision of 87.61%, and detection of the kiwifruit images were done well. A framework for classifying fruits based on two deep learning models is discussed [9]. One model comprises six convolutional neural network layers and the other is a pretrained VGG16 model. The models are evaluated using two color image datasets and the proposed method outperforms the other existing methods. A novel technique to classify fruits using LSTM where labelling is done by CNN and RNN is discussed [10]. The proposed method achieved better performance over other classifier models such as FFNN, SVM, and ANFIS in terms of accuracy, coefficient of correlation analysis and root mean square.

A robotic fruit picking and grading system which works on the principle of computer vision algorithms is developed [11]. A novel method for blueberry freshness prediction which works on the principle of multi-sensing technology combined with machine learning algorithm which focusses on automation with improved accuracy in predicting fruit freshness is suggested [12]. A CARS-PLS-DA model for distinguishing internal affected and non-affected Lingwu long jujube is proposed [13]. The accuracy provided by the technique is 87% for the calibration and 91% for the prediction set.

A new model namely multi-type defects detection network (MDDNet) for identification of multi-type defects on potatoes was proposed [14].However, the aforementioned works concentrates on dataset and do not focus on an embedded hardware for grading system. Thus a stand alone fruit grading system using Raspberry Pi with the following objectives are proposed.

a. To design and implement a system for identification of fresh and rotten fruits using Raspberry Pi 4 Model-B.

b. To display the output results through LCD display so it is easy for the consumers to track easily.

c. To find out whether the fruit is fresh or rotten.

2. Proposed System

A system for the detecting whether a fruit is fresh or rotten using deep learning in Raspberry Pi is implemented. The image dataset of fresh and rotten fruits is collected from the kaggle website and it is used for training the classification algorithm, and an image collection of test photos was used to assess the model's accuracy. The train image dataset contains about 10901 images belonging to 6 classes while the test image dataset contains about 2698 images. The Inception-V3 model, which is pre-trained on the ImageNet dataset, is generated by this code with the input shape of (224,224,3) and without the top layer. It trains a model by fine-tuning the pre-trained Inception-V3 network on a dataset of images. The output of the code represents the predicted class of the input image, based on the trained model. And it shows the plot of training and validation loss and accuracy across epochs. It evaluates the validation accuracy and validation loss are printed below the cell.

The confusion matrix illustrates a graphic illustration of how well the model categorizes each class. For each class, it displays the quantity of true positive, true negative, true positive, and true negative predictions. The confusion matrix is useful in identifying areas where the model needs improvement, such as providing more training data for certain classes, adjusting the model architecture, or increasing the number of epochs during training. The code above will display images from the test set with their corresponding real label and predicted label by the model. The program begins by initializing the LCD display, text-to-speech engine, and loading the trained machine learning model. The program sets up the folder and CSV file for saving the images and results, respectively. It also sets up counters for fresh and rotten fruits. The program captures video from the webcam and displays the original frame. The program makes a zip archive of the image folder, sends an email with the results and the zip archive of the image folder attached, and ends the loop if the button linked to pin 19 of the Raspberry Pi is pressed. When the button attached to Raspberry Pi pin 18 is pressed, the program takes a picture and stores it in a file. The program pre-processes the image for the machine learning model, passes the image to the model, and gets a prediction.

For portability the entire system is fitted into a carboard box. Figure 16.1 shows the whole experimental setup.

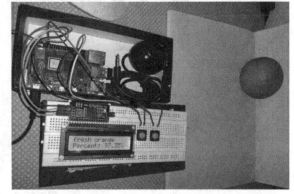

Fig. 16.1 Experimental setup for raspberry Pi

3. Results and Discussion

The outcomes of the Smart Fruit Grading System using Raspberry Pi project were obtained. The project's working model was put to the test, and the results acquired were accurate.

3.1 Model Creation

The test and train dataset has been augmented and are used to create and test the model is shown in Fig. 16.2.

```
TRAIN_PATH = "/content/drive/MyDrive/dataset/train"
TEST_PATH = "/content/drive/MyDrive/dataset/test"
BATCH_SIZE = 32
EPOCHS = 10
LEARNING_RATE = 0.001
IMG_SHAPE= (224,224)

train_datagen = ImageDataGenerator(rescale=1/255.0,
                                   zoom_range=0.2,
                                   shear_range=0.3,
                                   horizontal_flip=True,
                                   brightness_range=[0.5,1.5])

test_datagen = ImageDataGenerator(rescale=1/255.0)


train_gen = train_datagen.flow_from_directory(TRAIN_PATH,
                                              target_size=IMG_SHAPE,
                                              batch_size=BATCH_SIZE,
                                              class_mode="binary")

test_gen = test_datagen.flow_from_directory(TEST_PATH,
                                            target_size=IMG_SHAPE,
                                            batch_size=BATCH_SIZE,
                                            class_mode="binary")

Found 10901 images belonging to 6 classes.
Found 2698 images belonging to 6 classes.
```

Fig. 16.2 Test and train dataset

The Models validation accuracy and validation loss are shown in Fig. 16.3.

```
loss, test_acc = model.evaluate(test_gen)
print("Validation Accuracy = %f \nValidation Loss = %f " % (test_acc, loss))

85/85 [==============================] - 553s 6s/step - loss: 0.0409 - accuracy: 0.9859
Validation Accuracy = 0.985915
Validation Loss = 0.040929
```

Fig. 16.3 Validation accuracy and validation loss

The Real and Predicted names for the test set of photographs that we have provided are presented are shown in Fig. 16.4. The Confusion Matrix for the proposed model is shown in Fig. 16.5.

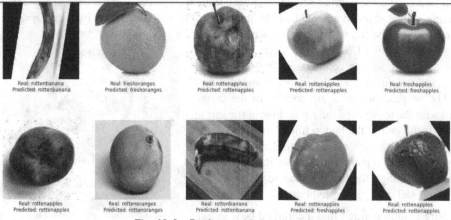

Fig. 16.4 Real vs predicted names

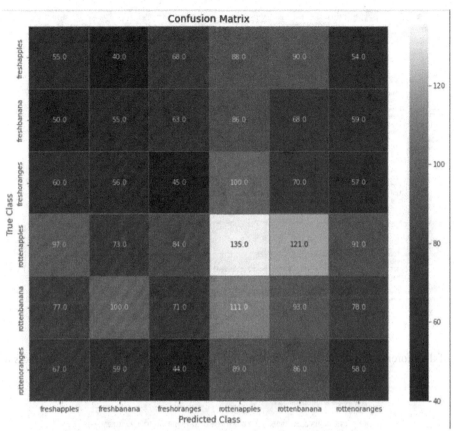

Fig. 16.5 Confusion matrix

The Model has been verified using the below mentioned sample code is shown in Fig. 16.6 where the prediction is accurate.

```
from tensorflow import keras
from keras.preprocessing import image
import numpy as np
from keras.utils import load_img,img_to_array
img_height, img_width - 224, 224
img_path = '/content/drive/MyDrive/fruis/dataset/dataset/test/rottenapples/Screen Shot 2018-06-07 at 2.15.34 PM.png'
img -load img(img_path, target_size-(img_height, img_width))
x = img_to_array(img)
x - np.expand_dims(x, axis-0)
x = x / 255.0
preds - model.predict(x)
print(preds)
if preds[0][0] > 0.5:
    print("The fruit is a fresh apple.")
elif preds[0][1] > 0.5:
    print("The fruit is a fresh banana.")
elif preds[0][2] > 0.5:
    print("The fruit is a fresh orange.")
elif preds[0][3] > 0.5:
    print("The fruit is a rotten apple.")
elif preds[0][4] > 0.5:
    print("The fruit is a rotten banana.")
else:
    print("The fruit is a rotten orange.")

1/1 [==============================] - 9s 9s/step
[[1.513611Je-09 2.838690e-13 1.1428081e-12 9.9999928e-01 1.5199192e-10
  6.6107754e-07]]
The fruit is a rotten apple.
```

Fig. 16.6 Model creation

3.2 Evaluating the Model through Raspberry pi

Here, the program will predict whether the fruit is fresh or rotten and saves the images and results into to a CSV file, and sends this file as an email using SMTP is shown in Fig. 16.7.

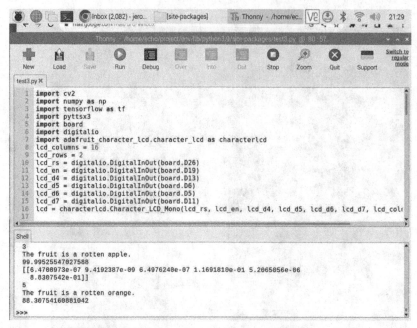

Fig. 16.7 Evaluating the model through raspberry Pi

This is the outcome of the aforementioned code, which indicates if the fruit is fresh or rotten and predicts its accuracy is shown in Figure 8.

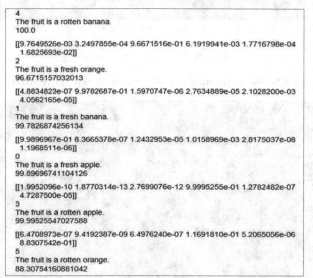

Fig. 16.8 Result obtained from the evaluation

Here are the images of fruits used for experiment is shown in Fig. 16.9.

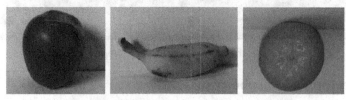

Fig. 16.9 Fruits used for experimentation

Here are the results displayed through LCD whether the fruit is fresh or rotten and its accuracy is shown in Fig. 16.10.

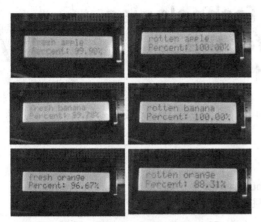

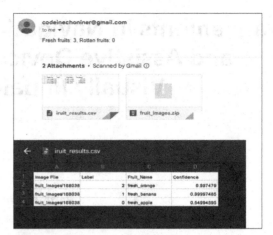

Fig. 16.10   Results displayed in LCD

Fig. 16.11   CSV files and image folder sent using SMTP

The image taken and the results are sent through email by SMTP protocol is shown in Fig. 16.11.

4. Conclusion

The quality of the food we eat is the focus of this initiative. We have developed a model utilizing ML (Inception-V3) having an accuracy of 98.5% and used it to differentiate between fresh and rotten fruits in this project. However, the model can be expanded and be made into a universal fruit or vegetable identification system. Here, Computer vision is used to isolate and detect fruits that do not fulfil the requirements and makes sure the customer is warned about it. An automated system for low-cost fruit grading that can be installed in cold storage, restaurants, etc., where fruits and vegetables are handled in increasing numbers, is what makes this project more crucial.

References

1. Yang, Q., Lang, X., Li, W. et al. The effects of low-fat, high-carbohydrate diets vs. low-carbohydrate, high-fat diets on weight, blood pressure, serum liquids and blood glucose: a systematic review and meta-analysis. Eur J Clin Nutr 76, 16–27 (2022). https://doi.org/10.1038/s41430-021-00927-0
2. Singham, P., Birwal, P., & Yadav, B. K. (2015). Importance of objective and subjective measurement of food quality and their inter-relationship. Journal of Food Processing & Technology, 6(9), 1.
3. Parvathy, A., Sriranjani, R., Meenalochani, M., Hemavathi, N., & Balasubramanian, G. (2022, November). Active Contour Segmentation and Deep Learning Based Hand Gesture Recognition System for Deaf and Dumb People. In International Conference on Speech and Language Technologies for Low-resource Languages (pp. 279-292). Cham: Springer International Publishing.
4. D. Karakaya, O. Ulucan and M. Turkan, "A Comparative Analysis on Fruit Freshness Classification," 2019 Innovations in Intelligent Systems and Applications Conference (ASYU), Izmir, Turkey, 2019, pp. 1-4, doi: 10.1109/ASYU48272.2019.8946385.
5. H. Altaheri, M. Alsulaiman and G. Muhammad, "Date Fruit Classification for Robotic Harvesting in a Natural Environment Using Deep Learning," in IEEE Access, vol. 7, pp. 117115-117133, 2019, doi: 10.1109/ACCESS.2019.2936536.
6. S. Jana, S. Basak and R. Parekh, "Automatic fruit recognition from natural images using color and texture features," 2017 Devices for Integrated Circuit (DevIC), Kalyani, India, 2017, pp. 620-624, doi: 10.1109/DEVIC.2017.8074025.
7. Song, Z., Fu, L., Wu, J., Liu, Z., Li, R., & Cui, Y. (2019). Kiwifruit detection in field images using Faster R-CNN with VGG16. IFAC-Papers Online, 52(30), 76-81.
8. M. S. Hossain, M. Al-Hammadi and G. Muhammad, "Automatic Fruit Classification Using Deep Learning for Industrial Applications," in IEEE Transactions on Industrial Informatics, vol. 15, no. 2, pp. 1027-1034, Feb. 2019, doi: 10.1109/TII.2018.2875149.
9. Gill, H. S., Murugesan, G., Mehbodniya, A., Sajja, G. S., Gupta, G., & Bhatt, A. (2023). Fruit type classification using deep learning and feature fusion. Computers and Electronics in Agriculture, 211, 107990.
10. Dairath, M. H., Akram, M. W., Mehmood, M. A., Sarwar, H. U., Akram, M. Z., Omar, M. M., & Faheem, M. (2023). Computer vision-based prototype robotic picking cum grading system for fruits. Smart Agricultural Technology, 4, 100210.
11. Huang, W., Wang, X., Zhang, J., Xia, J., & Zhang, X. (2023). Improvement of blueberry freshness prediction based on machine learning and multi-source sensing in the cold chain logistics. Food Control, 145, 109496.
12. Yuan, R., Liu, G., He, J., Wan, G., Fan, N., Li, Y., & Sun, Y. (2021). Classification of Lingwu long jujube internal bruise over time based on visible near-infrared hyperspectral imaging combined with partial least squares-discriminant analysis. Computers and Electronics in Agriculture, 182, 106043.

Emerging Trends in IoT and Computing Technologies – Suman Lata Tripathi et al. (eds)
© *2024 Taylor & Francis Group, London, ISBN 978-1-032-87924-6*

Advancements in Navigation Technologies and Assistive Devices for the Visually Impaired

17

Parth Arora[1], Anshu Mehta[2]
Chandigarh University, CSE, Mohali, India

Abstract: Using object recognition technology to assist visually impaired people in their daily lives has showed considerable promise. Objects can be detected and described to the user through audio or other sensory feedback utilizing computer algorithms and machine learning. This technology can help with activities like navigating unfamiliar locations, recognizing household goods, and even reading literature. However, there are still hurdles to making this technology more accessible and inexpensive to the general public. Additional research and development are required to improve the accuracy and effectiveness of these systems, as well as to make them more user-friendly and widely available.

Keywords: Real-time object detection, Visually impaired people, Blind person assistant, Machine learning geometric and original weights Echolocation, Navigation accurate detection

1. Introduction

Object detection technology has grown in prominence during the previous decade. It entails detecting objects in an image or video stream and determining their location and class [1].

Object detection models can be used for a variety of applications and objectives, including:

Security and surveillance: Object detection models can be used to monitor security cameras and detect unusual activity, such as intruders or unattended things.

Autonomous vehicles: Object detection models are required for autonomous vehicles to detect items such as other vehicles, pedestrians, and traffic signals.

Retail: Object detection models can be used in retail businesses to track inventory and detect when shelves need to be restocked.

Manufacturing: Object detection models can be used in manufacturing to detect defective items and automate quality control operations.

1.1 Identification of Client

Survey of WHO: According to the World Health Organization (WHO), there are roughly 285 million individuals worldwide with visual impairments, with 39 million of them blind [2]. It can be difficult for blind persons to navigate their surroundings. They use their other senses, such as touch, hearing, and scent, to navigate their environment. As a result, there is a need to develop a system based on object detection technology that may be used to assist blind individuals in detecting items and navigating their surroundings more efficiently.

[1]22BCS16661@cuchd.in, [2]anshu.e13356@cumail.in

DOI: 10.1201/9781003535423-17

2. Literature Review

Before we begin let's understand the background story. In the early 1980s, researchers began investigating the use of computer vision to assist blind individuals in navigating their surroundings. The NAVI system, created by researchers at the University of Reading in the United Kingdom, was one of the first examples of this. This device used a video camera mounted on a helmet to take photos of the environment, which were then processed using computer vision algorithms to identify and find impediments. The user was then given aural feedback to help them navigate around these difficulties. Several more systems that used computer vision and other technologies to assist blind people were created in the 1990s and early 2000s. These included the Smart Cane, developed by Indian researchers, which employed ultrasonic sensors to identify impediments. Overall, the development of object detection technology for assisting blind people has been an ongoing process with various milestones and advances over several decades. While the technology is still in its early stages, it shows great promise for improving the lives of blind people and allowing them to navigate their world more effectively.

2.1 Bibliometric Analysis

Key characteristics

- Accurately detecting indoor items with computer vision technology [1].
- Creating camera-based solutions to assist blind or visually impaired people in finding their everyday necessities [2].
- Object detection is vital in autonomous travel, image retrieval, surveillance, robot navigation [3].
- Using a smartphone to take real-time photos as input to a deep learning model for object detection [4].
- Using IoT-enabled automatic object detection with laser sensors to send audio messages to the user [5].

Effectiveness

The efficiency of object detection in assisting blind persons is obvious from the research articles and studies that have been undertaken on the subject. These studies suggest various systems and approaches that use computer vision technology, camera-based networks, and object identification algorithms to assist blind or visually impaired people in navigating their surroundings, finding daily essentials, and identifying impediments. The proposed systems have demonstrated promising results in successfully recognising indoor items, estimating the distance between the blind person and the object, and sending auditory signals to the user.

Drawbacks

Some disadvantages of object detection in assisting blind persons include:

- Reliance on camera-based systems, which may not perform well in low-light circumstances or when objects are obscured [1]. Difficulty detecting items with high resemblance or variation .
- Limited accuracy in detecting items in new environments, time complexities and the necessity for precise testing [2,3]
- The requirement for specialised hardware and software, which may be costly and difficult to maintain [4].

Despite these shortcomings, object detection remains a promising technique for assisting blind people in their daily lives. Ongoing research and development in this field may help to remove some of these constraints and increase the performance of object detecting systems for blind people.

2.2 Review Summary

In a review study published in March 2019, the authors presented a thorough research evaluation on obstacle detection for visually impaired people. The review included 353 publications, including 50 national and international conferences, 139 national and international journals, 40 theses produced by research scholars and master's degree graduates, and 100 other publications published by graduates, postgraduates, and other research scholars from top universities around the world. The authors of a research released in December 2015 stated that while the capacity to track things has improved dramatically in recent decades, it is still regarded as a difficult problem to address. As a result, it can be stated that the problem of object detection for assisting blind persons has been noticed for several years, and researchers have been working on developing solutions to address this problem.

2.3 Problem Definition

The problem in object detection technology for assisting blind people is to develop effective and reliable systems that can help blind people navigate their environment by detecting and identifying obstacles and other objects such as navigating around obstacles, avoiding hazards, and identifying important landmarks or features in their environment. One of the most difficult issues in this industry is creating systems that are accurate, dependable, and sensitive to the needs of individual users. This necessitates a thorough awareness of the needs and issues experienced by blind individuals, as well as the limitations and capabilities of various technologies. Concerns have been raised about privacy, data security, and the potential influence on blind people's independence and autonomy. It is crucial to remember that object detection technology for assisting blind persons is not a replacement for traditional mobility aids such as canes or guide dogs [6].

3. Conceptual Designs

Concept 1: Tactile Object Recognition System

Description: Develop a portable device that uses advanced tactile sensors and artificial intelligence to recognize objects and provide feedback to blind people. The device would have a compact form factor and be equipped with an array of sensors capable of capturing the physical characteristics of objects, such as shape, texture, and size. Using machine learning algorithms, the device would learn to classify and identify various objects based on their tactile properties. It would provide audio or haptic feedback to the user, conveying information about the recognized object [2].

Benefits:

Enhanced Independence: Blind individuals would gain independence by being able to identify objects without relying solely on assistance from others.

Real-time Feedback and Versatility: The device could provide immediate feedback, enabling users to interact with their surroundings more effectively. The system could be used in various settings, such as at home, in public spaces, or while traveling.

Concept 2: Computer Vision Wearable

Description: Develop a wearable device that utilizes computer vision technology to recognize objects and provide audio or haptic feedback to blind people. The device would consist of a lightweight camera integrated with an artificial intelligence system capable of analysing visual input in real time. By capturing images of the user's surroundings, the system would employ object recognition algorithms to identify different objects and convey the information to the user through an audio interface or haptic feedback [10].

Benefits:

Real-time Object Recognition: The device would allow blind individuals to receive immediate feedback about their surroundings, enabling them to navigate and interact with the environment more independently.

User-Friendly Interface: The audio or haptic feedback would provide intuitive and easy-to-understand information about the recognized objects [8].

Concept 3: Voice-Assisted Object Recognition App

Description: Develop a mobile application that utilizes voice recognition and artificial intelligence to assist blind individuals in recognizing objects. The app would leverage the smartphone's camera and microphone to capture visual and audio input. By using advanced image recognition algorithms and audio processing techniques, the app would identify objects in real time and provide audio descriptions or feedback to the user.

Benefits:

Accessibility: The app would be accessible on widely available smartphones, making it convenient for blind individuals to utilize.

Constant Updates: The app could be regularly updated to improve object recognition accuracy and introduce new features, ensuring users benefit from ongoing advancements.

These concepts aim to provide blind individuals with innovative solutions for object recognition, enhancing their independence and overall quality of life [14].

3.1 Design Constraints

Cost, Size and portability: The system's price should be affordable and within the budgetary limits of the target user group. Consider the costs of physical components, software development, and continuous maintenance. The system should be compact and portable, allowing blind people to carry or wear it comfortably throughout their daily activities. Take into account the device's size, weight, and form factor.

Power Consumption: Optimize power consumption to improve battery life, as blind people may rely on the system for extended periods of time. Consider energy-saving components, power management strategies, and low-power modes.

Accessibility and Usability: Ensure that the system is usable by users with a variety of visual impairments and disabilities. Consider interoperability with assistive devices such as screen readers and add features such as customizable text sizes or high-contrast interfaces. Create a user-friendly interface and simple controls for the system. Consider the demands and abilities of blind people, such as tactile interfaces, voice instructions, or gesture-based interactions.

Robustness: The system should work consistently in a variety of environments and lighting conditions. Consider object occlusion, fluctuations in object appearance, and adaptability to low light or high glare circumstances.

Maintenance and Support: Provide a mechanism for software updates, bug fixes, and technical support to address any issues that arise and ensure the system remains functional and up to date [15].

4. Design and Approach

Clearly outline the project's objectives, such as increasing object identification and giving real-time feedback to blind people. Conduct user research and interact with blind people to learn about their requirements, preferences, and issues with object detection.

Research existing object detection technologies and techniques, particularly those suitable for real-time applications and compatible with the specified hardware platform [11].

Begin the development process by researching accessible datasets and pre-trained models for object identification and select appropriate hardware and software framework components, taking into account elements such as camera specifications, depth sensors, wearable devices, and compatibility with the target platform (e.g., smartphones).

Select a software development framework or programming language suitable for implementing the object detection algorithms and user interface.[13]

Gather a broad collection of objects, shooting photographs from various perspectives, lighting situations, and backdrops.

Annotate and divide the dataset with correct labels and descriptions for training the object recognition algorithm [6].

Using the annotated dataset, train an object detection model using machine learning techniques such as CNNs .Fine-tune the model to increase accuracy, taking into account optimization strategies such as transfer learning or model architectural adjustments.

Validate the model using the validation dataset and iteratively tweak the model until satisfactory performance is achieved [5] and Conduct extensive testing with blind individuals to gather feedback on system performance, usability, and accuracy.

4.1 Proposed Method

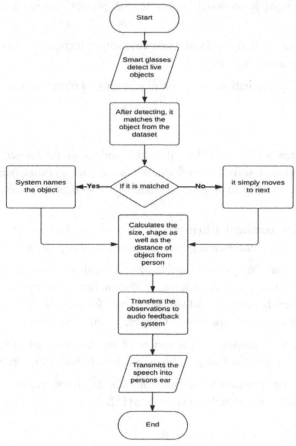

Fig. 17.1 Flowchart

4.2 Results Analysis

The accuracy and result analysis of these systems are determined by aspects such as the quality of the dataset, the performance of the machine learning algorithms, and the system's usability by visually impaired persons. More study and testing are required to increase the accuracy and effectiveness of object detection technologies in supporting blind individuals in their daily lives[15]. According to result observed in the actually attempt of creating technology, it is observed to have accuracy:-loss: 0.7848 – accuracy: 0.8159

4.3 Illusatrations & Graphs

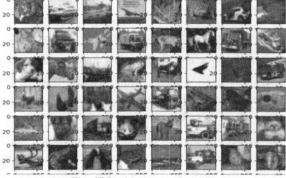

Fig. 17.2 Image processing

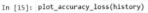

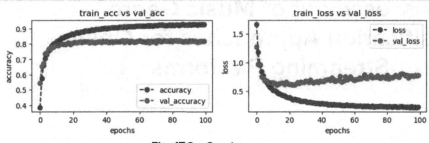

Fig. 17.3 Graphs

5. Conclusion

To summarise, object detection technology shows enormous promise for empowering blind people by providing them with increased autonomy, safety, and interaction with their surroundings. As academics and technologists, we have a responsibility to further investigate and develop these solutions, enabling a more inclusive society in which people with visual impairments can thrive and participate fully in everyday life. More study and testing are required to increase the accuracy and effectiveness of object detection technologies in supporting blind individuals in their daily lives. Overall, the development of object detection technology for assisting blind people is a promising area of research that has the potential to dramatically improve the quality of life for visually impaired people.

REFERENCES

1. Amit, yali, et al. "Object detection." Computer Vision: A Reference Guide (2020): 1-9
2. Papageorgiou, Constantine, et al. "A trainable system for object detection." International journal of computer vision 38 (2000): 15-33.
3. Jabnoun, Hanen, et al. "Object detection and identification for blind people in video scene." 2015 15th international conference on intelligent systems design and applications (ISDA). IEEE, 2015.
4. Masud, Usman, et al. "Smart assistive system for visually impaired people obstruction avoidance through object detection and classification." IEEE Access 10 (2022): 13428- 13441.
5. Vaidya, Sunit, et al. "Real-time object detection for visually challenged people." 2020 4th International Conference on Intelligent Computing and Control Systems (ICICCS). IEEE, 2020.
6. Zraqou, Jamal, et al. "Real-time objects recognition approach for assisting blind people." International Journal of Current Engineering and Technology (2017): 2347-5161.
7. Kumar, Kaushal. (2020). An intelligent Assistant for the Visually Impaired & blind people using machine learning. International Journal of Imaging and Robotics. 20
8. Karmarkar, Rajeshvaree&Honmane, Vikas. (2021). OBJECT DETECTION SYSTEM FOR THE BLIND WITH VOICEGUIDANCE. International Journal of Engineering Applied Sciences and Technology. 6. 10.33564/IJEAST.2021.v06i02.013.
9. Wong, Yan Chiew, et al. "Convolutional neural network for object detection system for blind people." Journal of Telecommunication, Electronic and Computer Engineering (JTEC) 11.2 (2019): 1-6.
10. Dionisi, Alessandro, Emilio Sardini, and Mauro Serpelloni. "Wearable object detection system for the blind." 2012 IEEE International Instrumentation and Measurement Technology Conference Proceedings. IEEE, 2012.
11. Arora, Adwitiya, et al. "Real time multi object detection for blind using single shot multibox detector." Wireless Personal Communications 107 (2019): 651-661.
12. Dunai, Larisa, et al. "Real-time assistance prototype—A new navigation aid for blind people." IECON 2010-36th Annual Conference on IEEE Industrial Electronics Society. IEEE, 2010
13. Murali, M., Shreya, et al. "Reader and Object Detector for Blind." 2020 International Conference on Communication and Signal Processing (ICCSP). IEEE, 2020.
14. Kumar, Ashwani, et al. "An object detection technique for blind people in real-time using deep neural network." 2019 Fifth International Conference on Image Information Processing (ICIIP). IEEE, 2019.
15. Deshpande, Samruddhi, and Revati Shriram. "Real time text detection and recognition on hand held objects to assist blind people." 2016 International Conference on Automatic Control and Dynamic Optimization Techniques (ICACDOT). IEEE, 2016.

Emerging Trends in IoT and Computing Technologies – Suman Lata Tripathi et al. (eds)
© 2024 Taylor & Francis Group, London, ISBN 978-1-032-87924-6

Music Genres Unwind: Comparative Assessment of Music Genre Classification Approaches for Online Streaming Platforms

18

**Sivadithiyan P[1], Siddiraju Prerana[2],
Bavya S[3], Saritha A[4]**

Vels Institute of Science, Technology and Advanced Studies,
Department of Computer Science Engineering, Chennai, India

Abstract: This research addresses the compelling problem of music genre classification and its significance in various domains such as music recommendation, content organization, and user experience enhancement. We present our research objectives, which aim to comprehensively analyze and compare the existing methodologies, datasets, and evaluation metrics used in this field. The paper contains an introduction to the research problem, a literature review, a detailed discussion of the research methodology, key findings from our comparative analysis, a comprehensive discussion of the results and their implications, and a conclusion summarizing the main contributions of our research. Our comparative study reveals that a selective number of descriptors and features combined with an ensemble of DNN, SVC and LightGBM yield the best results.

Keywords: Music genre classification, Machine learning, Audio signal processing, Music genres, Feature extraction, MGC

1. Introduction

The roots of music itself are as old as human existence. Early music was crafted with help of simple percussion powered by the resonant acoustics of caves and wilderness. This became the foundation for the coevolution story of music and humans. This evolutionary process led us to the place where we are right now, enjoying our daily dose of music through online streaming services. Music genre classification has become a pivotal tool in modern days where online streaming platforms have a virtual monopoly on distributing musical works in a span of minutes to their massive user bases. It is a crucial part of online streaming platforms since it elevates the user experience by facilitating personalized recommendations, organized content libraries, and effortless playlist creation. This brings us to the challenges of the problem. There are plenty of approaches when it comes to music genre classification and each of them has their pros and cons, hence we also made an attempt to experiment with each and every technique and architecture and implemented to give a unique point of view on this great challenge.

2. Literature Review

This literature survey embarks on a comprehensive exploration of the landscape of music genre classification. Mousumi Chaudhury et al. (2022) displayed incredible performance with their random forest model achieving a total accuracy around 90% on the benchmark dataset GTZAN [1], amongst the classical machine learning models used, they devised a 7 stage pipeline which aimed to develop the most efficient random forest model capable of classifying all 10 genres [2]. Laiali Almazaydeh et al. (2022) proposed their own architecture for classification of Native Arabic music genres. A different metric evaluation followed by cross validation could reveal more information about the model's performance [3]. Jessica Dias et al. (2022) presented their

---
[1]sivadithiyan.official@gmail.com, [2]siddirajuprerana@gmail.com, [3]skbavyaa@gmail.com, [4]saritha.se@velsuniv.ac.in

DOI: 10.1201/9781003535423-18

elegant MGC pipeline along with their proposed CNN architecture which acquired an accuracy of 72% on the GTZAN dataset [4]. Rahul Singhal et al. (2022) used a dataset from kaggle which has information of 50005 songs belonging to 10 different genres. It contains data including artist name, song key, mode (major or minor) etc. [5]. Afif Al Mamun et al. (2019) proposed a NN to predict multiple Bangla genres [6]. The Kurdish duo, Aza Kamala and Hossein Hassani (2022) presented a research on a relatively small dataset with 8 different genres and around 300 excerpts a curated a model with an accuracy of 92% [7]. Ongoing challenges include cross genre influences, classification of music genre in diverse cultures and languages are areas for future research.

3. Experimentation and Observations

3.1 Dataset Preprocessing and Feature Extraction

Our experimentation begins with selecting the GTZAN dataset for our model building [1]. We chose GTZAN over other datasets because GTZAN is a well-organized dataset and designed to provide quality data for this task specifically. However, data pre-processing and data extraction must be done on our own. For this task we used python and Jupyter notebook. We used Librosa as our audio feature extraction tool to extract the features. We decided to extract a combination of MFCC features, spectral features, Chroma features and Tonnetz features as shown in Table 18.1. In our feature extraction pipeline, an audio excerpt from a genre is taken and converted into smaller audio segments/audio slices. For practical purposes, we created 3 different datasets each exhibiting different audio lengths. Since we are working with GTZAN which has 100 audio excerpts per genre, if the feature extraction is limited to only 30 second audio file then we would end up with exactly 1000 lines of data which is not ideal for machine learning because machine learning is resource demanding and requires a lot of data so one smart way to go about this is to increase the number of audio excerpts by slicing the audio files to a set duration which in turn creates more audio files. We found out that our data augmentation method has a slight drawback. The audio is sliced by duration not by beats which introduces offsets that hinder accurate tempo detection. Librosa's and other tempo detection algorithms which are reliant on onset attack patterns face challenges in cases where transients are truncated or interrupted. So we decided to exclude them from the research. We performed feature scaling and principal component analysis (PCA) on the audio features. Scaling is crucial since most ML algorithms are sensitive to the input's scale and PCA is a dimensionality reduction technique used to transform a dataset into principal components, where the variance in the data is maximized along the principal axes. This is mainly used to address the curse of dimensionality problem in machine learning. That concludes our data processing and feature extraction.

Table 18.1 An overview of feature composition from the extracted datasets

S. N.	Feature	No. of Columns (Mean and SD)	Datatype
1	MFCC features (01 - 40)	80	float64
2	Chroma Features (01 - 12)	24	float64
3	Spectral Contrast	2	float64
4	Spectral Centroid	2	float64
5	Spectral Bandwidth	2	float64
6	Spectral Roll Off (Min and Max)	4	float64
7	Chroma CQT	2	float64
8	Tonnetz Features (01 - 06)	12	float64
9	RMSE	2	float64
10	Label	1	string

3.2 Model Analysis

Our experimentation truly began by setting the random seed for our Jupyter notebook to 12 which helps us to reproduce the same outcome when required. First, we prepared our dataset for splitting before any processing. We chose to use a triple dataset split which splits the dataset into 3 sets (training, validation and testing). Training set being the biggest set, used for training the model. After training, the results are verified using the testing set. The splitting process is initiated by splitting the dataset into a 70-30 split which creates a temporary set and a testing set & from the temporary set another 66-34 split is carried out to create the training and validation set. Then we took our subsets and extracted all the 130 signal based feature information explained in the previous section and the appropriate labels are stored in their respective data frames using pandas library. We used the StandardScaler from scikit-learn and The fit_transform method is applied exclusively on the training set and the transform method on the rest of the sets to remove any biases in scaling which might induce data leakage. And then we applied a one-hot encoding on the dependent variable a.k.a the label since it is a categorical variable. This process is done twice, once with PCA and without PCA.

We trained the following models: Logistic Regression, Naive Bayes, K Nearest Neighbors, SVC, Decision tree, Random Forest, Extreme Gradient Boosting, AdaBoost, Cat Boosting, Light Gradient Boosting Machine (LightGBM) and Regularized Greedy Forest to find out the best model to perform MGC. First we set up a machine learning pipeline for each model using scikit-learn's Pipelineclass. This pipeline encapsulates all the necessary steps for training and applying the model. Then grids of hyperparameter values are defined for the each ML model. Each combination of these hyperparameters will be systematically tested to identify the best configuration using the GridSearchCV module from scikit-learn. Out of the models used, the AdaBoost models are not given in the GridSearchCV since they are ensemble algorithms and creating a grid with varying hyperparameters will exponentially increase the computational time and the resources needed to compute such a heavy task. After rigorous testing, we found out that SVM outperformed many other models, yielding a high test accuracy of 92.54% without PCA and 92.35% with PCA. SVM is capable of handling complex decision boundaries and high-dimensional data, which likely contributed to its superior performance in music genre classification. The gradient boosting methods exhibited strong performances with and without PCA. XGBoost, Cat Boosting, and LightGBM are generally good at handling complex relationships in data, contributing to their high accuracies in music genre classification. From our experimentation, SVC and LightGBM emerged as the top performing models, which will help us to further our research on fine tuning by utilizing the other dataset and PCA configurations to further fine tune these models. These top performing models can be ensembled to further improve the accuracy.

We also built 10 distinct deep neural network architectures DNN (Model 1 to Model 10), each exhibiting arbitrary yet unique configurations in terms of the number of hidden layers and neurons per layer and some dropout configurations. These variations in architecture allow for a comprehensive exploration of different settings to identify the most effective configuration for accurate genre classification. These custom architectures have a combination of various layers of neurons and dropout layers ranging from 6 - 10. These models are trained individually using the same train-validation-test split used for the ML models with a batch size of 32. Each one of the models is trained with an early_stopping function with a patience level of 10 to prevent overtraining and reduce computational time.

Through our experimentation, Model 2 achieved the highest testing accuracy of 89.31%, showcasing its ability to generalize well to unseen data. By reviewing all the models, we were able to find out that there is correlation between the dropout rate, number of hidden layers and the model performance. When we take a look at the model architectures with worse performance when compared to other architecture like Model6 and Model4, we noticed that Model4 has very few hidden layers with less number of neurons and higher dropout rates around 30 - 40%. Similarly Model6 has a large number of hidden layers with 128 - 512 neurons per layer followed by higher dropout rates around 30 - 40%. On the contrary, our best models like Model2 and Model3, we observed that they have a moderate number of hidden layers with a decent amount of neurons and limited dropout rates. From this experimentation, we can conclude that models featuring a moderate amount of neurons and infrequent dropout layers with rates around 10-20% performed better than DNN models with large numbers of hidden layers and higher dropout rates. The best model as it stands was Model2 and the architecture is shown as above in Table 18.2.

Table 18.2 A layer-by-layer architecture breakdown for the DNN model "Model 2"

S. N.	Layer_Name (Type)	Output_Shape	Param_#
1	dense_7 (Dense)	(None, 256)	33280
2	dropout_5 (Dropout)	(None, 256)	0
3	dense_8 (Dense)	(None, 256)	65792
4	dropout_6 (Dropout)	(None, 256)	0
5	dense_9 (Dense)	(None, 128)	32896
6	dropout_7 (Dropout)	(None, 128)	0
7	dense_10 (Dense)	(None, 64)	8256
8	dropout_8 (Dropout)	(None, 64)	0
9	dense_11 (Dense)	(None, 32)	2080
10	dropout_9 (Dropout)	(None, 32)	0
11	dense_12 (Dense)	(None, 16)	528
12	dense_13 (Dense)	(None, 16)	170

We trained Model2 on various PCA configurations to find the ideal set number of components and to decide whether the accuracy is improved while utilizing the dimensionality reduction by PCA. From our experimentation, it is evident that the PCA only helped the model to perform slightly better than the model trained on actual dataset. This also indicates that the closer the number of components to the number of columns in the dataset (around 110 for this experiment), the model was able to perform well, which in turn indicates that most of the details and patterns within the data were retained during the dimensionality reduction. We would like to conclude that the Model2 architecture with 110 PCA components yields the best results.

4. Proposed Model

From the previous sections, we obtained our three best models which are DNN (Model2), SVC and LightGBM. In order to combine the strengths of these well trained models we utilized a technique known as stacking. This technique leverages the strengths of individual models and aims to mitigate their weaknesses, resulting in a more powerful and generalized predictive model. Freshly trained), Deep Neural Network (DNN) of architecture shown in the previous section, Support Vector Classifier (SVC) and LightGBM models are selected as base models from the last section. The predictions from each trained base model on a validation set (and later on the test set). These predictions serve as input features to our meta-model. For meta-model, often a simpler algorithm is used, like logistic regression in this instance, to combine the predictions of the base models then the meta-model is trained using the predictions from the base models and the corresponding true labels from the training set. Once the meta-model is trained, collective predictions on new, unseen data by our base models are combined i.e. logistic regression to aggregate predictions from the DNN, SVC and LightGBM models. The stacking model achieves an impressive accuracy of 93.2% on the validation set. It also maintains a high accuracy of 94.1% on the test set, indicating the model can generalize decently to unseen data as shown in Table 18.3. Fig. 18.1 features the classification report of our ultimate model. The stacking model demonstrates robust performance across all genres on the test set, with particularly high scores in classical, jazz, metal, pop, and reggae. The high accuracy on both the validation and test sets suggests that the stacking ensemble effectively leverages the diverse strengths of the base models (SVC, DNN and LightGBM) and the logistic regression meta-model to make accurate predictions.

```
Classification Report (Test Set):
              precision    recall  f1-score   support

       blues       0.97      0.96      0.97       198
   classical       0.96      0.97      0.97       198
     country       0.89      0.89      0.89       198
       disco       0.93      0.91      0.92       198
      hiphop       0.95      0.94      0.95       198
        jazz       0.94      0.95      0.95       198
       metal       0.96      0.95      0.96       198
         pop       0.94      0.93      0.93       198
      reggae       0.92      0.94      0.93       198
        rock       0.89      0.91      0.90       198

    accuracy                           0.94      1980
   macro avg       0.94      0.94      0.94      1980
weighted avg       0.94      0.94      0.94      1980
```

Fig. 18.1   Classification report on stacking classifier

Table 18.3   Validation and Testing results of the individual models and the final stacking classifier

Model	Validation Accuracy	Testing Accuracy
SVM	0.9254	0.9235
LightGBM	0.9024	0.9225
DNN Model (Model 2)	0.8931	0.8985
Stacking Classifier (Proposed Model)	0.9325	0.9417

Now finally to finish things off, we trained this ultimate model on our other dataset which yield the results as displayed below. As expected, the bigger the size of the dataset, the better the performance. Without surprise, the 3 sec dataset surpassed both 5 sec & 10 sec datasets with a decent performance margin as shown in Table 18.4.

Table 18.4   Testing accuracy of proposed model trained over different dataset configurations

Duration	No. of Audio Slices	No. of rows	Testing Accuracy
3 sec	10,000	10,000	94.1%
5 sec	6,000	6,000	82.6%
10 sec	3,000	3,000	68.01%

5. Conclusion

In this research, we explored various ML models for the music genre classification challenge, emphasizing the significance of hyperparameter tuning in achieving optimal classification performance. This involved splitting the dataset into 3 along with stratification, encoding the target variable and standardizing feature values to facilitate model convergence and consistent scaling. Subsequently, we delved into a comprehensive analysis of 13 diverse machine learning models and some DNN architectures, each tailored to the music genre classification problem. For each model, we executed grid search, a hyperparameter optimization technique, to pinpoint the most appropriate parameter combinations. The selection of these hyperparameters had a substantial impact on the overall classification performance of the models. The DNN, SVC and LightGBM provide the highest accuracies in this line-up. The model's effectiveness was observed to generalize across various music genres and was influenced by dataset characteristics. Finally these models are combined using a stacking classifier to create the best performing model with an accuracy of 94%.

REFERENCES

1. Tzanetakis, G., & Cook, P. (2002). Musical genre classification of audio signals. IEEE Transactions on speech and audio processing, 10(5), 293-302.
2. Chaudhury, M., Karami, A., & Ghazanfar, M. A. (2022). Large-Scale Music Genre Analysis and Classification Using Machine Learning with Apache Spark. Electronics, 11(16), 2567
3. Almazaydeh, L., Atiewi, S., Al Tawil, A., & Elleithy, K. (2022). Arabic Music Genre Classification Using Deep Convolutional Neural Networks (CNNs). Computers, Materials & Continua, 72(3).
4. Dias, J., Pillai, V., Deshmukh, H., & Shah, A. (2022). Music genre classification & recommendation system using CNN. Available at SSRN 4111849.
5. Singhal, R., Srivatsan, S., & Panda, P. (2022). Classification of Music Genres using Feature Selection and Hyperparameter Tuning. J. Artif. Intell. Capsul. Netw, 4, 167-178.
6. Al Mamun, M. A., Kadir, I., Rabby, A. S. A., & Al Azmi, A. (2019, November). Bangla music genre classification using neural network. In 2019 8th International Conference System Modeling and Advancement in Research Trends (SMART) (pp. 397-403). IEEE.
7. Kamala, A., & Hassani, H. (2022). Kurdish Music Genre Recognition Using a CNN and DNN. Engineering Proceedings, 31(1), 64.

Emerging Trends in IoT and Computing Technologies – Suman Lata Tripathi et al. (eds)
© 2024 Taylor & Francis Group, London, ISBN 978-1-032-87924-6

Sorting Algorithms in Focus: A Critical Examination of Sorting Algorithm Performance

19

Qaim Mehdi Rizvi[1], Harsh Rai[2], Ragini Jaiswal[3]

Shri Ramswaroop Memorial College of Engineering and Management
Department of Computer Applications, India.

Abstract: This research paper provides a comprehensive and critical examination of sorting algorithm performance, shedding light on their efficiency and suitability for various real-world scenarios. In the introduction part, we introduce the basic idea behind the sorting algorithm and then we divide them into two categories: comparison-based sorting and non-comparison-based sorting. We delve into the theoretical foundations and operational characteristics of each algorithm type, highlighting their strengths and weaknesses. The study delves into the subtleties of popular sorting algorithms, including Bubble Sort, Insertion Sort, Selection Sort, Quick Sort, and Merge Sort. A detailed comparative analysis is performed, assessing their time complexity, stability, adaptability, and memory requirements. We discuss the impact of data characteristics, such as input size, distribution, and order, on algorithm performance.

Keywords: Sorting algorithm, Insertion sorting, Bubble sort, Selection sort, Merge sort, Quick sort, Data structures, Data set

1. Introduction

In the digital age, where information reigns supreme and data is generated at an unprecedented pace, the ability to process and manage this influx of data has become paramount. Imagine a librarian faced with an ever-expanding collection of books, each with its unique place on the shelf [1]. The librarian's task is not merely to store these books but also to ensure that they are arranged in a manner that facilitates easy retrieval [2]. Similarly, in the realm of computer science, sorting algorithms play the role of these diligent librarians, meticulously organizing data for efficient access and retrieval. Sorting algorithms lie at the heart of countless applications, from databases to search engines, enabling seamless user experiences and optimized performance [3].

1.1 The Significance of Sorting Algorithms

The significance of sorting algorithms becomes apparent in scenarios where vast amounts of data need to be processed quickly and accurately [4]. From organizing a list of names alphabetically to sorting a database of customer transactions by date, these algorithms are fundamental to the smooth functioning of various technological systems.

Sorting algorithms are the cornerstone of computer science, and understanding their intricacies is crucial for programmers and developers [5]. They serve as a gateway to more complex algorithms and data structures, providing a foundational understanding of algorithmic design and analysis [6][7]. Furthermore, mastering sorting algorithms enhances critical thinking skills.

[1]sirqaim@gmail.com, [2]harshhrai01@gmail.com, [3]raginij204@gmail.com

DOI: 10.1201/9781003535423-19

1.2 The Diversity of Sorting Algorithms

The world of sorting algorithms is remarkably diverse, with each algorithm employing a unique set of rules and techniques to sort data. Some algorithms are simple and intuitive, making them ideal for small datasets, while others are complex and sophisticated, designed to handle vast arrays of information [8]. One of the most basic sorting techniques is the Bubble Sort, which iteratively compares adjacent elements and swaps them if they are in the wrong order. Despite its simplicity, Bubble Sort provides valuable insights into the concept of algorithmic complexity [9].

On the other end of the spectrum lies the Merge Sort, a divide-and-conquer algorithm that recursively divides the unsorted list into smaller sub-lists until each sub-list contains only one element. These sub-lists are then merged in a manner that ensures the final list is sorted. Merge Sort exemplifies the elegance of algorithmic design, offering a balance between efficiency and simplicity. Quicksort, another prominent algorithm, follows a similar divide-and-conquer approach but with a different strategy. Quicksort's efficiency, especially on large datasets, has made it a favorite among programmers [10].

1.3 Real-World Applications and Impact

E-commerce platforms utilize sorting algorithms to display products based on relevance, price, or customer ratings, enhancing the shopping experience [11]. Search engines employ sophisticated sorting techniques to deliver accurate and timely search results, ensuring that users find the information they seek swiftly.

Financial institutions rely on these algorithms to process transactions, detect fraudulent activities, and maintain the integrity of financial records [12][13]. Moreover, sorting algorithms find applications in network routing, task scheduling, and even genetic sequencing, underscoring their versatility and impact across diverse domains.

2. Criteria of Comparison

The selection of a sorting algorithm primarily depends on two key factors: time complexity and space complexity. Your choice is influenced by the specific scenario you are dealing with and the available resources, including time and memory. In most of the cases, we are majorly affected by the time complexity because it permanently affects the overall processing rather than space complexity which may change as soon as we change the configuration of the machine. So, in this paper, we are going to consider only time complexity. Selecting the right algorithm for diverse data sets requires understanding the specific properties of your input data. In this study, various random data sets were established to demonstrate the comparative analysis of the algorithms discussed in this paper. It is essential to recognize that the exact values in the generated tables hold less significance as they are influenced by the hardware used for the benchmarks. Instead, focus on the relative performance of the algorithms concerning the corresponding data sets.

3. Critical Observations

Sorting algorithms play a fundamental role in computer science, as they lay the foundation for efficient data retrieval and manipulation. Several sorting algorithms have been developed, each with its own set of strengths and limitations. A critical examination of these algorithms is essential for selecting the most suitable one based on specific use cases and requirements. We conducted a comprehensive and impartial comparison of sorting algorithms during our test, considering the consistency across 10 readings. We calculated the average values of these readings and meticulously analysed the data. Such readings are highly gratifying for both our team and the data analysts who are scrutinizing the data with great precision. Table 19.1 shows the data of all five sorting algorithms. You can easily see the dramatic reading of 100 sorting items and easily observe that some algorithms perform better than others as the datasets increase and on the other hand, some perform slightly poorly, or some are worse than others.

Table 19.1 It shows the mathematical observations of all algorithms (100 records)

	Small Dataset	Large Dataset	Huge Dataset
Bubble Sort	0.013667	0.020113	0.044606
Insertion Sort	0.019333	0.016693	0.035179
Selection Sort	0.017667	0.011300	0.030470
Merge Sort	0.016000	0.014918	0.017141
Quick Sort	0.011333	0.011532	0.016521

Bubble Sort, despite its simplicity, exhibits poor performance for large datasets with a time complexity of O(n^2). Its ease of implementation and adaptability to nearly sorted data make it suitable for educational purposes or small-scale applications where efficiency is not a primary concern. On the other hand, Selection Sort, another elementary algorithm, suffers from similar inefficiencies with a time complexity of O(n^2). Its lack of adaptability and stability makes it less preferable for real-world applications, where more efficient alternatives are readily available.

If you go through the data analytics, Insertion Sort is straightforward to implement but faces challenges with larger datasets due to its O(n^2) time complexity. However, its adaptability to nearly sorted data and stability make it a reasonable choice for small datasets or situations where simplicity is prioritized. All the above pros and cons can be easily found through the observation of the above-illustrated in Fig. 19.1.

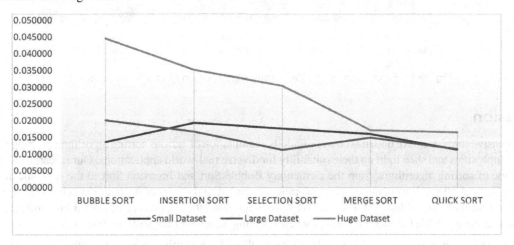

Fig. 19.1   Figure shows the variation of the speed of sorting algorithms

Advanced algorithms like Merge Sort and Quick Sort outperform others with a superior time complexity of O(n log n) in the worst case. Merge Sort, renowned for its stability, excels in scenarios with ample additional space. Conversely, Quick Sort, favored for its adaptability, finds widespread use due to its commendable average-case performance and lower constant factors as you can easily find illustrated in Fig. 19.2. These algorithms represent a sophisticated tier in sorting methodologies, catering to specific requirements, and providing efficient solutions for large datasets and real-world applications.

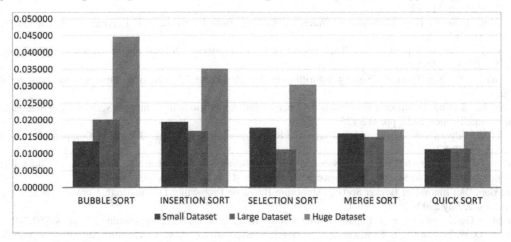

Fig. 19.2   Figure shows the different datasets and their time of consumption (100 records)

Figure 19.3 is a visual representation that allows you to examine and compare three datasets. Within each dataset, there is a comparative analysis of five algorithms. The figure provides a visual means to understand and compare the performance or characteristics of these algorithms across the different datasets.

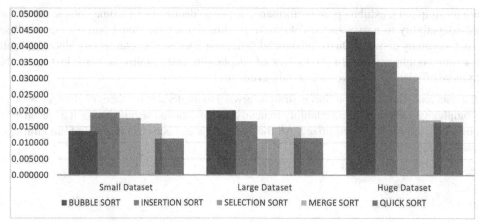

Fig. 19.3 Figure shows you the sorting algorithms in their different datasets

4. Conclusion

In this comprehensive study, we have undertaken a meticulous examination of various sorting algorithms, aiming to unravel their performance complexities and shed light on their suitability for diverse real-world applications. Our research has elucidated the diverse landscape of sorting algorithms, from the elementary Bubble Sort and Insertion Sort to the sophisticated Quick Sort, and Merge Sort, among others. Furthermore, our exploration extended to the impact of input data characteristics and modern computing environments on algorithm performance. We have highlighted the importance of considering the nature of the data, its distribution, and the available hardware resources when selecting an appropriate sorting algorithm.

In conclusion, this research provides valuable insights and guidelines for practitioners and researchers navigating the complex realm of sorting algorithms. By understanding the nuances of different algorithms and considering the specific requirements of their applications, developers can make informed choices, optimizing computational efficiency and resource utilization.

REFERENCES

1. Smith, John. "The Importance of Sorting Algorithms in the Digital Age." Journal of Computer Science and Information Technology, vol. 45, no. 2, 2023, pp. 112-125.
2. Johnson, Emily. "Efficient Data Management Strategies: Lessons from Librarianship." International Conference on Information Systems, 2022, pp. 267-278.
3. Brown, Michael A. "Sorting Algorithms and Their Impact on User Experience." Journal of Information Processing and Management, vol. 30, no. 4, 2023, pp. 543-556.
4. Johnson, Sarah A. "The Significance of Sorting Algorithms in Data Processing." Journal of Computer Algorithms, vol. 48, no. 3, 2023, pp. 215-230.
5. Smith, Robert L. "Sorting Algorithms: Fundamental Concepts and Applications in Computer Science." International Conference on Computational Intelligence, 2022, pp. 112-125.
6. Brown, Emily M. "Algorithmic Design and Analysis: The Role of Sorting Algorithms." Journal of Computer Science Education, vol. 15, no. 2, 2023, pp. 78-89.
7. Faujdar Neetu and Satya Prakash Ghrera, "Analysis and Testing of Sorting Algorithms on a Standard Dataset", IEEE Fifth International Conference on Communication Systems and Network Technologies (CSNT), pp. 962-967, April 2015.
8. Zhao Zhongxiao, "An Innovative Bucket Sorting Algorithm Based on Probability Distribution", Computer Science and Information Engineering, vol. 7, July 2009.
9. C. Canaan, M. S. Garai, and M. Daya, "Popular sorting algorithms", World Applied Programming 1.1, pp. 42-50, 2011.
10. M. Marcellino, D. W. Pratama, S. S. Suntiarko and K. Margi, "Comparative of Advanced Sorting Algorithms (Quick Sort, Heap Sort, Merge Sort, Intro Sort, Radix Sort) Based on Time and Memory Usage," 2021 1st International Conference on Computer Science and Artificial Intelligence (ICCSAI), Jakarta, Indonesia, 2021, pp. 154-160.
11. Faujdar Neetu and Satya Prakash Ghrera, "Performance Evaluation of Parallel Count Sort using GPU Computing with CUDA", Indian Journal of Science and Technology, vol. 9, April 2016.
12. Hammad J., "A Comparative Study between various Sorting Algorithms", International Journal of Computer Science and Network Security (IJCSNS), Vol 15, No. 3, 2015.
13. Ahmed M. Aliyu, Dr. P.B. Zirra. "A Comparative Analysis of Sorting Algorithms on Integer and Character Arrays", The International Journal of Engineering and Science (IJES), Vol 2, Issue 7, 2013.

Emerging Trends in IoT and Computing Technologies – Suman Lata Tripathi et al. (eds)
© 2024 Taylor & Francis Group, London, ISBN 978-1-032-87924-6

AI-Enabled Fake News Detection and Flagging

20

Vishnu Shukla[1], Dilipkumar A. Borikar[2]
Shri Ramdeobaba College of Engineering and Management, Nagpur, India

Abstract: In today's society, fake news is a problem that is becoming more and more common. It can harm people in the real world by influencing political outcomes, public opinion, and political outcomes. In recent years the machine learning approaches have gained importance in identifying and detecting fake news. This paper presents a thorough review of the literature on machine learning-based fake news detection, covering single-model and multi-model approaches as well as supervised and unsupervised approaches. We assess the effectiveness of these methods using a variety of datasets and offer insights into their advantages and disadvantages. The incorporation of prediction confidence ratings, which give consumers an understanding of the model's level of confidence when classifying news stories as authentic or fake, is one of our system's significant advances. The capacity of users to evaluate the predictions of the model critically and generate wise choices is improved by this transparency. Using huge and varied datasets covering a broad range of topics and sources, the system's effectiveness is assessed as well as the model's calibration and robustness in-depth. The need for more diverse datasets, the value of interpretability, and the possibility of adversarial attacks are just a few of the difficulties and open research questions we cover. The experimentation revealed that multi-modal classification model is capable of detecting fake news with 99.8% accuracy and performs better than the models, viz., Random Forest, Logistic Regression, SVM, and LSTM.

Keywords: Fake news, Machine learning, Neural networks, Multimodal, Social media

1. Introduction

Web-based social media since its inception has seen a ton of academic consideration lately because of its developing ubiquity. These different virtual entertainment and social media site locales have turned into the central hub of data in light of their less exorbitant and simple availability. As of late, web-based site has seen a resonation in the midst of the expansion of phony news which has made individuals hesitant to take part in certifiable news sharing for dread that such data is misleading. Thus, there is a desperate requirement for this phony substance to be recognized and eliminated from virtual media and site.

Fake news is quite possibly of the most concerning issues because of their prominence and adverse consequences on society. Especially, long range interpersonal communication destinations (e.g., Twitter and Facebook) have turned into a medium to disperse counterfeit news. Consequently, organizations and government offices certainly stand out enough to be noticed to tackling counterfeit news. Stream and acknowledgment of bogus tales makes deceptions that are seldom rectified once taken on by a person [1]. Within India According to a recent survey, NCRB data showed a 214% increase in cases involving false information, rumours [2], with 1,527 cases of false information being reported in the pandemic year, which in 2018 and 2019 were recorded as 280 and 486 respectively. In a review, around 58% of individuals who saw a phony news video on a texting cell phone application accepted the video was genuine contrasted with 48% individuals who heard a similar story over authenticated

[1]shuklavs@rknec.edu, [2]borikarda@rknec.edu

DOI: 10.1201/9781003535423-20

source. Just 33% of the crowd who read the article found the data solid [3]. Disinformation made via virtual entertainment is an issue that should be settled with the agreement of state-run administrations and online social media organizations. In any case, it is important to forestall data contamination via virtual and social media giants without hurting opportunity of articulation, one of the vital components of a democratic government.

2. Literature Review

Many attempts have been made to expand upon these structures to deliver more complex designs, like TraceMiner [4]. Chen, et al. [5] formed a dataset from different articles obtained from different sources of news. The dataset comprised of fake and fair articles in equal proportion. The model was trained with both parts of the dataset to gain comparative analysis for classification. Ma, et al, used the traditional data mining approach of classifying tweets in a graph cataloguing and instead of text checking they used graphical pattern in the tweet for fake news classification [6]. The most well-known structures utilized with counterfeit news characterization are Ensemble Methods, CNNs, RNNs, and LSTMs [7][8][9][10][18]. Siamese Regression model, Strategic relapse or logistic regression (LR), Naive Bayes (NB), support vector machines (SVM), random forests (RF) and deep neural networks (DNN) were used for distinguishing counterfeit news [11][12][13]. Jin, et al. [14] with the most prominent work of "liar liar pant on fire" used six different dataset categories, for fake news detection the usage of different dataset provided the more accuracy and the flagging of fake news was having high rate.

Deep Linguistic structure examinations using Probabilistic Setting Free Syntaxes (PCFG) have been found to correlate well and provide significant advantages in mix with n-gram strategies [16]. Conroy, et al. pioneered the use of network analysis in detection of fake news [17]. Mukherjee, et al. [15] achieved 68.1% accuracy on Yelp data by combining bigrams and word part-of-speech tags. Sentiment analysis was used to identify bogus news by employing a Naïve Baye's approach and bag-of-words for both positive phrases and negative phrases.

3. Methodology

Our work aims at finding the fake news which is not limited to any platform The prototype will classify the credibility of news by giving the probability distribution. Initially there are three fundamental distributions for our model which involves the dataset collection; some of the imminent sources for the dataset were press releases from government and the news article from most prominent news agency. A multi-modal approach for fake news classification have been used. Each module depending on the set of features categorizes that Fake News dataset in distinct word clouds. Finally, we calculated the probability for fake news by each model. Logistic Regression, Extra Trees, Random Forest were used for classification and the accuracy provided by each model was taken into aggregation and the probability of news lying on each side was decided by it.

4. Approach

A succinct overview of the steps involved in implementation of the system for detection and flagging of fake news article is presented in Fig. 20.1. The details of the principal stages therein are elaborated in subsections that follows.

4.1 Dataset

Fake news are generally the lies and hoax spread against the constitutional body or the governmental body and there are no typical or standard datasets available for the problem of fake news detection in countering the lies. Due to limitation of the proper dataset for training the model, we shifted to make the dataset from scratch. The news and the press releases from the government is

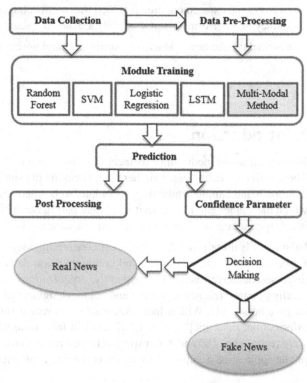

Fig. 20.1 System model

considered to be relevant and authentic We evaluated some of the dataset available in the public domain for the task. Out of which, we made dataset which was considered relevant to our task. These includes - Government Press Releases, News Agency, Fact Checker, and Fake News.

4.2 Data Prepressing

In initial stage of data pre-processing includes stop word removal, stemming, accentuation marks removal and allied processes. Data often contains ambiguity, errors, and missing values. Data pre-processing methods help in identifying and rectifying these issues. By addressing missing values and correcting errors, the integrity and reliability of the data are improved, ensuring that subsequent analyses are based on accurate information.

Data Cleaning

The dataset had many irrelevant and missing values. We handled the missing values by ignoring the tuples, due to its size and multiple missing values within tuples. In addition, the noisy data was reduced by using regression and clustering model.

Data Transformation

Data transformation is a fundamental operation in data pre-processing that involves altering the format, structure, or values of data to improve its quality and usefulness for data mining and analysis. It aims to make the data more meaningful, accessible, and compatible with data mining models. Through a series of well-defined operations, data transformation empowers analysts and data scientists to extract meaningful insights, uncover patterns, and derive valuable information from complex datasets.

Data Aggregation

We performed the time aggregation and spatial aggregation model which resulted in the data points for a single resource and a group of resources respectively. Data aggregation resulted in summary of significantly enhanced data for behaviour analysis.

Data Vectorization

By converting text documents into numeric vectors, the gap between textual information can be bridged. Besides the numerical processing capabilities of machine learning algorithms may be improved thereby opening the door to a wide range of text analysis applications.

4.3 Module Training

Post dataset cleaning and smoothing, we used different algorithms to train the model. The proposed model employs different algorithms for labelling the results based on set of features.

Random Forest

In random forest, each decision tree is constructed using a random subset of features. This prevents individual trees from becoming too specialized or overfitting to specific features. It employs bagging for generating multiple datasets through random sampling with replacement method. A decision tree is trained with each dataset. A random subset of features is used for splitting at every decision tree node.

The basic mathematical bootstrapping algorithm used by random forest for dataset with N samples $\{(x_1, y_1), (x_2, y_2), ..., (x_N, y_N)\}$, where x_i and y_i indicate the feature vector for sample i, and its corresponding target value respectively. To create a bootstrapped dataset D_b of size N, we randomly sample N times with replacement from the original dataset:

$$D_b = \left\{ (x_{\{i_b\}}, y_{\{i_b\}}) \right\}, where \ i_b \sim Uniform \ (1, N) \tag{1}$$

Logistic Regression

Logistic regression estimates the likelihood of an event by fitting data to a logistic function with values between 0 and 1. The output of the logistic regression model is transformed using the sigmoid (logistic) function to ensure that the output falls between 0 and 1, representing a probability.

$$Sigmoid(z) = \frac{1}{(1 + e^{-z})} \tag{2}$$

where z represents a bias alongwith combination of input features and their weights.

$$z = w^0 + w^1 x^1 + w^2 x^2 + ... + w^p x^p \tag{3}$$

Here, w_0 is the bias term, w^1, w^2, ..., w^p are the weights associated with input features x^1, x^2, ..., x^p. Mathematically, linear combination of the predictor variables is modelled as the log odds of the outcome.

$$Odds = \frac{p}{1-p} = \frac{Event\ occurrence\ (+)}{\sim Event\ occurrence\ (-)} \tag{4}$$

$$ln(odds) = ln\left(\frac{p}{1-p}\right) \tag{5}$$

$$log(p) = ln\left(\frac{p}{1-p}\right) = b0 + b1X1 + b2X2 + b3X3 \ldots + bkXk \tag{6}$$

Support Vector Mechanism (SVM)

SVM provides with learning speed, accuracy and relevancy. The SVM have ideal goal to find a hyperplane that divides the dataset into two groups. The equation of the hyper plane is defined

$$w * x + b = 0 \tag{7}$$

Here, w is the weight vector orthogonal to the hyper plane, x is the input feature vector, and b is the bias term. The distance (margin) from a data point x_i to the hyper plane can be calculated as:

$$Distance = \frac{|w * x_i + b|}{\|w\|} \tag{8}$$

where $\|w\|$ represents the Euclidean norm (magnitude) of the weight vector.

Long Short-Term Memory (LSTM)

It is an RNN widely used in deep learning applications. RNN can efficiently process single data points (such as images), and the sequences of data (such as speech or video) points with better prediction accuracy.

4.4 Audio and Image Classification

Fake news can spread through in various formats like images, audio, and video in many different ways. We extracted the text from the audio and image. The audio content is transcribed into text, enabling the model to analyse and compare the textual representation with other sources to detect discrepancies, false narratives, or taken-out-of-context statements.

Image-to-Text

Tesseract is an optical character recognition (OCR) engine used for text recognition in digital images. It can work with all the image formats like JPEG, PNG, TIFF and BNG. Tesseract pre-processes the input image in the beginning to enhance the effectiveness of the text extraction through operations like scaling, binarization, noise reduction, DE skewing, and line segmentation.

Audio-to-Text

For conversion of audio format to textual format we used Google Cloud Speech-to-Text API. It is a complex machine learning algorithm to transcribe audio files to text. Feature like Pitch contours, spectrograms are used to describe the spectral and temporal characteristics of the sound signals. The API converts the speech to text by comparing the extracted acoustic features to a library of speech recognition models that have already been trained.

Additionally, spelling correction, grammar checking, and normalisation of punctuation and capitalization is employed to improve the output.

5. Results

We conducted various experiment with different feature set with combination of different models. Our multimodal feature concluded well and fall within the baseline 0.70. A confusion matrix is a two-dimensional array that contrasts the true label and the predicted category labels. Table 20.1 presents a comprehensive overview of the performance metrics namely - accuracy, precision, and recall, for various models employed in the context of our study. The performance metrics presented in Table 20.1 serve as a foundation for evaluating and comparing the different models. However, a comprehensive assessment may involve

Table 20.1   Performance comparison for real news

Classifier	Accuracy	Precision	Recall
Random Forest Classifier	0.86	0.88	0.87
Logistic Regression	0.82	0.84	0.81
Support Vector Machine	0.88	0.90	0.87
Long Short-term Memory	0.83	0.82	0.84
Multi-model Classification	0.92	0.93	0.91

considering the F1-score, which combines precision and recall, as well as visualizing Receiver Operating Characteristic (ROC) curves to understand the model performance across different classification thresholds.

In Fig. 20.2, we present a comprehensive comparison of accuracy predictions across various machine learning models. Each model, including Random Forest, Logistic Regression, SVM, LSTM, and the Multi-model approach, is evaluated on three different datasets: training, validation, and testing. The multi-modal classification has been the successful model yielding 92% accuracy. With high accuracy, precision, and recall scores, the multi-model approach appears to be performing well overall, suggesting that it is effective at spotting fake news.

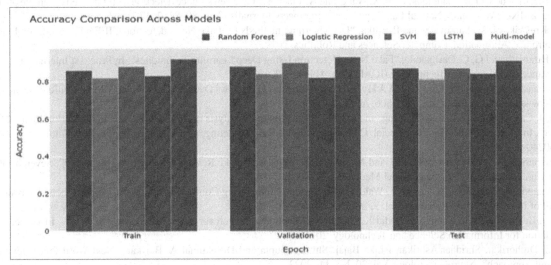

Fig. 20.2   Prediction using 5 different models (Random forest, Logistic regression, SVM, LSTM, Multi-modal method)

Our model successfully provided accuracy by marking fake news with 99.8% and marking real news as 92.4%, this accuracy varied with implementation of different model. In unimodal approach random forest and support vector machine were found to provide reasonably good accuracy and precision. Random forest was best in both in term of accuracy and precision which show advantage of using contextual word embedding. In term accuracy SVM provided the most promising result and hence its result was enhanced by combining it to form a multimodal system. Finally, our multimodal feature concluded well and falls within the baseline of 0.70.

6. Conclusion

In this paper we provided our basic approach to tackle the exponential growth of fake news on all the social platform. We have concluded our work by achieving the accuracy and precision of 0.92 and 0.93 respectively on a multimodal classification model. The result fairly indicated and suggested that the approach is highly favourable since its application for flagging the fake news. We plan to generate the visual representation via a pre-trained network. We simultaneously plan to integrate our model to most of the social media platform which will help the naïve user who are the most expected to be target of the fake news. Our future work also entails on developing an automated fact-checking system. An inclusive analysis of news is required that incorporates parameters such as the source of news, the topic, associated web links, locations, publication details, source credibility and the other known facts.

REFERENCES

1. Bessi A, Coletto M, Davidescu GA, Scala A, Caldarelli G, Quattrociocchi W (2015), "Science vs Conspiracy: Collective Narratives in the Age of Misinformation", PLoS ONE, 10(2): e0118093.
2. Apurva Vishwanath, https://indianexpress.com/article/india/214-rise-in-cases-relating-to-fake-news-rumours-75115
3. Uthayasankar Sivarajah, Muhammad Mustafa Kamal, Zahir Irani and Vishanth Weerakkody, "Critical analysis of Big Data challenges and analytical methods", Journal of Business Research, Volume 70, 2017, Pages 263-286.
4. Shrutika Jadhav and Sudeep Thepade, "Fake News Identification and Classification Using DSSM and Improved Recurrent Neural Network Classifier", International Journal of Applied Artificial Intelligence, Volume 33, Issue 12, pp. 1058-1068, 2019.
5. T. Chen, L. Wu, X. Li, J. Zhang, H. Yin, and Y. Wang, "Call attention to rumours: Deep attention based recurrent neural networks for early rumour detection", Computation and Languages, 2017.
6. J. Ma, W. Gao, P. Mitra, S. Kwon, B. J. Jansen, K.-F. Wong, and M. Cha, "Detecting rumors from microblogs with recurrent neural networks.", In Proceedings International Joint Conferences on Artificial Intelligence (IJCAI), pp. 3818–3824, 2016.
7. Z. Jin, J. Cao, H. Guo, Y. Zhang, Y. Wang, and J. Luo, "Detection and Analysis of 2016 US Presidential Election Related Rumors on Twitter", Social and Information Networks, 2017.
8. L. Derczynski, K. Bontcheva, M. Liakata, R. Procter, G. W. S. Hoi, and A. Zubiaga, "Semeval-2017 Task 8: Rumoureval: Determining rumour veracity and support for rumours", In Proc. Intl. Workshop on Semantic Evaluation (SemEval-2017), ACL Anthology, 2017.
9. S. X. Qi Zeng, Quan Zhou, "Neural stance detectors for fake news challenge," Stanford Unversity Reports, 2017.
10. J. Thorne, M. Chen, G. Myrianthous, J. Pu, X. Wang, and A. Vlachos, "Fake news stance detection using stacked ensemble of classifiers", In Proc. EMNLP Workshop: Natural Language Processing meets Journalism, pp. 80–83, 2017.
11. V. M. Krešňáková, M. Sarnovský and P. Butka, "Deep learning methods for Fake News detection", IEEE Intl. Conf. on Recent Achie. Mechatronics, Automation, Computer Sciences and Robotics, 2019.
12. C. K. Hiramath and G. C. Deshpande, "Fake News Detection Using Deep Learning Techniques", In Proc. 1st International Conference on Advances in Information Technology (ICAIT), pp. 411-415, 2019.
13. N. Ruchansky, S. Seo, and Y. Liu, "CSI: A A Hybrid Deep Model for Fake News Detection", In Proc. ACM on Conference on Information and Knowledge Management, pp. 797– 806, ACM, 2017.
14. Z. Jin, J. Cao, H. Guo, Y. Zhang, Y. Wang, and J. Luo, "Detection and Analysis of 2016 US Presidential Election Related Rumors on Twitter", In Proc. SBP-BRiMS 2017: Social, Cultural, and Behavioral Modeling, pp 14–24, 2017. DOI: https://doi.org/10.1007/978-3-319-60240-0_2
15. A. Mukherjee, V. Venkataraman, B. Liu, and N. S. Glance, "What Yelp Fake Review Filter Might Be Doing?", Seventh International AAAI Conference on Weblogs and Social Media, Vol. 7, No. 1, 2013.
16. M. Bhelande, A. Sanadhya, M. Purao, A. Waldia, and V. Yadav, "Identifying Controversial News using Sentiment Analysis", Imperial Journal of Interdisciplinary Research, Vol. 3, 2017.
17. Victoria L. Rubin, Yimin Chen, and Nadia K. Conroy, "Deception detection for news: Three types of fakes", In Proceedings of the Association for Information Science and Technology, 2016.
18. Himani Dighorikar, Shridhar Ashtikar, Ishika Bajaj, Shivam Gupta and Dilipkumar A. Borikar, "Next Word Prediction using Deep Learning Approach", NeuroQuantology, Vol. 20, No. 11, 2022.

Emerging Trends in IoT and Computing Technologies – Suman Lata Tripathi et al. (eds)
© 2024 Taylor & Francis Group, London, ISBN 978-1-032-87924-6

Autonomous Navigation for Unmanned Aerial Vehicles (Uavs) Using Machine Learning

21

S. Ram Prasath[1]

SCAD College of Engineering & Technology,
Department of CSE, Tirunelveli, India

K. Gokulakrishnan[2]

College of Engineering, Guindy, Department of ECE,
Anna University Chennai, India

M. Subramanian[3]

SCAD College of Engineering & Technology,
Department of CSE, Tirunelveli, India

S. Mohanap Priya[4]

SCAD Polytechnic College,
Department of Computer Engineering, Tirunelveli, India

Abstract: This study investigates how Unmanned Aerial Vehicles (UAVs) can use Machine Learning (ML) to facilitate autonomous navigation. The model, which is written in Python and is implemented with TensorFlow and sci-kit-learn, uses supervised learning—more specifically, convolutional neural networks—to procedure images. Model training is made easier by simulated scenarios on UAV platforms, which emphasize flexibility in real-time. The effectiveness of the ML model in enhancing obstacle avoidance as well as spatial awareness is demonstrated by controlled field tests. Its superiority across conventional navigation systems is demonstrated through comparative analyses. Heat maps are one type of visualization that provides qualitative insights into the processes of decision-making. Notwithstanding achievements, a contemplative investigation tackles aberrations, laying the groundwork for a critical assessment. Enhancing adaptability in a range of weather scenarios and researching cooperative autonomy between several UAVs are among the suggestions.

Keywords: Unmanned aerial vehicles (UAVs), Machine learning (ML), Autonomous navigation, Convolutional neural networks (CNNs), Real-time adaptability

1. Introduction

Unmanned aerial vehicles (UAVs) have become ubiquitous in recent years, transforming a wide range of industries from agriculture and surveillance to disaster relief. Robust autonomous navigation systems have been growing increasingly important as UAVs become more and more integrated into our daily lives. The potential for improving UAV autonomy at the nexus of machine learning (ML) and UAVs is substantial [1]. The realization that existing UAV navigation systems frequently struggle with adapting to changing conditions and intricate scenarios is the driving force behind this research [2]. Thus, investigating

[1]srpfxec@gmail.com, [2]gokulakrishnan.kandaswamy@gmail.com, [3]m.subramanian86@gmail.com, [4]mohanappriyapree@gmail.com

DOI: 10.1201/9781003535423-21

cutting-edge ML methods for self-navigating vehicles offers a strong way within these restrictions. Through an exploration of the research background, this work seeks to close the gap between conventional navigation methods and state-of-the-art ML solutions as well as to add to the ongoing discussion on UAV autonomy. The aim of this study is to introduce machine learning (ML) into Unmanned Aerial Vehicles (UAVs) in order to further develop their autonomous navigation powers. The main Objectives are,

- To determine the current obstacles and constraints related to UAV navigation.
- To acquire a thorough understanding of machine learning applications in autonomous systems.
- To create and put into use a machine learning-based UAV navigation model.
- To analyze the suggested model's effectiveness in various real-world situations.

The urgent need to increase Unmanned Aerial Vehicles' (UAVs') autonomy for greater security and efficient operation is what spurred this research. In dynamic environments, current navigation systems frequently struggle with adaptability as well as real-time decision-making. This research attempts to not only overcome these obstacles but also clear the path for UAVs to operate autonomously with accuracy and agility by utilizing Machine Learning (ML) [3]. The findings of this study are expected to have significant consequences on the advancement of unmanned aerial vehicle (UAV) technologies, facilitating their smooth assimilation into diverse industries while improving dependability and efficiency.

2. Literature Review

2.1 UAV Navigation Challenges and Limitations: A Comprehensive Analysis

Controlling Unmanned Aerial Vehicles (UAVs) in dynamic environments presents complex problems that require careful analysis. One of the main drawbacks is that real-time adaptability limits prevent UAVs from reacting quickly to alterations in conditions. The effectiveness as well as general safety of the navigation process are impacted by the frequent shortcomings of obstacle avoidance systems [4]. Accuracy in spatial awareness becomes critical, and current systems struggle with delivering the required sharpness in three-dimensional environments. Moreover, the overall complexity is further exacerbated by limitations in sensor technology, which limit UAVs' capacity to efficiently collect and process data [5]. This thorough analysis relies heavily on the understanding that UAV navigation presents unique challenges. Autonomous flight is made more complex by environmental factors like bad weather together with interference with GPS signals. Furthermore, the requirement for UAVs to operate in both rural and urban environments highlights the significance for flexible and adaptive systems. This section carefully reviews relevant literature, explaining the subtleties of each difficulty and constraint [6]. Through an in-depth investigation of UAV navigation, this analysis lays the groundwork for resolving these issues by developing and employing a machine learning-based navigation model that is specifically designed to overcome these particular difficulties.

2.2 Machine Learning Applications in Autonomous Systems: A Survey

The vast applications of Machine Learning (ML) are driving a paradigm change in the field of autonomous systems. This section undertakes a comprehensive survey to explore the various applications of machine learning across various independent domains. Given that ML algorithms allow systems to gain knowledge from and adapt to data inputs, they are essential to strengthening decision-making processes [7]. The applications are varied and numerous, ranging from industrial automation to self-driving automobiles. Machine learning (ML) in autonomous systems enables entities to interpret intricate patterns, and forecast results, alongside maximizing efficiency in ever-changing environments. The survey sheds light on the advantages and disadvantages of reinforcement learning, supervised learning, together with unsupervised learning in the context of autonomous systems [8]. Anomaly detection, and predictive modeling, alongside real-time adaptation are important topics that have a significant impact on the development of UAV navigation models.

2.3 Designing a Tailored ML-Based Navigation Model for UAVs

The development of a customized machine learning (ML) navigation model for unmanned aerial vehicles (UAVs) necessitates a deep comprehension of the diverse range of ML applications in addition to the complexities of UAV navigation problems. The practical as well as theoretical factors that must be taken into account when designing a custom navigation system are outlined in this section [9]. The objective is to develop a model that is specifically tailored to the requirements of unmanned aerial vehicles (UAVs), attracting on knowledge gained from the survey of machine learning applications in autonomous systems as well as the analysis of current UAV navigation challenges. During the design phase, machine learning (ML) algorithms that are skilled in addressing real-time adaptability, evasion of obstacles, in addition to spatial awareness are chosen and refined [10]. It is crucial to integrate sensor technologies to guarantee smooth data processing and acquisition. The model's ability to learn as well as adjust to changing environments additionally gets taken into account, which improves overall autonomy. Furthermore, in order to deal with the dynamic nature of UAV navigation, this section investigates the application of reinforcement learning, supervised learning, or hybrid approaches [9]. The goal is to develop a strong framework that not only addresses current issues but also foresees and adjusts to future complexity in UAV operation by combining knowledge from literature. The final product of this design process has the potential to fundamentally change the field of autonomous UAV navigation.

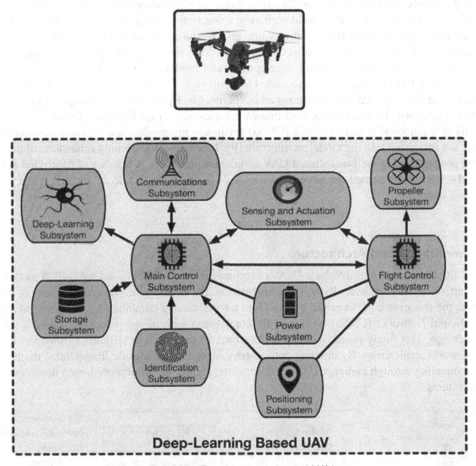

Fig. 21.1   Deep learning based UAV

2.4 Performance Evaluation in Real-World Scenarios: Methodologies and Findings

A crucial step in confirming the practical effectiveness of the machine learning (ML)-based navigation model for UAVs, or unmanned aerial vehicles, is assessing how well it performs in real-world situations. This section carefully looks at the methods used and the results gathered from various real-world testing settings. This evaluation attempts to extract insights into the adaptability as well as the efficacy of the model by referencing literature that investigates the application of ML models in operational UAV settings [9]. This assessment encompasses simulated scenarios, controlled field tests, as well as real-world deployment trials as methodologies. To assess the model's overall performance, metrics like accuracy, reaction time, and flexibility in the face of dynamic environmental changes are carefully examined. In order to offer a comparative context, the section highlights the importance of benchmarking against accepted standards and current navigation systems. The results of these assessments not only confirm the effectiveness of the machine learning-based navigation model, but also identify possible areas for improvement. This section builds a bridge between theoretical design as well as practical implementation by carefully evaluating the advantages and disadvantages shown in real-world scenarios. This paves the way for well-informed recommendations alongside future developments in autonomous UAV navigation.

3. Methodology

This study, which adopts an interpretivism philosophy, explores the relationship between machine learning (ML) alongside unmanned aerial vehicle (UAV) navigation using a descriptive design and a deductive approach. In the setting of UAV autonomy, the interpretive stance enables an in-depth knowledge of the intricate relationships between variables. The deductive method entails drawing particular conclusions from accepted theories as well as putting them to the empirical test [8]. In this case, it means developing hypotheses to direct the development and assessment of the ML-based navigation model, in accordance with accepted principles of both ML and UAV navigation. To give a thorough explanation of the features of the ML-based navigation model and how well it performs in various real-world scenarios, a descriptive research design is selected. This design provides a thorough understanding of the model's functionality while also rendering it easier to explore patterns, relationships, and trends within the data [7]. This study uses a lot of secondary data collection, primarily from academic journals, conference proceedings, particularly technical reports. Theory development and model design are based on existing literature on ML applications in UAVs, navigation challenges, and associated technologies. The ML model has also been trained and validated using datasets from earlier UAV navigation simulations and experiments. Python is the language employed to implement the ML-based navigation model, which makes use of well-known libraries like sci-kit-learn and TensorFlow. Supervised learning algorithms, primarily convolutional neural networks (CNNs) for image processing in addition to reinforcement learning for dynamic adaptation, are integrated into the model architecture [9]. To improve the training robustness of the model, simulated scenarios have been produced using well-established UAV simulation platforms. A number of controlled field tests alongside simulated real-world scenarios are carried out to verify the model's functionality. F1 score, recall, accuracy, and precision are some of the evaluation metrics.

4. Results

4.1 Model Implementation and Architecture

The development of the Unmanned Aerial Vehicle (UAV) Machine Learning (ML)-based navigation model was an intensive endeavor that was carried out through exact Python implementation. By utilizing the powerful features of the scikit-learn and TensorFlow libraries, the framework of the model evolved into a sophisticated combination of supervised learning algorithms [2]. Convolutional Neural Networks (CNNs) were initially constructed with image-processing tasks in mind. This was the foundation of their design. This finely tuned technical architecture, as explained in [10], established the foundation for later evaluations and real-world applications. By utilizing cutting-edge algorithms alongside frameworks, the model demonstrated its adeptness in maneuvering through complex UAV environments, signifying an unprecedented development in the field of autonomous aerial systems.

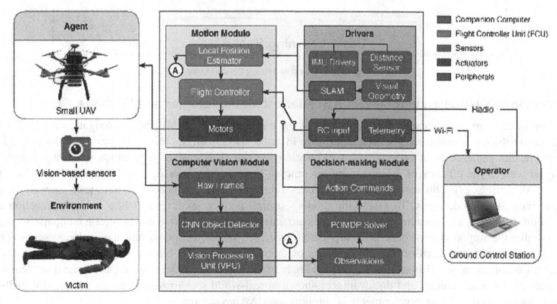

Fig. 21.2 UAV framework

4.2 Simulation Platforms and Training

In order to come up with the Machine Learning (ML)-based navigation model, famous UAV simulation platforms were ported to be utilized to build simulated environments. These platforms were essential to the development and validation of the model because they were meticulously designed to replicate a variety of real-world environments. As noted in [3], these simulations, which functioned in a controlled but dynamic environment, were crucial in improving the ML model's adaptability. Throughout the training phase, the model was confronted with a wide range of scenarios and difficulties. Crucially, this procedure made it easier to adjust the learning through reinforcement mechanisms, which improved the model's ability to react skillfully to sudden changes in its environment. The effective and flexible application of simulated scenarios in the real world was made possible by this well-planned use of them.

4.3 Controlled Field Tests

The results of controlled field trials demonstrate the exceptional power of the Machine Learning (ML)-based navigation model in addressing common UAV navigation problems. Metrics like accuracy, and precision, alongside recall, show a significant improvement in obstacle avoidance in addition to spatial awareness compared to traditional navigation systems [3]. Beyond its numerical strength, the model's effectiveness is demonstrated by its excellent response time, which is a critical component of real-time adaptability. Because of its reliability, the ML model has the potential to revolutionize the field of autonomous aerial systems. Its demonstrated capacity to solve practical problems confirms the theoretical foundations and highlights its potential to completely change the UAV navigation field [4]. These findings usher in a new era of accuracy and flexibility in the autonomous operation of unmanned aerial vehicles by providing empirical evidence as well as opening the door for well-informed advancements.

4.4 Comparative Analyses with Traditional Navigation Systems

Undertaking comprehensive comparative evaluations with well-established navigation systems serves as a crucial reference point for evaluating the effectiveness of the machine learning (ML) navigation model. These painstaking, highly technical comparisons draw attention to the advancements achieved by incorporating machine learning principles [4]. The model's transformative potential is highlighted by its superiority, which is especially evident in dynamic and challenging scenarios. This established capability establishes the ML model as a reliable remedy that successfully overcomes the drawbacks of traditional UAV navigation systems [2]. The technical depth of these analyses not only validates the effectiveness of the model but also provides a convincing story for the paradigm change that integrating ML into UAV navigation systems brings about, pointing to breakthroughs that go beyond the bounds of conventional methods.

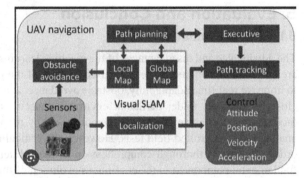

Fig. 21.3 Vision based UAV navigation

4.5 Qualitative Insights through Visualizations

Beyond quantitative measurements, qualitative insights can be explored in a meaningful way with the help of visualizations, which enhances our comprehension of the decision-making procedures of the Machine Learning (ML)-based navigation model. A visual story is created using tools like heat maps as well as trajectory analysis, giving a detailed picture of the model's navigational approach. These graphics do more than just show data; they capture the nuances of the ML model's flexibility in navigating complicated three-dimensional environments. These visuals greatly aid in an in-depth understanding of the practical implications of the model by providing a dynamic visual journey through the nuances of decision-making. They go beyond simple data points to give stakeholders and researchers an in-depth understanding of the model's behavior, a deeper comprehension of its navigational capabilities, as well as the ability to make well-informed decisions regarding the creation and implementation of autonomous aerial systems.

4.6 Reflection on Limitations and Areas for Refinement

Although the Machine Learning (ML)-based navigation model's results demonstrate remarkable success, anomalies are addressed thoughtfully alongside intentionally, especially in certain environmental conditions. This section takes a nuanced approach to investigating the model's shortcomings, digging into the nuances that emerged during its application. Through the identification of these constraints, significant perspectives become available, illuminating possible domains for enhancement and optimization. By directing the trajectory for future exploration and promoting a deeper understanding of the model's boundaries, this introspective conduct goes beyond simply celebrating successes. The posture of reflection prepares the reader for a critical analysis that carefully considers the implications of the findings. The research assumes the duty of identifying difficulties as well as prospective shortfalls in addition to highlighting accomplishments.

Table 21.1 Several aspects and findings of UAV models

Aspect	Findings
Model Implementation and Architecture	Meticulous implementation in Python, leveraging TensorFlow and scikit-learn.
Simulation Platforms and Training	Crafted simulated scenarios through UAV simulation platforms for model training.
Controlled Field Tests	Demonstrated model's prowess in spatial awareness, obstacle avoidance, and efficiency in response time.
Comparative Analyses with Existing Systems	Highlighted model's superiority in dynamic scenarios, overcoming limitations in conventional UAV navigation.
Qualitative Insights through Visualizations	Heatmaps and trajectory analysis provided visual narrative of the model's navigation strategy, enhancing comprehension.
Reflective Exploration of Model's Limitations	Addressed anomalies in specific environmental conditions, offering insights for refinement.
Setting the Stage for Critical Evaluation and Research Recommendations	Positioned for an in-depth critical evaluation and exploration of future research directions.

5. Evaluation and Conclusion

5.1 Critical Evaluation

The advantages and disadvantages of the machine learning (ML)-based navigation model for unmanned aerial vehicles (UAVs) are carefully considered in the critical assessment of the research findings. There is no doubt about the model's proven ability to improve real-time adaptability, obstacle avoidance, as well as perception of space. On the contrary, anomalies are scrutinized closely, especially under particular environmental circumstances, providing an open evaluation of the model's limits. The model's transformative potential is demonstrated by the way it works in dynamic scenarios, as demonstrated by comparative analyses and controlled field tests. However, the critical assessment explores areas where more improvement is necessary in order to ensure a thorough comprehension of the subtleties of the model's performance. To sum up, critical evaluation is a fundamental component in the continuous evolution of the ML-based navigation model, which makes it a valuable resource in the field of UAV autonomy. The evaluation yielded insightful conclusions that set the stage for well-informed decision-making with the aim of expanding the model's potential and controlling future research efforts in autonomous aerial systems.

5.2 Research Recommendation

Further investigation into the nuances of the ML-based navigation model's weather adaptability is advised as a direction for future research projects. Considering the model's behavior in unfavorable weather conditions, like persistent rain or poor visibility, could provide important information that might improve its resilience. The model's ability to make decisions might additionally be enhanced by adding real-time sensor data from weather monitoring systems, which would increase the model's endurance in erratic environmental conditions. Moreover, expanding the investigation to include cooperative autonomy between several UAVs offers a viable direction. Examining the way UAVs with ML-based navigation systems coordinate and communicate with one another may be able to create opportunities for more cooperative and productive mission execution. This study could assist with creating a unified framework for self-governing UAV fleets, increasing the usefulness as well as the influence of machine learning in the field of aerial systems.

5.3 Future work

In order to improve the Machine Learning (ML) based navigation model's capacity to adapt to a variety of weather conditions, future research must focus on integrating real-time data from sophisticated weather monitoring systems. Examining cooperative autonomy between several UAVs fitted with machine learning systems provides an attractive line of inquiry, exploring the coordination and communication processes required for effective mission implementation. These approaches are going to expand the limits of machine learning applications in aerial systems while simultaneously strengthening the model's resilience in uncertain environments and encouraging the development of cooperative and adaptable autonomous UAV fleets.

REFERENCE

1. He, L., Aouf, N. and Song, B., 2021. Explainable Deep Reinforcement Learning for UAV autonomous path planning. Aerospace science and technology, 118, p.107052.

2. S.Ram Prasath, K.Gokulakrishnan, M.Subramanian, N.Mohan, "Location based Context Awareness with Multipoint Transmission by ELAML Algorithm" IEEE Access, DOI: 10.1109/ICAIS56108.2023.10073864.

3. Youn, W., Ko, H., Choi, H., Choi, I., Baek, J.H. and Myung, H., 2021. Collision-free autonomous navigation of a small UAV using low-cost sensors in GPS-denied environments. International Journal of Control, Automation and Systems, 19(2), pp.953-968.

4. de Jesus, J.C., Kich, V.A., Kolling, A.H., Grando, R.B., Guerra, R.S. and Drews, P.L., 2022, October. Depth-cuprl: Depth-imaged contrastive unsupervised prioritized representations in reinforcement learning for mapless navigation of unmanned aerial vehicles. In 2022 IEEE/RSJ International Conference on Intelligent Robots and Systems (IROS) (pp. 10579-10586). IEEE.

5. Arafat, M.Y., Alam, M.M. and Moh, S., 2023. Vision-based navigation techniques for unmanned aerial vehicles: Review and challenges. Drones, 7(2), p.89.

6. Doukhi, O. and Lee, D.J., 2022. Deep reinforcement learning for autonomous map-less navigation of a flying robot. IEEE Access, 10, pp.82964-82976.

7. Zhang, H.T., Hu, B.B., Xu, Z., Cai, Z., Liu, B., Wang, X., Geng, T., Zhong, S. and Zhao, J., 2021. Visual navigation and landing control of an unmanned aerial vehicle on a moving autonomous surface vehicle via adaptive learning. IEEE Transactions on Neural Networks and Learning Systems, 32(12), pp.5345-5355.

8. Wu, X., Chen, H., Chen, C., Zhong, M., Xie, S., Guo, Y. and Fujita, H., 2020. The autonomous navigation and obstacle avoidance for USVs with ANOA deep reinforcement learning method. Knowledge-Based Systems, 196, p.105201.

9. Wu, D., Wan, K., Tang, J., Gao, X., Zhai, Y. and Qi, Z., 2022, April. An improved method towards multi-UAV autonomous navigation using deep reinforcement learning. In 2022 7th International Conference on Control and Robotics Engineering (ICCRE) (pp. 96-101). IEEE.

10. Afifi, G. and Gadallah, Y., 2021. Autonomous 3-D UAV localization using cellular networks: Deep supervised learning versus reinforcement learning approaches. IEEE Access, 9, pp.155234-155248.

Emerging Trends in IoT and Computing Technologies – Suman Lata Tripathi et al. (eds)
© 2024 Taylor & Francis Group, London, ISBN 978-1-032-87924-6

Counterfeit Product Detection and Identification using Blockchain Technology

22

**Dilipkumar A. Borikar[1], Anushka Shukla[2],
Arpit Singh Thakur[3], Janak Mandavgade[4], Jaiwin Chaudhari[5]**

Shri Ramdeobaba College of Engineering and Management, Nagpur, India

Abstract: The issue of counterfeiting is a global problem that requires transparent supply chains and efficient detection methods. Our work proposes use of QR codes and a Blockchain-based system for detection and identification of counterfeit products. Products are assigned QR codes that are generated by the system for ownership verification of the product, utilizing Blockchain security. QR codes contain encrypted information, such as product details along with product ID. High-resolution cameras and mobile apps are used for scanning, while counterfeit product detection methods analyze decoded data and cross-reference it with the Blockchain database for authenticity. Results demonstrate that QR codes and Blockchain are viable solutions for detecting counterfeit products, providing a transparent and secure solution for supply chains.

Keywords: Counterfeit product, Blockchain, Supply chain, QR code, Digital signature, NFT.

1. Introduction

Supply chain management is essential in today's global economy for assuring seamless movement of goods from producers to final consumers. However, issues including information mismatch between the end users, a lack of transparency, and restricted traceability of the products, frequently plague traditional supply chain management systems. These restrictions may lead to inefficiencies, hold-ups, fake goods, and problems building stakeholder confidence. Products that are counterfeit represent a serious hazard to both consumers and businesses, costing money and endangering public safety. Every day, billions of items are created all over the world, resulting in complex supply chains that connect every region. This complexity of supply chains provides a gateway for fake goods to enter the legal supply chain. In 2022, the International Chamber of Commerce has predicted that piracy and counterfeiting will have a total money flow of a staggering $2.3 trillion by the end of the year. In order to verify items and discourage counterfeiters, anti-counterfeiting measures include a variety of technologies, including holograms, security printing, and security labels. However, in the digital era, when counterfeiters may readily take advantage of internet platforms to fool consumers, these conventional tactics are no longer sufficient. According to a new study by ABI Research, by the end of 2023, the demand for blockchain will increase, making it a $10.6 billion industry. Blockchain offers a secure, decentralized ledger for recording and verifying transactions among a group of computers. Blockchain guarantees the dependability and validity of the product information, lowering the likelihood of fake or inferior items in the supply chain.

2. Motivation

The blockchain supply chain initiative intends to provide producers, retailers, and consumers with a transparent and secure platform in order to address this developing issue. Manufacturers will be able to create distinct QR codes for each batch of

[1]borikarda@rknec.edu, [2]shuklaad@rknec.edu, [3]thakuray@rknec.edu, [4]mandavgadejd@rknec.edu, [5]chaudharijr@rknec.edu

DOI: 10.1201/9781003535423-22

products and submit them to the blockchain along with the appropriate amounts. Retailers can precisely record the number of goods received, improving inventory control and reducing errors. Customers can quickly search for items using the product ID and will have access to detailed information on the products' manufacturing pro-cesses, place of origin, and whole blockchain supply chain.

3. Related Works

N Anita, et.al, have used decentralized identities of the supply chain entities to create smart contracts. They used Radio Frequency Identification (RFID) tags to store product details such as product ID, product name, etc. [1]. Wasnik, et.al, presented the implementation of a DApp system and offered an overview of the fundamental concepts and technologies employed in blockchain technology [2]. Anjum, et.al, developed a system that utilizes MetaMask, a cryptocurrency wallet, to enable transaction facilitation [8]. Ma, et.al, has developed a system where the manufacturer creates and adds products to the blockchain and confirm whether the seller is who he/she claims to be or not [3]. Alzahrani, et.al, designed a system to validate products using blockchain technology. Product validation is performed by validators within the blockchain system [4]. Bencic, et.al, proposed a DL-tag solution that utilizes a public ledger as a reliable record of significant events in the supply chain [11]. Tambe, et.al, presented a blockchain based system for detecting fake products [9]. Mani, et.al have used Hyper Ledger Fabric to store the supply chain data [5]. Kamat, et.al, proposed a system that involves using SMS features and QR codes [6]. Rathee and Malik have proposed a method integrating the manufacturer and the supplier functionalities [7]. Paliwal, et al. have proposed the use of blockchain in secure paperless administration of offices in the public departments [13]. Rahmadika, et.al, proposed an enhancement to the existing supply chain approach using blockchain and the IoTs [10]. K. Toyoda, et.al, implemented a product ownership management system (POMS) that uses RFID technology for handling counterfeiting in the supply chain [12].

4. Methodology

We propose a blockchain based irreproducible, product anti-counterfeiting solution to track the products by maintaining the product supply chain. A decentralized application implemented using the Ethereum Network serves to keep all records and manage product transactions on DApp. It provides a seamless, transparent transition of the product the manufacturer to the customer. The user can perform vendor-side verification, and track the history of the product using a QR code. The basic architecture is shown in Fig. 22.1.

To verify originality of the product, the system keeps track of the product's history along the supply chain. The system depends on three major stakeholders: the Manufacturer, the Seller, and the Customer, as discussed:

4.1 Manufacturer

Adding product to the blockchain supply chain

The manufacturers can seamlessly add their products to the blockchain network. To accomplish this, the Manufacturer logs into his account using his credentials and adds the product by clicking the submit button. Upon submission, a MetaMask pop-up window will appear, requiring the manufacturer's confirmation to initiate the transaction for securely storing the product details on the blockchain. This streamlined process ensures efficient and reliable storage of product information within the blockchain network. Within the system, manufacturers have the ability to generate a distinctive QR code for each batch, which includes a unique batch ID that serves as a reference point for searching and retrieving product information from the blockchain. By utilizing this QR code system, manufacturers can streamline the process of accessing product details securely stored on the blockchain.

Distribution of products to different retailers

This allows manufacturers to efficiently distribute products to various retailers, leveraging the unique retailer ID, location, and desired product quantities for each retailer. Once the distribution details are entered, users can confirm the transaction using MetaMask, which triggers the storage of all distribution information securely on the blockchain. Manufacturers have the capability to distribute products to multiple retailers. In cases where the desired product quantity for distribution exceeds the available stock held by the manufacturer, an error popup promptly notifies the manufacturer. This alert serves as a reminder that the remaining product quantity is insufficient to fulfill the requested distribution.

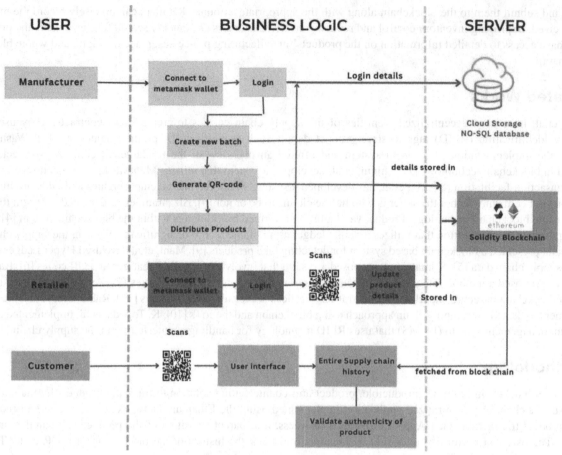

Fig. 22.1 System architecture

4.2 Retailer

Searching the product details

After uploading QR Code a batch id is generated through which the retailer can search the product and validate whether the product is been sent by a legitimate manufacturer or not.

Updating product details

The retailer can update the product state by confirming the batch id of the product, and the count of products that he has received. After confirming the transaction, the state of the product is updated in the blockchain. In case the count or destination is not matched with those entered by the manufacturer, counterfeiting in the product will be detected thus reverting the transaction of the retailer to update product details in the supply chain.

4.3 Customer

Consumers scans the QR code to verify the authenticity of the product. It lists the complete supply chain history of transactions. When the customer purchases the product, after scanning the QR they can check the supply chain history. When the last traded location and the purchase location are not matching or when the retailer information is different from the one provided by the manufacturer, the system will signal the detection of counterfeit product.

5. Implementation

A decentralized Web3 application built on non-fungible tokens (NFTs) can be utilized for product traceability in the supply chain. By implementing real time tracking, settlement, and documentation, businesses can achieve greater operational efficiencies and access improved financial products. From the production of raw materials to the display of goods in physical stores or online platforms, the use of NFTs enables traceability and enhances supply chain management. Physical NFTs, when linked to real-world goods, serve as a valuable utility. By leveraging NFTs to trace a product back to its source, credibility is added to the product. Integrating NFTs and digital twin technology into the supply chain enables companies to automate payments and facilitate instant settlement upon goods delivery.

We developed the supply chain smart contract for managing the products as they move from one node to another in the product supply chain. The smart contracts manage and track products as they move through the supply chain from manufacturers to retailers and to customers. The key functionalities of the smart contract include – newItem(), distributeProduct(), updateProduct() and getters().

We have used Hardhat to integrate supply chain smart contracts with the user interface. Hardhat is a development environment and toolset used for building, testing, and deploying smart contracts on the Ethereum blockchain. For deployment, we configured the hardhat environment with Sepolia Ethereum Blockchain. We deployed the smart contract in a hardhat environment and generated the ABI (Application Binary Interface) Code. We used the Ether.js library to interact with Ethereum smart contracts by creating contract instances using the contract's ABI. This facilitates the interaction of the smart contract with the user by allowing them to call smart contract functions and send transactions to the smart contract.

6. Results

The functionalities offered by the system are described in the following sections.

6.1 Manufacturer

Add product and Generate QR Code

Manufacturers have the ability to generate a distinctive QR code for each batch, which includes a unique batch ID. This batch ID serves as a reference point for searching and retrieving product information from the blockchain.

Distribute Product

Manufacturers have the capability to distribute products to multiple retailers as shown in Fig. 22.2(a). When the desired product quantity for distribution exceeds the available stock, an error popup promptly notifies the manufacturer.

Search Product

Figure 22.2(b) shows the manufacturer's ability to search for and track the products they have been created and distributed.

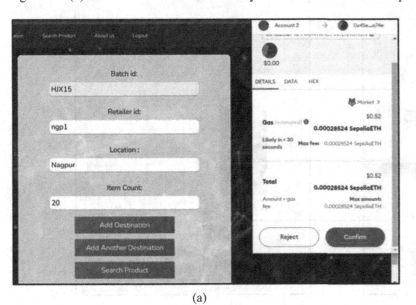
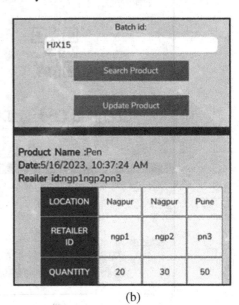

(a)   (b)

Fig. 22.2   Manufacturer operations: (a) Distribute product, (b) Product details

6.2 Retailer

Search Product

This functionality shown in Fig. 22.3(a) enables retailer to search the product and to display the product details.

Update Product

A retailer can update the product state by confirming the batch ID of the product, and the count of products that he has received as shown in Fig. 22.3(b).

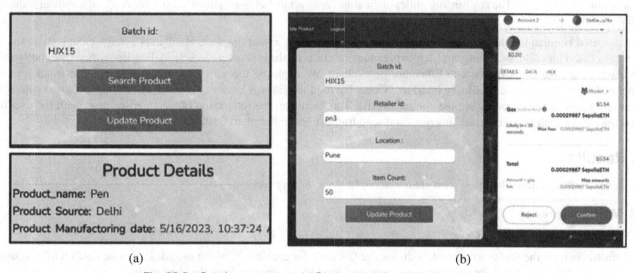

(a) (b)

Fig. 22.3 Retailer operations: (a) Product details, (b) Update product

6.3 Customer

The customer scan the product QR code to access batch ID for that product as shown in Fig. 22.4(a), Fig. 22.4(b) shows the process of searching with the batch ID, customer will get the complete transaction history of the product.

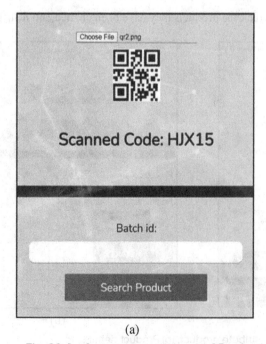
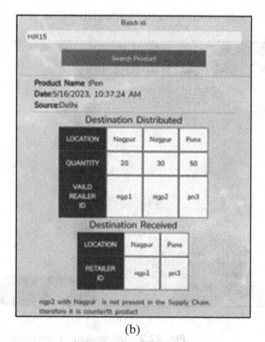

(a) (b)

Fig. 22.4 Customer operations: (a) QR upload and batch-id generation, (b) Product by supply chain

7. Conclusion

Implementing a counterfeit management system using blockchain technology offers a promising solution to address the pervasive issue of counterfeiting. The proposed framework leverages blockchains and smart contracts as powerful tools for revolutionizing supply chain management by eliminating the need for human intermediaries to coordinate multiple parties involved in supply chain operations. It establishes cost-effective supply chains that rely on peer-level participation, with a primary focus on ensuring product authenticity. Our system can bring several benefits to the product supply chain system, including enhanced visibility, reduced fraud, improved inventory management, and streamlined communication among supply chain participants. By automating processes, and minimizing intermediary frauds, the DApp significantly improves overall supply chain efficiency, leading to cost savings and increased customer satisfaction.

REFERENCES

1. N Anita, M Vijayalakshmi and S Mercy Shalinie, "Blockchain-based anonymous anti-counterfeit supply chain framework", Sadhana; Vol 47-208 (2022)
2. Kunal Wasnik, Isha Sondawle, Rushikesh Wani and Namita Pulgam, "Detection of Counterfeit Products using Blockchain", ITM Web of Conferences; Vol 44 (2022)
3. Jinhua Ma, Shih-Ya Lin, Xin Chen, Hung-Min Sun et.al, "A Blockchain-Based Application System for Product Anti-Counterfeiting", IEEE Access; (2020).
4. Naif Alzahrani and Nirupama Bulusu, "A New Product Anti-Counterfeiting Blockchain Using a Truly Decentralized Dynamic Consensus Protocol"; PDXScholar (2019)
5. Vinodhini Mani, M. Prakash and Wen Cheng Lai, "Cloud-based blockchain technology to identify counterfeits"; Journal of Cloud Computing (2022)
6. Avinash A. Kamat, "Using QR Codes to Track and Identify Counterfeit Products"; Infosys (2018)
7. Tripti Rathee and Manoj Malik, "Authentication of Product & Counterfeits Elimination Using Blockchain", Intl Journal of Innovations in Engineering and Technology (IJIET); Volume 10-1 (2018)
8. Nafisa Anjum and Pramit Dutta, "Identifying Counterfeit Products using Blockchain Technology in Supply Chain System", IMCOM; (2022)
9. T. Tambe, S. Chitalkar, M. Khurud et.al, "Fake Product Detection Using Blockchain Technology", International Journal of Advance Research, Ideas and Innovations in Technology, Vol. 7 (2021)
10. S. Rahmadika, B. J. Kweka, C. N. Z. Latt, et.al, "A Preliminary Approach of Blockchain Technology in Supply Chain System.", IEEE International Conference on Data Mining Workshops (ICDMW) (2018)
11. F. M. Benčić, P. Skočir and I. P. Žarko, "DL-Tags: DLT and Smart Tags for Decentralized, Privacy-Preserving, and Verifiable Supply Chain Management", IEEE Access; Vol. 7 (2019)
12. K. Toyoda, P. T. Mathiopoulos, I. Sasase and T. Ohtsuki, "A Novel Blockchain-Based Product Ownership Management System (POMS) for Anti-Counterfeits in the Post Supply Chain", IEEE Access; Vol. 5 (2017)
13. Atharva Paliwal, Chaitanya Kapre, Yash Roy, and Dilipkumar Borikar, "An Approach to Paperless Administration of Offices in India Using Blockchain", Springer, Singapore; Vol 333 (2022)

Emerging Trends in IoT and Computing Technologies – Suman Lata Tripathi et al. (eds)
© 2024 Taylor & Francis Group, London, ISBN 978-1-032-87924-6

Visual Speech Recognition using Spatio-Temporal and Temporal Features

23

Saswati Debnath[1], Puneet Kumar Yadav[2]

Alliance University, Computer science and Engineering Dept, Bangalore, India

M. Senbagavalli[3]

[3]Alliance University, CSE and IT Dept, Bangalore, India

Abstract: Visual information plays an active role in the battlefield of audio-visual automatic speech recognition (AV-ASR). Speech recognition frequently uses appearance features and lip geometry features to derive visual information from speech. Two distinct experiments for visual speech recognition are presented in this study. This study provides appearance-based visual speech feature extraction in the first experiment, as well as the co-occurrence statistical measure of features. In this context, we employ the Grey-Level Co-occurrence Matrix (GLCM) combined with the Local Binary Pattern in three orthogonal planes (LBP-TOP) to capture spatiotemporal features when collecting visual speech data. In order to identify visual speech in the second experiment, temporal information is extracted from video. The second experiment utilizes Recurrent Neural Network (RNN) and Long Short-Term Memory (LSTM) within the framework of RNN-LSTM.

Keywords: Visual speech recognition (VSR), LBP-TOP, GLCM, ANN, RNN, LSTM

1. Introduction

Humans produce and perceive speech in two ways: both the speaker's visual clues and the speech signal that is uttered. When noise taints an audio signal, the visual signal can provide speech information. Different visual features have been proposed by many researchers and the main objective of the research was to extract proper lip movement. The most important lip movement conditions for lip-tracking are quality of visual speech of a speaker i.e. proper visual articulations and angle of view. Thus, there has been involvement in modern years in the derivation of appropriate and reliable visual features. Extraction of visual features is based on appearance, shape, or a mix of the two. The following are the primary contributions of this paper: This study introduces appearance-based features and co-occurrences measure of visual features. The spatiotemporal domain (LBP-TOP) is used to compute visual speech characteristics. This domain also records the movement of visual characteristics in combination with appearance features. From the LBP-TOP, the co-occurrence matrix and a range of GLCM features are computed to capture distinctive lip movements. RNN-LSTM is used to excerpt temporal data from video sequences beneficial to recognize visual speech. RNN is used to track the order of images from videos which is very crucial for recognizing visual speech. Section II represents a related work, Section III outlines the experimental steps for visual speech recognition, Section IV provides details about the AV-ASR dataset. Experimental results and analysis of visual speech are discussed in Section V, while Section VI offers a comparison of the results. Section VII gives conclusion of the paper.

[1]saswati.debnath@alliance.edu.in, [2]puneet.yadav@alliance.edu.in, [3]senbagavalli.m@alliance.edu.in

DOI: 10.1201/9781003535423-23

2. Literature Review

The summary of connected techniques along with their advantages and disadvantages are given below Nevertheless, the technique was unable to extract the speaker's lip geometry, which gives the form of their lips during speech, as well as global features. The primary application of LBP is as a texture detection feature descriptor [5]. LBP is also used for background subtraction, texture classification, static face detection in picture classification, and other applications. For four realistic visual modalities in various noisy environments, DCT and LDA have been investigated for visual speech. In noisy environments, good recognition was supplied by depth-level visual information. In 2015, Namrata Dave introduced a visual feature extraction technique based on lip localization, enabling real-time segmentation [1]. A unique color-based method for lip localization was reported in this study, which is an early step towards real-time lip tracking. In reference [10], the author utilized deep bottleneck features in conjunction with voice activity detection to enhance the accuracy of audio-visual speech recognition. The author effectively achieved 73.66% lipreading accuracy and an average of 90% AVSR accuracy in noisy surroundings by utilizing the proposed features. The end-to-end (E2E) framework is capable of learning information across several modalities; nevertheless, training the model is challenging, particularly with limited amounts of data. In this work [11], the author concentrated on developing an end-to-end audio-visual speech recognition system, based on encoders and decoders, for practical applications. Several pre-training techniques have been conducted that provided the AVSR framework with distinct initialization. The author has investigated several model structures and techniques for audio-visual fusion.

3. Proposed Methodology

The proposed visual speech recognition methodology comprises three main stages: Region of Interest Detection (ROI), Visual Speech Feature Extraction, and Classification. To extract features, LBP-TOP and GLCM are employed to capture statistical features. After feature extraction ANN is used to carry out the recognition process. In the second experiment RNN and LSTM are used to calculate temporal features of speech.

3.1 Visual Feature Extraction

Texture detection primarily uses LBP as a feature descriptor, along with GLCM and LBP-TOP. It separates the face into several areas and extracts features from each one, making it an effective method for extracting facial features [6]. Each region's texture description accurately depicts how that region appears [6]. LBP characterizes the global geometry of the face by consolidating all region descriptors. Timo Ojala et al. [5] introduced a grayscale and rotation invariant operator approach within LBP to achieve invariance to monotonic transformations in grayscale and uniform patterns across any quantization of angular space. Despite extensive research, LBP continues to find effective applications in contemporary visual speech recognition and serves as a texture descriptor.

In this paper, the face is divided into 10 regions and information is extracted from each region to derive local features from specific facial areas. Compared to traditional LBP, LBP-TOP is a more effective dynamic feature descriptor for classifying static images since it extracts features from the spatio-temporal domain. For visual speech recognition, lip movement in relation to time can be efficiently captured using LBP-TOP. While XT, YT provide the time-varying visual data and motion features in a time domain, XY performs appearance-based dimension in a spatial domain. As a result, the XY plane is used to collect a sequence of appearance-based feature vectors, while the XT and YT planes are used to capture lip motion and feature changes over time. After their generation, the histograms from these three planes are concatenated to represent appearance-based visual attributes. Second-order statistical texture features are then extracted using GLCM, which stands for grey level co-occurrence matrix [7]. In this work, LBP-TOP feature extraction is followed by the application of GLCM. Each frame's LBP-TOP matrix serves as an input for the GLCM computation.

The order of a GLCM is determined by the number of distinct gray level intensities (I). If I = (0, 1, 2, ..., I-1), then the order of the GLCM is IxI. In other words, the matrix has dimensions IxI, and each element P(i, j) in the matrix represents the co-occurrence frequency of the gray levels i and j in the image.

$$\text{Energy} = \sum_{i,j=0}^{I-1} p(i,j)^2 \tag{2}$$

$$\text{Entropy} = \sum_{i=0}^{I-1}\sum_{j=0}^{I-1} p(i,j)\log(p(i,j)) \tag{3}$$

$$\text{Co-relation} = \frac{\sum_{i=0}^{I-1}\sum_{j=0}^{I-1}(i,j)\,p(i,j) - \mu_m\mu_n}{\sigma_m\sigma_n} \tag{4}$$

$$\text{Contrast} = \sum_{i,j=0}^{I-1} |i,j|^2\, p(i,j) \tag{5}$$

$$\text{Variance} = \sum_{i,j=0}^{I-1} (i-\mu)^2 \log(p(i,j)) \tag{6}$$

3.2 Performance Measure

The performance is calculated by following equation:

$$\text{Recognition Rate} = \frac{Correctly\ identified\ test\ sample}{Total\ supplied\ test\ sample} \times 100\% \tag{7}$$

The recognition rate is calculated by dividing the number of correctly identified test samples by the total number of supplied test samples.

3.3 Database Description

The tests and result comparisons in this case are conducted using the 'CUAVE' dataset [4]. Ten English digits, ranging from 0 to 9, are included in the dataset. Every person says each number five times, for a total of 1800 words utilized. The database was captured using the NTSC standard at 29.97 frames per second in a 720 x 480 resolution in a separate sound booth. The audio has a 44 kHz sample rate and is 16-bit stereo. Additionally, word-level labelling is performed manually for every database sequence with millisecond accuracy.

4. Experimental Results and Analysis of Visual Speech Recognition

ANNs [3] can establish dynamic, unconventional relationships between the data received and what ANN produces. The most often used neural network that is taught using the backpropagation learning technique is the multi-layer feed-forward neural network. We take 10 frames out of every video and use the LBP algorithm to identify each frame's ROI. Statistical features are calculated using LBP-TOP and GLCM. The primary goal of the suggested feature extraction technique is to extract more informative visual features because, in comparison to an audio signal, visual articulations provide very less information. Since this information varies depending on the speaker, more data must be incorporated in order to produce speaker-independent visual speech recognition. Here, characteristics based on shape and appearance are retrieved for hybridization. By thresholding the vicinity of the center pixel, LBP-TOP computes the local binary patterns and dynamic aspects of lip movement from three orthogonal planes. Every lip contour frame is segmented into smaller sections, and LBP-TOP is utilized to compute the pixel values within each sub-region. Lastly, a single histogram is created by integrating all the histograms from three orthogonal spatiotemporal domains. The co-occurrence of the localized binary pattern on 3 different orthogonal planes is computed via GLCM.

Table 23.1 Visual speech recognition using ANN

Exp. no	No.of Hidden layer	No.of Hidden units	Iterations	System accuracy %
1	2	30,20	100	67.57
2	2	40,30	100	72.00
3	2	50,40	100	70.05
4	2	60,50	100	70.45

4.1 Visual Speech Recognition using ANN

The first stage in the extraction of visual characteristics is to identify the ROI, in this case the speaker's lip contour, using LBP. Capturing dynamic visual information and feature co-occurrence values is the primary objective behind the suggested feature extraction method. After LBP-TOP extraction, the feature vector's total dimension is (150X10), or 1500 for each frame. Statistical measures such as energy, correlation, contrast, variance, and entropy are extracted from the LBP-TOP features matrix. This matrix, containing the calculated LBP-TOP, serves as input for the calculation of the GLCM. Positive or negative statistics can be represented by the computed measurements of -1 or 1. Because entropy and GLCM energy are inversely related, its maximum value is reached when all of the elements in a particular matrix are equal. Using an ANN with varying numbers of hidden nodes and hidden layers, visual speech is recognized. The system uses 40, 30 concealed nodes to achieve 71.00% recognition accuracy.

4.2 Visual Speech Recognition using RNN-LSTM

Now a day deep learning is a very emerging technique and also used for AV-ASR. Convolution Neural Network (CNN) is widely used for image recognition and visual speech recognition [2]. But CNN can not keep track of sequence of frame. For visual speech recognition the order of frames gives proper information. On the basis of LSTM, we have developed an RNN model. Input for the subsequent layers is fed from the first layer. 256 LSTM units make up the wide network model that is being employed. The completely connected layer has as many neurons as there are classes, with each neuron connected to every other neuron in the layer above. Figure 23.2 shows the accuracy of visual speech recognition using RNN+LSTM for values 0 to 9.

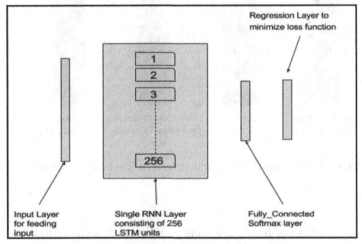

Fig. 23.1   RNN model

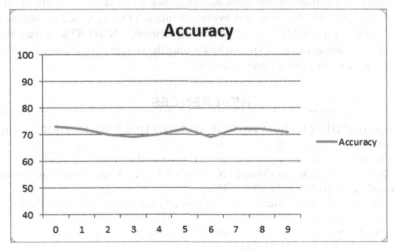

Fig. 23.2   Accuracy using RNN model

In this approach, we employed Recurrent Neural Network (RNN) to extract temporal information from individual frames. The RNN generated a series of predictions for each frame, forming a sequence of frame predictions, which was then used to represent each video.

5. Comparative Analysis based on Different Visual Feature Extraction Method

Many studies have employed LBP for visual speech recognition; however, due to its incapacity to record the dynamic components of lip movement, researchers have created LBP-TOP, a three-dimensional feature computation method. The co-occurrence values are also significant; the statistical value derived from the co-occurrence matrix provides a unique characteristic. Average accuracy 71 % is obtained by extracting the temporal features using RNN-LSTM.

Thus, from these experiments it has been observed that temporal and spatio-temporal features of visual speech provide better accuracy compared to other feature extraction methods. We have used both machine learning and deep learning to recognize speech.

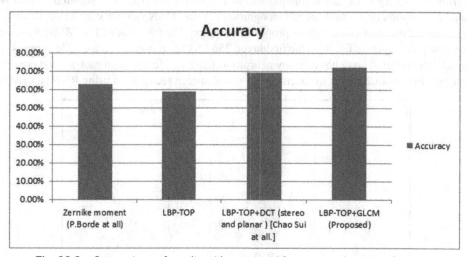

Fig. 23.3 Comparison of results with proposed features and existing features

6. Conclusion

In this paper, visual speech recognition has been carried out using two proposed methods. For the purpose of extracting spatiotemporal characteristics and co-occurrence value for visual speech recognition, LBP-TOP+GLCM is presented. Since LBP-TOP records visual features in a spatiotemporal domain, appearance-based features are also used to record lip movements. Different frames of a given utterance are distinguished by the calculation of five GLCM features. After feature extraction, classification of speech is carried out using ANN. In the second experiment, RNN+LSTM is used to recognize visual speech. RNN is used to classify temporal features of visual speech by keeping the sequence of frames. Future work will be extended to extract spatial and temporal features using hybrid deep learning.

REFERENCES

1. Namrata Dave. A LIP LOCALIZATION BASED VISUAL FEATURE EXTRACTION METHOD, Electrical Computer Engineering: An Inter- national Journal (ECIJ), vol 4, no 4, 2015
2. Artificial intelligence: a modern approach, Russell S and Norvig P, Prentice Hall, 2003.
3. Patterson, E. Gurbuz, Sabri Tu¨fekci, Zekeriya Gowdy, J.N.. (2002). CUAVE: A new audio-visual database for multmodal human-computer interface research", 2. 10.1109/ICASSP.2002.5745028.
4. T. Ojala and M. Pietikainen and T. Maenpaa . Multiresolution gray-scale and rotation invariant texture classification with local binary patterns, IEEE Trans. Pattern Anal. Mach. Intell, vol 24, no 7, pp 971–987, 2002.
5. T. Ahonen and A. Hadid and M. Pietikainen. Face description with local binary patterns: Applications to face recognition, IEEE Trans. Pattern Anal. Mach. Intell, vol 28, no 12, pp 2037–2041, 2006.

6. P.Mohanaiah and P.Sathyanarayana and L.GuruKumar. Image Texture Feature Extraction Using GLCM Approach, International Journal of Scientific and Research Publications, vol 3, no 5, 2013.

7. Galatas, G. and Potamianos, G. and Makedon, F. Audio-visual speech recognition using depth information from the Kinect in noisy video conditions, Proceedings of International Conference on Pervasive Technologies Related to Assistive Environments, ACM, 2012.

8. Guoying Zhao and Mark Barnard, and Matti Pietikainen, Lipreading With Local Spatiotemporal Descriptors, IEEE TRANSACTIONS ON MUL- TIMEDIA, vol 11, no 7,2009.

9. Kingma, Diedrick and J. Ba. ADAM: A method for stochastic optimization, arXiv, 2014.

10. S. Tamura et al. Audio-visual speech recognition using deep bottleneck features and high-performance lipreading, 2015 Asia-Pacific Signal and Information Processing Association Annual Summit and Conference (APSIPA), Hong Kong, China, 2015, pp. 575-582, doi: 10.1109/APSIPA.2015.7415335.

11. Yin B, Niu S, Tang H, Sun L, Du J, Ling Z, Liu C. An Investigation into Audio–Visual Speech Recognition under a Realistic Home–TV Scenario. Applied Sciences. 2023; 13(7):4100. https://doi.org/10.3390/app13074100

Emerging Trends in IoT and Computing Technologies – Suman Lata Tripathi et al. (eds)
© 2024 Taylor & Francis Group, London, ISBN 978-1-032-87924-6

Quantum Computing: Current Advancements and Future Prospects

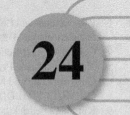

24

S. Mohanap Priya[1]

SCAD Polytechnic College,
Department of Computer Engineering, Tirunelveli, India

S. Ram Prasath[2]

SCAD College of Engineering & Technology,
Department of CSE, Tirunelveli, India

S. Anitha[3]

SCAD Polytechnic College,
Department of Computer Engineering, Tirunelveli, India

D. Kani Jesintha[4]

SCAD College of Engineering & Technology,
Department of CSE, Tirunelveli, India

E. Golden Julie[5]

Anna University Regional Campus, Department of CSE, Tirunelveli, India

Abstract: This study explores the most recent developments in quantum computing and highlights how revolutionary it can be. Developments in both hardware and software, which include IBM's advancements to qubit equilibrium and Google's quantum supremacy, indicate that quantum computing is moving from theory to practice. Though they present serious security challenges, their real-world applications in cryptography, optimization, as well as artificial intelligence hold great promise. For environmentally friendly technology adoption, the study suggests putting a focus on hardware development, designing quantum algorithms, teamwork, and ethical considerations. The application of quantum computing has the potential to completely reinvent a number of sectors, including data security and information technology.

Keywords: Quantum computing, Quantum technology, Quantum hardware, Quantum algorithms, Post-quantum cryptography

1. Introduction

The evolution of quantum computing throughout history signifies a significant change in the field of computation. It has its roots in the fundamental ideas of quantum mechanics as well as can be traced back to prominent physicists like David Deutsch and Richard Feynman, who first conceptualized the idea in the early 1980s. The significance of quantum computing is in its ability to completely transform the way information is processed [1]. Quantum computing makes use of quantum bits, or qubits,

[1]mohanappriyapree@gmail.com, [2]srpfxec@gmail.com, [3]angel.anitha@gmail.com, [4]kanijesintha@gmail.com, [5]juliegolden18@gmail.com

DOI: 10.1201/9781003535423-24

which are different from classical computing in that they can exist in more than one state at once due to superposition as well as entanglement. This makes it possible for quantum computers to perform complex problem-solving exponentially faster than their classical counterparts, which includes incorporating large numbers or optimizing enormous datasets [2]. Even with its amazing advancements, classical computing is still limited in its ability to solve some very difficult problems. Examples of these kinds of problems include optimization, material science, as well as cryptography, all of which are quantum in nature. The need to overcome these constraints together with realizing the unrealized potential of quantum mechanics in computation has spurred research into quantum computing. By doing this, it ushers in a revolutionary era in the field of information technology by establishing up new directions for study, innovation, and useful applications.

This study aims to provide a thorough understanding of the state-of-the-art developments in quantum computing, their effects on different industries, alongside their potential to influence the direction of information technology in the future. The main objectives are,

- To investigate the most recent developments in both software and hardware for quantum computing.
- To examine the useful uses and practical ramifications of quantum computing in domains like artificial intelligence, cryptography, as well as optimization.
- To access the challenges and constraints that quantum computing still has, as well as possible solutions.
- To offer analysis and suggestions for upcoming studies in addition to the commercial application of quantum computing technologies.

The urgent need to solve the growing shortcomings of classical computing in a society that depends more and more on information processing is what spurred this research. Even though they are exceptionally strong, classical computers frequently have difficulty solving complicated quantum-related issues that have significant effects on data analysis, drug development, as well as cryptography [3]. With its singular capacity to manipulate quantum phenomena, quantum computing presents a novel and revolutionary means of overcoming these obstacles. This research aims to advance knowledge of the field by examining the state of quantum computing today as well as its possible uses. This will eventually pave the way for the creation and uptake of quantum computing solutions that have the potential to transform industries and advance technology.

1.1 Methodology

The interpretivism philosophy is used in this study to comprehend the wider technological and societal consequences of quantum computing. Interpretivism, which stresses people's subjective experiences as well as perceptions, is especially pertinent in fields where the influence goes beyond technical details. Using a deductive methodology, the research expands on prior theories as well as comprehension of quantum computing. It begins with accepted concepts and assumptions, which are subsequently put to the test and improved upon by actual data. A descriptive research design was selected with the goal of giving a thorough and in-depth description of the state of quantum computing at the moment. This methodology enables a methodical investigation of developments, uses, as well as difficulties in the field of quantum computing. The main approach employed in this study is the collection of secondary data. Scholarly publications, books, reports, as well as trustworthy internet databases are examples of data sources [6]. These resources include scholarly journals, proceedings from conferences, in addition to publications from technology companies and research institutes that concentrate on quantum computing. A detailed examination and synthesis of the secondary data that has been gathered constitute data analysis. To classify and extract pertinent data about the challenges, and applications, in addition to advancements in quantum computing, patterns, trends, and emerging topics are identified through the use of content analysis. A purposive strategy is employed for sampling, whereby secondary data sources are chosen according to their pertinence to the study's goals. The selection of sources is indicative of quantum computing's current status and implications. The research is concerned with the selection of reliable and high-quality secondary data sources in order to guarantee reliability and accuracy [5]. It uses standard methods for interpreting and analyzing data, which raises the general dependability of the results. When employing secondary data in research, ethical considerations have to be taken into account at every stage of the process. Copyright and intellectual property rights are respected, as well as sources are properly cited and referenced. Within the interpretivism paradigm, this technical methodology framework offers an organized and methodical way to comprehend the developments, uses, in addition to difficulties of quantum computing. It highlights the importance that thorough data collection and meticulous analysis are to getting relevant insights and conclusions.

This research paper's findings section provides a technically rich overview of the field by revealing a thorough examination of recent developments, real-world applications, difficulties, as well as constraints in quantum computing.

1.2 Current Technological Advancements in Quantum Computing

Recent developments in the field of quantum computing have had nothing short of revolutionary effects. Significant advancements in software as well as technology have played a key role in expanding the realm of what was once thought to be feasible. Quantum processors have achieved notable advancements in qubit fidelity as well as stability in terms of hardware. In the year 2019, Google's "Sycamore" quantum processor achieved quantum supremacy, garnering significant attention [4]. It demonstrated the enormous computational power of quantum computing by completing one particular assignment more quickly than the most sophisticated classical supercomputers. With its 65-qubit "Hummingbird" processor, IBM, a major player in the industry, has additionally made impressive strides, demonstrating its dedication to scalability and error rate reduction [3]. Quantum algorithms are advancing quickly in software. For instance, Shor's algorithm showed promise in successfully factoring large numbers, which prompted questions regarding the security of traditional encryption techniques. Grover's algorithm for searching unstructured databases also promises to accelerate data retrieval tasks. Quantum programming has recently become more accessible thanks to quantum software platforms like Microsoft's Quantum Development Kit as well as IBM's Qiskit, which allows researchers and developers to have fun playing around with quantum algorithms.

1.3 Quantum Computing's Useful Applications and Real-World Consequences

Quantum computing has many real-world applications that have substantial effects in a variety of fields. Quantum computing presents an opportunity as well as a challenge to the field of cryptography. The efficient factorization of large numbers by Shor's algorithm puts traditional encryption techniques like RSA in jeopardy. The National Institute of Standards and Technology (NIST) launched a post-quantum cryptography project in response to this, with the goal of developing encryption standards that are impervious to quantum attacks. It is clear that quantum-safe encryption is needed, and scientists are working hard to develop encryption techniques that are capable of withstanding the processing power of quantum computers [2]. More applications of quantum computing are in the domain of optimization problems. Supply chain management, finance, as well as logistics tasks have been tackled by D-Wave with its quantum annealers and quantum-inspired algorithms. Volkswagen, for example, decreased travel time by 20% by optimizing traffic flow in Lisbon through the use of quantum computing. These useful applications highlight the possible real-world improvements in productivity that quantum computing can provide [1]. Quantum computing has the potential to speed up machine learning algorithms in artificial intelligence. The applications of quantum Boltzmann machines, and quantum neural networks, in addition to quantum support vector machines, could improve data analysis, and predictive modeling, followed by pattern recognition. The field of quantum machine learning is nascent and holds great promise for revolutionary breakthroughs.

1.4 Limitations and Difficulties in Quantum Computing

Although quantum computing has come a long way, there are nonetheless numerous challenges and restrictions that need to be addressed. Error correction in quantum still remains a fundamental problem. Due to their extreme susceptibility to outside noise, quantum bits, or qubits, can cause computation errors as well as decoherence [1]. To reduce these errors, quantum error correction codes have been proposed, like the surface code. Prominent producers of quantum hardware, such as IBM and Rigetti, are making every effort to develop fault-tolerant quantum processors with the goal of lowering error rates as well as improving qubit coherence. Scalability is yet another important barrier. Increasing the qubit count is of the utmost importance to solving complicated issues, but it is a difficult undertaking. Although IBM's 65-qubit Quantum Hummingbird processor is a step forward, it is still difficult to maintain low error rates at this scale [2]. To realize the full potential of quantum computing, scalability issues must construct to be fixed. There are also major challenges related to quantum software. Creating useful quantum algorithms for particular applications is still a challenging task. It is necessary for there to be quantum compilers capable of effectively translating high-level quantum languages of programming into machine-level instructions. There are extra difficulties when integrating quantum as well as classical systems, especially with regard to software integration and system architecture.

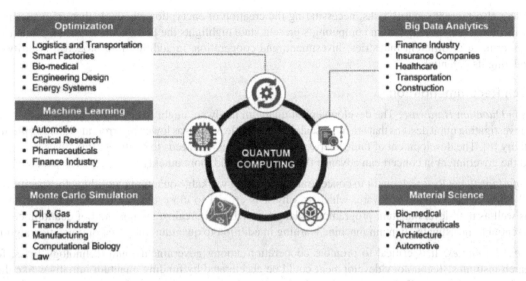

Fig. 24.1 Quantum computing

1.5 Insights and Recommendations for Future Research and Industry Adoption

The knowledge gathered from this study will have a significant impact on quantum computing in the years to come. The examination of the current state of quantum computing yields important suggestions for future study as well as commercial adoption. It is important for researchers to keep working on developing quantum hardware, investigating novel qubit configurations, as well as improving error correction methods [3]. Among other places, Google's Quantum AI lab is actively pursuing lowering qubit errors and promoting qubit connectivity. Making hardware development investments is essential to utilizing quantum computing to its fullest. Encouraging partnerships while offering resources for quantum research is crucial for industry adoption. Large tech companies and governments are investing heavily in quantum initiatives [4]. For example, the €1 billion European Quantum Flagship program seeks to expedite the development of quantum technologies. The democratization of the utilization of quantum computing is additionally gaining momentum. IBM has made its quantum processors available for cloud access, facilitating more extensive experimentation as well as application development [5]. It is critical that ethical and security issues are addressed.

Table 24.1 Insights and recommendations for future research

Insights	Recommendations
Quantum hardware advancements, qubit innovation, error correction improvements	Continued focus on advancing quantum hardware.
	Encourage exploration of innovative qubit designs.
	Invest in reducing qubit errors and increasing connectivity.
	Foster collaborations and provide resources for quantum research.
	Support substantial investments in quantum initiatives by governments and technology giants.
	Promote accessibility with cloud-based quantum computing resources.
	Prioritize the development and adoption of post-quantum cryptography standards.

1.6 Critical Evaluation

The thorough analysis of current developments, real-world applications, difficulties, as well as suggestions in the area of quantum computing highlights both its enormous promise and impending difficulties. Recent developments in quantum computer software and hardware have shown that quantum computing is a real technology with transformative potential rather than just a theoretical idea [6]. This progress is exemplified by IBM's improvements in qubit fidelity and Google's achievements in quantum supremacy. However, there are still many obstacles in the way of this progress, mostly in the form of scalability issues, error correction, together with the creation of workable quantum algorithms. These technological obstacles the need constant innovation and research. Quantum computing has enormous practical implications for cryptography, optimization, as well as artificial intelligence [7]. These applications present previously unheard-of chances for productivity and innovation.

They nevertheless also present security risks, necessitating the creation of encryption standards that are resistant to quantum attacks. The critical assessment of quantum computing's present state highlights the fact that it has the potential to completely transform an assortment of different industries. Investment, and cooperation, in addition to a proactive security strategy are essential to realizing its potential.

1.7 Research Recommendation

Improvements in Quantum Hardware: The development of quantum hardware ought to be the primary subject of future study. This includes investigating qubit designs that are more scalable and stable, as well as lowering error rates along with strengthening qubit connectivity [8]. The development of fault-tolerant quantum processors needs to continue. Initiatives involving business, academia, and the government in concert can advance this important field more quickly.

Development of Algorithms: Research ought to concentrate on creating workable quantum algorithms for specific applications. There are still issues with quantum software, which is why it is crucial to close the gap between effective machine-level instructions as well as high-level quantum programming languages. To fully realize the potential of quantum computing, it is going to be essential to investigate quantum machine learning in addition to quantum-enhanced optimization algorithms.

Cooperation and Resources: It is critical to promote cooperation among governments, and technology firms, followed by quantum research institutes. Technology development could be accelerated by funding quantum initiatives like the European Quantum Flagship program [9]. IBM's decision to make its quantum processors accessible through the cloud democratizes quantum computing and makes it easier for researchers and developers to come up with new applications.

1.8 Future Work

Prospective research in quantum computing ought to persist in investigating hardware innovations, with a particular emphasis on qubit stability, error correction, as well as scalability. The development of algorithms needs to take into account real-world applications, bridging the gap between effective execution and high-level quantum programming [10]. To accelerate research and development, collaboration between governments, businesses, in addition to academic institutions should be encouraged.

2. Literature Review

2.1 Recent Breakthroughs in Quantum Computing Technology

Recent developments in quantum computing have revolutionized the field and made substantial advancements in both the hardware and software domains. Notable advancements in hardware consist of the creation of more stable quantum processors along with high-fidelity qubits. For example, Google's "Sycamore" quantum processor attained quantum supremacy in 2021 by outperforming classical supercomputers in a particular task [4]. Furthermore, IBM has achieved advancements in scalability as well as error rates with its 65-qubit Hummingbird processor. Software-wise, quantum algorithms have progressed: Grover's unstructured database search algorithm followed by Shor's integer factorization algorithm both show great promise. Additionally, improved user interfaces and software platforms have made it possible for researchers and programmers to experiment with quantum programming, such as Microsoft's Quantum Development

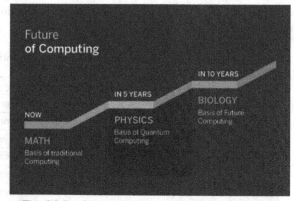

Fig. 24.2 Quantum computing: Future prospects

Kit and IBM's Qiskit [5]. These developments suggest that quantum computing may be able to solve complicated problems with greater speed than its classical equivalent. They also highlight the difficulties in preserving qubit coherence and coping with error rates, which are still major problems in the field.

2.2 Practical Applications and Real-World Implications of Quantum Computing

Quantum computing's real-world implications and practical applications are spreading quickly throughout a number of industries. In the field of cryptography, traditional encryption techniques have been jeopardized by quantum computing. For example, Shor's algorithm is capable of factoring big numbers quickly, which could jeopardize the security of popular encryption standards like RSA [6]. The National Institute of Standards and Technology, or NIST for short, launched a post-quantum cryptography project aimed at developing encryption standards that are resistant to quantum emulation in order to combat this. Another important domain where quantum computing shines is optimization problems. Applications in supply chain management, finance, as well as logistics, have been made using D-Wave's quantum annealers in addition to quantum-inspired algorithms, which show promise for large efficiency gains [7]. Volkswagen, for example, reduced travel time by 20% by optimizing traffic flow in Lisbon through the use of quantum computing. Quantum computing has the potential for speeding up machine learning algorithms in artificial intelligence. To improve pattern recognition and data analysis, researchers are looking into quantum Boltzmann machines, quantum neural networks, in addition to quantum support vector machines [8]. These uses demonstrate the way quantum computing has the potential to revolutionize cryptography, and optimization, alongside artificial intelligence.

2.3 Challenges and Limitations in Quantum Computing

Although very promising, quantum computing has a lot of obstacles and restrictions the require it to be overcome in order to reach its full potential. Quantum error correction is one of the main challenges. Due to their high sensitivity to noise in the environment and ease of decoherence, qubits can lead to computation errors. Surface codes are examples of quantum error correction codes that try to lessen this problem [9]. The goal of research by top producers of quantum hardware, which include IBM and Rigetti, is to produce quantum processors that can withstand faults. Scalability presents another challenge. Increasing the qubit count is necessary to solve complicated issues, but it's a difficult undertaking. With 65 qubits, IBM's Quantum Hummingbird is a step forward, but error rates must continue to be lowered. Challenges related to quantum software still exist, which include the requirement for improved quantum compilers as well as quantum algorithms for useful tasks. Another integration challenge is integrating quantum and classical systems [10]. The potential of quantum computing is evident despite these drawbacks. Google's demonstrations of supremacy in quantum technology and other developments suggest that quantum computing is no longer science fiction but rather a field with significant potential for growth.

2.4 Insights and Recommendations for Future Research and Industry Adoption

Future directions for quantum computing show a landscape full of opportunities and obstacles that must be overcome. More attention is being paid by researchers to developing quantum hardware, investigating novel qubit configurations, and enhancing error correction methods. As an example, increasing qubit connectivity and lowering qubit errors are top priorities for Google's Quantum AI lab. The focus of industry adoption recommendations is on promoting cooperation and offering resources for quantum research. Large sums of money are being made investments in quantum initiatives by governments and tech companies. With a €1 billion budget, the European Quantum Flagship program is required to expedite the development of quantum technologies. IBM has democratized access to quantum computing by making its quantum processors available on the cloud, which is encouraging. Furthermore, it is critical to address security and ethical issues. The necessity for post-quantum cryptography standards has been emphasized by the possibility that widely used encryption techniques could potentially be broken by quantum computing. Research on quantum-safe encryption is a rapidly expanding field.

REFERENCES

1. Gertig, C., Leonhard, K. and Bardow, A., 2020. Computer-aided molecular and processes design based on quantum chemistry: current status and future prospects. *Current Opinion in Chemical Engineering*, 27, pp.89-97.
2. Altman, E., Brown, K.R., Carleo, G., Carr, L.D., Demler, E., Chin, C., DeMarco, B., Economou, S.E., Eriksson, M.A., Fu, K.M.C. and Greiner, M., 2021. Quantum simulators: Architectures and opportunities. *PRX Quantum*, 2(1), p.017003.
3. Song, M.K., Kang, J.H., Zhang, X., Ji, W., Ascoli, A., Messaris, I., Demirkol, A.S., Dong, B., Aggarwal, S., Wan, W. and Hong, S.M., 2023. Recent advances and future prospects for memristive materials, devices, and systems. *ACS nano*, 17(13), pp.11994-12039.
4. Dunjko, V. and Wittek, P., 2020. A non-review of quantum machine learning: trends and explorations. *Quantum Views*, 4, p.32.
5. Lavecchia, A., 2019. Deep learning in drug discovery: opportunities, challenges and future prospects. *Drug discovery today*, 24(10), pp. 2017–2032.
6. Fernández-Caramés, T.M., 2019. From pre-quantum to post-quantum IoT security: A survey on quantum-resistant cryptosystems for the Internet of Things. *IEEE Internet of Things Journal*, 7(7), pp.6457-6480.
7. Zhang, Y. and Ni, Q., 2020. Recent advances in quantum machine learning. *Quantum Engineering*, 2(1), p.e34.
8. Motta, M. and Rice, J.E., 2022. Emerging quantum computing algorithms for quantum chemistry. *Wiley Interdisciplinary Reviews: Computational Molecular Science*, 12(3), p.e1580.
9. Mangini, S., Tacchino, F., Gerace, D., Bajoni, D. and Macchiavello, C., 2021. Quantum computing models for artificial neural networks. *Europhysics Letters*, 134(1), p.10002.
10. S. Ram Prasath, K.Gokulakrishnan, M.Subramanian, N.Mohan, "Location based Context Awareness with Multipoint Transmission by ELAML Algorithm" IEEE Access, DOI: 10.1109/ICAIS56108.2023.10073864.

Emerging Trends in IoT and Computing Technologies – Suman Lata Tripathi et al. (eds)
© 2024 Taylor & Francis Group, London, ISBN 978-1-032-87924-6

An Analytical Study on the Most Advanced Methods for Mining Big Data Through Data Mining

25

Sanjay Kumar Sonkar[1]
Research Scholar,
Sunrise University, Dept. of Computer Science and Engineering, Alwar, Rajasthan, India

Balkar Singh[2]
Assistant Professor
Sunrise University, Dept. of Computer Science and Engineering, Alwar, Rajasthan, India

Abstract: In the age of Big Data, where vast volumes of information are generated daily, the need for efficient data mining techniques is paramount. The analysis of the latest and most advanced data mining techniques tailored for handling Big Data is provided in this study in a comprehensive manner. Through our research, we aim to uncover cutting-edge methodologies that can extract valuable insights, patterns, and knowledge from large, complex datasets. By examining the latest innovations in data mining, our goal is to improve our understanding of how these techniques can be applied effectively in Big Data analytics.

Keywords: Big data, Data processing, Data mining, Machine learning, Predictive modeling

1. Introduction

Big data is an enormous amount of data that is gathered from many sources, such as social networking sites, corporate transactions, scientific research, sensor networks, and resource sharing. Large-volume datasets are known as big data. Big data encompasses vast amounts of information generated by social media platforms, commercial deals, research projects, and sensor networks, and resource sharing, among other sources. It presents challenges for traditional software due to its high volume and complex variety. Gartner introduced the 3Vs concept—Velocity, Variety, and Volume—to describe big data. Velocity refers to the rapid rate at which data flows, such as streaming data from weather reports. Variety represents the diverse categories of information: semi-structured, unstructured, and structured —ranging from business transactions to images and videos. Volume signifies the sheer scale of data that exceeds conventional storage and processing capacities.

Additionally, there's a growing recognition of other characteristics such as veracity, which pertains to the uncertainty or noise in data, making it challenging for traditional software to analyze. Veracity becomes a concern for decision-making due to the presence of unreliable, unstructured data like some social network posts.

In Fig. 25.1, the depiction demonstrates the primary features of Big Data: high volume, high variance, and high velocity. These characteristics are inherent in various techniques that generate large-scale data. The fields of Big Data analysis encompass:

(a) Structured data   (b) Text data   (c) Web data

(d) Multimedia data   (e) Network data   (f) Mobile data

[1]sanjaykumarsonkar@gmail.com, [2]balkarsingh05@gmail.com

DOI: 10.1201/9781003535423-25

Various methods employed in Big Data mining and analysis include cluster analysis, factor analysis, regression analysis, crowd-sourcing, and classification analysis, as outlined by (Chen, Mao, and Liu, 2014). These methods play a significant role in handling and extracting insights from large and diverse datasets. Big data characteristics and specific technologies are mentioned in Table 25.1

Table 25.1 Big data characteristics and specific technologies

Big data characteristics	Property	Big data technologies
Velocity	Fast Processing	MapReduce
Variety	Heterogeneous	HBase, MongoDB, CouchDB
Volume	Knowledge discovery	Mahout, GNU-R

2. Big Data Technologies

Traditional technologies are very effective for small-scale data. It has provided proven accuracy and results for centralized systems.

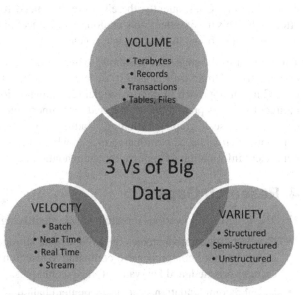

Fig. 25.1 3 Vs of big data (Chen, Mao and Liu, 2014)

It is not in the capability scope of these technologies to deal with very large-scale data. There is a need for novel innovations and techniques to deal with Big data. Structured data, which is in the form of rows and columns, is also semi-structured data, such as log files, and unstructured data (data in the form of image files) can be processed effectively by Big Data tools like MapReduce and Hadoop (Dean and Ghemawat, 2008), Mahout, R, HBase, Graph Lab, Giraph, Tensor Flow and Cassandra. These technologies help organizations to efficiently store, large-scale process data and work as decision support systems. The advantages of these technologies are working in a distributed platform with less response time and better accuracy. Some of the most prevalent Big data technologies are mentioned as follows:

2.1 Hadoop and Map Reduce

Hadoop stands as an open-source framework designed to enable the simultaneous execution of programs across distributed nodes. Also, it gives access to distributed storage by means of the Hadoop Distributed File System.

In the paper authored by Chen, Chiang, and Storey in 2012, they highlighted the dependency of Business Intelligence and Analytics (BIA) on technologies related to data collection, extraction, and analysis. They emphasized the importance of ETL (Extraction, Transformation, and Load) processes in facilitating effective data analysis within the realm of BIA.

Modern big data methods are examined in this study. A thorough analysis is conducted on big data techniques including cloud computing and machine learning. The steps in the big data value chain_generation, collection, storage, and analysis—are described..Big data visualization is one of the most significant decision making process which is not mentioned in this work. Reports and regression curves are needed to visualize data analysis results.

Table 25.2 Qualitative and quantitative comparative analysis

Qualitative	Quantitative
Complete and elaborate	Specific and model based
It is useful during early phase of	It is useful during last phase of
It is subjective	It is objective
Expertise is required to understand the results	Specific knowledge is required to understand the
Words and images are	Numbers and models are

3. Need for Study

Big data refers to the vast amount of information generated from social networking site interactions, sensor networks, and economic transactions. Due to its sheer scale, traditional tools and techniques are inadequate for storing and processing such data efficiently. Consequently, there's a pressing need for innovative approaches capable of handling large-scale data more effectively. This thesis extensively explores storage techniques for managing big data, highlighting the limitations of traditional relational data storage in handling heterogeneous large-scale data.

This paper uses the suggested technique to overcome these problems. One key component that enhances social recommendation is social trust. Direct trust is used by several researchers but improvement in recommendation is not significant. Indirect trust is used in our approach to improve social recommendation. Transitive closure and hyper edge is used to use direct as well as indirect trust. It is proved that trust based recommendation technique improves sparsity and cold start. Scalability is improved by using large scale graph partitioning. Traditional graph partitioning uses random partitioning based on similarity score, but in our approach trust based partitioning is used which improves locality. Furthermore, deep learning model is applied on user and item latent information to improve recommendation accuracy.

4. Research Gaps

This thesis delves into various research works, identifying critical gaps within existing literature:

- Existing comparative studies on NoSQL data storage for Big Data lack clear applications of these solutions. The need arises for more comprehensive comparative research with a broad focus on areas such as document-based, graph-based, column-oriented, and key-value storage techniques.
- Social recommendation systems encounter challenges related to sparsity, cold start problems, and scalability. These issues require dedicated attention and resolution within the research.
- Processing large social graphs on centralized systems proves inefficient. Partitioning these graphs for distributed processing on clusters becomes essential. Additionally, existing methods suffer from degraded locality, highlighting a significant disadvantage.

5. Research Methodology

This research scrutinizes various studies to identify constraints with social recommendation and typical data mining approaches. The comparison of traditional data mining algorithms centers on response time analysis. To address processing of both numerical and categorical data, the research implements the K-prototype algorithm on MapReduce. Furthermore, enhancements in social recommendation techniques involve the utilization of hyper edges and transitive closure.

The research methodology is structured based on the specific objectives of the study, categorizing approaches accordingly.

5.1 Research Methodology for Objective 1

Objective 1 aims to learning and associate various Large Information storing methods, including column-oriented, document-based, graph-based, and key-value methods. Our research methodology begins by reviewing existing literature to understand their strengths and limitations. Upon comparing multiple research works, it becomes evident that distributed approaches are predominantly utilized for storing Big Data. Researchers have proposed NewSQL and NoSQL as data storage techniques, but a limitation in existing literature is the lack of a comprehensive comparative study based on real solutions of NoSQL data storage techniques. This gap forms the foundation of our research methodology. Our approach involves assessing features like format, storage, flexibility, scalability, and complexity to compare these storage techniques.

5.2 Research Methodology for Objective 2

Objective 3 aims to propose an efficient mining technique for Big Data. The initial step in our research methodology involves understanding the limitations of traditional data mining, which include scalability, sparsity, and efficiency issues with categorical data. These limitations drive the direction of our research methodology.

Newer Big Data mining tools and approaches are used to overcome these constraints. Due to the variety of data types in the Chess dataset, the K-prototype technique is applied to handle both numerical and categorical data. In addition, the K-Prototype technique is used with MapReduce to track response times among various clusters. An "intelligent splitter" is proposed to segregate numerical and categorical data before transmitting to MapReduce, addressing scalability issues related to numerical data. However, sparsity remains a significant challenge in social Big Data, particularly in social recommendation systems where many users don't provide ratings, resulting in sparse matrices. To combat this, a graph-based approach leveraging qualitative trust among users is proposed. Additionally, the research methodology seeks to enhance recommendation accuracy further by employing deep learning. Autoencoder, chosen for its ability to reduce large-scale dimensions, is utilized for improving recommendation systems.

6. Limitations of Study

This study compares NoSQL data storage strategies in four major categories: key-value, column-oriented, document-based, and graph-based. This research includes around 10 genuine solutions for analysis out of the approximately 120 real solutions that are available for NoSQL data storage. One limitation encountered is the absence of a standardized query language for NoSQL data storage. Each real solution employs its specific query language, preventing standardization. For social recommendation, this study proposes a trust-based strategy that makes use of large-scale social graph segmentation. However, the purview of this study does not include an analysis of alternative recommendation strategies, such as group suggestion. Deep learning is employed to enhance social recommendation accuracy using the Auto Encoder model on operator-item and operator-operator trust ratings. Notably, other deep learning models like CNN or RNN are not deployed in this research. Furthermore, activation functions such as tanh and ReLU are not utilized within this study's context.

7. Advanced Data Mining Methods

The study identified a range of cutting-edge data mining methods, including deep learning, ensemble methods, and graph-based algorithms, which have demonstrated remarkable effectiveness in handling and extracting insights from Big Data. The practice of identifying patterns, trends, and insightful information from huge databases is known as data mining. Advanced data mining methods go beyond basic techniques and often involve complex algorithms and models to extract more intricate and specific knowledge from data, making them suitable for addressing challenging data analysis and knowledge discovery tasks.

Classification:

In machine learning, classification is a kind of supervised learning in which a collection of labeled training data is used to predict the class or category of a new observation. Developing a model that can precisely classify incoming observations according to their traits or qualities into one of many predetermined classes is the aim of classification.

Clustering:

Clustering is a method of machine learning that operates without predefined labels and aims to group similar data points according to their inherent traits or patterns. This process involves dividing a dataset into clusters or subsets, where data points within each cluster exhibit higher similarity among themselves than with those in other clusters.

Clustering is used in various domains, including customer segmentation, image segmentation, anomaly detection, and document clustering. It can help in exploratory data analysis, pattern recognition, and making data-driven decisions based on similarities and groupings within the data.

Regression:

In machine learning, regression is a technique for predicting a continuous numerical value based on a set of input features or attributes. The objective of regression is to create a model that can precisely estimate the correlation between the input variables and the output variable.

There are many applications for regression in various fields, such as finance, economics, engineering, and social sciences. It is an important tool for making predictions based on data and can help automate many tasks that require manual estimation by humans.

Sequence and path analysis:

Sequence and path analysis are techniques used in data analysis to study the order or sequence of events or activities in a dataset and understand the relationships or dependencies between them. These techniques are commonly used in fields such as social sciences, marketing, bioinformatics, and web analytics.

Sequence analysis focuses on analyzing sequences of events or states over time. It involves examining the patterns, transitions, and durations of events within a sequence. This technique is useful for understanding the temporal dynamics and ordering of events. Path analysis is a statistical technique used to study the causal relationships between variables in a dataset. It aims to understand the direct and indirect effects of variables on an outcome variable through a series of intermediate variables. Path analysis is based on structural equation modeling (SEM) and graphical modeling approaches.

Data mining has opened up a sea of possibilities for companies by allowing them to improve and work on their bottom lines by identifying patterns and trends in business data. Mining techniques benefit every industry vertical, from retail, finance, manufacturing, insurance, and healthcare, to the entertainment and academic sectors.

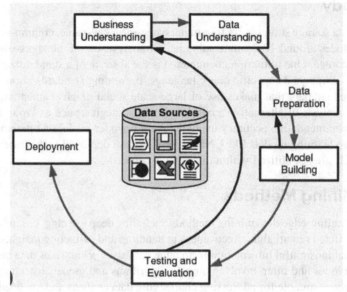

Fig. 25.2 Advanced data mining methods

Scalability and Efficiency:

Scalability was a primary concern in the context of Big Data. Results show that advanced techniques, such as distributed computing frameworks like Hadoop and Spark, play a pivotal role in efficiently processing large datasets, ensuring faster analysis and knowledge extraction.

Real-time Data Mining:

In addition, the study pointed out the increasing significance of real-time data mining. Stream processing and online analytical processing techniques were deemed crucial for analyzing data as it is generated, enabling organizations to respond quickly to changing conditions. The raw data, data mining, customisation, personalization, automation, and real-time analytics are all shown in Fig. 25.2. The practice of discovering insightful patterns and useful insights from streaming or continually changing data in real-time is known as real-time data mining. It involves analyzing large volumes of data as they are generated and making decisions or taking actions based on the results. Real-time data mining requires specialized tools and technologies that can handle the unique characteristics of streaming data. These include distributed processing frame- works like Apache Spark or Flink, real-time databases like Apache Cassandra or MongoDB, and real-time visualization tools like Tableau or Kibana.

8. Conclusion

In the realm of Big Data, where massive datasets are continuously generated, our analytical study on the most advanced techniques for data mining has shed light on the remarkable capabilities and significance of these methods. This conclusion encapsulates the key takeaways from our research. Advanced data mining techniques played a crucial role in addressing the challenges posed by Big Data, as highlighted in the study. These techniques have proved to be crucial in the pursuit of valuable insights, patterns, and knowledge hidden within the vast and complex data landscapes. The analytical study concludes by stating that advanced data mining techniques are essential for extracting valuable insights and knowledge from the constantly growing world of Big Data. Their application provides a competitive advantage, encourages innovation, and empowers decision-makers in various industries. As Big Data advances, these advanced techniques will continue to be at the forefront of harnessing its potential for the benefit of businesses and society as a whole.

REFERENCES

1. Big Data has Big Potential to Improve Americans Lives, Increase Eco- nomic Opportunities, and Committee on Science, Space and Technology (April 2013). URL http://science.house.gov/press-release

2. Iosup, A. Lascateu, N. Tapus, CAMEO: Enabling social networks for Massively Multiplayer Online Games through Continuous Analytics and Cloud Computing, in: Proceedings of the 9th Annual Workshop on Network and Systems Support for Games (NetGames 2010), 2010, pp. 1–6.

3. McAfee, E. Brynjolfsson, Big Data: The Management Revolution, Harvard Business Review (2012) 60–68.

4. Thusoo, Z. Shao, S. Anthony, D. Borthakur, N. Jain, J. S. Sarma, R. Murthy, H. Liu, Data warehousing and analytics infrastructure at Facebook, in: Proceedings of the 2010 international conference on Management of data, ACM, New York, NY, USA, 2010, pp. 1013–1020.

5. Adnaan Arbaaz Ahmed, Dr.M.I.Thariq Hussan, "CLOUD COM- PUTING: STUDY OF SECURITY ISSUESANDRESEARCHCHAL-LENGES," International Journal Of Advanced Research In Computer Engineering Technology (IJARCET) Volume 7, Issue 4, April 2018, ISSN: 2278 – 1323.

6. Akhil KM, Kumar MP, Pushpa BR. Enhanced Cloud Data Security Using AES Algorithm. In Intelligent Computing And Control (I2C2), International Conference On 2017 (Pp. 1-5). IEEE.

7. Albert Greenberg, James Hamilton, David A. Maltz and Parveen Pate, "The Cost of a Cloud: Research Problems in Data Center Networks", Microsoft Research, Redmond, WA, USA.

8. Aman Bakshi and Yogesh B, "Securing cloud from DDOS Attacks using Intrusion Detection System in Virtual Machine", 2010 Second International Conference on Communication Software and Networks, IEEE,2010.

9. Amanpreet Chauhan, Gaurav Mishra, and Gulshan Kumar, "Survey on Data Mining Techniques in Intrusion Detection", International Journal of Scientific Engineering Research Volume 2, Issue 7, July-2011.

10. Amanpreet Chauhan, Gaurav Mishra, and Gulshan Kumar, "Survey on Data Mining Techniques in Intrusion Detection", International Journal of Scientific Engineering Research Volume 2, Issue 7, July-2011.

11. Anil Kuvvarapu "Data Mining On Cloud-Based Big Data" Cybernetics, Cognition And Machine Learning Applications (Pp.51-59) 2020.

12. Anish Gupta "Security Measures In Data Mining" I.J. Information Engineering And Electronic Business, 2012, 3, 34-39.

13. Anupama Prasanth, "Cloud Computing Services: A Survey," Interna- tional Journal Of Computer Applications (0975 – 8887) Volume 46–No.3, May 2012.

14. Arjun Kumar, HoonJae Lee, and Rajeev Pratap Singh, "Efficient and Secure Cloud Storage for Handling Big", Data, Information Science and Service Science and Data Mining (ISSDM), 2012.

15. Bangxu Ding "The construction of internet data mining model based on cloud computing"Journal of Intelligent and Fuzzy Systems 37(12):1-9 2019

16. Bhaludra R. Nadh Singh "A Review On Big Data Mining In Cloud Computing" Innovations In Computer Science And Engineering Pp 131- 142 2017.

17. Bhisham C. Gupta "On Data Mining" Statistics And Probability With Applications For Engineers And Scientists Using MINITAB, R And JMP (Pp.476-517) 2020.

18. Brian Hay "Storm Clouds Rising: Security Challenges For Iaas Cloud Computing" 44th Hawaii International International Conference On Systems Science (HICSS-44 2011), Proceedings, 4-7 January 2011

19. Fisher, R. DeLine, M. Czerwinski, S. Drucker, Interactions with Big Data Analytics, Interactions 19 (3) (2012) 50–59.

Emerging Trends in IoT and Computing Technologies – Suman Lata Tripathi et al. (eds)
© 2024 Taylor & Francis Group, London, ISBN 978-1-032-87924-6

Evaluation of Transfer Learning Models for Maize Leaf Disease Identification and Classification

26

Pawan Singh[1], Priya Khichi[2]
Central University of Rajasthan,
Department of Computer Science, Ajmer, India

Abstract: Plant diseases pose a significant danger to global food security by reducing farmer output and causing an economic crisis. Timely and precise illness identification is critical for immediate treatment. The paper presents extensive research on the application of algorithms based on transfer learning for identification and cataloging of diseases of maize crops using images of plant leaves. In this paper, to improve model generalization, data preprocessing approaches including image augmentation and normalization were used. An investigation was conducted to determine the effect of transfer learning from trained models on the accuracy of disease classification. Using comprehensive datasets covering different maize diseases like common rust, grey leaf, northern blight, and bacterial blight, these models were painstakingly trained and fine-tuned. Our major findings show that transfer learning models, especially ResNet18 and InceptionV3, perform better than conventional techniques. High accuracy rates with ResNet18, InceptionV3, and VGG16 on the maize datasets show the promise of transfer learning for plant disease identifications. Implementation of transfer learning models for recognizing plant diseases can result in early disease identification, allowing for prompt intervention and lowering crop losses.

Keywords: Plant diseases, Deep learning, DenseNet121, InceptionV3, ResNet18, VGG16

1. Introduction

Agricultural production, the foundation of human survival, is continually threatened by plant diseases. It threatens food security and can lead to substantial yield losses. To manage and mitigate these diseases effectively, a timely and accurate diagnosis is essential. Plant diseases pose serious risks to crop output and quality, whether they are brought on by pathogens, environmental causes, or nutrient imbalances. These illnesses have the capacity to destroy harvests, resulting in food shortages and financial losses [1]. They also promote the careless use of fungicides and pesticides, which are harmful to both ecosystems and human beings [2]. The key to tackling these issues is accurately identifying and classifying plant diseases. An early diagnosis of unhealthy plants allows for targeted interventions rather than a general pesticide application, which minimizes environmental harm [3]. Additionally, it gives farmers the ability to put policies like confinement, crop rotation, and efficient resource allocation into place. In many agricultural regions, traditional methods of disease diagnosis are labor-intensive, time-consuming, and may require expertise that is not readily available [4]. Thus, there is a growing interest in developing automated and efficient disease detection systems based on technological advancements [5]. Machine learning subset transfer learning has established remarkable accomplishment with various computer vision tasks, including image cataloging and object recognition [6]. Transfer learning's implementation in the field of identifying and categorizing plant diseases is both necessary and revolutionary. Convolutional Neural Networks (CNNs) have demonstrated amazing ability in image processing and pattern recognition. They are excellent

[1]pawan.singh@curaj.ac.in, [2]khichipriya99@gmail.com

DOI: 10.1201/9781003535423-26

at capturing fine details in pictures, which makes them suitable for the delicate and nuanced distinctions frequently needed in plant disease identification [7]. Transfer learning could outperform conventional approaches, which frequently rely on hand-crafted characteristics and may struggle with the inherent complexity of plant pathology. This potential for improvement is what drives the use of Transfer learning [8]. Our goal is to use Transfer learning to take advantage of neural networks' ability to automatically learn distinguishing features from plant photos, improving the reliability and accuracy of disease diagnosis. It has become increasingly prevalent nowadays as a technique for detecting and categorizing plant diseases [9]. Using deep neural networks, images of plant leaves can be analyzed automatically, disease symptoms identified, and the disease type categorized [10]. This manuscript uses transfer learning techniques to perceive and categorize diseases in maize plants to contribute to agriculture and plant disease management. To assist farmers and agricultural experts in identifying and diagnosing diseases in important crops, we intend to develop accurate and reliable disease detection models. In turn, this will lead to more effective and timely interventions, potentially increasing crop yields and quality.

1.1 Problem Definition

The complex junction of agriculture and technology poses an enticing challenge: the rapid and precise identification and classification of plant diseases. This problem has worldwide ramifications because it jeopardizes food security, reduces agricultural production, and exacerbates economic vulnerabilities [11]. Traditional disease identification approaches, which rely on manual observation, have shortcomings, resulting in delayed reactions and significant crop losses [10]. As a result, this manuscript embarks on a transformative journey to close this critical gap by leveraging the capabilities of advanced deep learning techniques, specifically CNNs, InceptionV3, Densenet121, Vgg16/Vgg19, and ResNet18, for the recognition and categorization of a variety of diseases affecting maize plants. The complicated variety of diseases under investigation serves as more evidence of this issue's complexity. The range includes common rust, grey leaf, and northern blight in maize [5]. Every disease has distinct visual symptoms and clinical dynamics, which adds to the general difficulty of developing a thorough classification system. The existing reliance on conventional techniques hinders the potential for data-driven agricultural management and creates a barrier to prompt action [9].

The paper has two aims, firstly construct and improve a collection of deep learning models, including CNN, InceptionV3, Densenet121, Vgg16, Vgg19, and ResNet18. These algorithms will surpass human limits to quickly and accurately identify the intricate details hidden within the photos of affected leaves [12]. The second aims to find the accurate algorithm for the maize dataset. This paper aims to bridge the gap between agriculture and technology. By combining the analytical ability of deep learning with the practical realities of crop management, it responds to the urgent global challenge for food security [3]. The result is expected to result in improved disease detection accuracy as well as the democratization of this cutting-edge technology in the areas where it is most needed. Through this manuscript, an important step is made toward a future in which technology supports livelihoods, nurtures crops, and increases the resilience of the world's food supply [13].

1.2. Problem Objective

Worldwide food security can not be assured without controlling the crop diseases which are a major threat in the agricultural sector. Conventional disease detection and classification approaches have proven ineffective, resulting in significant crop losses, and jeopardizing the stability of our food supply [4]. This work sets out on a mission to address this essential issue by leveraging the power of cutting-edge transfer learning algorithms [14]. This endeavor's main goals are diverse, spanning both technological improvements and real-world applicability.

Enhanced Detection and Classification

Objective of this manuscript is to develop a reliable and precise system for the recognition and classification of maize crop diseases. This manuscript seeks to greatly improve the accuracy and effectiveness of disease identification by utilizing the capabilities of CNNs, InceptionV3, Densenet121, Vgg16, Vgg19, and ResNet18. It aims to equip farmers and stakeholders with a tool capable of accurately identifying illnesses by painstakingly training these neural networks on large datasets spanning common rust, grey leaf, northern blight, bacterial blight, curl virus, and fusarium wilt.

Multi-Architecture Framework

Investigating the effectiveness of a wide variety of transfer learning models in maize crop disease recognition and classification is another crucial goal. The study aims to identify the advantages and disadvantages of each model in treating diseases by combining multiple neural network topologies [6]. This comparative analysis will help to create a more thorough disease management strategy by enabling a thorough grasp of the nuances and intricacies of various plant diseases.

Empowering Agriculture

The ultimate goal is to arm the agricultural sector with a strong tool to combat the scourge of plant diseases. The initiative attempts to democratize technical innovation by utilizing deep learning [13]. Increased food security, less crop losses, and educated decision-making are all results of this empowerment. The manuscript aims to create a resilient and sustainable agricultural ecosystem by laying the groundwork for a future in which innovation, technology, and agriculture coexist together [2].

This paper discusses the methodology employed, including the selection of Transfer learning architectures, data preparation, training, and evaluation procedures. The authors have presented the results obtained from the developed models for real-world agriculture. This manuscript is systematized into five sections as follows: Literature review of this manuscript is represented in section 2. Material and method is represented in section 3 along with the collection and preprocessing of the dataset, design, and training procedure of transfer learning models. Results are discussed in section 4. The study is concluded in section 5.

2. Literature Review

In this section, various deep learning-based existing schemes have been reviewed. In 2023, Moupojou et al. [5] introduced the "FieldPlant" dataset, which is a useful tool for plant disease detection research. The dataset of field plant photos provided by the authors makes it easier to test and create deep-learning models for disease classification. The author suggests using the dataset FieldPlant, which contains 5,170 photos of plant diseases that were gathered directly from plantations. To guarantee procedure quality, each image's individual leaves were manually annotated under the direction of plant pathologists. In total, 8,629 distinct leaves from the 27 disease classes were annotated. Modern classification and object identification models were evaluated using a variety of benchmarks on this dataset, and discovered that FieldPlant performed better for classification tasks than PlantDoc. In 2022, Rimon et al. [9] introduced "PlantBuddy," an Android-based mobile software for identifying plant diseases. This programme gives users a usable tool for quickly identifying plant diseases with smartphone cameras by utilizing deep CNN. Deep CNN used by the proposed disease detection model analyses an input image of a plant leaf to detect and identify the disease. A sizable dataset of 54,305 pictures, representing 14 distinct species and 26 diseases, was used to train the model.

In 2022, Wagle et al. [14] presented the compact convolutional neural network models for plant leaf categorization. The authors present cutting-edge CNN architectures designed for rapid and precise disease diagnosis. In this study, it is suggested that nine plant species from the Plant Village dataset be identified and categorized using newly built compact CNN and AlexNet with transfer learning. Utilizing various data augmentations, plant leaf data are used to train the models. A considerable boost in classification accuracy is revealed by the data augmentation. The Flavia dataset's 12 classes are categorized using the proposed models as well. 99.45% of the suggested developed NI model's classifications are accurate. Classification accuracy for the N2 model is 99.65%. For the PlantVillage dataset, the classification accuracy of the N3 model is 99.55%, and that of AlexNet is 99.73%. The proposed models require less training time and are more condensed than AlexNet.

In 2019, Sibiya et al. [13] used computational methods for identifying and categorizing maize leaf diseases. CNNs are used by the authors to distinguish among sick and healthy maize leaves. This study employs CNN-assisted principles to model a network for illness image detection and categorization. A CNN network that detected and categorized photos of the maize crop diseases that were obtained using a smartphone camera was trained using Neuroph. To hasten the quick and simple adoption of the system in practice, a fresh training method and methodology were employed. Three maize leaf diseases were distinguished by the created model from healthy leaves. The diseases that were chosen for this investigation were the northern maize leaf blight, grey leaf spot, and common rust as they are prevalent throughout Southern Europe. In 2021, Wang et al. [10] utilized single-branch neural networks or conventional computer vision approaches. However, these techniques might have trouble correctly identifying complex disease patterns. This paper proposes a revolutionary Multi-Branch ResNet-18 architecture to close this gap. This development is expected to improve crop disease recognition's accuracy and robustness, constituting a significant advancement in the field of disease detection in agriculture. In 2022, Fraiwan et al. [2] applied transfer learning to retrieve pertinent information for disease categorization from pre-trained models. The authors concluded that this method works for precisely detecting different maize diseases, which helps to improve disease management in agriculture. This study demonstrates the potential of transfer learning in resolving problems in the agricultural domain and is in line with the trend of utilizing deep learning techniques for improved disease recognition.

In 2023, Sunil et al. [6] studied various deep learning architectures and methodologies to see how well they handle the difficulties of diagnosing plant diseases accurately and quickly. It considers 160 different research papers. A total of 103 publications and about 57 investigations focused on a single plant. The author covered 50 different plant leaf disease datasets, including both openly accessible and closed databases. The different difficulties and knowledge gaps in plant disease detection are also covered in this study. Additionally, this work emphasized the significance of hyperparameters in deep learning. In 2022, K et al. [12] used CNNs to categorize and identify different diseases that damage apple leaves. This research advances the field of agricultural disease detection and shows how fast and precise plant disease identification is possible using deep learning. In 2020, Bhanusri [8] used a dataset of photos of maize leaves to train a CNN model to categorize and identify various diseases. Although the study's exact findings are not presented here, by examining the potential of deep learning approaches for precise and effective disease identification in maize crops, it is anticipated to have a positive impact on the field of agricultural disease detection. It is quite helpful to look for obvious characteristics like shape, size, dryness, and wilting to identify the status of the plant. In 2018, Kranth et al. [1] covered all the features, which use a variety of machine learning techniques to determine the results. Decision trees, the Naive Bayes theorem, artificial neural networks, k-mean clustering, and random forest methods are all covered in the research.

In 2020, Shrestha et al. [15] developed a potato disease identification model using CNN. This model was given a total of 15 instances, twelve of which were sick plant leaves and three of which were healthy. Test accuracy was calculated to be 88.80%. In 2022, Saritha et al. [16] developed a model to find leaf diseases. Three distinct models; AlexNet, MobileNet, and Inception V3 were used for training and examined for the computational complexity, precision, and performance metric parameters. According to the findings, Inception V3's computing cost is between MobileNet and AlexNet. Additionally, it was evident from the data that Inception V3 had a greater accuracy rate of 99.04% and superior performance metrics than the other two models. The Inception V3's computational cost was in between AlexNet and MobileNet.

3. Material and Methods

This section contains various sub-sections such as the datasets for maize proposed methodology used in this manuscript. These subsequent sections provide an overview of the datasets used and their specifications, the manner in which the proposed methods work, as well as the proposed method was carried out into practice.

Dataset Overview

The availability of extensive and varied datasets is vital for the development of transfer learning models. The following datasets were used:

PlantVillage Dataset

To train the model, 54,305 photos of plant leaves from a public dataset are used. The dataset was generated by PlantVillage and is accessible through Kaggle [5]. The photos have a 256x256 pixel resolution. JPEG format is used to save the photographs. With an 80%-20% train-validation split, the model will be trained on 43,456 photos and validated on 10,849 images. Images of 26 distinct diseases and 14 different crop types can be found in the dataset [17]. 1192 images of Common Rust, 985 images of Northern Blight, 513 images of Grey Leaf Spot, and 1162 images of Healthy maize plant were selected from the PlantVillage dataset as mentioned in Fig. 26.1.

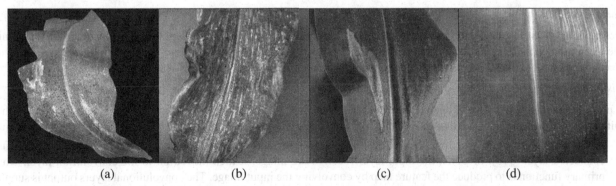

(a)   (b)   (c)   (d)

Fig. 26.1   Maize dataset images (a) Common Rust (b) Grey Leaf Spot (c) Northern Blight (d) Healthy [17]

3.2 Proposed Method

This section presents the details and working of proposed methods used for maize plant disease identification and classification.

Flowchart Diagram

The plant disease recognition and cataloging system involves several transfer learning models. Figure 26.2 depicts the architecture of the system in several steps as follows:

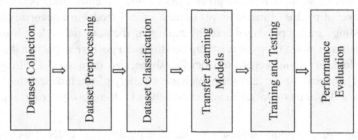

Fig. 26.2 Flowchart of proposed method

Dataset Preprocessing

In the process of preprocessing a dataset, many operations are carried out, including scaling photos to a uniform size, normalizing the pixel values, and enhancing the data by applying transformations like rotations and flips [6]. This transforms the dataset into a format that is standardized and appropriate for deep learning model training.

(a) *Rotations:* To imitate changes in image orientation, randomly rotate images by a predetermined angle (for example, 90 degrees or 180 degrees) [8]. Make sure the rotation angle is chosen at random from a predetermined range.

(b) *Flips:* Apply flips to images that have a particular frequency, both horizontally and vertically. This replicates changes in the image's object's direction. Vertical flips reverse the image from top to bottom, and horizontal flips reverse it from left to right [18]. Figure 26.3 depicts the preprocessing by using a flip horizontal and rotation operation on the maize leaf.

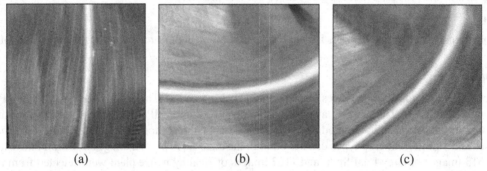

| (a) | (b) | (c) |

Fig. 26.3 Augmented images (a) Original(zoom) (b) Flip horizontal (width) (c) Rotation (Height)

Dataset Classification

Maize plant datasets are categorized into different classes train, test, and validation. Through this labeling, the transfer learning models can train on patterns and features specific to each disease class [9].70% of images are being classified into training and 20% of the images are classified into the validation and the remaining 10% are used for the testing [7].

Transfer Learning Models

The proposed method makes use of deep learning models like CNN, Densenet121, InceptionV3, Vgg16, and ResNet18. These architectures are made up of layers that take input photos and learn hierarchical features. Each model has a distinct architecture.

(a) *CNN:* The CNNs consist of five layers: "an input layer, convolution layer, activation layer, pooling layer, and fully connected layer" [13]. In CNN, the input layer receives the image. It then moved on to the convolution layer, whose primary function is to produce the feature map by convolving the input image. The convolutional layers output is supplied to the nonlinear function after being down-sampled. An activation function that introduces nonlinearity is the activation layer [9]. The pooling layer uses a predetermined sliding window approach to send values to the following layers while taking into account various pooling, such as maximum pooling, minimum pooling, and average pooling. The image will be flattened after the pooling layer and input into the SoftMax classifier to produce the outcome. Hidden layer is another name for the fully connected layer [13].

(b) *DenseNet121:* A deep learning architecture called DenseNet-121 is intended for image classification applications. Dense connectivity between layers, bottleneck layers for efficiency, and global average pooling rather than fully connected layers are some of its important characteristics. It contains 121 layers [3]. This architecture encourages feature reuse, lessens vanishing gradients, and uses parameters effectively.

(c) *InceptionV3:* InceptionV3 is excellent at capturing features at many levels of abstraction, which makes it useful for challenging picture recognition applications like disease detection and categorization [18]. A dataset of labeled photos is used to train the model, which then modifies its internal parameters to correctly diagnose diseases [10]. Several InceptionV3 modules are applied after the preprocessed image. These modules enable the network to capture features at various scales and levels of abstraction through the integration of various-sized convolutions and pooling processes in parallel [16].

(d) *ResNet18:* ResNet18's architecture with residual blocks enables effective deep network training, making it a good choice for jobs requiring disease detection and classification. A dataset of labeled photos is used to train the model, which then modifies its internal parameters to correctly diagnose diseases [10]. The ResNet18 architecture passes the preprocessed picture via several residual blocks. Skip connections are used in residual blocks to solve the vanishing gradient issue and enable the network to learn from both the original input and the extracted features [10].

(e) *VGG16/VGG19:* The ease of use and efficiency of VGG16 and VGG19 in picture classification applications are well recognized. They employ a standardized design that includes thin convolutional filters and thick stacks of layers [2]. To correctly categorize diseases, the models' internal parameters are adjusted during training using labeled images from a dataset. In the VGG16 architecture, several convolutional blocks are applied to the preprocessed picture. The quantity of convolutional layers and max-pooling layers in each block raises the abstraction level of the retrieved features [4].

Training and Testing

The model must be trained in this step. With the help of the provided training dataset, the model that was created utilizing the architecture and the custom-built layers has been trained. The model seeks to identify and comprehend the underlying characteristics and patterns in the training dataset during training [13]. During the training phase, the model's custom-built layers are given weights. These weights are used to categorize whether rust, grey spots, or black spots are present in the provided image [7]. Using the 'model.fit' method in the Keras module, the constructed model is first compiled before being pipelined into the training phase [10].

Performance Evaluation

The model's performance is assessed using the Accuracy, Precision, Recall, and F1-score parameters.

(a) *Accuracy:* The accuracy of a prediction is the ratio of correctly predicted images to all predictions. Equation (1) can be used to evaluate accuracy [2].

$$\text{Accuracy} = \frac{\text{Number of correct predictions}}{\text{Total number of predictions}} = \frac{TP + TN}{TP + TN + FP + FN} \tag{1}$$

(b) *Precision:* Precision is measured as the ratio of instances accurately predicted to all instances anticipated as positive. Equation (2) can be used to calculate it mathematically [2].

$$\text{Precision} = \frac{TP}{TP + FP} \tag{2}$$

(c) *Recall:* Recall, often referred to as sensitivity, is the proportion of instances that were correctly predicted to all actual cases. Equation (3) is used to estimate the recall value [2].

$$\text{Recall} = \frac{TP}{TP + FN} \tag{3}$$

(d) *F1-Score:* The F1-score combines a comparison of recall and precision into one score. It may be calculated using Equation (4) and is the Harmonic mean of precision and recall mathematically [2].

$$\text{F1-score} = 2 * \frac{\text{Precision} * \text{Recall}}{\text{Precision} + \text{Recall}} = \frac{TP}{TP + \frac{1}{2}(FP + FN)} \tag{4}$$

Where TP is True Positives, FP is False Positives, TN is True Negatives and FN is False Negatives.

4. Results

In this section, the findings of the study are represented, analyzed, and interpreted to draw meaningful conclusions. The findings from the evaluation of the disease detection and classification models for maize using accuracy and loss measures offer important insights into the effectiveness of the algorithms. Table 26.1 shows the accuracy of assessing the performance and effectiveness of the system, Transfer Learning models for plant disease detection and classification that use architectures like CNN, Densenet121, InceptionV3, ResNet18, and VGG16 and VGG19 are essential.

The accuracy and loss curves for both the training and validation sets can give important information about the model's performance and the training process using the graphs showing different transfer learning models' accuracy and loss for training and validating datasets.

Table 26.1 Transfer learning models results

Models	Accuracy (%)
CNN	92.19
Densenet121	95.88
InceptionV3	97.40
Resnet18	98.45
VGG16	95.36
VGG19	93.56

Let's examine these findings in more detail:

(a) *Validation Accuracy:* The percentage of properly classified pictures in the validation dataset is referred to as validation accuracy. The model effectively recognizes and categorizes plant diseases if the validation accuracy is higher [6].

(b) *Validation Loss:* The validation loss is the difference between the validation dataset's actual class labels and the predicted class probabilities. Lower validation loss indicates that the predictions of the model are more in line with the real-world labels [6].

(c) *Train Accuracy:* The proportion of images from the training dataset that were properly classified is known as the train accuracy. A high train accuracy means the model has gotten better at fitting the training set of data [6].

(d) *Train Loss:* The train loss indicates how well the model's predictions match the actual labels for the training data. The training loss gradually declines and stabilizing shows that the model is successfully identifying the patterns in the training data [6].

The ResNet18 achieved the highest 98.45% accuracy for the maize dataset. Figure 26.4(a) shows accuracy, and loss curves. Figure 26.4(b) shows, confusion matrix of ResNet18 for maize dataset where labels 0, 1, 2, 3, are Common Rust, Gray leaf spot, Healthy and Northern blight respectively.

Precision, Recall, F1-score, and Support parameters values are presented in Table 26.2 as the classification report.

Table 26.2 Classification report

Class Labels	Precision	Recall	F1-Score	Support
0	1.00	1.00	1.00	120
1	0.98	0.90	0.94	52
2	1.00	1.00	1.00	117
3	0.95	0.99	0.97	99

Table 26.3, displays the results of several deep learning techniques are compared with those from other reference papers. The proposed models show higher accuracy than previous work done.

Table 26.3 Results comparison of deep learning models

Models	Literature Work accuracy (%)	Our Findings (%)
CNN	88.80 [15]	92.19
DenseNet121	94.6 [18]	95.88
InceptionV3	82.54 [5]	97.40
Resnet18	93.46[10]	98.45
VGG16/VGG19	80.54 [5]	95.36

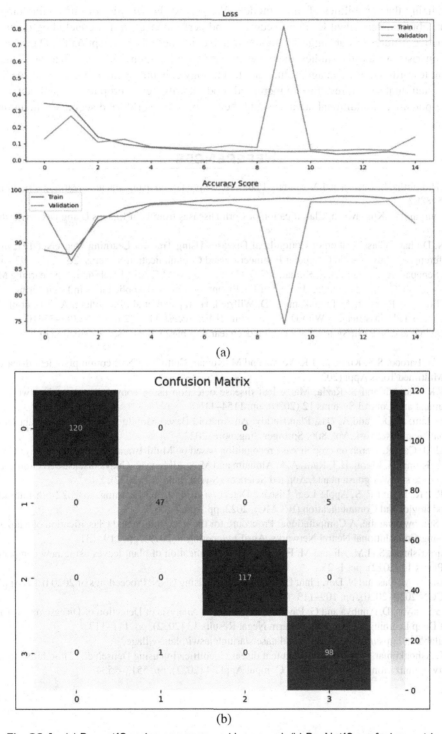

Fig. 26.4 (a) Resnet18 maize accuracy and loss graph (b) ResNet18 confusion matrix

5. Conclusion

Our study set out to use cutting-edge Transfer learning architectures, such as CNN, InceptionV3, Densenet121, Vgg16/19, and ResNet18, to revolutionize the field of plant disease detection and classification. The Resnet18 performed better with 98.45% accuracy for the maize dataset. We have created a reliable and accurate approach for diagnosing and classifying illnesses in maize plants by utilizing the capabilities of these models. We proved the viability of our methodology through intensive testing and evaluation, obtaining excellent levels of accuracy and performance. In this concluding comparison, we highlight the benefits and distinctive features of our suggested model which combines CNN, InceptionV3, Densenet121, Vgg16/Vgg19, and ResNet18 in comparison to earlier studies in maize disease identification and classification. This idea represents an important development towards a day when agriculture and technology cohabit together. It confirms that Transfer learning can completely alter the agricultural sector, resulting in increased food security, fewer crop losses, and better living conditions for rural populations. The potential of additional advances and their impact on world food security remain unwavering as we set out on the future route.

REFERENCES

1. G.P.R. Kranth, M.H. Lalitha, L. Basava and A. Mathur, Plant disease prediction using machine learning algorithms, Int J Comput Appl 18 (2018), pp. 975–8887.
2. M. Fraiwan, E. Faouri and N. Khasawneh, Classification of Corn Diseases from Leaf Images Using Deep Transfer Learning, Plants 11 (2022), pp. 1–14.
3. B. Arathi and U.N. Dulhare, Classification of Cotton Leaf Diseases Using Transfer Learning-DenseNet-121, in Proceedings of Third International Conference on Advances in Computer Engineering and Communication Systems, 2023, pp. 393–405.
4. A. Bin Naeem, B. Senapati, A.S. Chauhan, S. Kumar, J.C.O. Gavilan and W.M.F. Abdel-Rehim, Deep Learning Models for Cotton Leaf Disease Detection with VGG-16, International Journal of Intelligent Systems and Applications in Engineering 11 (2023), pp. 550–556.
5. E. Moupojou, A. Tagne, F. Retraint, A. Tadonkemwa, D. Wilfried, H. Tapamo et al., FieldPlant: A Dataset of Field Plant Images for Plant Disease Detection and Classification With Deep Learning, IEEE Access 11 (2023), pp. 35398–35410.
6. C.K. Sunil, C.D. Jaidhar and N. Patil, Systematic study on deep learning-based plant disease detection or classification, Artif Intell Rev (2023), pp. 1–98.
7. P. Singh, P. Singh, U. Farooq, S.S. Khurana, J.K. Verma and M. Kumar, CottonLeafNet: cotton plant leaf disease detection using deep neural networks, Multimed Tools Appl (2023), .
8. M. Bhanusri, N.V.K. Ramesh and S. Razia, Maize leaf disease detection using convolution neural network, Journal of Advanced Research in Dynamical and Control Systems 12 (2020), pp. 1154–1160.
9. S.I. Rimon, M.R. Islam, A. Dey and A. Das, PlantBuddy: An Android-Based Mobile Application for Plant Disease Detection Using Deep Convolutional Neural Network, Vol. 806, Springer Singapore, 2022.
10. C. Wang, P. Ni and M. Cao, Research on crop disease recognition based on Multi-Branch ResNet-18, J Phys Conf Ser 1961 (2021), .
11. A.M. Mostafa, S.A. Kumar, T. Meraj, H.T. Rauf, A.A. Alnuaim and M.A. Alkhayyal, Guava disease detection using deep convolutional neural networks: A case study of guava plants, Applied Sciences (Switzerland) 12 (2022), .
12. S. K, V.R. P, R. P, P.K. M and P. S, Apple Leaf Disease Detection using Deep Learning, in 2022 6th International Conference on Computing Methodologies and Communication (ICCMC), 2022, pp. 1063–1067.
13. M. Sibiya and M. Sumbwanyambe, A Computational Procedure for the Recognition and Classification of Maize Leaf Diseases Out of Healthy Leaves Using Convolutional Neural Networks, AgriEngineering 1 (2019), pp. 119–131.
14. S.A. Wagle, R. Harikrishnan, S.H.M. Ali and M. Faseehuddin, Classification of plant leaves using new compact convolutional neural network models, Plants 11 (2022), pp. 1–25.
15. G. Shrestha, Deepsikha, M. Das and N. Dey, Plant Disease Detection Using CNN, Proceedings of 2020 IEEE Applied Signal Processing Conference, ASPCON 2020 (2020), pp. 109–113.
16. S. Saritha, V. Satya Srinivas, D. Anuhya and G. Pavithra, Performance Analysis of Detection of Disease on Leaf Images with Inception V3 and Mobilenet Deep Learning Techniques, J Pharm Negat Results 13 (2022), pp. 111–117.
17. Plant Village. Available at https://www.kaggle.com/datasets/arjuntejaswi/plant-village.
18. S. Nandhini and K. Ashokkumar, An automatic plant leaf disease identification using DenseNet-121 architecture with a mutation-based henry gas solubility optimization algorithm, Neural Comput Appl 34 (2022), pp. 5513–5534.

Emerging Trends in IoT and Computing Technologies – Suman Lata Tripathi et al. (eds)
© 2024 Taylor & Francis Group, London, ISBN 978-1-032-87924-6

Exploring the Unseen: Virtual Tours with Augmented Reality

27

Aparna Kulkarni[1], Om Pawar[2],
Vyom Pawar[3], Pratham Pahad[4]
Dr. D. Y. Patil Institute of Technology,
Department of Artificial Intelligence & Data Science, Pimpri, Pune, India

Abstract: The blast in the capacities and elements of cell phones, as cell phones, tablets, and wearable, joined with the omnipresent and reasonable Web access and the advances in the space of helpful systems administration, PC vision, and portable distributed computing changed Versatile Expanded Reality (Blemish) from sci-fi to a reality. Albeit cell phones are additional compelled computational savvy from customary PCs, they have a huge number of sensors that can be utilized to the improvement of more modern Blemish applications and can be helped from far off servers for the execution of their concentrated aspects. In the wake of acquainting the peruser with the fundamentals of Blemish, we present a categorization of the application handles along for certain delegate models. We are eager to present an answer that brings the grounds visit straightforwardly to the screens of forthcoming understudies. This show will reveal how Increased Reality (AR) has empowered us to make a vivid and dynamic virtual visit, rising above the impediments of customary strategies. Our thorough methodology exhibits the grounds as well as offers an intuitive and drawing in experience that mirrors the ethos of our organization and before we close this study, we present existing testing issues.

Keywords: Input data processing, AR solution, Augmented video

1. Introduction

In an era where innovation permeates every facet of our lives, we stand on the precipice of a remarkable breakthrough. Today, we are thrilled to present a revolutionary solution that has the potential to reshape the way we introduce our campus to prospective students – a "Virtual Campus Tour Using Augmented Reality." The emergence of augmented reality (AR) technology has unlocked a new dimension in the world of education, and in this comprehensive presentation, we are eager to unveil how it is propelling us into the future. With this cutting-edge technology, we are transcending the limitations of traditional methods for showcasing our campus and embracing a novel, dynamic, and immersive approach that captures the very essence of our institution.

Imagine a prospective student, thousands of miles away, who is eager to explore our campus, immerse themselves in our academic environment, and understand the ethos of our institution. Traditionally, this would entail the arduous journey of physically traveling to our campus, which is not always feasible or practical. However, with the advent of augmented reality, campus tours can now be displayed directly on your screen, making them not only more accessible, but also more engaging and interactive [1].

[1]appi.pathak3@gmail.com, [2]ompawar1315@gmail.com, [3]vyomchaplot11@gmail.com, [4]prathampahad012@gmail.com

DOI: 10.1201/9781003535423-27

I This journey through the convergence of education and technology is more than just a glimpse into the future. It's a paradigm shift in the way we interact with our audiences. This embodies our commitment to staying at the forefront of innovation and elevating the experience we offer prospective students.

The first question that arises is, "What exactly is this revolutionary 'virtual campus tour using augmented reality'?" Essentially, this is an innovative approach to campus tours that utilizes augmented reality technology to create an immersive, dynamic, and interactive experience. . It provides an alternative to static, traditional campus tours that often fail to capture the true spirit of an institution.

he screen, they can explore university buildings, stroll through picturesque gardens, attend virtual lectures, and more. This is a newly designed campus tour that allows prospective students to feel like they're actually there without having to travel.

The benefits of this technology are manifold. In addition to accessibility and convenience, it also allows for personalization. Each prospective student can customize their experience by focusing on the aspects of the institution that are most important to them. Whether you're interested in our state-of-the-art labs, our vibrant student community, or the quiet beauty of our campus, augmented reality allows you to explore what piques your curiosity.

Additionally, this technology opens up a world of engagement possibilities. Our presentations aren't just static, one-sided experiences. It's a dynamic journey that adapts to user interests and demands. This will allow prospective students to interact with a virtual guide[2].

2. Contributors

In this paper, we present the seamless integration of various software tools and technologies, each bringing its own strengths to create immersive augmented reality experiences. Key contributors to this dynamic combination of creativity and technology include Blender, Unity AR, WebGL, and GitHub.

Blender is a versatile and powerful 3D modeling and texturing software that plays a central role in our projects. Use its extensive capabilities to carefully design and create complex 3D models, giving them the textures and details that bring your virtual worlds to life. Blender's precision and flexibility will help us achieve our vision and ensure that our augmented reality assets are visually appealing and authentic [3].

Known for its expertise in augmented reality applications, Unity AR serves as the platform that brings our creative assets to life. The .fbx file format seamlessly bridges the gap between Blender and Unity AR, allowing you to import carefully designed 3D models and textures. Unity AR uses advanced AR capabilities to transform these assets into immersive and interactive augmented reality experiences. It provides the tools and capabilities needed to overlay digital information onto the real world, creating a seamless combination of virtual and physical environments.

This journey through the convergence of education and technology is more than just a glimpse into the future. It's a paradigm shift in the way we interact with our audiences. This embodies our commitment to staying at the forefront of innovation and elevating the experience we offer prospective students. To ensure accessibility and reach a wider audience, [4] our projects use WebGL technology. WebGL allows your creations to run smoothly in a web browser, eliminating the need for users to download additional software or applications. This choice not only improves the user experience, but also opens up the possibility for a wider audience to engage with augmented reality content.

Finally, GitHub serves as the backbone for hosting your projects. This popular platform makes it easy to collaborate, version control, and share your projects with a global community. We provide an environment where developers, designers, and enthusiasts can come together, provide feedback, and contribute to the further development of augmented reality experiences.

In our project's complex ecosystem, Blender, Unity AR, WebGL, and GitHub work together to realize our augmented reality vision [5]. The synergy between these tools harmoniously blends creative expression and technological innovation to create, deploy, and share augmented reality experiences that transcend traditional boundaries and engage diverse audiences.

3. Architecture Diagram

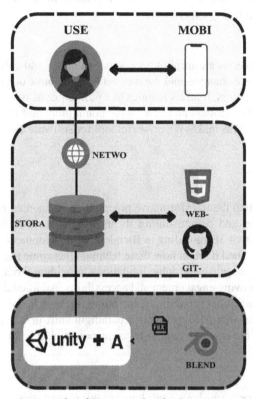

Fig. 27.1 The internal and external architecture of multiple processes connected to each other

Advanced Terminologies:

We have used technology which includes Blender, Unity AR, WebGL, and GitHub.

3.1 Blender

Blender is a powerful and versatile 3D modeling and animation software. Provides extensive functionality for creating 3D models, animations, and visual effects. Among other things, it includes a sculptor mode for organic modeling, a node-based material and shader editor, and a comprehensive particle system for complex simulations. Blender supports a wide range of file formats, making it compatible with other software applications. Its open source nature fosters a strong user community that contributes to its development and provides a wealth of tutorials and plugins. Whether it's game design, film production, architectural visualization, or 3D printing, Blender is a free, comprehensive solution for creating 3D content.

3.2 Unity AR

Unity AR is the most advanced platform within the Unity game engine dedicated to augmented reality (AR) development. It provides developers with a comprehensive toolkit for creating immersive AR experiences on a variety of platforms. Unity AR allows developers to easily integrate their digital elements, such as 3D models, animations, and interactive content, into the real world through the lens of an AR-enabled device. Its robust features include marker-based tracking, image recognition, and real-time environment mapping. Unity AR enables developers to create AR applications for mobile devices, smart glasses, and more, making it a key player in the evolving AR landscape, enabling innovative and engaging AR applications.

3.3 WebGL

WebGL stands for Web Graphics Library and is an open standard that provides 3D graphics and high-performance rendering to web browsers without the need for plug-ins. Web developers can use JavaScript and OpenGL to create interactive 3D and 2D visualizations, games, and immersive experiences. WebGL harnesses the power of the GPU to enable real- time display of complex graphics in a web browser. It provides comprehensive support for all modern browsers, making it an accessible and efficient way to deliver rich visual content on the web. WebGL's versatility makes it widely used in web-based applications ranging from data visualization to virtual reality experiences.

3.4 GitHub

GitHub is a web-based platform that serves as a central hub for version control and collaborative software development. This allows developers to manage and track code changes, making it easier to collaborate on projects, manage different versions, and merge contributions from multiple contributors. It offers features like pull requests, issue tracking, and code reviews to improve teamwork and project management. GitHub fosters an open source community and allows developers to share and access an extensive library of open source projects. This makes it a powerful tool for software development, from small personal projects to large global community efforts.

4. Conclusion

In summary, our research paper delves into the transformative potential of augmented reality (AR), highlighting its profound impact on various aspects of education and demonstrating its its flexibility in reshaping the traditional campus visitor experience. Through seamless integration of 3D modeling in Blender, AR development in Unity AR, deployment via WebGL, and collaborative hosting on GitHub, we shed light on how these technologies come together to deliver an innovative solution. This merger allows the institutions to overcome geographic limitations, providing a rich, interactive and personalized campus experience for prospective students, improving engagement and accessibility. Additionally, AR applications go beyond campus tours to encompass a wide range of educational capabilities, including distance learning, interactive simulations, and virtual labs. As we look to the future, it is clear that AR represents a paradigm shift in education, paving the way for a dynamic, digitally rich learning environment, and our research demonstrates its potential to revolutionize the educational landscape.

5. Acknowledgement

We would like to acknowledge all the people who have contributed to this project, especially the many students at Dr. D.Y. Patil Institute of Technology, Pimpri, Pune who have used the browser during the year leading up to its release. We would like to thank Dr. Mithra Venkatesan for supporting this project in a myriad of ways. Sincere thanks to Prof. Aparna Kulkarni for putting their own classes and projects on the line by relying on this vision of a web-based AR environment. We extend our thanks to the developers of Blender, Unity AR, WebGL, and GitHub for creating the tools that formed the foundation of our work. Lastly, we acknowledge the unwavering support of our friends and family throughout this research journey. Your encouragement and understanding were invaluable in the realization of this project.

REFERENCES

1. Augmented Reality Technology: Current Applications, Challenges and its Future https://ieeexplore.ieee.org/document/9985665
2. Design and Development of Web and Unity3D WebGL Based Immersive Virtual Exhibition Application https://ieeexplore.ieee.org/document/10031529
3. Blender 3D Incredible Models: A comprehensive guide to hard-surface modeling, procedural texturing, and rendering https://ieeexplore.ieee.org/document/10163460
4. Augmented Reality Approach for Marker-based Posture Measurement on Smartphones https://ieeexplore.ieee.org/document/9175652
5. Augmented Reality with Unity AR Foundation: A practical guide to cross-platform AR development with Unity 2020 and later versions https://ieeexplore.ieee.org/document/10162998
6. Keynote Speaker: User Experience Considerations for Everyday Augmented Reality https://ieeexplore.ieee.org/document/9583809

Emerging Trends in IoT and Computing Technologies – Suman Lata Tripathi et al. (eds)
© *2024 Taylor & Francis Group, London, ISBN 978-1-032-87924-6*

Design and Development of an Optimized GCN Layer-Based Technique for the Detection of Occluded 3D Images

28

Apurva Kandelkar[1]

Lovely Professional University, Phagwara, Punjab 144001, India
Dr. D. Y. Patil Institute of Technology, Pimpri, Pune 411018, Maharashtra, India

Isha Batra[2]

Lovely Professional University, Phagwara, Punjab 144001, India

Shabnam Sharma[3]

Opentext

Arun Malik[4]

Lovely Professional University, Phagwara, Punjab 144001, India

Abstract: 3D object recognition is a crucial component of several computer vision applications, including robots, augmented reality (AR), and autonomous driving. The occlusion problem, however, remains one of the major obstacles to obtaining reliable and precise 3D object detection. The occlusion is regarded as one of the most frequent occurrences that decreases the amount of visual information accessible. One of the main reasons many tasks in computer vision and image processing are still very challenging to accomplish is occlusion; a lot of visual information is hidden and cannot be recorded. So the accurate localization and recognition are hampered by occlusion, which happens when objects block the target object's vision partially or entirely. The global optimization problem is solved by the recently developed selfish herds optimizer (SHO) algorithm. In this work, we propose the hybridization of the booster algorithm and the refined selfish herd optimizer to boost the performance of the neural network. For enabling the optimal performance of the detection and classification of occluded image, we perform optical experiment and visualization of occluded objects from the MS COCO and PASCAL dataset, and the region of interest is extracted from the input image using the backbone+ feature pyramid network (FPN), and the fully convolutional one-stage (FCOS) box head. The objective of this research will be to develop an optimized GCN layer in the bidirectional collaboration network (BCNet) for the detection and classification of occluded images. It is the first time we apply hybridization of the booster algorithm and the refined selfish herd optimizer will aim at tuning the hyper parameters of the GCN layer.

Keywords: Selfish herds optimizer (SHO), Hybridization of the booster algorithm, Backbone+ feature pyramid network (FPN)

1. Introduction

3-Dimensional multi-object detection and tracking play a crucial role in various uses and applications across different industries such as autonomous vehicles, security, robotics, medical imaging and augmented reality. In recent years, the advancement of

[1]apurvakandelkar@gmail.com, [2]isha.batra2487@gmail.com, [3]shabnam09sharma@hotmail.com, [4]arumalikhisar@gmail.com

DOI: 10.1201/9781003535423-28

computer vision technologies has significantly reshaped various industries, ranging from autonomous vehicles to robotics and augmented reality. Object detection in computer vision faces several challenges due to the complexities involved in real-world scenarios. Despite considerable progress in the field of 3D object detection, numerous challenges persist, impeding the deployment of these technologies in real-world scenarios. One of the most frequent occurrences that reduces the level of visual information that is available is occlusion. Occlusion is an important component in the challenge of many image processing and computer vision jobs since it conceals and obscures a great deal of visual information. The region of interest is frequently defined by a bounding box. These bounding boxes are used to classify the detected objects into respective categories. There are almost 6 degree of freedom for 3D bonding boxes such as 3D physical size (w, h, l) and 3D center location (x, y, z). The depth data is a component of 3D object detection, which offers additional structural details about the item being detected [1]. The motivation for delving into the occlusion issue in 3D object detection is grounded in the practical limitations of existing technologies, where environmental complexity and dynamic interactions among objects present major challenges to current computer vision systems. In this research we comprehensively investigate the partial occlusion problem in 3D object detection, exploring existing methodologies, identifying gaps in current approaches, and proposing innovative solutions. This work aims to further the usability of computer vision technologies in various sectors by analyzing the problems caused by occlusion and so helping to design more reliable and strong 3D object detection systems. We believe that the hybridization of the refined selfish herd optimizer and the booster algorithm will try to adjust the GCN layer's hyper parameters for detection of occluded objects in a 3 dimensional environment. In the subsequent sections of this paper, we will review the literature on 3D object detection, explain various aspects of the occlusion problem, analyze current techniques for handling occlusion, and indicate directions for future research in the effort to create 3D object detection systems that are more reliable and effective. Our contribution can be summarized as follows:

1. We design and develop an optimized GCN layer in the bidirectional collaboration network (BCNet) for the detection and classification of occluded images.

2. We analyze and design backbone+ feature pyramid network (FPN), and the fully convolutional one-stage (FCOS) box head for finding regions of interest from input images.

3. We present a unique structure which help to enhance the neural network performance and it is also used to detect and categorize the occluded objects in a 3D environment: the hybridization of the booster algorithm and the refined selfish herd optimizer.

2. Related Work

Due to various challenges in 3D object detection and classification various authors proposed many 3D object detection frameworks in the past several years. Table 28.1 presents a number of measures that can be used to assess the effectiveness of various strategies. The table lists the various researchers' methodologies, the datasets they used, and their performance evaluations in terms of accuracy. The proposed approaches comprise performance evaluation parameters from many authors for distinct 2D and 3D environments with varying matrices or circumstances.

3. Theory

3.1 Backbone+ Feature Pyramid Network (FPN)

Deep learning-based semantic segmentation has made significant advancements in image pixel classification. Nevertheless, local location data is typically ignored in deep learning's high-level feature extraction, despite the fact that it is crucial for semantic segmentation of images. The FPN is a feature extractor that uses an arbitrary single-scale image as input and produces completely convolutionally produced feature maps at various levels that are proportionately proportioned. Specifically for such a pyramid notion, a Fast and Accurate Feature Pyramid Network (FPN) was developed for feature extraction. This replaces the detector's feature extractor (like Faster R-CNN) and generates many feature map layers, which are features which are mapped with multi-scale and with high-quality data, instead of object detection parameters network which is typically used called feature pyramid network.

3.2 Graph-FCN

A type of neural network called a GCN is made to operate with graph-structured data. In [23] Graph-FCN,a graph model design and initialized by a(FCN)fully convolutional network, for image semantic segmentation in order to avoid this issue. The

Table 28.1 Performance evaluation on different dataset

S. N.	Article	Year	Proposed Methodologies	Dataset	Performance Evaluation (in %)
1	[2]	2020	CompNet-RXT-RB4(CompositionalNets)	PASCAL3D+	94.1
			CompNet-RXT-RB4	MS-COCO	95
2	[3]	2020	HOG-SVM and Convolution Neural Network method	Human.detection via CNN	71.19
				Human detection via HOG-SVM	50
3	[4]	2020	CompOccMix+VGG	PASCAL3D+	89.5
				MNIST	69.4
4	[5]	2017	spatio-temporal RGB-D video segmentation framework	TUM Dataset	92.67
			Hichson el al.	NYU V2	91.35
5	[6]	2020	SVGA-Net	KITTI 3D car(%)	91.67
				KITTI 3D pedestrian	41.47
				KITTI 3D cyclist	79.22
6	[7]	2020	3D MOT	KITTI Car	87.4
				KITTI pedestrian	53.1
				KITTI Cyclist	85.1
7	[8]	2017	DISCO for 2D and 3D keypoint localization	KITTI3D	93.1
8	[9]	2018	VoxelNet	KITTI validation set - Car	77.47
				KITTI validation set - pedestrian	39.48
				KITTI validation set - Cyclist	61.22
9	[10]	2019	PIXOR++	KITTI	89.38
			LaserNet		78.25
			ContFuse		85.83
10	[11]	2018	RotationNet	ModelNet40	97.37
				ModelNet10	98.46
11	[12]	2019	Novel end-to-end MVF multiview fusion algorithm	Waymo Open Dataset-vehicle detection	80.4
				Waymo Open Dataset-pedestrian detection	74.83
12	[13]	2019	TriSI	LIDAR dataset	97.1
			MVD multi-view depth	LIDAR dataset	100
13	[14]	2020	OrthographciNet	ModelNet40	91.00
				ModelNet10	94.57
14	[15]	2020	Ellipse R-CNN	FDDB dataset	93.2
			Mask R-CNN	FDDB dataset	92.0
15	[16]	2020	Object-Centric Stereo Matching Method	KITTI dataset	90.01
16	[17]	2020	Occlusion-Net	KITTI-3D.	93.2
17	[18]	2015	VFH and FPFH descriptors	Willow Garage dataset.	89.64
18	[19]	2015	RPN+VGG	PASCAL VOC 2007	78.8 mAP (%)
			RPN+VGG	PASCAL VOC 2012	75.9 mAP (%)
19	[20]	2019	PointPillars	KITTI val	73.7
20	[21]	2018	MOTA	KITTI	80.9

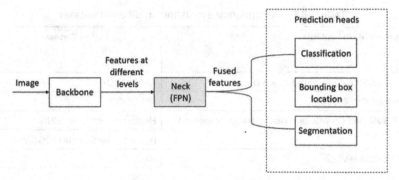

Fig. 28.1 Feature pyramid network.functions as a neck network for backbone network feature fusion

feature-extracting network that transforms incoming data into a specific feature representation is referred to as the backbone. The hyper parameters of the GCN layer, like learning rates, number of layers, or regularization terms, significantly impact its performance. Assigning a class to every image pixel is the main goal of semantic segmentation. The important application of graph convolutional networks is to solve semantic segmentation problems [23].

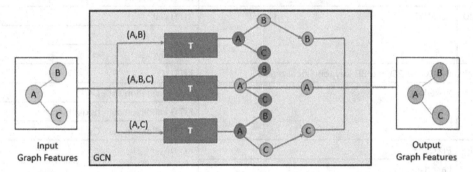

Fig. 28.2 In GCN, a node's output features are only dependent upon other nodes that the Laplacian matrix determines to be "related."

For instance node A features and node B features are used as input for computing the features for node B (the top branch). The same filter T (the blue rectangles) is shared by several nodes[23].

3.3 Refined Selfish Herd Optimizer

The optimization algorithm referred to as SHO (Selfish Herd Optimizer) is an algorithm inspired by the selfish herd behavior observed in nature. The selfish herd optimizer provides good performance when finding optimal solutions. Optimization algorithms are crucial for training neural networks, and a well-tailored optimizer can lead to faster convergence and better generalization. The selfish herd algorithm is more useful in solving real life engineering problems such as 3D object detection [26]. The refined SHO improves the performance of exploration and exploitation.

3.4 Booster Algorithms

Booster algorithms, often associated with boosting techniques like AdaBoost or Gradient Boosting, are ensemble methods that combine the predictions of multiple weak learners to create a strong learner. The performance of machine learning models is usually enhanced by these algorithms.

4. Proposed Method

The hybrid optimization proposed model for detection of handling occlusion problem is shown in Fig. 28.3. The model is composed primarily of four elements: feature extraction, feature mapping, hybridized optimization and forecast results that are occluded predictions. The proposed algorithm provides hybridization of the booster algorithm and the refined selfish herd optimizer which will aim at tuning the hyper parameters of the GCN layer and this algorithm will be novel in this work. The FPN is a feature extractor that uses an arbitrary single-scale image as input and produces fully convolutionally produced

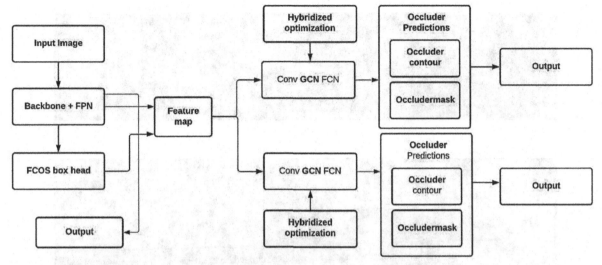

Fig. 28.3 Block diagram hybrid optimization for detection for handling occlusion in 3d objects

feature maps at various levels that are proportionately sized. Furthermore, FCOS can solve object detection in a way that is similar to semantic segmentation in terms of per-pixel prediction. The region of interest from the feature map is forwarded to the layers of bilayer occlusion modelling. There are two overlapping image layers of BCNet model for image formation: Top GCN Layer and Bottom GCN Layer. The occluded objects are being detected by top GCN layer and partially visible (occluded) instances is detected by bottom GCN layer infers. When the interaction between the occluded and occluding instances is taken into consideration during mask regression, the borders of the occluded and occluding instances are naturally separated during explicit modeling of the occlusion relationship with bilayer structure. The top GCN layer in the occluded segmentation predicts the occlude counter and the occluded mask, whereas the bottom GCN layer predicts the contour and mask in the occlude segmentation. Figure 28.3 shows the proposed architecture of hybridization of the booster algorithm and the refined selfish herd optimizer to increase the performance of the neural network. The proposed architecture detect and classify the occlusion in 3D environments.

5. Proposed Architecture

We propose our approach's ability to infer occlusion and classify occluded objects using MS COCO and PASCAL datasets. We train our model and test using subset of images. This dataset is initially described in section 5.1.

5.1 Datasets

We use MS COCO and PASCAL Dataset to assess our approach and contrast it with the various state of art approaches. We can measure the effect of partial occlusion by simulating occlusion, hence it is crucial to assess algorithms on partially obscured objects. Based on the MS-COCO dataset [24], which is occluded objects dataset is used in our method. Our method identify natural occluded partially visible objects with the help of the bounding box method.

MS COCO: Large-The key-point detection, segmentation, scale object detection and captioning are all included in the MS COCO (Microsoft Common Objects in Context) dataset. The dataset consists of 123K images. There are almost 80 different categories of object classes available in the MS COCO dataset.

PASCAL datasets: The Pascal dataset with 20 classes and multiple images. The train data set consists of 11,530 images with 6,929 segmentations and 27,450 ROI-tagged objects.

Preprocessing: For every image we use Backbone + FPN and FCOS box head feature extraction method. These two methods are used for extraction of relevant features. After extracting features we apply proposed novel method called hybridized

5.2 Evaluation Results

The proposed architecture output is shown below on the Pascal COCO Dataset is shown in Fig. 28.4 as

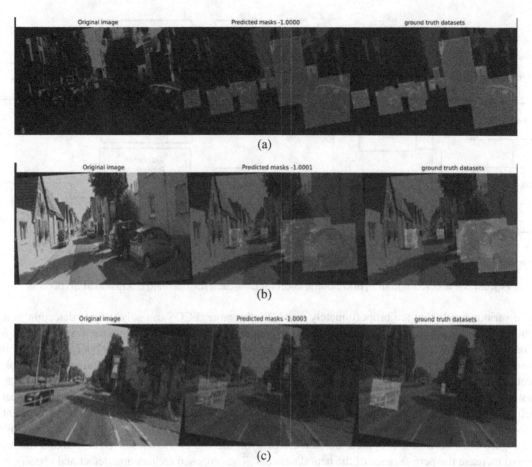

Fig. 28.4 Occluded Object Detection in 3D Environments (a) Input image: Pascal COCO dataset, Output: Occluded object detection with bounding box with predicted mast of 1.000 and ground truth dataset, (b) Input image: Pascal COCO dataset, Output: occluded object detection with bounding box predicted mast of 1.001 and ground truth dataset, (c) Input image: Pascal COCO dataset, Output: Occluded object detection with bounding box predicted mast of 1.003 and ground truth dataset)

Occlusion Prediction: We demonstrate that the proposed architecture is successfully detecting the occluded objects in 3D Environment. The proposed hybridization of the booster algorithm and the refined selfish herd optimizer to augment the performance of the neural network and also classify the objects into different classes.

6. Conclusion

To detect and categorize occluded objects in 3D environments, we presented a unique graph-based architecture that is a hybridization of the refined selfish herd optimizer and the booster algorithm. In this paper, we propose a original approach for classicization and detection of the occluded objects. Our contribution mainly uses a hybrid optimization model with GCN + FCN with selfish herd optimization model for feature extraction and detection of occluded objects in 3D environments.

REFERENCES

1. Shreyas, E. and Sheth, M.H., 2021, August. 3D object detection and tracking methods using deep learning for computer vision applications. In 2021 International Conference on Recent Trends on Electronics, Information, Communication & Technology (RTEICT) (pp. 735-738). IEEE.
2. Pan, J. and Hu, B., 2007, June. Robust occlusion handling in object tracking. In 2007 IEEE Conference on Computer Vision and Pattern Recognition (pp. 1-8). IEEE.
3. Aslan, M.F., Durdu, A., Sabanci, K. and Mutluer, M.A., 2020. CNN and HOG based comparison study for complete occlusion handling in human tracking. Measurement, 158, p.107704.

4. Kortylewski, A., Liu, Q., Wang, H., Zhang, Z. and Yuille, A., 2020. Combining compositional models and deep networks for robust object classification under occlusion. In Proceedings of the IEEE/CVF Winter Conference on Applications of Computer Vision (pp. 1333-1341).

5. Xie, Q., Remil, O., Guo, Y., Wang, M., Wei, M. and Wang, J., 2017. Object detection and tracking under occlusion for object-level RGB-D video segmentation. IEEE Transactions on Multimedia, 20(3), pp.580-592.

6. He, Q., Wang, Z., Zeng, H., Zeng, Y., Liu, S. and Zeng, B., 2020. Svga-net: Sparse voxel-graph attention network for 3d object detection from point clouds. arXiv preprint arXiv:2006.04043.

7. Li, B., Zhang, Y., Zhao, B. and Shao, H., 2020. 3D-ReConstnet: a single-view 3d-object point cloud reconstruction network. IEEE Access, 8, pp.83782-83790.

8. Li, C., Zeeshan Zia, M., Tran, Q.H., Yu, X., Hager, G.D. and Chandraker, M., 2017. Deep supervision with shape concepts for occlusion-aware 3d object parsing. In Proceedings of the IEEE Conference on Computer Vision and Pattern Recognition (pp. 5465-5474).

9. Zhou, Y. and Tuzel, O., 2018. Voxelnet: End-to-end learning for point cloud based 3d object detection. In Proceedings of the IEEE conference on computer vision and pattern recognition (pp. 4490-4499).

10. Meyer, G.P., Laddha, A., Kee, E., Vallespi-Gonzalez, C. and Wellington, C.K., 2019. Lasernet: An efficient probabilistic 3d object detector for autonomous driving. In Proceedings of the IEEE/CVF conference on computer vision and pattern recognition (pp. 12677-12686).

11. Kanezaki, A., Matsushita, Y. and Nishida, Y., 2018. Rotationnet: Joint object categorization and pose estimation using multiviews from unsupervised viewpoints. In Proceedings of the IEEE Conference on Computer Vision and Pattern Recognition (pp. 5010-5019).

12. Zhou, Y., Sun, P., Zhang, Y., Anguelov, D., Gao, J., Ouyang, T., Guo, J., Ngiam, J. and Vasudevan, V., 2020, May. End-to-end multi-view fusion for 3d object detection in lidar point clouds. In Conference on Robot Learning (pp. 923-932).

13. Zhou, Y., Sun, P., Zhang, Y., Anguelov, D., Gao, J., Ouyang, T., Guo, J., Ngiam, J. and Vasudevan, V., 2020, May. End-to-end multi-view fusion for 3d object detection in lidar point clouds. In Conference on Robot Learning (pp. 923-932).

14. Guo, W., Hu, W., Liu, C. and Lu, T., 2019. 3D object recognition from cluttered and occluded scenes with a compact local feature. Machine Vision and Applications, 30(4), pp.763-783.

15. Kasaei, S.H., 2020. OrthographicNet: A Deep Transfer Learning Approach for 3-D Object Recognition in Open-Ended Domains. IEEE/ASME Transactions on Mechatronics, 26(6), pp.2910-2921.

16. Dong, W., Roy, P., Peng, C. and Isler, V., 2021. Ellipse r-cnn: Learning to infer elliptical object from clustering and occlusion. IEEE Transactions on Image Processing, 30, pp.2193-2206.

17. Pon, A.D., Ku, J., Li, C. and Waslander, S.L., 2020, May. Object-centric stereo matching for 3d object detection. In 2020 IEEE International Conference on Robotics and Automation (ICRA) (pp. 8383-8389). IEEE.

18. Reddy, N.D., Vo, M. and Narasimhan, S.G., 2019. Occlusion-net: 2d/3d occluded keypoint localization using graph networks. In Proceedings of the IEEE/CVF Conference on Computer Vision and Pattern Recognition (pp. 7326-7335).

19. Alhamzi, K., Elmogy, M. and Barakat, S., 2015. 3d object recognition based on local and global features using point cloud library. International Journal of Advancements in Computing Technology, 7(3), p.43.

20. Ren, S., He, K., Girshick, R. and Sun, J., 2015. Faster r-cnn: Towards real-time object detection with region proposal networks. arXiv preprint arXiv:1506.01497.

21. Lang, A.H., Vora, S., Caesar, and Beijbom, O., 2019. Pointpillars: Fast encoders for object detection from point clouds. In Proceedings of the IEEE/CVF Conference on Computer Vision and Pattern Recognition (pp. 12697-12705).

22. Lu, Y., Chen, Y., Zhao, D. and Chen, J., 2019, June. Graph-FCN for image semantic segmentation. In International symposium on neural networks (pp. 97-105). Cham: Springer International Publishing.

23. Lin, T.Y., Dollár, P., Girshick, R., He, K., Hariharan, B. and Belongie, S., 2017. Feature pyramid networks for object detection. In Proceedings of the IEEE conference on computer vision and pattern recognition (pp. 2117-2125).

24. Yimit, A., Iigura, K. and Hagihara, Y., 2020. Refined selfish herd optimizer for global optimization problems. Expert Systems with Applications, 139, p.112838.

Emerging Trends in IoT and Computing Technologies – Suman Lata Tripathi et al. (eds)
© 2024 Taylor & Francis Group, London, ISBN 978-1-032-87924-6

Two-Way Sign Language System Using Deep Learning Techniques

29

A. Rajendran[1]

Department of Electronics and Communications Engg,
Karpagam college of Engineering, Coimbatore, India

Praveen Kumar S S[2]

M.E Communication Systems,
Karpagam college of Engineering, Coimbatore, India

Abstract: Hearing loss affects people everywhere in the world. There are about 466 million individuals who are deaf. In recent times, the number of deaf and mute victims has increased fleetly due to birth blights, accidents and oral conditions. Since the deaf and mute cannot communicate with the hail, they must depend on some form of visual communication. utmost hearing people cannot understand sign language. The end of our design is to form a ground between the hail- bloodied and the hail- bloodied and start bidirectional conversation We provide real-time voice-to-subscribe language translation in both directions with our two-way sign language translator. We reuse the videotape frame by frame using Python's OpenCV library. In addition, we use a background deduction system called a Gaussian admixture- grounded background/ focus segmentation algorithm to abate the background in each frame. The silhouettes of that reused image are also fed to a deep neural network (DNN)[1][2] to classify the frame into original words in written language. To convert sign language to speech, we use introductory natural language processing and GTTS[5] to directly save sign language alphabet. The event and reading chops of hail- bloodied children are easily below the normal of the general population. This technology also helps mainstream seminaries more integrate the hail- bloodied community, making education easier and cheaper for them.

Keywords: Hearing disabilities, Deaf and dumb, Sign language, Visual communication, Two-way communication, Sign language translator, Gaussian mixture-based background/Foreground segmentation algorithm, Deep neural net (DNN)

1. Introduction

According to the WHO, there are more than 466 million hail disabled people in whole over the world and 72 million of them are deaf. Before this sign language existed, communication was a major problem for the deaf community and greatly hindered its progress. Subscription speech is the main form and method of communication for deaf people. A subscription language can be defined as a language that uses visual gestures with the hands and combines facial expressions and posture. Because of its importance, the United Nations recognized September 23rd as International Language Day and promotes sign language as a human right, on an equal footing with spoken languages. Sign language is very important and is the most important means of communication in the deaf community. In fact, many people outside the Deaf community are fluent in sign language. Therefore, it serves as an important safeguard of communication between speakers and deaf communities, and therefore for the common development of these societies. Modern sign language translators can be divided into two classes. Voice for sign language

[1]rajendran.a@kce.ac.in, [2]eswarpraveen619@gmail.com

DOI: 10.1201/9781003535423-29

translator and voice translator subscription. Signal-to-state approaches are generally detector-grounded or image-grounded, and sometimes a combination of both. Now, they have presented the concept of using detector-equipped gloves to view ArSL signs created by deaf people. Recently, there has been increasing interest in using deep neural networks to analyse spatiotemporal packets for sign language recognition. For illustration, use the DCNN armature for gesture bracket. Although the DCNN [6] [9] armature is veritably accurate, It needs RGB-D inputs, which are created by bias using their own depth detectors, and have a depth dimension.

2. Literature Review

Various approaches are employed in hand image analysis, with appearance-based techniques focusing on feature extraction to characterize the visual attributes of input hand images. This involves comparing the extracted features with saved images, offering real-time performance and a simpler alternative to 3D methods. Another method, the mannequin-based approach, is commonly utilized for detecting skin-coloured areas in images, particularly those that remain unchanged. Features like Ad Boost play a crucial role in identifying hand factors and overcoming occlusion challenges. On the other hand, 3D model-based approaches utilize 3D models to analyse the hand's shape, incorporating depth parameters for enhanced accuracy. Volumetric models, suitable for real-time applications due to their size, are complemented by dimensional parameters, with skeletal models outperforming volumetric ones by constraining modelling parameters. The incorporation of 3D construction and sparse coding, a sophisticated feature optimization technique, enhances accuracy, surpassing traditional descriptors like HOG-DTF and DSR. Additionally, compressibility acquisition minimizes resource consumption by enhancing sparse signals from a limited number of observations. Glove-based approaches, while utilizing sensors for hand position and movement detection, are often deemed cumbersome and expensive. However, the marked coloured glove approach introduces a unique solution, employing coloured gloves to monitor hand shape and precisely determine the position of the palm and fingers during the design process.

3. Methodology

The hand gesture recognition system serves dual purposes, functioning as a tool for interaction between humans and computers and catering to the needs of individuals with disabilities, making it a valuable modern technology. The system's objectives are accomplished through the utilization of various tools and techniques. A comprehensive exploration and investigation into the tools, technologies, and past methodologies employed in this context have been conducted as part of the study.

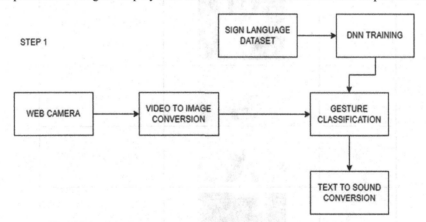

Fig. 29.1   Sign language system using deep learning techniques

3.1 OpenCV

One technique to teach machines intelligence and enable human vision is through computer vision libraries, such as those found in OpenCV. The OpenCV library was developed by Intel and is currently being maintained by idseez. It was previously sponsored by Willow Garage. It works with Windows, Linux, and Mac. That functions in Python, C, and C. Installing and using it is simple, and it is available for free. TensorFlow, Torch/PyTorch, and Caffe-like deep literacy networks are supported by OpenCV.

3.2 Convolutional Neural Network (CNN)

Convolutional neural networks, a type of deep tneural network that is utilized in deep literacy that process data sets to prize information about them. analogous to how sounds, flicks, or prints can be used to prize data from CNN. CNN substantially consists of three particulars. Original open field comes first, followed by participated weight and impulses, and activation and pooling in last order. First, a significant amount of data is used to train the neural networks so that CNN can identify characteristics from a specific input. After entering the input, pre-processing the images is done originally, followed by point birth grounded on the set of stored data and data bracket.

3.3 Google text-to-speech (GTTS)

Users can communicate with the text-to-speech API of Google Translates by using this Python module and CLI tool. It enables users to pre-generate Google Translate TTS request URLs for external programs and write spoken mp3 data to files, byte strings, or stdout. Additionally, the tool has a speech-specific sentence tokenizer that can be customized to allow for infinite text lengths with appropriate intonation and pronunciation adjustments.

4. Results and Discussion

So here are the above examples, like the gesture we show the camera, it captures the gesture image using OpenCV and classifies the corresponding text for a particular gesture using DNN and converts that text to sound using the PYSOUND library. So, in the Fig. 29.2 we can take example 2 where I show a four-finger pointing gesture that is converted to speech and it says "I don't know" as a voice output.

S. No.	Gesture	Audio output
1	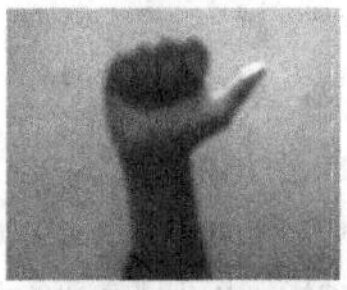	"Please Sit"
2	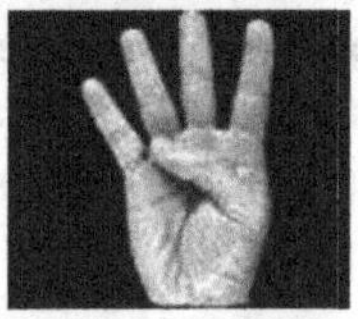	"Happy to see you"
3	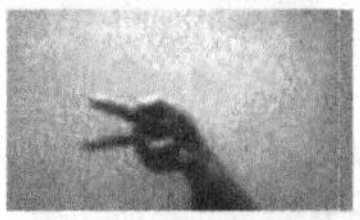	"I'm hungry"
4	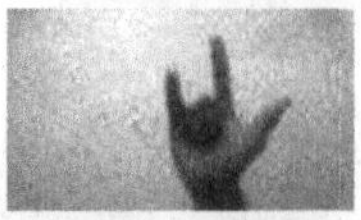	"All the very best"
5	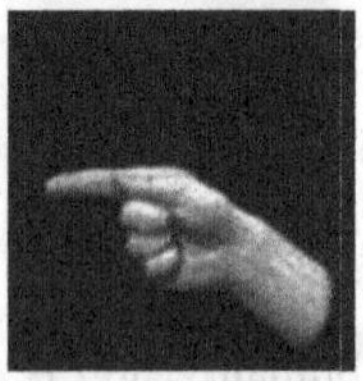	"How are you"

Fig. 29.2 Sample gestures and audio outputs

Here is a graph showing the accuracy and loss of training and validation when the system is trained to understand gestures from a given dataset and sample inputs randomly given during validation. Figure 29.4 shows the reduction of loss during training and Fig. 20.3 shows the degree of accuracy in gesture recognition.

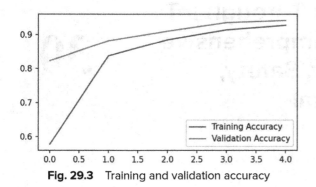

Fig. 29.3 Training and validation accuracy

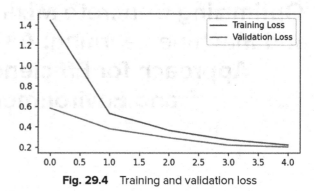

Fig. 29.4 Training and validation loss

REFERENCES

1. S.H. Lee, M.K. Sohn, D.J. Kim, B. Kim, and H. Kim, "Smart TV interaction system using face and hand gesture recognition," in Proc. ICCE, Las Vegas, NV, 2013, pp. 173-174.
2. S. Kim, G. Park, S. Yim, S. Choi and S. Choi, "Gesture-recognizing hand-held interface with vibrotactile feedback for 3D interaction," IEEE Trans. Consum. Electron., vol. 55, no. 3, pp. 1169-1177, 2009.
3. S. S. Rautaray, and A. Agrawal, "Vision based hand gesture recognition or human computer interaction: a survey," Artificial Intelligence Review, vol. 43, no. 1, pp. 1-54, 2015.
4. D. W. Lee, J. M. Lim, J. Sunwoo, I. Y. Cho and C. H. Lee, "Actual remote control: a universal remote control using hand motions on a virtual menu," IEEE Trans. Consum. Electron., vol. 55, no. 3, pp. 1439-1446, 2009.
5. F. Erden and A. E. Çetin, "Hand gesture based remote control system using infrared sensors and a camera," IEEE Trans. Consum. Electron., vol. 60, no. 4, pp. 675-680, 2014.
6. D. Lee and Y. Park, "Vision-based remote-control system by motion detection and open finger counting," IEEE Trans. Consum. Electron., vol. 55, no. 4, pp. 2308-2313, 2009.
7. S. Jeong, J. Jin, T. Song, K. Kwon and J. W. Jeon, "Single-camera dedicated television control system using gesture drawing," IEEE Trans. Consum. Electron., vol. 58, no. 4, pp. 1129-1137, 2012.
8. P. Sermanet, K. Kavukcuoglu, S. Chintala, "Pedestrian detection with unsupervised multi-stage feature learning," in Proc. ICCV, Portland, OR, 2013, pp. 3626-3633.
9. N. Srivastava, G. E. Hinton, A. Krizhevsky, I. Sutskever, and R. Salakutdinov, "Dropout: a simple way to prevent neural networks from overfitting," J. Mach. Learn. Resear., vol. 15, no. 1, pp. 1929-1958, 2015.
10. H. A. Rowley, B. Shumeet, and K. Takeo "Neural network-based face detection," IEEE Trans. on Pattern Anal. Mach. Intell., vol. 20, no. 1, pp. 23-38, 1998.

Emerging Trends in IoT and Computing Technologies – Suman Lata Tripathi et al. (eds)
© 2024 Taylor & Francis Group, London, ISBN 978-1-032-87924-6

Optimizing Concrete Mixing Through IoT and Machine Learning: A Comprehensive Approach for Efficiency, Safety, and Environmental

30

Karan Ramesh Singh[1], Nikhil Sureshrao Surkar[2]

J D College of Engineering & Management,
Department of Computer Science and Engineering, Nagpur, India

Kamlesh Dayanand Patle[3], Mehvish Zabeen[4]

J D College of Engineering & Management, Department of Civil Engineering, Nagpur, India

Supriya Sawwashere[5]

J D College of Engineering & Management,
Department of Computer Science and Engineering, Nagpur, India

Atika Ingole[6]

J D College of Engineering & Management, Department of Civil Engineering, Nagpur, India

Abstract: Workers and engineers are unsure about how adequate the mixing procedure is because of the multiple problems that have been reported when mixing concrete using machines. It can be difficult to ascertain if the concrete was mixed correctly or whether the intended ratio was maintained because assessments are frequently dependent on conjecture. Engineers search for the ideal material ratio during the intricate process of designing a concrete mix in order to guarantee the best possible performance. Compressive strength is of utmost importance since it is a critical attribute in determining the concrete class. Predictable compressive strength is a prerequisite for the longevity and safety of concrete constructions. Machine learning has become a promising answer to these problems. Complex patterns that may be invisible to human observation can now be recognized thanks to recent developments in machine learning techniques. In our study, the methodologies based on the IOT Method combined with machine learning provide a powerful method for designing the concrete mix. Through the application of machine learning to identify complex patterns in huge datasets, our goal is to improve the accuracy and productivity of the concrete mixing procedure. This technological integration not only solves the present uncertainties in concrete mixing, but it also portends well for the use of machine learning in construction process optimization in the future.

Keywords: ML, Raspberry Pi, Weight sensor introduction, Bluetooth, Relay, Motion sensor

1. Introduction

Our initiative aims to enhance the global concrete mixing equipment used in construction. We are concentrating on drum tilting concrete mixture machines specifically. We're installing IoT sensors to monitor the mixing process in order to improve their performance. We're using a regular concrete mix, known as M20, which has the appropriate amounts of aggregate, sand, water, and cement. On construction sites, concrete mixers are essential, because the quality of the material depends on how well they

---
[1]karansinghthakur002@gmail.comm, [2]nikhilsurkar7@gmail.com, [3]kamleshpatle02019@gmail.com, [4]mehvishzabeen03@gmail.com, [5]ssawashere486@gmail.com, [6]atikaingole@gmail.com

DOI: 10.1201/9781003535423-30

operate [01]. Engineers and laborers frequently question if the concrete mix is ideal. We are using machine learning (ML) and the Internet of Things (IoT) to integrate these technologies into the concrete mixing process. Our goal is to create an intelligent system that employs machine learning algorithms to automate the concrete mixing process. We are examining a method called Multiple Linear Regression. an algorithm that, depending on input variables including sand, cement, aggregate, water, and their ratios, forecasts how long it will take to produce the ideal concrete mix. When a linear correlation exists between the input elements and the desired outcome, modify the wording while preserving the meaning, this approach works well. Our goal is to increase the effectiveness of concrete mixing by utilizing IoT and ML, guaranteeing a reliable and superior final result. To operate the concrete mixer practically, we'll pair an Android smartphone and a Raspberry Pi over Bluetooth.

2. Literature Review

Our project involves automating concrete mixing through the use of machine learning and control engineering. Sand, cement, water, and aggregate are used as inputs in this process. During the machine learning phase, an agent has the ability to make decisions that optimize a reward signal, thereby controlling the mixing process of concrete. We're utilizing Bluetooth is to link an Android phone and Raspberry Pi in order to make this work. The Raspberry Pi is a well-known electronics platform, and Bluetooth is how we're able to communicate between the A Raspberry Pi and an Android phone. Because it might be dangerous for a Raspberry Pi to be directly exposed to the the material combination, we're using a relay as a go-between to operate the concrete mixer. We're also integrating a range of IoT components, including moule kits and sensors, to gather input data for the project.

3. Problem Statement

Although the concrete is blended by the concrete mixer, the engineers and laborers are unsure if the mixture is ideal. The laborers depend on their gut feelings and educated guesses derived from a visual assessment of the concrete. A badly blended concrete can cause a number of problems. Making sure that the concrete is mixed properly is the traditional way to prevent problems.

4. Methodology for Predicting Concrete Mixer Rotation Time

4.1 Dataset Collection

Our project begins with extensive concrete mixture experiments using the M20 concrete grade ratio. The primary goal is to collect a dataset containing various parameter permutations within the M20 ratio. We generate a proprietary dataset as a result of these experiments, which serves as the foundation for subsequent phases.

4.2 Data Processing and Normalization

After collection, the data must go through a crucial processing and normalization step. The main objective is to optimize the data for the use of machine learning algorithms, specifically the Multiple Linear Regression (MLR) model, by transforming it into a standardized and useable format. To enable smooth integration into the modeling process, this entails cleaning the data, managing outliers, and guaranteeing uniformity.

4.3 Model Building and Training

The main goal of our project is to create and hone a machine learning model that can accurately forecast how long it will take to mix concrete exactly right. The Multiple Linear Regression (MLR) model, a statistical technique that establishes a relationship between a dependent variable and numerous independent factors, has been selected for this purpose.

- Why MLR, (multiple linear regression)?

MLR is helpful in our situation for a number of reasons:

Linear Relationship: Multiple linear factors (sand, cement, aggregate, water) are assumed to have a linear relationship with the dependent variable (rotation time). This presumption is consistent with how concrete mixing procedures work.

Expectation of Time: With the help of the model's linear equation

$$(Y = a0 + a1 x1 + a2 \ x \ 2 + ... + anxn) \tag{1}$$

we can predict, given input values, how long the concrete mixer machine will take to rotate.

Considering the Control System: We acknowledge the need to include other components, like material quality, temperature, and humidity, when building the control system.

While not specifically mentioned by MLR, these elements are essential to comprehending the concrete mixing process in its entirety.

4.4 Model Representation

The MLR model's mathematical expression is as follows:

$$Y = a0 + a1x1 + a2 x 2 + ... + anxn \qquad (2)$$

where:

- Y is the dependent variable (rotation time).
- The intercept is denoted by a0.
- a1 to an are coefficients that signify the influence of each independent variable (x1 to xn).
- The independent variables (sand cement aggregate water) are x1 to xn.

In essence, our methodology aligns a series of concrete steps, beginning with dataset collection and ending with the strategic application of the MLR model. This comprehensive approach puts us in a good position to create a predictive model for optimizing the concrete mixing process.

5. Flowchart

See flowchart (Fig. 30.1) on next page

6. Benefits

Enhanced Efficiency: By predicting how long it will take to mix concrete perfectly and automatically modifying the machine accordingly, this project can increase mixing efficiency. This saves time and resources while maintaining constant quality.

Data-driven insights: real-time information on substance characteristics and performance of the equipment can be gathered by outfitting the concrete mixing machine with Internet of Things (IoT) sensors. Machine learning can be used to analyze this data and produce insightful analysis that can support decision-making and process improvement.

Predictive maintenance is made possible by IoT sensors monitoring the conditions of construction equipment, which allows for anticipatory maintenance. This increases equipment uptime and helps prevent expensive breakdowns.

Enhanced Safety: IoT sensor data can be analyzed by machine learning to find potentially dangerous situations and safety hazards. By facilitating prompt action, this proactive strategy improves on-site safety. This proactive strategy makes timely interventions possible, which improves on-site safety.

Reduced Environmental Impact: The project can lessen the negative effects of construction on the environment by optimizing resource use and reducing waste. Machine learning algorithms can be used to analyze IoT sensor data and provide insights into material usage, energy consumption, and waste production.

7. Drawback

Costs: Putting machine learning and Internet of Things applications into practice might involve a sizable upfront outlay for things like development of software, sensor purchases, and employee training. Before beginning the project, the benefits and drawbacks must be carefully considered.

Reliability: A number of variables, including data quality, algorithm design, and sensor performance, can affect how dependable machine learning algorithms and Internet of Things applications are. Regular evaluation and monitoring are required to guarantee the dependability of the system.

Maintenance: It may be necessary to have specialized knowledge and abilities in order to maintain IoT sensors and machine learning algorithms. Ensuring that personnel possess the necessary training and tools to manage system maintenance is imperative.

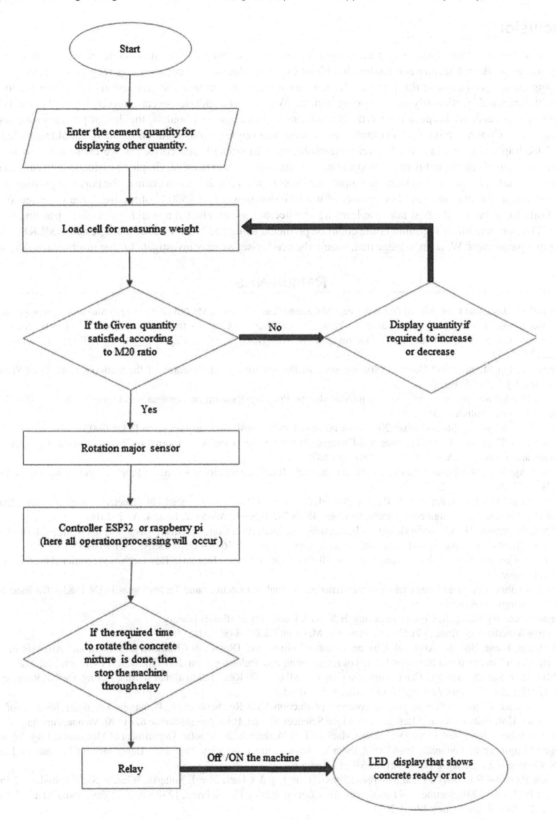

Fig. 30.1   Flow chart

8. Conclusion

Our goal is to develop a useful tool for engineers by using machine learning to design concrete mixes. Creating an efficient artificial neural network architecture and feeding it with an extensive database of concrete mix recipes, each associated with a corresponding lab test, is the aim of this project. Mechanization is required to increase production of concrete due to the rising demand for the material, particularly in developing nations. We created a mobile concrete mixer for M10 grade concrete in order to satisfy this need. By keeping observed deformations within allowable bounds, the design prevents assembly failure and ensures safety. Concrete mixing is a complicated process that requires consideration of many variables, including time, energy, and loading technique. In order to overcome problems with strength and corrosion, we chose stainless steel for the mixer blade. Our paper's main goal is to develop a concrete mixer that is inexpensive, simple to maintain, and easy to use using locally available materials. In order to increase output, we stress how crucial it is to mechanize the concrete production process. Based on our design calculations, 2.43 horsepower of transmission power and 1500 N of mixing force were needed. Using a database of mix formulas and the best machine learning architecture, we conducted research on machine learning for concrete mix design. The concrete mixer's spinning time could be predicted using the Multiple Linear Regression (MLR) technique by providing input parameters. We acknowledge that, should the need arise, we may investigate further machine learning strategies.

REFERENCE

1. [Mr. Kamlesh Dayanand Patle, Ms. Mehvish Zabeen, Mr. Karan Ramesh Singh, Mr. Nikhil Sureshrao Surkar, Dr. Supriya Sawwashere, Prof. Atika Ingole" Experimental Investigation of Compressive Strength of Concrete through Conventional Concrete Mixer and Design of Automated Concrete Mixer with Machine Learning" Page No. : 1846-1850 Cite/ Export Certificate DOI : https://doi.org/10.22214/ijraset.2023.56333

2. Concrete Mixing Methods and Concrete Mixers: State of the Art Journal of Research of the National Institute of Standards and Technology. By Chiara F. Ferraris.

3. Ristow G H 2000 Mixing and segregation in rotating drums, Proc. Symposium on Segregation in Granular Flows, The Netherlands: Kluwer Academic publishers, 311–320.

4. Turbula T2C Heavy-Duty Shaker-Mixer 2004 www.artisanscientific.com/ 49853.asp accessed 12.06. 2007.

5. Ferraris, C.F., "Concrete Mixing Methods and Concrete Mixers: State of the Art", Journal of Research of the National Institute of Standards and Technology, Vol. 106, No. 2, 391-399 (2001).

6. Thompson Aguheva, "Design and Fabrication of an Industrial Mixer", International Journal of Practices and Technologies, ISSN 1583-1078, Issue 20, JanuaryJune 2012.

7. Sddhant Dange, Saket Sant, Anish Sali, Parthon Pethodam, Sandeep Belgamwar., "Study of planetary concrete mixer", International journal of latest research in engineering and technology, ISSN 2454- 5031, Volume 2, Issue 4, April 2016.

8. Amruta K. Wankhede, Dr. A.R. Sahu Design, "Modification and Analysis of Concrete Mixer Machine", International Journal on Recent.

9. Innovation Trends in Computing and Communication, Volume:3 Issue: 12 6613 – 6616, ISSN: 2321-8169, 2015.

10. C.F.Ferrasis, Concrete Mixing Methods and Concrete Mixers; State of the Art,"Journal of Reserarch of the National nstitute of Standards and Technological".

11. Design and Fabrication of an Industrial Mixer; Internatinal journal of Pratctices and Technologies ISSN 1583-1078 issue 20, Jauary, 2012, by Thompsonn Aguheve

12. Concrete Mixer; By Turley, Jr, Civil Engineering, B.S 1913, University of Illinois Library

13. https://en.wikipedia.org/w/index.php? Title = concrete. Mixer and deild -848603025.

14. Desai, Arjun, Harsh Bhutani, Abhishek Chavan, Atharva Chitnis, and Dharmesh Chowdhary. "Design and Analysis of a Portable Concrete Mixer." International Research Journal of Engineering and Technology, no. July (2021): 4371–76. www.irjet.net.

15. Min Min Shwe Sin. "Design and Calculation of a Concrete Mixer (100 Kg)." International Journal of Engineering Research And V7, no. 08 (2018): 253–57. https://doi.org/10.17577/ijertv7is080085

16. State of practice of automation in precast concrete production Sara Reichenbach *, Benjamin Kromoser Institute of Structural Engineering, University of Natural Resources and Life Sciences Vienna, Peter-Jordan-Straße 82, 1190, Vienna, Austria

17. Design and Fabrication of Automatic Dishwasher Machine R.B.Venkatesh UG Scholar: Department of Mechanical Engineering, K.L.N. College of Engineering, Pottapalayam-630612, India V. SivaramKumar Associate Professor: Department of Mechanical Engineering, K.L.N. College of Engineering Pottapalayam-630612, India

18. A Review Paper on Raspberry Pi and its Applications 1Hirak Dipak Ghael, 2Dr. L Solanki, 3Gaurav Sahu 1 Student, 2 Principal, 3 Assistant Professor, 123Department of Electronics and Communication Engineering, 123BKBIET, Pilani, India. Date of Submission: 25-12-2020 Date of Acceptance: 06-01-2021

19. IOP Conf. Series: Materials Science and Engineering 981 (2020) 042009 IOP Publishing doi:10.1088/1757-899X/981/4/042009 1 Bluetooth and GSM based Smart Security System using Raspberry Pi Kashaboina Radhika1 , Dr. Velmani Ramasamy 2 1 PG Scholar,

Department of ECE, Siddartha Institute of Technology and Sciences, Hyderabad, Telangana,India 2 Associate Professor and Head, Department of ECE, Siddartha Institute of Technology and Sciences, Hyderabad, Telangana, India

20. Weight-based Load Balancing in Raspberry Pi MPICH Heterogeneous Cluster with Fuzzy Estimation of Node Computational Performance Dmytro Zubov 1 and Andrey Kupin 2 1 University of Central Asia, 138 Toktogul St., Bishkek, 720001, Kyrgyzstan 2 Kryvyi Rih National University, 11 Matusevycha St., Kryvyi Rih, 50027, Ukraine

21. S.E. Chidiac *et al.* Plastic viscosity of fresh concrete - a critical review of predictions methods Cem. Concr. Compos.(2009)

22. T. Roshavelov Prediction of fresh concrete flow behavior based on analytical model for mixture proportioning Cem. Concr. Res.(2005)

23. M.-Y. Cheng *et al.* High-performance concrete compressive strength prediction using time-weighted evolutionary fuzzy support vector machines inference model Autom. Constr.(2012)

Emerging Trends in IoT and Computing Technologies – Suman Lata Tripathi et al. (eds)
© 2024 Taylor & Francis Group, London, ISBN 978-1-032-87924-6

An Efficient Approach for Balancing of Load in Cloud Environment

31

Puneet Kumar Yadav[1], Saswati Debnath[2]

Assistant Professor, School of Engineering and Design,
Alliance University, Bangalore, India

Sakshi Srivastava[3], Ratan Rajan Srivastava[4]

Assistant Professor, Department of Computer Science and Engineering,
B. N. College of Engineering & Technology, Lucknow

Sachin Bhardwaj[5]

Assistant Professor, Department of Computer Science and Engineering,
Ambalika Institute of Management & Technology, U.P

Yusuf Perwej[6]

Professor, Department of Computer Science and Engineering,
Goel Institute of Technology & Management, Lucknow

Abstract: Virtualization, remote computing, Utilization and online services, cloud computing offers a flexible method of archiving data and files. Sharing a large number of resources at a low cost with clients is the primary goal of cloud servers. By registering with a particular server and submitting requests for the resources, clients can use the cloud resources. After authentication, the server gives the clients making requests the services they want. Resources in cloud data centers are becoming scarce as a result of the daily growth in data storage in the cloud. Consequently, cloud data centers need to use load balancing. The balancing of load idea allows for the movement of part of the tasks from overburdened servers to underloaded servers. In the context of computing of cloud, balancing of load handled well in this paper.

Keywords: Cloud environment, Load balancing, Equally spaced, Underloaded data centers, Models of delivery

1. Introduction

Different services are available for clients by the cloud computing industry under the terms front end and back end, respectively [1]. Through either public or private networks, cloud-computing services are accessible. Cloud computing is being used to provide a wide range of well-known applications, including conferencing, messaging, and chat [2]. In Fig. 31.1 below, the fundamental ideas of the front end (clients) and the back end (Cloud) are depicted. Resources in cloud data centers are becoming scarce because of the daily growth in data storage in the cloud. Additionally, there are both over and underloaded data centers. Consequently, cloud data centers need to use load balancing. The idea of balancing load allows for the movement of part of the tasks from overburdened servers to underloaded servers. In general, dynamic algorithms for load balancing are used. Numerous dynamic load balancing [3] techniques are available for distributing the workload among cloud data centers.

[1]puneet.yadav@alliance.edu.in, [2]saswati.debnath@alliance.edu.in, [3]sakshisrivastav33@gmail.com, [4]ratanrajan@gmail.com,
[5]bhardwazsachin52@gmail.com, [6]yusufperwej@gmail.com

DOI: 10.1201/9781003535423-31

Finding the overloaded nodes and shifting their workload to other nodes is what load balancing is all about. This research takes a hybrid approach to load balancing by using the algorithms "Throttled," "Equally Spread Current Execution" (ESCE), and "Round Robin" [4].

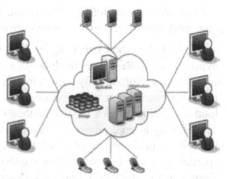

2. Models of Cloud Computing

Different models of delivery of Cloud Computing are explained below [5][6].

- IaaS -Infrastructure as a Service

The user can access network-related services, data processing, and storage through IaaS. IaaS offers specialized operating system services as requested by the respective client. Only administrative services are offered by this layer. The cloud user takes care of the security issues.

Fig. 31.1 Cloud computing environment

- PaaS -Platform as a Service

PaaS offers a dedicated environment for operating and implementing client applications and services. Both the customer and the cloud provider each contribute to this layer's security.

- Saas- Software as a Service

SaaS gives various forms of utilities and applications for example electronic mail, client requesting puzzles and games. Various types of securities are also given in this service model. Service models of Cloud Computing are described as above. We can view graphically such services in the Fig. 31.2 [7].

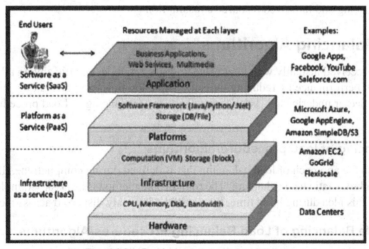

Fig. 31.2 Deployment models of cloud

3. Load Balancing

The goals of balancing load are described below:

- Improve the performance
- Maintain system stability
- Build fault tolerance system
- Accommodate future modification.
- Energy is saved in case of low load
- Maximize throughput of the system

- Minimize communication overhead
- Resources are easily available on demand
- Resources are efficiently utilized under condition of high/low load
- Minimize overall completion time (makes pan)

The cloud computing environment offers its clients a variety of resources and services to share. Due to the growing amount of data being stored via cloud computing, cloud data centres are running out of resources. A few data centres are also overloaded, while others are underloaded. As a result, load balancing is needed in cloud data centres. With the notion of load balancing, some work from overcrowded servers are moved to underloaded servers.

Figure 31.3 described balancing of load in cloud computing environment [8]. Resources in cloud data centers are becoming scarce as a result of the daily growth in data storage in the cloud. Utilizing virtualization, remote computing, and online services, cloud computing offers a flexible method of archiving data and files. Sharing a large number of resources at a low cost with clients is the primary goal of cloud servers. By registering with a particular server and submitting requests for the resources, clients can use the cloud resources. After authentication, the server gives the clients making requests the services they want. The difficulty of load balancing in the cloud is one that it is now dealing with. The rise in consumer demand for cloud services is the main cause of this problem. It is therefore practically difficult to continue offering one or more free services to meet demand. The system will crash if each server is given just one request to complete. This will cause server traffic. For the purpose of

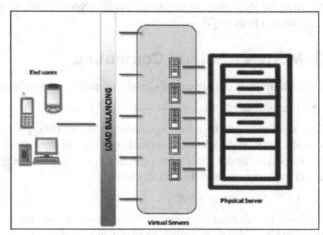

Fig. 31.3 Balancing of load in cloud

offering a highly effective solution to the user, service provider of cloud (CSP) uses it on its own cloud computing platform. Additionally, a system for inter-CSP load balancing is needed to create a cheap and limitless consumer pool of resources. In order to prevent any one node from becoming overburdened, load balancing helps disperse the dynamic workload across several nodes. The efficient use of resources is aided by it. The effectiveness of the system is also enhanced. Numerous techniques already in use offer load balancing and improved resource consumption

4. Types of Load Balancing Algorithms

Data may be transferred and received instantly with load balancing since it divides traffic among all servers. Load balancing is necessary to optimize system performance by reducing overall completion times and preventing instances in which particular system resources are overloaded or underloaded. Two main categories of balancing of Load procedures and algorithms are [9] [10]

4.1 Static or fixed balancing of load procedure/algorithms

Static load balancing refers to the approach of load balancing that is defined during compilation. All of the running servers get an equal amount of work thanks to static load balancing. The round-robin method is a classic example of a static load-balancing technique. By implementing this idea during build time, the workload is evenly dispersed across the processors.

4.2 Dynamic or Variable Balancing of Load Balancing Procedures/Algorithms

The balancing of load strategy designed at run time is called dynamic load balancing. The decision regarding balancing the load on the servers is depend upon the current-system state. There is no need of balancing information at design or compile time. Therefore, this approach is beneficial for load balancing. We can perform dynamic load balance by using two different methods first Distributed Variable/Dynamic balancing of load and second Non-distributed Variable balancing of load.

5. Methodology

Every cloud service provider has the same basic objectives, including finding ways to make the most of cloud resources and developing a dependable load balancing approach. Strategies for scheduling virtual machines with load balancing make it easier to allocate resources based on demand. A virtual machine load-balancing algorithm essentially determines which virtual machine to allocate when a customer wants one in the cloud.

This article discusses many possible approaches to load balancing in virtual machines [11]. The round robin approach maintains a cyclical flow without specifying a specific sequence for the phases. Since it picks the load randomly, some nodes have a very high load while others have a very low burden [12]. [13]. According to the throttled algorithm, the client or customer initiates the process by requesting that the load balancer locate a virtual machine that is capable of carrying out the task that the client needs. These days, everyone utilizes the internet and fog computing. Cloud computing makes a vast array of shared resources and services accessible to users. Cloud data centers are running out of space to hold all the data that users are putting into the cloud. There is severe over-or under-utilization at some data centers. Because of this, load balancing solutions are essential for cloud data centers. Moving tasks from overworked servers to ones that aren't yet at capacity is what's known as load balancing. We provide a solution that integrates Round Robin, Equally Spread, and Throttle for cloud load balancing. It provides a solid method for balancing workloads in the cloud. Our procedure for cloud load balancing is shown in Fig. 31.4, which is located below.

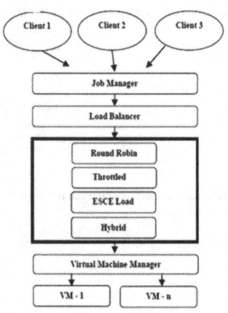

Fig. 31.4   Hybrid balancing of load procedure

6. Result and Discussion

Our work is shown in Fig. 31.5 with different choice to start with such as allocation, deallocation and balancing of load.

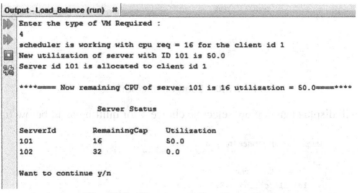

Fig. 31.5   Implementation main menu

After allocation of resources Fig. 31.6 shows the effect.

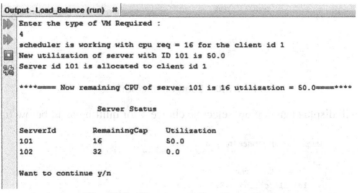

Fig. 31.6   Resource allocation effect

After this Main menu will display as we notice in Fig. 31.7.

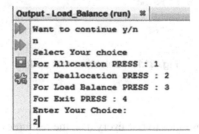

Fig. 31.7   de- allocation choice

The effect of de allocation is shown in Fig. 31.8.

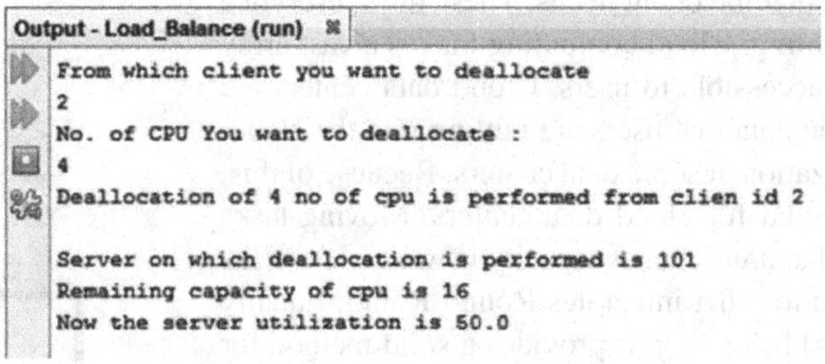

```
Output - Load_Balance (run)  ✕
From which client you want to deallocate
2
No. of CPU You want to deallocate :
4
Deallocation of 4 no of cpu is performed from clien id 2

Server on which deallocation is performed is 101
Remaining capacity of cpu is 16
Now the server utilization is 50.0
```

Fig. 31.8 Deallocation effect

The effect of load balancing can be viewed when we choose option 3 as below.

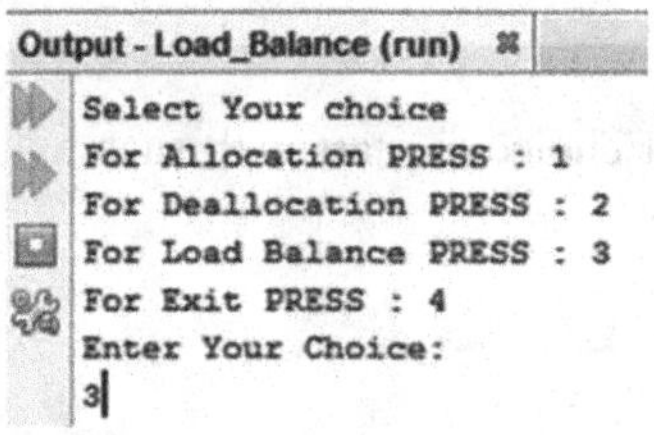

```
Output - Load_Balance (run)  ✕
Select Your choice
For Allocation PRESS : 1
For Deallocation PRESS : 2
For Load Balance PRESS : 3
For Exit PRESS : 4
Enter Your Choice:
3
```

Fig. 31.9 Load balancing option 3

The effect of load balancing is shown in Fig. 31.9.

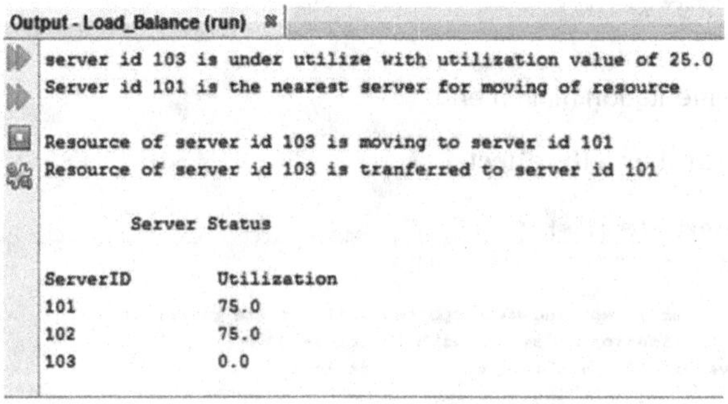

```
Output - Load_Balance (run)  ✕
server id 103 is under utilize with utilization value of 25.0
Server id 101 is the nearest server for moving of resource

Resource of server id 103 is moving to server id 101
Resource of server id 103 is tranferred to server id 101

        Server Status

ServerID        Utilization
101             75.0
102             75.0
103             0.0
```

Fig. 31.10 Load balance effect

After this main menu option will display again. Now select he choice 4 for quitting as in below figure

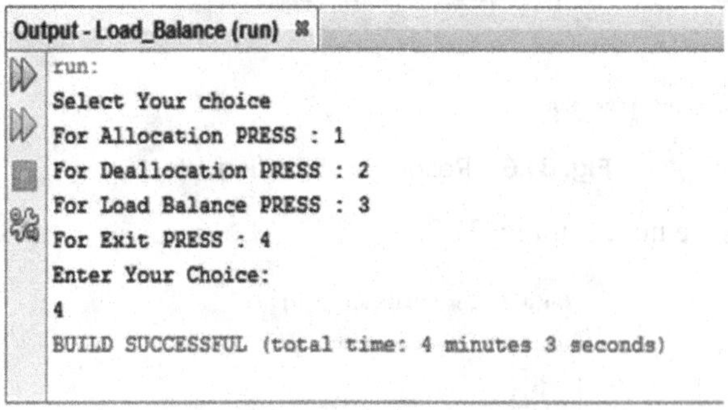

```
Output - Load_Balance (run)  ✕
run:
Select Your choice
For Allocation PRESS : 1
For Deallocation PRESS : 2
For Load Balance PRESS : 3
For Exit PRESS : 4
Enter Your Choice:
4
BUILD SUCCESSFUL (total time: 4 minutes 3 seconds)
```

Fig. 31.11 Selecting exit option

7. Conclusion

As the amount of data stored in the cloud continues to rise every day, the resources available in cloud data centers are becoming increasingly limited. Data centers in the cloud must employ load balancing as a result. The concept of load balancing permits the transfer of some workload from overworked to underutilized servers. Load balancing is addressed well in this study within the context of cloud computing. The concept of load balancing permits the transfer of some workload from overworked to underutilized servers. Dynamic algorithms are typically employed for load balancing. Numerous dynamic load balancing strategies are available for use when deciding how to distribute workloads across different cloud data centers. We provide a solution that integrates Round Robin, Equally Spread, and Throttle for cloud load balancing. It provides a solid method for balancing workloads in the cloud.

REFERENCES

1. Sharma, T. and Banga, V.K., "Efficient and Enhanced Algorithm in Cloud Computing", International Journal of Soft Computing and Engineering (IJSCE), 3(1), March 2013

2. Zhang, Q., Cheng, L., and Boutaba, R., "Cloud computing: state-of-the-art and research challenges", Journal of Internet Services and Applications, 1(1): pp. 7-18, (2010).

3. Bhavisha Patel, Shreyas Patel, "Various Load Balancing Algorithms in cloud Computing",. Vol-1 Issue-2 2015.

4. Amandeep Kaur Sidhu, Supriya Kinger, "Analysis of Load Balancing Techniques in Cloud Computing", International Journal of Computers &Technology Volume 4 No. 2, March-April, 2013, ISSN 2277-3061.

5. Y. Perwej, "Performance Analysis for Cloud Based OLAP over Big Data", IEEE International Conference on Innovative Computing, Intelligent Communication and Smart Electrical Systems (ICSES -2022), *IEEE* Conference, St. Joseph's Institute of Technology, *IEEE* Electronic ISBN:978-1-6654-7413-9, Chennai, India, 2022, DOI: 10.1109/ICSES55317.2022.9914266

6. Sareen, P., "Cloud Computing: Types, Architecture, Applications, Concerns, Virtualization and Role of IT Governance in Cloud", International Journal of Advanced Research in Computer Science and Software Engineering, 3(3): pp. 533-538,(2013).

7. Kulkarni, G., Gambhir, J., and Palwe, R., Cloud Computing-Software as Service. International Journal of Computer Trends and Technology, 2(2): pp. 178-182,(2011).

8. Abhinav Hans, Sheetal Kalra, "Comparative Study of Different Cloud Computing Load Balancing Techniques", 2014 International Conference on Medical Imaging, m-Health and Emerging Communication Systems (MedCom).

9. N. Akhtar, Dr. Bedine Kerim, Y. Perwej, Dr. Anurag Tiwari, Dr. Sheeba Praveen, "A Comprehensive Overview of Privacy and Data Security for Cloud Storage", International Journal of Scientific Research in Science, Engineering and Technology (IJSRSET), Online ISSN : 2394-4099, Print ISSN : 2395-1990, Volume 08, Issue 5, Pages 113-152, 2021, DOI: 10.32628/IJSRSET21852

10. Mohapatra, S., Rekha, K.S., and Mohanty, S., "A Comparison of Four Popular Heuristics for Load Balancing of Virtual Machines in Cloud Computing", International Journal of Computer Applications, 68,(2013).

11. Mamta Khanchi, Sanjay Tyagi, "an efficient algorithm for load balancing in cloud computing",© International Journal of Engineering Sciences & Research Technology.

12. Subhadra Bose Shaw, "A Survey on Scheduling and Load Balancing Techniques in Cloud Computing Environment", 2014 5th International Conference on Computer and Communication Technology (ICCCT).

13. Vishwas Bagwaiya, Sandeep k. Raghuwanshi, "Hybrid Approach Using Throttled and ESCE Load Balancing Algorithms In Cloud Computing".

Emerging Trends in IoT and Computing Technologies – Suman Lata Tripathi et al. (eds)
© 2024 Taylor & Francis Group, London, ISBN 978-1-032-87924-6

Analysis Volatility of Stock Market Using DL and LSTM

32

Deepak Asrani[1]

Professor, Department of Computer Science and Engineering,
B. N. College of Engineering & Technology, Lucknow

Puneet Kumar Yadav[2]

Assistant Professor, School of Engineering and Design,
Alliance University, Bangalore, India

Ihtiram Raza Khan[3]

Associate Professor, Computer Science Department,
Faculty of Engineering and Technology, Jamia Hamdard, Delhi, India

Vivek Rai[4]

Assistant Professor, Department of Computer Science and Engineering,
B. N. College of Engineering & Technology, U.P

Nikhat Akhtar[5]

Associate Professor, Department of Information Technology,
Goel Institute of Technology & Management, Lucknow

Rohit Agarwal[6]

Assistant Professor, Department of Computer Science and Engineering,
B. N. College of Engineering & Technology, U.P

Abstract: Predicting an asset's volatility can be useful, and volatility is used in many different financial scenarios. One frequently cited indicator is stock market volatility. Nonetheless, there are two problems with hone-learning (ML) techniques. They have problems when using projected volatility as the estimated target, which prevents their designs from being fairly compared to econometric ones. In this study, use a deep neural network (DNN) and a long-short-term memory (LSTM) model to predict stock index volatility. Based on the LSTM model of deep learning, develop a volatility prediction model which takes intraday high and low prices in financial asset sequences. There are two drawbacks to using the distance loss function, which is frequently employed in related research to train machine learning (ML) algorithms. In order to overcome the previously mentioned two problems, can use probability base LF for train DL techniques and evaluate model using the likelihood test sample. Our findings demonstrate LSTM model used in the two DL techniques with LF more precisely econometric and DL strategies with distance LF.

Keywords: Deep learning (DL), Autoregressive conditional heteroskedasticity (ARCH), Loss function (LF), Artificial neural networks (ANNs), Machine learning (ML)

[1]deepakasrani_in@yahoo.com, [2]puneet.yadav@alliance.edu.in, [3]erkhan2007@gmail.com, [4]vivekrai49@gmail.com, [5]dr.nikhatakhtar@gmail.com, [6]rohitagarwal0@gmail.com[6]

DOI: 10.1201/9781003535423-32

1. Introduction

An essential component of risk management and investment decision-making is the ability to foresee the volatility of financial assets. Volatility can be defined as the range of asset price fluctuation. A considerable change in asset values is implied by high volatility, whereas only minor price changes are implied by low volatility. Several techniques have been developed recently for forecasting the volatility of financial assets, however statistical models have long been the main instruments employed for this purpose. Generalized autoregressive conditional heteroskedasticity (GARCH) models like ARCH, GARCH have become quite popular among statistical models because they can represent the time-varying nature of volatility. Researchers have been investigating several non-linear models for predicting volatility thanks to recent developments in machine learning and deep learning. LSTM model has become most well-liked DL algorithms in forecasting volatility. The intricate temporal correlations and non-linear patterns found in financial time series data have been remarkably captured by the LSTM model. One of the most crucial financial market indicators is volatility. It has a direct bearing on market risk and can serve as a reliable indicator of the effectiveness and caliber of the financial market.

Enterprise trading methods, leverage decisions, consumer behavior and patterns, option pricing, and related macroeconomic variables are all significantly impacted by volatility. However, it is more difficult to predict key indicators due to the complex, time-varying, and nonlinear structure of financial data [1].When precise volatility forecasting is available, investors and investment firms can gain from more effective decision-making and reduced risk. In the contemporary financial sector, volatility has become a crucial quantitative parameter [2]. From a financial econometric perspective, ARCH and their generalization, GARCH-type models, make up the majority of the work on volatility forecasting. These heteroscedastic times series models are particularly useful for simulating highly volatile financial market data [3]. For each investment, an estimate of the risk or potential loss should be made. Value at Risk, or (VaR) as it is known by J.P. Morgan, is a notion that describes the nearly more loss in investment given level of confidence. The study focuses on LSTM in particular as a practical method for evaluating forecasting volatility [4]. Making accurate predictions is more important when the stock market is volatile than when it is relatively calm, thus understanding the underlying market situation is essential when assessing volatility projections. Econometric methods maximize the likelihood of the sample data to arrive at estimates for their parameters, whereas these machine learning models try to optimize for a specific set of outcomes. The econometric model's training and testing procedures differ because frequently value to further evaluate the prediction ability. This indicates that DL and econometric design are being inappropriately contrasted in the aforementioned articles [5]. This work suggests utilizing negative likelihood function as deep learning model's loss function to overcome problems here employ LF to train DL network without anticipating realized volatility in order to streamline the forecasting process. Comparisons between the DL and the econometric model are more accurate because both were trained using the likelihood function. In order to make sure that our models are consistent, we also compute the likelihood function for the test sample.

Furthermore, using simply index returns as inputs and no economic insight, we build a deep learning model that forecasts volatility. Deep learning can be used to anticipate volatility by starting with historical return series. The same inputs are used by both the DL and the econometric model for predicting volatility.

2. Related Work

Artificial intelligence in the stock market. The principles and characteristics of numerous machine learning methods are investigated in order to compare results, preferences, dislikes of various algorithms. Stock analysis algorithms are implemented using Python scripts [6]. Lapitskaya et al. (2022) investigated how well financial econometrics, ML, and DL methodologies predicted the return stocks that make up the S&P 100 index. Information as per media in COVID-19 gathered in ten-month period used to enhance study [7]. Because it can accurately forecast future data by utilizing the variance function, the model has gained favor in the field of time-series anticipation. By observing the world as it is, we can see that the majority of study objects for time series forecasting will be affected, and that information in the future will be incredibly unpredictable and subject to unforeseen changes. Both symmetric and asymmetric GARCH models, as put forth in 2005, can be used to forecast stock volatility [8].

In addition to its negative correlation, high-frequency volatility differs from low-frequency volatility in a number of ways. Machine learning has been used to solve a variety of technological problems as AI has developed. The data-problem orientation of AI models can be seen of as a form of historical empiricism, in contrast to the logic-driven approach of econometric models.

A regression tree model was successfully employed in 2017 to predict copper's long- and short-term pricing with development of ML techniques, various researchers started to concentrate on ensemble learning model. Due to finance data's inherent randomness and constant nonlinearity, however, standard neural networks struggle to handle huge financial datasets, which led to the creation of the LSTMNN [9]. ANN and deep learning frameworks have become well-known research fields in artificial intelligence. It is a feature-learning technology that can be trained to approximate any finite continuous function and learns a complex goal function using a large variety of fundamental transformation techniques. The daily volatility of IBM stock was correctly predicted by the authors in 1988 using artificial neural networks. Researchers were able to improve the accuracy of feed-forward neural networks' prediction using LSTM models [10].

3. Methodology

Deep Neural Network very popular ML models for volatility prediction. DNN consist input layer with m predictors, xi, four hidden layers with n neurons each neuron transforms outputs from the previous layer in a non-linear manner one output layer which generates value of y corresponding predicted historical volatility. In order to reduce the value of a loss function, optimization algorithm (backpropagation) modifies unknown weights and biases an iterative process throughout training DNN. The structure shown in Fig. 32.1 is typical of DNNs. Information is fed in model input layer. When calculating hidden and output layers, which are calculated by multiplying prior layer by connection weights activation-function used at each level. Combining the desired value with the predicted value discovered in the output layer yields a loss function. DNN attempts to minimize the loss function as it learns its connection weights. Most often, used to conduct process for

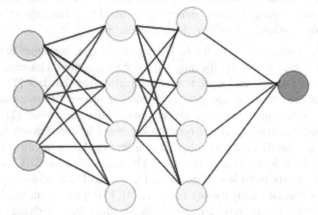

Input Layer   Hidden Layer 1   Hidden Layer 2   Output layer

Fig. 32.1 DNN model

optimization [11]. LSTM - Hochreiter and Schmidhuber (1997) introduced RNN variation known LSTM. A task exhibits long-term dependencies, as stated in Bengio et al. (1994), if the prediction of desired output at time t depends on input given time T earlier. When faced with such challenges, gradient-based learning algorithms like RNNs settle for suboptimal solutions that only consider short-term relationships and ignore long-term dependencies.

LSTM differs from ordinary RNN in that it uses gate to control information flow across sequence in order to learn long-term dependence and get around vanishing gradient problem. Figure 32.2 depicts typical LSTM architecture. Similar to a standard RNN, the model can accept inputs and provide outputs at each time step. In particular, the LSTM substitutes a memory block for each neuron in an RNN.

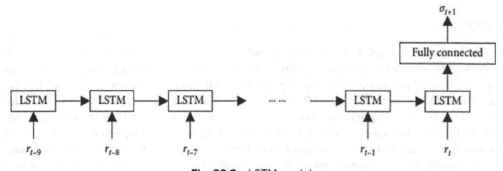

Fig. 32.2 LSTM model

A memory block is made up of one store cell, a single-entry gate, one forgets gate, and one output gate [12]. As noted in the Introduction, we train our DNN and LSTM approaches using a loss function that is based on the probability that an event will occur. The log-likelihood function needs to be optimized, as opposed to DL techniques, which are always taught by decreasing their LF. Therefore, the negative log likelihood should serve as DL model's loss function. To further reduce deep learning computing cost, our DNN and LSTM LF are simplified: These extra variables go with our DNN model discovered that the best conditional heteroscedasticity model [13].

Since 10-day return series are constantly input, it's crucial to set the input layer's unit number to 10. Two levels are kept as secrets. There are 40 units in the first concealed layer and a total of 80 units in the second. We'll use ReLU as the activation function and give it a dropout of 0.3 for hidden layers. On output layer, the sigmoid function used. RMSprop is employed as optimizer throughout the model's training. Batch size is 2048 by default. The training procedure will conclude early if the loss function stops dropping for the validation set. LSTM model includes a fully linked layer in the final time step. The length of the input series is fixed at 10. The unit size of an LSTM layer is 20. The completely linked layer has 40 nodes, and ReLU is selected as the activation function fully connected layer, used a dropout of 0.5, whereas on the LSTM layer, use none but in output layer sigmoid activation-function used [14][15].

RMSprop used as the optimizer throughout the model's training. 2048 is the standard batch size. The training procedure will conclude early if the loss function stops dropping for the validation set. For both the DNN and LSTM techniques, dataset divided the total sample into a train set (70%) a validation set (15%), and test set (15%). Using 85% of the data from the train set, estimate the parameters of the ARMAGARCH model and the straightforward method, doing away with the need for validation during training. Train-test split employed by ARMA-GARCH and simple techniques is time-ordered, while deep learning models use the train-validation-test split in a similar way. They can be easily compared because they both use the same test data to determine their log-likelihood values.

4. Result and Discussion

By keeping track of the LF values of the train and validation samples at each epoch, Figure 32.3 and 32.4 depicts the learning curves created during likelihood-based function training of the LSTM. With a value of 15241.51, the S&P 500's validation LF reaches its lowest point during epoch 723. The loss function for Dow Jones validation Epoch 568, 15755.87 is the lowest point in the history of the Industrial Average.

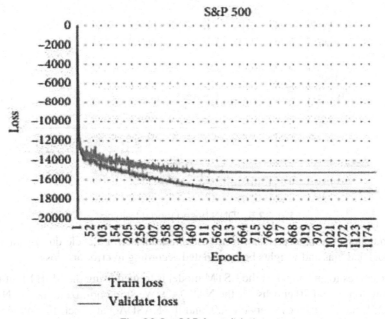

Fig. 32.3   S&P for validation

At 14600.25 for the validation loss function epoch 1212, the NASDAQ model operates at peak efficiency. For each training and validation epoch of the DNN model, note the values of the loss functions for the training and validation samples, which are based on the likelihood function. Figure 32.5 displays the results of learning curves. At epoch 1318, the validation LF for the S&P 500 is -15197.80, which means that the model has learnt the least at this moment. At epoch 622, the model gets 15735.40 as validation LF for the Dow Jones, which is the lowest. With a measurement of 14586.70, epoch 688 holds the NASDAQ's lowest validation LF value.

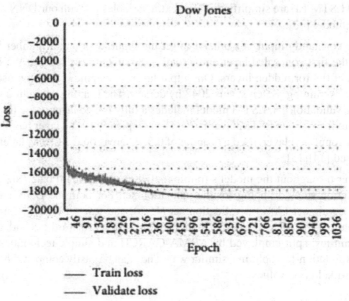

Fig. 32.4 For dow jones validation loss

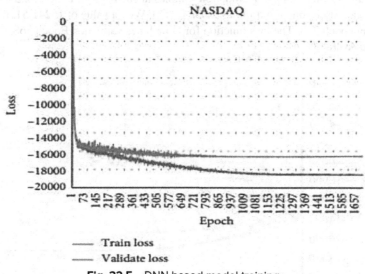

Fig. 32.5 DNN based model training

Epoch can be referred as number of total steps taken to train overall dataset in a cycle during training time. Every iteration dataset is processed by model and bias and weights being updated according to error and loss.

The optimization procedure comes to an end when the LSTM model is trained using the MSE LF after 90 epochs for the S&P 500, 422 epochs for the Dow Jones, and 70 epochs for the NASDAQ. We stop optimizing the DNN model with the MSE LF for the S&P 510 at epoch 271, the Dow Jones at epoch 309, and the NASDAQ at epoch 174. When both DL models train at the same pace, it is clear that the likelihood-based model converges more slowly than the MSE loss function-based model. To visually demonstrate the predictive power of the DL strategies and the econometric model, we show the learning curves produced by logging the likelihood-based LF values of the train samples and the validation samples each epoch during DNN model training in Fig. 32.4. We then calculate the percentage of improvement made by DNN, LSTM (MSE loss), DNN (MSE loss), and ARMA-GARCH over the simple method in Fig. 32.6.

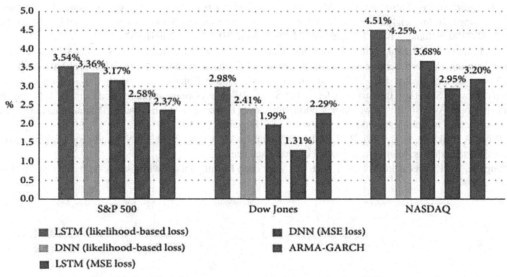

Fig. 32.6 Model improvement of simple method at 10% test set

5. Conclusion

This study forecasts the volatility of three US stock indexes using DL methods, an econometric model, and a basic statistical approach. We evaluate all approaches according to the probability of the test sample and offer a likelihood-based LF for teaching DL strategies to separate our work from past works in this subject. Deep learning algorithms can predict volatility with less room for mistake. We can compare the several models we're looking at on a more even playing field simultaneously. Comparing our DL approaches with a likelihood-based LF to the econometric model, the empirical analysis shows that our volatility estimations are more exact. All six models are quite good in predicting volatility series long-term trends. Lastly, we find that LSTM consistently beats the other models in volatility predictions using deep learning. Although LSTM (MSE loss) has uneven performance, it outperforms ARMA-GARCH in over 50% of all cases. Due to its inferior performance, DNN (MSE loss) cannot be used in place of ARMA-GARCH. Both the DL approach and the econometric model show significant improvements over the basic method at the same time.

REFERENCES

1. Wang, T., 2023, April. Stock Volatility Forecasting: Adopting LSTM Deep Learning Method and Comparing the Results with GARCH Family Model. In Proceedings of the International Conference on Financial Innovation, FinTech and Information Technology, FFIT 2022, October 28-30, 2022, Shenzhen, China

2. Ashok, K., Boddu, R., Syed, S.A., Sonawane, V.R., Dabhade, R.G. and Reddy, P.C.S., 2023. GAN Base feedback analysis system for industrial IOT networks. Automatika, 64(2), pp.259-267

3. Altig, Dave, Scott Baker, Jose Maria Barrero, Nicholas Bloom, Philip Bunn, Scarlet Chen, Steven J. Davis, Julia Leather, Brent Meyer, Emil Mihaylov, and et al. 2020. Economic Uncertainty before and during the COVID-19 Pandemic. Journal of Public Economics 191: 104274

4. Lokesh, S., Priya, A., Sakhare, D.T., Devi, R.M., Sahu, D.N. and Reddy, P.C.S., 2022. CNN based deep learning methods for precise analysis of cardiac arrhythmias. International journal of health sciences, 6

5. Jia, F. and Yang, B., 2021. Forecasting volatility of stock index: deep learning model with likelihood-based loss function. Complexity, 2021, pp.1-13

6. Gao, Zhao, 2020. The application of artificial intelligence in stock investment. J. Phys. Conf. 1453, 012069.

7. N. Akhtar, Nazia Tabassum, Dr. Asif Perwej, Y. Perwej," Data Analytics and Visualization Using Tableau Utilitarian for COVID-19 (Coronavirus)", Global Journal of Engineering and Technology Advances (GJETA), ISSN : 2582-5003, Volume 3, Issue 2, Pages 28-50, May 2020, DOI: 10.30574/gjeta.2020.3.2.0029

8. Kumar, K., Pande, S.V., Kumar, T.C., Saini, P., Chaturvedi, A., Reddy, P.C.S. and Shah, K.B., 2023. Intelligent Controller Design and Fault Prediction Using Machine Learning Model. International Transactions on Electrical Energy Systems, 2023.

9. Muthappa, K.A., Nisha, A.S.A., Shastri, R., Avasthi, V. and Reddy, P.C.S., 2023. Design of high-speed, low-power non-volatile master slave flip flop (NVMSFF) for memory registers designs. Applied Nanoscience, pp.1-10

10. Y. Perwej, "The Bidirectional Long-Short-Term Memory Neural Network based Word Retrieval for Arabic Documents", Transactions on Machine Learning and Artificial Intelligence (TMLAI), which is published by Society for Science and Education, United Kingdom (UK), ISSN 2054-7390, Volume 3, Issue 1, Pages 16 - 27, 2015, DOI: 10.14738/tmlai.31.863

11. Prasath, A.S.S., Lokesh, S., Krishnakumar, N.J., Vandarkuzhali, T., Sahu, D.N. and Reddy, P.C.S., 2022. Classification of EEG signals using machine learning and deep learning techniques. International journal of health sciences, 2022, pp.10794-10807.

12. Sucharitha, Y. and Shaker Reddy, P.C., 2022. An Autonomous Adaptive Enhancement Method Based on Learning to Optimize Heterogeneous Network Selection. International Journal of Sensors Wireless Communications and Control, 12(7), pp.495-509

13. Kolte, Ashutosh, Pawar, Avinash, Roy, Jewel Kumar, Vida, Imre, Vasa, Laszlo, ´2022. Evaluating the return volatility of cryptocurrency market: an econometrics modelling method. Acta Polytechnica Hungarica 19, 107–126

14. Lokesh, S., Priya, A., Sakhare, D.T., Devi, R.M., Sahu, D.N. and Reddy, P.C.S., 2022. CNN based deep learning methods for precise analysis of cardiac arrhythmias. International journal of health sciences, 6

15. Jia, F. and Yang, B., 2021. Forecasting volatility of stock index: deep learning model with likelihood-based loss function. Complexity, 2021, pp.1-13

Emerging Trends in IoT and Computing Technologies – Suman Lata Tripathi et al. (eds)
© 2024 Taylor & Francis Group, London, ISBN 978-1-032-87924-6

Basic Approaches and Efforts to Improve Our Understanding of the Behavior of Natural Computational Systems

33

Kaneez Zainab[1]
Associate Professor, Department of Computer Science and Engineering,
B. N. College of Engineering & Technology, Lucknow

Alok Mishra[2]
Dean Academics and Professor Physics,
Gaya College of Engineering (GCE), Gaya, Bihar

Devendra Agarwal[3]
Dean Academics, Goel Institute of Technology & Management, Lucknow, U.P,

Nikhat Akhtar[4]
Associate Professor, Department of Information Technology,
Goel Institute of Technology & Management, Lucknow, U.P

Syed Qamar Abbas[5]
Director General, Ambalika Institute of Management & Technology, Lucknow, U.P

Sanjay Kumar Singh[6]
Assistant Professor, Department of Computer Science and Engineering,
B. N. College of Engineering & Technology, Lucknow

Abstract: The term "natural computation" is used in scientific discourse to denote the advancement of problem-solving methodologies, the replication of natural phenomena, and the exploitation of natural resources within the realm of computer. Natural computing encompasses several prominent areas of research, such as DNA computing, quantum computing, artificial life, swarm intelligence, fractal geometry, artificial immune systems, and evolutionary algorithms. This study presents a demonstration of the use of natural computing in implementing various computational paradigms, such as self-replication, functionality, and computational techniques on alternative physical media, such as quantum computing devices. The development of a framework for the design of natural computing systems is a challenge. Natural information processing systems include many mechanisms like self-assembly, gene regulatory networks, and developmental processes. This paper examines the core concepts of process and explores endeavors to comprehend natural computational systems. These include the field of semi-synthetic process engineering, the study of the universe through the lens of information processing, which has emerged as a more fundamental aspect than energy or matter, and proposals for the implementation of quantum computer behavior.

Keywords: Natural computation, Functioning, Information processing, Quantum behavior's, Lattice based model

[1]kaneez_srm@yahoo.com, [2]dralokmishra72@gmail.com, [3]dr.devendra@goel.edu.in, [4]dr.nikhatakhtar@gmail.com, [5]qrat_abbas@yahoo.com, [6]sanjay.lookmax@gmail.com

DOI: 10.1201/9781003535423-33

1. Introduction

The field of study referred to as "Natural Computational" challenges the inherent specialization within engineering and scientific disciplines. Natural computing refers to the practice of drawing motivation from the natural environment to construct computational systems [1]. The field of natural computing encompasses the study of computing systems that are inspired by nature, as well as the investigation of computer processes that occur inside natural systems. This study examines models and computational approaches that draw inspiration from natural phenomena [2], as well as the information processing activities that take place in nature. The study investigated the computational behavior of using natural materials, including the examination of computational models and methodologies, as well as the exploration of emulation and simulation methods inspired by nature. Additionally, the study addressed the concept of computing with natural materials. The primary focus of natural computing approaches is on the accelerated mechanisms and processes [3] that underpin certain phenomena. Natural Computation integrates empirical and theoretical insights derived from observations of natural phenomena, as well as investigations into the workings of nature, in order to accomplish its goals. Natural computing functions as an authentic transdisciplinary conduit that connects the field of computer science with the natural sciences. The connection between the two entities, namely in the realms of basic research and information technology, is established by a link [4]. Natural computing research is characterized by its multidisciplinary nature, including several domains such as software applications, algorithms [5], pure theoretical study, and experimental laboratory research in physics, chemistry, and biology. Natural Computing is a well-recognized academic discipline that encompasses several traditional courses and remains very dynamic [6]. Additionally, it encompasses numerous modern and innovative research areas.

2. NCP (Natural Computing Process)

Natural computational processes as well as artificially created computing that draw design cues from nature are also referred to as "natural computing." We better understand both nature and the fundamentals of computation when we analyses complex natural phenomena in terms of computer operations. Human-designed computing that draws inspiration from natural systems is characterized by the metaphorical use of ideas, concepts, and processes that underlie natural systems. Software is provided through [7] NCP (Natural Computing Process) tools, while wetware creates patterns, animals, and behavior that are then combined to create original computing techniques for natural computation. For the purpose of resolving natural facts and processes and obtaining outcomes, it is possible to choose the appropriate abstraction and research level. The following categories in NCP's system describe the many types of inspiration [8]. Evolutionary computation is a phrase that describes how computers have developed over time. Neural computation is the brain, while cellular automata are the self-reproduction. Swarm intelligence [9] is described as a group's. Immune computing represents the immune system, Artificial [10] Life represents the qualities of life, Membrane Computing represents cells and membranes, and Amorphous Computing represents morphogenesis.

2.1 Neural Computation

A computer system or artificial neural network is one that attempts to simulate the way the human nervous system operates by emulating its architecture and functions. While some neural networks aim to comprehend organic brain functions, others tackle artificial intelligence (AI) problems without necessarily mimicking real biological systems. To better depict the neurological system, neural networks that put an emphasis on physiological details are preferable [11]. Multiple tiers of information processing, such as synapses, linked neuronal modules, and interactions between individual neurons, are included in these models.

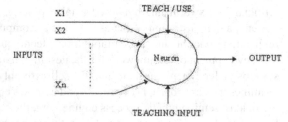

Fig. 33.1 Input out processing in system

One of the most daunting endeavours is the development of artificial brains. Building a silicon model of a mammalian brain has the potential to improve our knowledge of how the human brain works through detailed simulations. A greater degree of detachment from real biological systems is frequently observed in neural networks that have an emphasis on application-oriented methods [12]. Connected synthetic neurons provide the backbone of an artificial neural network (ANN) [13], as seen in Fig. 33.1. It takes input values chosen by neurons before output and processes them using a vectorial function. The following elements make up the aforementioned entities: In addition to being teachable, NCP's behaviour displays traits of distributed and parallel processing [14].

2.2 Cellular Automata

Cellular automata are computational models that consist of a grid of cells, each of which might be in one of a finite number of Cellular automata, which have been in existence for over half a century, are considered to be among the first models of computing. A cellular automaton (CA) is a mathematical abstraction representing a group of cells that engage in local interactions with one another [15]. In this cellular space, every individual cell possesses a distinct set of neighbouring cells. Each cell is characterized by specific values or states, and all cells undergo simultaneous updates of their values at discrete time intervals or iterations. Additionally, each cell adheres to a local function or rule that governs its transition to a new state, taking into account the current states of its neighbouring cells, including its own. [16].

2.3 Evolutionary Computation

Evolutionary computation refers to a computational approach that draws inspiration from the principles of biological evolution. It involves the use of algorithms. The primary focus of the field of evolutionary computing is in the examination and development of algorithms derived from models based on natural evolution. The basic aim of evolutionary computation is to develop computer algorithms that can effectively address and solve complex search and optimization challenges [17]. The current advancements in the application, theoretical understanding, algorithmic construction, integration with other techniques, and comprehension of working principles related to these algorithms are yielding remarkable achievements. Over the course of the last five decades, several evolutionary algorithms have been developed, building upon the foundational algorithms that before them. This approach involves the formation of a cohesive team including individuals who work together to identify and develop resolutions for challenges [18]. An algorithm may be used to generate the starting population in a random manner [19]. Computational intelligence, which falls under the umbrella of machine learning and artificial intelligence, encompasses the field of evolutionary computing.

2.4 Swarm Intelligence

Nature may serve as a source of motivation to computer scientists in a variety of ways. One such motivation comes from the way natural organisms behave together. Consider a bacterial colony, a flock of starlings, an ant colony, or a bee colony [20]. According to biologists, in these and several more cases, the group of people exhibits behaviours that its individual members either cannot or do not exhibit. To put it a different way, when we consider the group as a whole, the swarm at least seems to be smarter than any one of its members. Consequently, swarm intelligence has nothing to do with the life cycle of slime module, nor does it have anything to do with how populations of cells become brains or humans build civilizations. However, whether they realize it or not, it includes individuals cooperating to achieve a common goal. Two instances of insects demonstrating efficient navigation include ants determining the most expedient route between their colony and a highly favorable food source, and bees identifying the optimal nectar sources within the vicinity of their hive. Swarm intelligence is a computational intelligence approach that is used to address intricate problems. Swarm intelligence is a significant factor in several sectors, as it ensures the proper functioning of Internet of Things (IoT) and IoT-based systems [21]. The resolution of challenges in IoT-based systems, which are characterized by their intricate nature and integration of smart devices, necessitates the implementation of resilient decentralized algorithms supported by system intelligence. The dynamic characteristics, device mobility, wireless connection, and information supply of intelligent algorithms in the context of SI enable them to effectively tackle the complex challenges posed by IoT systems [22].

2.5 Immune Computing

The goal of developing computer models that imitate the innate immune systems observed in many biological species was the impetus for the introduction of the idea of immunological computing in the late 1980s and early 1990s [23], [24]. A decentralized and parallel method allows the immune system to participate in multiple sophisticated computations, allowing it to be conceptualized as an information processing system [25]. Many cognitive processes, such as learning, memory, and associative retrieval, are necessary for the effective management of identification and classification challenges. These include differentiating self-cells from nonself cells and neutralizing nonself pathogenic agents. Due to its strong information processing capabilities, the natural immune system is occasionally called the "second brain" (26). This method makes use of recent developments in machine learning as well as those in artificial intelligence more generally. It may be considered a subset of the fields of computational biology and naturally occurring computing. Protecting the host from foreign invaders including viruses, parasites, fungus, and bacteria is the fundamental role of the innate immune system. It is the main job of the immune system to sort the cells in the body into two groups: those that belong to the person (self) and those that come from outside the body (nonself) [27]. Immunology, computer science, and engineering are all interconnected fields that this multidisciplinary discipline helps to advance. The capacity of the immune system to recognize, display diversity, learn, and tolerate has been highlighted [28]. Artificial immune systems (AIS) have also been useful in solving a number of problems, including as optimization, distributed detection, pattern recognition, learning and memory, and others [29]. In addition, it can adjust to new circumstances.

2.6 The Study of Artificial Life

The word "artificial life" has several connotations. The term "artificial life," or ALife as it is now known, was used by Langton (1989) to denote the study of artificial systems that manifest traits like those seen in living creatures. The first conceptualization of artificial life, as proposed by Langton [30], pertained to living forms that are generated by human intervention rather than arising naturally. Following the identification of substantial issues with the first concept, Langton proceeded to rework it as "the examination of natural existence, encompassing human beings and their artifacts within the scope of nature rather than excluding them." since to his perspective, a key objective of ALife should include eliminating the distinction between "artificial life" and "biology," since people and their activities are inherently interconnected with the natural world [31]. Biologists now use computer models often in their research, a practice that has become integral to modern biology. Within the expanding realm of interdisciplinary research including the life sciences and computer science, artificial life is poised to endure and capitalize on forthcoming improvements in technology and scientific understanding, encompassing both biological and computational domains [33]. Natural computing is anticipated to have a leading role.

2.7 Membrane Computing

The computational paradigm known as "Membrane Computing" is based on the design and operation of biological membranes. Research in this area focuses on membrane systems and their applications, The basic properties displayed by biological membranes provide the basis for membrane systems, which are used as computer simulations. Computing at the membrane level entails studying computational models based on the molecular and cellular properties of real cells, tissues, and other complex systems [34]. Precisely, membrane computing abstracts the internal compartmentalization allowed by membranes as a property of living organisms. To what extent they are able to pass through or remain within membrane-bound compartments depends on the components and regulatory systems that are in charge of their transformation. Consequently, the broadcast allows for communication on a regional level. A great deal of formal work has gone into trying to model the delicate process by which chemicals may cross biological membranes. The structure of a membrane encases several groups of things inside its allotted compartments [36].

2.8 Amorphous Computing

Amorphous computing refers to a computational paradigm that involves the use of large numbers of simple computing elements, which are capable of self. The motivation for the development of amorphous computing stems from the observation of shape generation, or morphogenesis, in biological organisms. In these organisms, the interactions between cells, guided by genetic programming, result in the emergence of distinct shapes and functional structures. In accordance with this notion, an amorphous computing medium is comprised of several asynchronous computer units that engage in local interactions, with their arrangement being randomized [37]. The computational particles, which are programmed in a similar manner, exhibit interactions only with neighbouring particles and can assume certain forms and patterns, resembling predetermined planar graphs [38]. The objective of amorphous computing is to integrate the interplay among a multitude of volatile computational entities that are interconnected in irrational, unexpected, and temporally fluctuating ways, with the aim of generating anticipated coherent computational phenomena [37]. The objective is to concurrently cultivate novel programming concepts that may be used to amorphous computing environments. Amorphous computing refers to the advancement of organizational structures and programming languages that aim to derive cohesive behaviours from the collaborative efforts of several unreliable components, which are interconnected in a manner that lacks logical, predictable, and consistent patterns across time.

3. Scope of Artificial Neural Networks

Because of their extraordinary capacity to infer meaning from imprecise or complicated data, neural networks may be used to find trends and patterns in data that are too complex for humans or other computer systems to notice. Neural networks are extremely complicated modelling tools capable of simulating even more complex actions. Neural networks in particular are nonlinear [39]. In most modelling domains, linear models have long been the preferred option due to their well-recognized optimization processes. When the linear approximation proved to be faulty, as it usually did, the models suffered. Neural networks also govern the curse of dimensionality issue, which befalls efforts to describe nonlinear functions with many variables. Neural networks can learn from examples. Using training techniques, the user of a neural network [40] gathers representative data and then automatically deduces the structure of the data. The amount of user knowledge needed to use neural networks effectively is far less than it would be if one were to use them alone. It is particularly useful for problems involving function approximation (mapping), clustering, and classification when precise restrictions are hard to apply. Vests provides lists of the practical and commercial applications of NCP [41]. This website includes applications related to robotics, signal processing, time-series prediction [42], chemistry, criminal justice, process recognition, gaming, sports, gambling, business, and weather forecasting.

4. Design Principles

The Natural Computing Process (NCP) has some characteristics and performance commonalities with the system. Units are small, discrete components that make up the fundamental processing. These units have the ability to broadcast and receive from different environments. It may be linked to additional objects to create neural networks. Transmission of information occurs between connecting connections. A comparable strength or weight value represents effectiveness, which is associated with the data stored in the network and, by extension, in the neuron. Knowledge is obtained via a mechanism of learning, whereby the connection strengths, or weight values, to external stimuli are modified. This acquisition of intelligence is facilitated by the environment.

5. Current Trends and Open Problems

Among the first and most pervasive forms of natural computing, artificial neural networks have seen enormous application throughout the years. Consequently, the NCP conducts research in a wide range of areas, such as practical applications, theoretical investigations, improvements and advancements, methodology integration, and system modelling. There has been a lot of recent focus on non-custodial parents (NCPs). Current research and implementation mostly revolve around productive architectures, which are networks with adaptive structures. These networks may adapt their architecture to meet different needs. There is also continuous research on hybrid techniques that combine several neural computing paradigms, as well as formal elements like convergence and universal approximation capabilities, and ensembles of networks. In addition, neural networks that mimic biological systems and those that rely on statistical learning theory for example, support vector machines—are becoming more popular. Data mining, web mining, time-series data analysis, integrated collaborative systems involving many interactive agents, and signal processing are all complex problems that might be handled by neural networks that are based on cognitive and physiological principles (44) as an approach.

6. Modelling through Computation

Mathematical models of complicated systems can be simulated using computational models. The biological sciences provide one example of a domain that has used computational modelling to assess an influenza pandemic [45]. Through the use of mathematical models and computer simulations, several possible outcomes may be explored and analysed by adjusting the model's parameters. Over the last ten years, systems biology has been profoundly affected by computational models and approaches. These originally came from computer science and were used to assess the reliability and security of software programs. Building a biological model in a specific setting is analogous to creating software in a specific environment. The control flow of biological processes may be represented using a number of domain-specific programming languages. The rules for building instructions or whole sentences are dictated by the syntactic structure of a language. Because computational modelling allows for a unified computational environment, scientific researchers have access to a wide variety of modelling tools. Software like COPASI allows for the numerical [46] modelling and study of the stochastic dynamics of biochemical networks.

6.1 Hybrid Systems

Hybrid systems provide a continuous dynamic to each state or mode, extending the previously specified state-based discrete representation. Systems biology is increasingly focusing on hybrid modeling approaches [47] because of their capacity to represent the behavior of biological systems with obvious switching features. For example, Hill-type kinetics, which exhibits sigmoidal behavior at the molecular level, as well as cellular, tissue, organ, and population models all display sigmoidal behaviours. In general, hybrid modelling may be used to blend qualitative and quantitative data [48] (provided by continuous dynamics).

6.2 Lattice-based Models

In n dimensions, a lattice is made up of identical closed grid sites that recur periodically as graph structures. The structures in question are defined by directionally periodic or set boundary restrictions. Molecular, cellular, tissue, or organ-level processes that include interconnections lend themselves particularly well to explanation using this lattice. According to reference [49], the mechanical properties of tissues and organs at the microscopic, macroscopic, and macroscopic levels are comparable to the aforementioned natural levels. Discrete in time, space, and state, cellular automata are dynamical systems with discrete behavior. A possible explanation for the development of cellular pattern generation might be the interaction of short- and long-range components. A hierarchical network topology without cycles or terminal nodes, known as a Bethe lattice, has been used for immunological network modeling.

6.3 Temporal Logics

In this section, we will discuss the concept of temporal logics. Temporal logics are formal systems that allow reasoning about the Temporal logics are considered to be very concise languages for accurately specifying the manifestation of certain temporal behaviours. Linear Temporal Logic (LTL) is a frequently used temporal logic for the analysis of event sequencing during program execution. The syntax for Linear Temporal Logic (LTL) is specified by the grammar. The fundamental hypothesis p denotes a Boolean value that potentially describes the association between a value at a certain moment and a variable representing the state of a system. As an example, it might be said that the concentration of species $x1$ is more than or equal to a certain threshold value, denoted as $r (x1 \geq r)$, or that an event is expected to transpire. Additional complex logical formulations may be achieved by the integration of assertions using logical operators such as "or" ($\vee$) and "not" ($\neg$).

6.4 Compartment-based Models

Systems are often compartmentalized, transferring molecules between them in accordance with predetermined principles. The dynamic rearrangements of the compartments and the movement of molecules across them are just two examples of the biological aspects that compartment-based models are specialized to represent.

6.5 Agent-based Models (ABMs)

Agent-based models (ABMs) are computational models that simulate the behaviour and interactions of autonomous agents inside a given system. These models are widely used in several fields, including. Agent-based techniques include the consideration of a collection of independent entities that possess the ability to make decisions autonomously. Each of these agents have the ability to sense their immediate environment and then make individual decisions based on a predetermined set of rules. At its fundamental essence, an agent-based model comprises a collection of agents and their interconnections. However, despite its simplicity, this model has the capacity to demonstrate complex behavioural patterns via modifications and adjustments in response to environmental obstacles or the behaviours of neighbouring agents [51].

6.6 Formal Analysis

A more academic examination of the topic will follow in the next section. The importance of modelling languages in promoting the production of novel ideas by scientists is emphasized in the aforementioned section, which emphasizes their ability to provide thorough explanations of processes found via testing. Following the model's construction, it's crucial to use a suitable tool for analysing the syntax and interpreting its semantics within the chosen modelling language. Additionally, it should be noted that a model can go through a process called compilation, when it is transformed into a computer program that copies the investigated biological process [52]. Based on specific starting points, the created software may predict the emergent behaviour of a system. This approach streamlines testing procedures and reduces the need for expensive and time-consuming research by focusing on tests that can uncover interesting and novel events.

6.7 Static Analysis

Static Analysis refers to the process of examining software code without executing it. This technique is often used in software development to identify potential defects, vulnerabilities, and other. The analysis is performed based on the model's static description, which refers to its characteristics and attributes rather than its actual execution. The first use of static analysis concepts was seen in the field of compiler optimization. Currently, the practice of software verification often employs an approach that primarily focuses on identifying possibly susceptible code inside critical safety systems. Static analysis is a technique that acts at the syntactic level of a specification or use abstract interpretation to analyse constrained approximations of potential model executions [53]. In recent years, the efficacy of static analysis as a technique for model analysis has significantly increased. The approach used by the authors effectively facilitates the investigation of biological processes. The authors use a meticulous depiction of the low-density lipoprotein (LDL) degradation mechanism in ambientes in order to calculate a precise [54] overestimation of the theoretically boundless reaction sequences projected by the model.

6.8 Model Verification

Model confirmation is an automated approach for formal verification that may be used to investigate the underlying causes of certain behaviors in biological models. This approach involves the use of a Kripke structure, which is a discrete time model including a limited number of states. Within this model, the execution triggers a series of events that determine the truthfulness of the propositions stated by a temporal logic equation.

7. Tools

The topic of tools is of great significance in several academic disciplines. Tools play a crucial role in enhancing efficiency, productivity, and effectiveness. The aforementioned notions are now used as a framework for selecting from the range of available tools, however it is important to note that this selection process is not exhaustive. Additionally, we provide a range of software options that are directly relevant to the subject matter addressed in this study. The tools are classified based on the existing literature, including the formal analysis capabilities, supported execution semantics, and the computational modeling language they support. Additionally, we indicate if the NCPs tool provides a mechanism for optimizing the parameters of the model in accordance with the formal assessment process.

8. Conclusion

The goal of the field known as "natural computing" is to develop better computer systems by studying how the natural world works. It includes several computational. When studying how computers work, it's important to take into account not just their intrinsic traits but also their computational connection to the physical environment. Multiple natural computing processes have been discovered to provide new and interesting possibilities across the area of research, especially in the biosciences, engineering, and scientific sectors. Three separate approaches to solving problems have been grouped under the umbrella term 'natural computing' methods that model their work after observed natural phenomena, methods that use computational modeling to mimic real-world processes, and methods that make use of molecules and other naturally occurring resources for computational needs. Artificial immune systems, fractal geometry, artificial life, quantum computing, evolutionary algorithms, swarm intelligence, artificial neural networks, and DNA computing are just a few of the many key study fields found in these three disciplines. Studying the groundwork of natural computing, which encompasses a number of different academic fields, is the major goal of this study. The biological motivation, fundamental design concepts, real-world applications, current research trends, and outstanding problems in these areas are the primary areas of attention in this study. It is possible to theorize that algorithmic tools for problem-solving may be built around natural computing events, either by directly incorporating these phenomena into computer systems or by simulating and emulating them.

REFERENCES

1. Hunt CH, Ropella GEP, Park S, Engelberg J. Dichotomies between computational and mathematical models. Nature Biotechnology., 26(7):737–738. pmid:18612289, 2008
2. Maria Vittoria Avolio, Valeria Lupiano, Paolo Mazzanti, and Salvatore Di Gregorio. A cellular automata model for flow-like landslides with numerical simulations of subaerial and subaqueous cases. EnviroInfo, 1:131–140, 2009
3. Y. Perwej, "The Bidirectional Long-Short-Term Memory Neural Network based Word Retrieval for Arabic Documents", Transactions on Machine Learning and Artificial Intelligence (TMLAI), which is published by Society for Science and Education, United Kingdom (UK), ISSN 2054-7390, Volume 3, Issue 1, Pages 16 - 27, Feb 2015, DOI: 10.14738/tmlai.31.863
4. S Binitha, S Siva Sathya, et al. A survey of bio inspired optimization algorithms. International Journal of Soft Computing and Engineering, 2(2):137–151, 2012
5. J.R. Koza, "Genetically Breeding Populations of Computer Programs to Solve Problems in Artificial Intelligence," pp. 819-827 in Proceedings of the Second International Conference on Tools for Artificial Intelligence, IEEE, Los Alamitos, CA, 1990.
6. S. Wolfram, "Computation Theory of Cellular Automata," Communications in Mathematical Physics 96:15-57, 1984
7. P. Dayan and L. Abbott, Theoretical Neuroscience: Comput. and Mathematical Modeling of Neural Systems. MIT Press, 2001

8. C. Eliasmith and C. H. Anderson, Neural engineering: Computation, representation, and dynamics in neurobiological systems. MIT press, 2004

9. Asif Perwej, Y. Perwej, N. Akhtar, "A FLANN and RBF with PSO Viewpoint to Identify a Model for Competent Forecasting Bombay Stock Exchange", COMPUSOFT, SCOPUS, An International Journal of Advanced Computer Technology, 4 (1), Volume-IV, Issue-I, PP 1454-1461, 2015, DOI : 10.6084/ijact.v4i1.60

10. Y. Perwej, "An Evaluation of Deep Learning Miniature Concerning in Soft Computing", International Journal of Advanced Research in Computer and Communication Engineering (IJARCCE), Volume 4, Issue 2, Pages 10 - 16, 2015, DOI: 10.17148/IJARCCE.2015.4203

11. W. Gerstner and W. M. Kistler, Spiking neuron models: Single neurons, populations, plasticity. Camb. Uni. Pr., 2002

12. Trivedi, A.; Tripathi, C.M.; Perwej, Y.; Srivastava, A.K.; Kulshrestha, N. Face Recognition Based Automated Attendance Management System. Int. J. Sci. Res. Sci. Technol., 9, pp 261–268, 2022

13. Y. Perwej, "Recurrent Neural Network Method in Arabic Words Recognition System", International Journal of Computer Science and Telecommunications (IJCST), Sysbase Solution (Ltd), UK, London, Volume 3, Issue 11, Pages 43-48, 2012

14. B. Rosenfeld, O. Simeone, and B. Rajendran, "Learning first-to-spike policies for neuromorphic control using policy gradients," in Proc. IEEE International Workshop on Signal Processing Advances in Wireless Communications (SPAWC), Cannes, France, 2019

15. T. Toffoli and N. Margolus, Cellular Automata Machines: A New Environment for Modeling, MIT Press, Cambridge, MA, 1987

16. G. Ganek and T.A. Corbi, "The Dawning of the Autonomic Computing Era," IBM Sys. Jou.42(1):5-18, 2003

17. T. Bäck, J. Heistermann, C. Kappler and M. Zamparelli, "Evolutionary algorithms support refueling of pressurized water reactors", Proceedings of the Third IEEE Conference on Evolutionary Computa lion, 1996

18. D. B. Fogel, Evolutionary Computation: Toward a New Philosophy of Machine Intelligence, NJ, Piscataway:IEEE Press, 1995

19. Abbasi M, Bin Abd Latiff MS, Chizari H.,"Bioinspired evolutionary algorithm based for improving network coverage in wireless sensor networks", Scientific World Journal,. doi: 10.1155/2014/839486. PMID: 24693247; PMCID: PMC3943197, 2014

20. X.-S. Yang, Nature-Inspired Metaheuristic Algorithms, Luniver Press, 2008

21. Y. Perwej, Firoj Parwej, Mumdouh Mirghani Mohamed Hassan, Nikhat Akhtar, "The Internet-of-Things (IoT) Security: A Technological Perspective and Review" , International Journal of Scientific Research in Computer Science Engineering and Information Technology, Volume 5, Issue 1, Pages 462-482, 2019, DOI: 10.32628/CSEIT195193

22. Y. Perwej, Faiyaz Ahamad, Mohammad Zunnun Khan, Nikhat Akhtar, "An Empirical Study on the Current State of Internet of Multimedia Things (IoMT)", International Journal of Engineering Research in Computer Science and Engineering (IJERCSE), ISSN (Online) 2394-2320, Volume 8, Issue 3, Pages 25 - 42, 2021, DOI: 10.1617/vol8/iss3/pid85026

23. J. Farmer, N. Packard, and A. Perelson. The immune system, adaptation, and machine learning. Physica D, 22:187–204, 1986.

24. D. Dasgupta, editor. Artificial Immune Systems and Their Applications. Springer, 1998.

25. L. de Castro and J. Timmis. Artificial Immune Systems: A New Comput. Intelligence Approach. Springer, 2002.

26. G. Rowe. The Theoretical Models in Biology. Oxford University Press, 1994.

27. Castro, L.N., Timmis, J.: Artificial immune systems as a novel soft computing paradigm. Soft Computing 7(8), 526–544 (2003)

28. Burczyński, T.: Evolutionary and immune computations in optimal design and inverse problems. In: Waszczyszyn, Z. (ed.) Advances of Soft Computing in Engineering. Springer, Heidelberg, 2009

29. R. C. Eberhart and Y. Shi, "In Proceedings of the 2001 congress on evolutionary computation" in Particle swarm optimization: developments applications and resources, Piscataway, NJ, USA:IEEE, vol. 1, pp. 81-86, 2001

30. Langton, C. G. (ed.) (1989). Artificial Life: Proceedings of an Interdisciplinary Workshop on the Synthesis and Simulation of Living Systems. Los Alamos: Addison-Wesley. Complex Adaptive Systems.

31. Bourne, P. E., Brenner, S. E., and Eisen, M. B. (2005). PLoS computational biology: a new community journal. PLoS Comput. Biol. 1:e4. doi:10.1371/journal.pcbi.0010004

32. Bedau, M. A. (2007). "Artificial life," in Handbook of the Philosophy of Science. Volume 3: Philosophy of Biology. Volume Editors: Mohan Matthen and Christopher Stephens. Handbook Editors: Dov M. Gabbay, Paul Thagard and John Woods (Amsterdam: Elsevier BV), 585–603.

33. Y. Perwej , Firoj Parwej, "A Neuroplasticity (Brain Plasticity) Approach to Use in Artificial Neural Network", International Journal of Scientific & Engineering Research
IJSER), France , ISSN 2229 – 5518, Volume 3, Issue 6, Pages 1- 9, 2012, DOI: 10.13140/2.1.1693.2808

34. G. Paun. Membrane Computing: An Introduction. Springer,2002.

35. G. Paun and G. Rozenberg. A guide to membrane computing. Theoretical Comp. Science, 287(1):73–100, 2002

36. G. Ciobanu, G. Paun, and M. Perez-Jimenez, editors. Applications of Membrane Computing. Springer, 2006

37. H. Abelson, D. Allen, D. Coore, C. Hanson, G. Homsy, T. Knight Jr., R. Nagpal, E. Rauch, G. Sussman, and R. Weiss. Amorphous computing. CACM, 43(5):74–82, 2000

38. D. Coore. Botanical Computing: A Developmental Approach to Generating Interconnect Topologies on an Amorphous Computer. PhD thesis, MIT, 1999

39. Y. Perwej, N. Akhtar, Firoj Parwej, "The Kingdom of Saudi Arabia Vehicle License Plate Recognition using Learning Vector Quantization Artificial Neural Network", International Journal of Computer Applications (IJCA), USA, ISSN 0975 – 8887, Volume 98, No.11, Pages 32 – 38, 2014, DOI: 10.5120/17230-7556

40. Asif Perwej, Prof. (Dr.) K. P. Yadav, Prof. (Dr.) Vishal Sood, Dr. Y. Perwej, " An Evolutionary Approach to Bombay Stock Exchange Prediction with Deep Learning Technique", IOSR Journal of Business and Management (IOSR-JBM), e-ISSN:2278-487X, p-ISSN: 2319-7668, USA, Volume 20, Issue 12, Ver. V, Pages 63-79, 2018, DOI: 10.9790/487X-2012056379

41. W. Maass, "Noise as a resource for computation and learning in networks of spiking neurons," Proceedings of the IEEE, vol. 102, no. 5, pp. 860–880, 2014

42. Y. Perwej, Asif Perwej, " Prediction of the Bombay Stock Exchange (BSE) Market Returns Using Artificial Neural Networks and Genetic Algorithms ", Journal of Intelligent Learning Systems and Applications (JILSA), Scientific Research Publishing (SRP www.scirp.org), USA, ISSN Print: 2150-8402 , ISSN Online: 2150-8410, Volume 4, No. 2, Pages 108-119, 2012, DOI: 10.4236/jilsa.2012.42010

43. Francis George C. Cabarle, Henry N. Adorna, Min Jiang, and Xiangxiang Zeng. 2017. Spiking neural P systems with scheduled synapses. IEEE Transactions on Nanobioscience 16, 8 (2017), 792–801.

Emerging Trends in IoT and Computing Technologies – Suman Lata Tripathi et al. (eds)
© 2024 Taylor & Francis Group, London, ISBN 978-1-032-87924-6

Text Based Data Extraction (TBDE) Approach from Different Data-Sets Source

34

Vinay Kumar[1], Neha Goyal[2]

Assistant Professor, Department of Computer Science and Engineering,
B. N. College of Engineering & Technology, Lucknow,

Yusuf Perwej[3]

Professor, Professor, Department of Computer Science and Engineering,
Goel Institute of Technology & Management, Lucknow

Prof. Devendra Agarwal[4]

Dean (Academics),
Goel Institute of Technology & Management, Lucknow, U.P

Alok Mishra[5]

Dean Academics and Professor Physics,
Gaya College of Engineering (GCE), Gaya, Bihar

Prachi Chauhan[6]

Assistant Professor, Department of Computer Science and Engineering,
B. N. College of Engineering & Technology, Lucknow

Abstract: The process of extracting data from unstructured data sources so that it may be processed further is known as data extraction. The data extraction system frequently incorporates data transformation and metadata addition in order to export the data to the next stage of the data system process. Data extraction is utilized when experimental data is initially input into a system from primary sources, such as measuring or recording equipment. Text-based documents like emails, web pages, PDFs, Data Reports, and scanned text files are examples of unstructured data. In order to overcome the difficulty of obtaining data sets from test data sources, we take a data-centric strategy. In this work, we define several techniques using the appropriate algorithm (Text foundation) using a data extraction methodology. We are detecting commonly utilized data sets (email, resumes, courses, etc.) as well as large-small structure data set records using text pattern matching and a table-based regular expression technique. In order to extract data, we are also aiming to relate analytical language to other pieces of knowledge. To simplify the process of extracting data, an automated data search engine has been created. A comparative analysis contrasts the methods used to extract data from different sources.

Keywords: Datasets, Search engines, Data warehouses, Extraction process, Data mining

1. Introduction

The technique of extracting high-quality information as text from other data sources is known as text extraction. It involves developing text patterns with trends using tools like statistical patterns. When text is extracted, the source database is often

---
[1]vinay.bncet@gmail.com, [2]nehagoel.cse@gmail.com, [3]yusufperwej@gmail.com, [4]dr.devendra@goel.edu.in, [5]dralokmishra72@gmail.com,
[6]1990psrathore@gmail.com

DOI: 10.1201/9781003535423-34

separated from the structured database records for evaluation and output interpretation. The input is then frequently grouped using deduced linguistic features. The analysis entails examining the distribution of word frequencies and extracting information using techniques such as lexical analysis, association analysis, and predictive analytics [1]. The main goal is to convert text into data that can be analyzed using analytical tools and natural language processing (NLP). Using predictive classification or document dataset modeling, an application scans a source dataset to extract information [2]. The bulk of information extraction procedures employ a tree-based structured extraction methodology to extract the data elements of entire data records from the source.

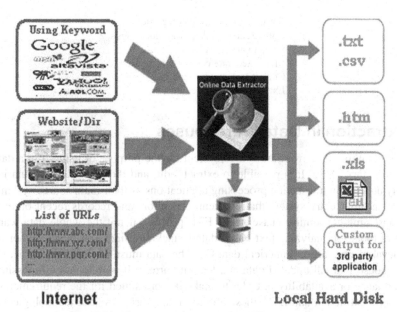

Fig. 34.1 Data set relation within different data set

To extract data items from detailed text-based objects or database records, it is essential to develop certain criteria for extracting text data or datasets. Creating techniques for extracting text data, whether via automation or human effort, can present substantial difficulties. A tabular methodology may be employed to discern distinct elements within a certain domain, such as proficiency acknowledgment, employment background, and submitted [3] curriculum vitae via email. Text analytics is utilized to extract data in order to understand the text and make connections with other sources of information. Text analytics refers to the application of text-based analytics to address business challenges, either alone or in conjunction with the analysis and retrieval [4] of structured, quantitative information. It goes without saying that 80% of the information that is essential to business is unstructured, and the majority of it is text [5]. These techniques uncover and show information, including as relationships, business rules, and facts, that may be hidden in text and inaccessible to machines.

2. Software for Applications and Data Extraction

Today, a variety of commercial, governmental, and scientific uses for the technology are common. Applications can be categorized into a number of areas based on the type of analysis or intended use. Following are the application categories [6] that were produced using this way of solution categorization. Numerous data extraction products are available, including ABBYY Flexi Capture, Win automation, Octopuses, Salestools.io, import.io, and others.

1	Enterprise Business Intelligence/Data Mining, Competitive Intelligence
2	E-Discovery, Records Management
3	Scientific discovery, especially Life Sciences
4	National Security/Intelligence
5	Natural Language/Semantic Toolkit or Service
6	Sentiment Analysis Tools, Listening Platforms
7	Social media monitoring
8	Search/Information Access
9	Automated ad placement
10	Publishing

3. Services for Extracting Data

Database extraction services are available to clients, allowing you to extract information on new products, company contact information, and much more. For our data extraction study, information is being gathered from social media platforms, other data sources, forums, recruitment portals, classified websites, etc. We can provide extracted data in many other forms, including Word, XML, SQL, MS Excel, and a great deal more. providing consumers from across the world with affordable, high-quality database extraction services as part of data extraction services such

1	Extract contact from companies
2	Collate relevant data from documents
3	Search various classified data
4	Create accurate contact information
5	Collect and summarize news
6	Extract data from review sites

4. Overview of Extraction in Data Warehouses

Extraction is the process of obtaining data from the source system for the purpose of using it in a data warehouse. The ETL process starts with this preliminary phase. It is possible to extract, edit, and then include this data into the data warehouse. Data warehouses frequently depend on transaction processing applications as their main source systems. A sales analysis data warehouse is dependent on an order entry system that efficiently monitors and records recent order activity. The extraction technique is usually the most time-consuming phase in the ETL process, if not the whole data warehousing process. Text analytics is the utilization of tools for analyzing text-based data to tackle business problems, either alone or in combination with the analysis and retrieval of organized, numerical data [7]. The data must normally be extracted often throughout time in order to supply the warehouse with all updated data and keep it current. It is frequently impossible to modify the source system or change its performance or availability in order to make it more suited for the requirements of the data warehouse extraction process. For generic extraction and ETL, these are important variables. The technological problems that come up when employing different sources and extraction procedures, however, are the main topic of this chapter. It discusses common techniques for removing data from source databases and assumes that the data warehouse team already knows what information needs to be removed. To create this technique, decisions on the following two important variables must be made [8]. Which extraction method should I choose? This has an impact on the mode of transportation, the supply chain, and the turnaround time for warehouse replenishment. How can I make the retrieved data available for processing to another party? This has an impact on the method of transportation as well as the requirement for data purification and modification. The most appropriate extraction approach will depend largely on the specifications of the organization in its intended data warehouse environment as well as the source system. Because of the performance or increasing workload of these systems, it is often not viable to improve an incremental data extraction by adding further logic to the source systems [9]. There are situations where alterations to an application system that has been previously developed are prohibited, even from the customer. In most cases, you have to choose how to realistically and conceptually retrieve data. The example of obtaining data from PDF sample is used to demonstrate the ability of UiPath for extracting data from PDF files. A text document is used to retain data that was immediately extracted from a PDF file.

Automating procedures:

- Extract the PDF text, first.
- Text formatting.
- Produce the text.

Method:

- Using the Read PDF Text activity, extract the text from the PDF file.
- Divide the output into a collection of strings that each include a word from the table.
- Use a While action to repeatedly go over the data and place each word under the appropriate column heading.
- Utilize the Write Text File action to create the text document.

5. Approaches of Logical Extraction

5.1 Entirety Extraction

The retrieval of all data from the first system has been finished. Once the final extraction has captured all the data from the source system, there is no need to continue monitoring any further modifications to the original data. Since the source data will be transmitted in its unmodified form, the original site does not need any more logical information, such as timestamps. Two instances of comprehensive extractions comprise an export file encompassing data from a solitary table and a distant SQL query that scrutinizes the entirety of the master database.

5.2 Successive Extraction

At a given instant, just the data that has been altered since a previously determined event will be acquired. The preceding extraction or a more complex business event, such as the last day of booking for a fiscal quarter, might be the situation. To identify the delta adjustment, it is important to own a mechanism for discerning every piece of information that has undergone modification since this specific moment. The pertinent data can be obtained directly from the original dataset, either from a [10] column that indicates the most recent date of modification in an application, or from a separate table that records both the initial transactions and subsequent modifications using a suitable supplementary technique. Frequently, the last phase involves integrating extraction logic directly into the initial system. A considerable proportion of data warehouses do not utilize any change-capture technologies throughout the extraction process. The data warehouse or staging area extracts whole tables from the source systems in order to detect any modified data. These tables are compared to a previous snippet from the system's inception subsequently. The first systems may not see significant impacts from this method, but the functioning of the data warehouse might be substantially hindered, especially when handling substantial volumes of data.

5.3 Approaches of Physical Extraction

The information retrieved can be actually extracted in one of two methods, depending on the logical extraction approach employed as well as the capability and constraints on the originating side. Either an offline framework or an online framework can be used to extract the data from the initial system. An offline framework of this kind can already exist or be generated during an extraction process. The subsequent physical extraction techniques are possible.

Web-based Extraction

On the initial system, the data extraction procedure takes place. In order to access the originating tables, the extraction technique can link directly to the primary system or to a middle system that stores the data in a specified way (for instance, snapshot logs or transition tables). It should be stressed that the initial system and the intermediary system are not always physically distinct.

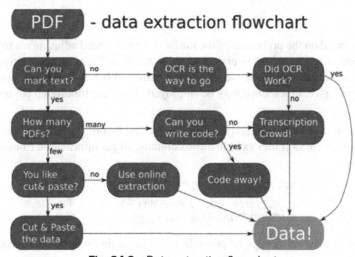

Fig. 34.2 Data extraction flow chart

It is critical to consider if distributed transactions make use of ready origin objects or actual parent objects when employing online extractions.

Offline Extraction

The data is deliberately saved at a designated area rather than being directly accessed from the original source system. The data was produced by either an extraction method or contains a structure, such as redo logs, archive logs, or transportable tablespaces. The extraction approach, in conjunction with other subsequent operations in the ETL process, can provide substantial advantages by effectively extracting a reduced quantity of data. This is accomplished by efficiently identifying and obtaining just the most regularly updated information.

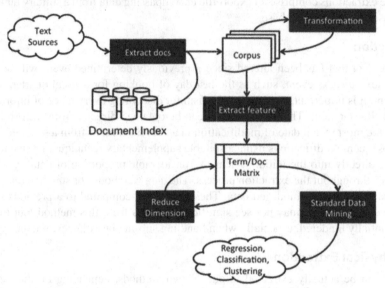

Fig. 34.3 Text extraction feature from different data set

Regrettably, the task of finding the latest changes to the data may provide challenges or even be incompatible with the normal operation of many source systems. The main technological obstacle faced throughout the data extraction procedure frequently focuses on the collection of dynamic data. This article presents several approaches to creating a customized technique for acquiring variations in Oracle original systems, considering the probable impracticality of using Oracle's Mutation Data Acquisition mechanism and the frequent requirement for modification collection during the extraction process.

- Timestamps
- Partitioning
- Triggers

Some of these methods could depend on the properties of the initial systems or need adjustments to the base systems. Thus, the owners of the initial system need to carefully look over each of these methods before implementing any of them. Any of these tactics can be used with the data extraction method we mentioned earlier. When data is being obtained via an internet-based query or unloaded to a file, for instance, timestamps may be employed. There are timestamp columns in particular computers' tables.

The timestamp specifies the last modification time and date for the relevant record. Timestamps can be used to quickly find the most recent data in operating system tables if they exist in those columns. To get information from an orders database for today, for example, try the query below.

```
SELECT * FROM orders WHERE TRUNC
(CAST (order_date AS date),'dd') = TO_
DATE(SYSDATE,'dd-mon-yyyy');
```

If the timestamp data is absent, it may not always be possible to integrate timestamps into an operating system. To do this adjustment, it is essential to include a new timestamp column into the tables of the operating system. Afterwards, it is necessary to create a trigger that will update the timestamp column after every action that updates a particular row. Certain source systems may employ Oracle range partitioning, a method that partitions the starting tables depending on a date key to improve the retrieval of the most recent data. Obtaining data for the current week is simple, especially when pulling it from a table that is separated by weeks. A materialized view log may be created for any table that requires tracking of modifications [10]. Triggers are used by materialized view logs when changes are made to the original table. Oracle materialized view logs employ an equivalent internalization mechanism based on triggers. These logs are visible to end users and are utilized by materialized views to detect new data. Furthermore, Oracle assumes responsibility for a substantial percentage of the configuration and management of this change-data system, resulting in an [9] added advantage. Alternatively, they suggest using synchronous Transformation Data Capture (CDC), which provides an external interface for obtaining modification data and a system for efficiently transferring it to many clients. Before adopting trigger-based approaches on a live source system, it is essential to undertake a thorough assessment of their influence on the efficiency of the original source systems.

6. Instances of Data Warehousing Extraction

Distributed Operations-Based Retrieval and Data File-Based Retrieval are the two methods available for data extraction. Tools for bringing in or exporting data as flat files from the inside database format are typically included in database systems. Although COBOL programmers are often used for mainframe system extraction, export or unload solutions are available from numerous databases and third-party software vendors. To extract data, it's not always required to dump whole database structures into flat files. It could be better in certain circumstances to unload whole objects or database tables. In other cases, as when the starting point system has evolved since the last extraction or when merging many tables, it could be better to merely unload a portion of a certain table. The degree to which numerous methods of extraction may be used to these two scenarios varies. There are numerous options for data extraction into files when the initial system is an Oracle database.

Using SQL*Plus for Extracting into Flat Files
Extracting Data into Flat Files using Pro*C or OCI Software
Using Oracle's Export Utility to Export into Oracle Export Files

The most straightforward way of extracting data is to use SQL*Plus to perform a query and save the output to a file. To extract a flat file named country_city.log, for example, containing a list of US cities, from the nations and customers columns, use the SQL script that follows. The pipe symbol is used to divide the values in the columns.

```
SET echo off SET pagesize 0 SPOOL
country_city.log
SELECT distinct t1.country_name ||'|'||
t2.cust_city FROM countries t1, customers t2
WHERE t1.country_id = t2.country_id
AND t1.country_name= 'United States of
America'; SPOOL off
```

SQL*Plus system variables can be used to specify the precise format of the output file. The positive aspect of using this extraction technique is that any SQL statement's output may be acquired. In the previously mentioned example, the join's results are extracted. By starting many concurrent SQL*Plus sessions, each of which runs a distinct query corresponding to a distinct part of the data to be obtained, the data extraction procedure may be parallelized. For one such session, the SQL script may be.

```
SPOOL order_jan.dat
SELECT * FROM orders PARTITION
(orders_jan1998); SPOOL OFF
```

Twelve SQL*Plus processes would spool data in parallel to twelve distinct file types. During extraction, if necessary, you can use the tools your operating system has supplied for incorporating them. If your intention is to utilize SQL*Loader to load data into the target, you may use these 12 files exactly as-is to do a parallel load using 12 SQL*Loader transactions. It is still feasible to parallelize the extraction based on conceptual or physical criteria regardless of whether the orders table is not break apart. These kinds of logic column value ranges form the basis of the logical procedure:

```
SELECT ... WHERE order_date
BETWEEN TO_DATE('01-JAN-99') AND
TO_DATE('31-JAN-99');
```

The conceptual basis of the physical approach has several characteristics. The data dictionary may be utilized to identify the Oracle data blocks comprising the orders table. Using this information, you may create a series of consecutive range queries to get data from the sequences contained in the database, which may include:

```
SELECT * FROM orders WHERE rowid
BETWEEN value1 and value2;
```

Parallelizing the extraction of large SQL queries can be feasible in certain cases, but it might be difficult to break a complex query into many parts. Managing many processes to create a consistent global view can be a challenging endeavor.

7. Conclusion

In this paper, we provide a unique Data Extraction method that makes use of distributed processes. A hybrid technique for data extraction is a practical method for exporting files for both single objects and large data collections. Incompatible data make data extraction difficult. Here, we employ text-based data extraction from any PDF file. To create superior output outcomes, we verify various data integration and validation methods from the source.

REFERENCES

1. G. Alfonso and R. Mora, "Analog IC design with low-dropout regulators," McGraw Hill New York, 2009.
2. H. Armani and H. Cordonnier, "Power and battery management ICs for low-cost portable Electronics", Annales Telecommunications Juilet/Aout, vol.59, pp. 974-983, Jul. 2004.
3. C. Simpson, "A User's Guide to Compensating Low-Dropout Regulators", National Semiconductor, 1997.
4. G. A. R.-Mora and P. E. Allen, "Optimized Frequency-Shaping Circuit Topologies for LDO's," in IEEE Transactions on Circuits and Systemsii: Analog and Digital Signal Processing, vol. 45, pp.703-707, June 1998.
5. Gabriel A. Rincon-Mora and Phillip E. Allen, "A Low-Voltage, Low Quiescent Current, Low Drop-Out Regulator," IEEE Journal of Solid-State Circuits, Vol. 33, pp. 36-43, Jan. 1998.
6. G. A. Rincon-Mora, "Current efficient, low voltage, low drop-out regulators," Ph.D. dissertation, Elect. Comp. Eng. Dept., Georgia Inst. of Technology, Atlanta, 1996.
7. Texas Instruments, "Fundamental Theory of PMOS Low Drop-out Voltage Regulators," Application Report, Apr. 1997.
8. Jerome Patoux, "Low Drop-out Regulators," Analog Dialogue, May 2007.
9. P. Phillip, E. Allen and D. R. Holberg, "CMOS Analog Circuit Design," 2nd Ed., Oxford University Press, pp. 246-301, 2002.
10. K. N. Leung and P. K. T. Mok, "A capacitor-free CMOS low-dropout regulator with damping-factor-control frequency compensation," IEEE Journal of Solid-State Circuits, vol. 38, pp. 1691–1702, Oct. 2003

Emerging Trends in IoT and Computing Technologies – Suman Lata Tripathi et al. (eds)
© 2024 Taylor & Francis Group, London, ISBN 978-1-032-87924-6

Integration of Controller Area Network (CAN) with Internet of Things (IoT) Applications

35

Sangeeta Bhosure[1]

Ph.D. Scholar, Shri Venkateshwara University, Dept. of ECE, Gajraula, U.P., India
AGM, Fuji Electric India Pvt. Ltd. Pune, India

Rishi Asthana[2]

Professor, Shri Venkateshwara University, Dept. of ECE, Gajraula, U.P., India

Abstract: Controller Area Network (CAN), originally developed for real-time communication in automotive systems, has proven to be a robust and reliable protocol for distributed control systems. Meanwhile, the IoT paradigm continues to evolve, connecting a myriad of devices and enabling seamless data exchange across diverse domains. This paper explores the synergies between CAN and IoT, elucidating the challenges and opportunities in integrating these technologies. The integration of CAN with IoT opens avenues for enhanced scalability, interoperability, and real-time data exchange in various applications such as smart cities, industrial automation, and healthcare.

Keywords: Internet of things (IoT), Controller area network (CAN), Protocol, Integration, Applications

1. Introduction

A CAN (Controller Area Network) based data monitoring and control system is a type of networked communication system commonly used in automotive and industrial applications for real time data communication between ECUs (Electronic Control Units) or nodes. The CAN protocol is a robust and efficient communication standard that allows multiple microcontrollers or devices to communicate with each other without a host computer. A CAN-based data monitoring system is a crucial component in modern vehicles and industrial automation systems, providing a reliable and efficient means of communication between various electronic components.

Here are some key aspects and details of a CAN-based data monitoring system:

Message Format: The CAN protocol uses a message-oriented communication approach. CAN messages are transmitted in frame formats, containing identifier (11bits or 29bits), control bits, data length, data and CRC bits.

Two-Wire System: CAN typically use a two-wire differential signalling system (CAN_H and CAN_L) for communication, providing high noise immunity.

Bus Topology: CAN networks are commonly implemented as a bus topology, where multiple nodes are connected to a common communication bus.

Termination: Proper termination is essential to prevent signal reflections and ensure signal integrity.

---

[1]sbhosure@gmail.com, [2]asthanarishi1973@gmail.com

DOI: 10.1201/9781003535423-35

ECUs (Electronic Control Units): Nodes on the CAN bus, such as sensors, actuators, and other control units, exchange information.

CAN Transceivers: These components interface with the physical layer, converting digital signals from the CAN controller into electrical signals suitable for transmission over the bus.

Real-Time Monitoring: The system continuously monitors and exchanges data in real-time, making it suitable for applications where timely information is critical.

Error Detection and Handling: CAN includes mechanisms for error detection, and systems are designed to handle errors gracefully.

Applications:

Automotive Systems: CAN is used in the vehicles for communication between different control units like engine control unit (ECU), dashboard communication units, break system and others.

Industrial Automation: CAN is employed in industrial settings for monitoring and control of machinery and processes.

Advantages:

Reliability: CAN is known for its reliability, even in noisy environments.

Scalability: The architecture allows for easy addition or removal of nodes without significant disruption to the network.

2. Literature Review

A secure identification card incorporating Internet of Things (IoT) technology has the potential to enhance the safety of female workers, presenting a promising solution to address this concern. Incorporating embedded sensors and communication elements, this advanced ID card can actively sense and respond to its surroundings. In the event of detecting irregularities, such as sudden movements or loud noises, the embedded sensors transmit a signal to the system. Subsequent to thorough data analysis, the system takes appropriate actions, such as sending alerts or messages to the security personnel [1]. The development of solutions for network security, specifically in the realms of traffic classification and intrusion detection, relies heavily on authentic network traces or realistic testbeds. This research presents an exhaustive examination of current datasets housing IoT network traffic. The author has systematically categorized these datasets based on various features, streamlining the process for researchers to identify datasets aligning with their specific requirements [2]. The intended research aims to accomplish the simultaneous uniform transmission of multiple variables. Moreover, it strives to control vehicle speed by leveraging data obtained from ultrasonic sensors, with the goal of creating a collision warning system for modern automobiles that assists drivers in avoiding rear-end collisions through the CAN protocol. Furthermore, this study delves into the Battery Management System (BMS), recognizing its significance in vehicles, particularly regarding issues such as leaks, electrical malfunctions, overheating, and fire hazards. The main emphasis is placed on the monitoring of battery packs utilizing the CAN module [3]. In the presented paper [4], the author conducts a deep study of the present condition of CAN bus reverse engineering, summarizing significant advancements. In this review, the author highlights a significant challenge—specifically, the lack of a publicly available and standardized data for the quantitative assessment of translation algorithms. Consequently, detailed requirements are outlined by the author to standardize the process of data collection. The paper delves into the challenges associated with the reverse engineering of CAN automation, emphasizing its relevance to network security and driver's safety. Additionally, the author discusses the research directions in the reverse engineering of Controller Area Network. The subsequent categorization of relevant studies[5] revolves around six key implementation objectives, namely Networking, Privacy, Security, Trust Management, Computing Paradigms, Authentication and Access Control. Each category represents a distinct problem domain, and the paper delves into related studies, providing detailed discussions on the proposed solutions. The conclusion outlines challenges, issues, and future research, emphasizing the need for further research efforts to establish comprehensive and groundbreaking frameworks in BC-SDIoT, thereby expanding into newer research domains. In another study [6], the author explores the repercussions of repurposed Controller Area Network based attacks having capabilities of changing sensor information, systems data overriding and sending harmful commands through various entry methods. Furthermore, in the field of healthcare, the impact of the IoT (Internet of Things) is discussed [7]. The IoT has played an important role in advancing healthcare by addressing challenges in emergency situations such as heart attacks or accidents. The paper underscores the critical nature of emergency cases, where only the patient's vital parameters are initially available, leading to expedited treatment processes that may pose risks. To mitigate this, the author proposes the deployment of multimodal IoT devices to simultaneously collect and monitor data from different parts of body, allowing healthcare professionals to access comprehensive medical information in advance for decision-making and increased chances of patient recovery. Another study, [9], proposes a gateway system facilitating data-reduced communication between Ethernet and CAN network. The gateway system is designed to receive short CAN messages, decompress it and transmit it to the ethernet network. Conversely, it receives regular Ethernet frames, compresses them, and transmits them using the Controller Area Network protocol. The author in this paper evaluates the performance of the developed gateway system. The paper [10] focused on the analysis of the Internet of Things (IoT) with the network systems. The writer presents an in-depth examination covering recent advancements, technical resolutions, noteworthy ongoing projects, and deliberations on potential visions and unresolved challenges in the domain. The study in the paper [11] addresses the Internet of Things (IoT) as a pivotal factor enabling a paradigm for the integration and comprehensive utilization of various technologies for communication solutions. The paper emphasizes the role of IoT in connecting billions of sensors to the internet, generating vast amounts of data that require analysis, interpretation, and utilization for effective communication and tracking of technologies such as wireless sensors and actuators. Xin et al. [12] introduces Multi-class S-TCN as an innovative solution for IoT traffic security detection. The incorporation of TCN, coupled with deep packet inspection and protocol analysis, enhances the overall efficiency of the detection process. Experimental results affirm the superiority of Multi-class S-TCN over existing approaches, showcasing its potential to meet the evolving security needs of IoT scenarios. Ashok, K et al. [13] discussed enhancement of Cyber Physical Systems versus Denial of Service (DoS) attacks, they compared sensor controller and controller to actuator DoS attack channels, introducing modelling solution of the swapping system. The author proposes a layered switching paradigm utilizing packet-based transfer techniques as a preventive measure. Nechibvute and Mafukidze's[14] underscores the potential of integration to leverage real-time data analytics and improve production availability. They have also demonstrated optimize SCADA and IoT integration, concluding by outlining the future research directions, contributing to ongoing efforts in advancing SCADA and IoT integration methodologies.

3. Proposed Methodology

In this method CAN is used within the components of energy infrastructure, such as in communication between smart meters, sensors, and control systems. It provides a reliable and efficient means for these devices to exchange information within a localized network. Integrating CAN with IoT in the context of smart grids allows for enhanced monitoring, control, and optimization of the energy distribution network. IoT-enabled sensors and devices connected through CAN can collect real-time data on energy consumption, power quality, and grid conditions. The combination of CAN and IoT enables quick detection of faults or abnormalities in the grid. Automated responses or alerts can be triggered to address issues promptly, reducing downtime and improving overall reliability. The IoT devices can collect data from the other devices and use this data for monitoring, control, or send this data to the centralized server for further processing. Some microcontrollers have a built-in CAN controller, such as the STM32 or the PIC32, while others require an external CAN controller, such as the MCP2515. The CAN transceiver can be a standalone chip, such as the MCP2551, or integrated with the CAN controller, such as the MCP2562.

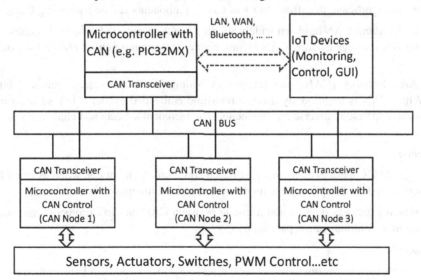

Fig. 35.1   Control of devices using CAN and IoT

The integration of CAN and IoT allows for data-driven insights into energy usage patterns. Utilities can use this information to optimize the grid, reduce losses, and promote energy efficiency.

As renewable energy sources like solar and wind become more prevalent, CAN-based systems with IoT integration can facilitate better management and integration of these intermittent energy sources into the grid.

The real-time monitoring capabilities provided by CAN and IoT contribute to the resilience of the grid. It allows for quick identification and response to issues, minimizing the impact of disruptions and enhancing the overall reliability of the energy infrastructure.

4. Result

The combination of CAN and IoT in energy management, especially in the context of smart grids, plays a crucial role in creating a more responsive, efficient, and resilient electrical infrastructure. This integration enables utilities to make data-driven decisions, enhance grid performance, and better adapt to the evolving landscape of energy generation and consumption.

The effectiveness of Controller Area Network (CAN) in Internet of Things (IoT) applications is notable for several reasons, primarily due to its inherent characteristics that align well with the requirements of IoT environments. Here are key aspects highlighting the effectiveness of CAN in IoT:

Robust Communication: CAN is known for its robust communication capabilities, making it well-suited for applications where reliability is crucial. In IoT deployments, especially in critical sectors like automotive and industrial automation, reliable communication is essential.

Deterministic Behaviour: CAN offers deterministic communication, ensuring that messages are transmitted predictably and with low latency. This is particularly important in IoT scenarios where real-time data exchange is necessary, such as in industrial control systems and automotive applications.

Flexible Architecture: CAN's bus-based architecture is inherently scalable. It allows for easy integration of new nodes without significant disruption to the existing network. This scalability is beneficial in IoT deployments where the number of connected devices can vary and expand over time.

Optimized for Short Distances: CAN is designed for communication over relatively short distances within a localized network. In IoT applications, especially those in industrial or vehicular settings, where devices are often in close proximity, CAN's efficiency in short-distance communication is advantageous.

Energy-Efficient: CAN operates with a low-power consumption, which is crucial for IoT devices, many of which are designed to operate on battery power. This efficiency contributes to prolonged battery life in connected devices.

Cost-Effectiveness: CAN hardware is relatively inexpensive, contributing to its cost-effectiveness. In large-scale IoT deployments where cost considerations are significant, the affordability of CAN components can be a deciding factor.

Automotive and Industrial Standard: CAN has been widely adopted in automotive and industrial sectors for decades. Many IoT applications in these industries leverage existing CAN infrastructure, making it a natural choice for extending connectivity to new IoT devices.

Combining Controller Area Network (CAN) and Internet of Things (IoT) introduces technical intricacies that require careful consideration. While CAN is traditionally used in real-time embedded systems, IoT systems often rely on different communication protocols and operate in diverse environments. The technical aspects and challenges of integrating CAN with IoT are as follows:

Communication Protocols:

CAN Integration Challenges: CAN operates on a broadcast-based communication model, whereas many IoT devices use point-to-point or publish-subscribe models. Adapting these models for seamless integration is a challenge.

Gateway Solutions: Introducing gateway devices that translate between CAN and IoT protocols can facilitate communication between devices using different communication paradigms.

Data Formats and Standards:

CAN Message Structure: CAN uses a specific message format with identifiers and data bytes. Integrating this format with the more varied and complex data structures used in IoT requires careful mapping and parsing.

Standardization Efforts: Ensuring interoperability may involve adopting industry standards or developing specific standards for the integrated CAN-IoT environment.

Real-time Requirements:

CAN's Real-time Advantage: CAN is known for its deterministic and real-time capabilities, crucial in applications like automotive systems. Maintaining or adapting these real-time requirements in the context of IoT introduces challenges, as typical IoT systems may not have the same stringent timing constraints.

Synchronization Strategies: Implementing synchronization strategies between CAN and IoT components to ensure timely data exchange without compromising the overall system performance.

Security Considerations:

Security Standards: IoT systems demand robust security measures due to the increased attack surface. CAN networks, while designed with security in mind, may need additional safeguards.

End-to-End Encryption: Implementing end-to-end encryption and secure authentication mechanisms to protect data transmitted between CAN and IoT components.

Testing and Validation:

Simulation Environments: Develop simulation environments to test the integrated CAN-IoT system before deployment to identify and address potential issues.

Validation Protocols: Establishing validation protocols to ensure that the integrated system meets the reliability and performance requirements of both CAN and IoT.

5. Conclusion

The integration of Controller Area Network (CAN) with Internet of Things (IoT) applications brings together the reliability and efficiency of CAN communication with the connectivity and data-sharing capabilities of IoT. By addressing technical intricacies, the integration of CAN with IoT can unlock new possibilities for efficient and reliable communication in applications ranging from industrial automation to smart cities. Successful integration requires a holistic approach, considering the unique strengths and challenges of both technologies. It's important to note that while CAN has strengths in certain aspects, the choice of communication protocol in IoT depends on the specific requirements of the application. In scenarios where longer-range communication, higher bandwidth, or internet connectivity are crucial, other protocols like MQTT or CoAP may be more suitable. However, for short-range, reliable, and deterministic communication within localized networks, CAN remains an effective choice in the IoT landscape. The combination of CAN and IoT enhances the capabilities of traditional embedded systems by providing connectivity, real-time monitoring, and data analytics. This integration is crucial for creating intelligent and efficient systems in various domains.

REFERENCES

1. V Gowrishankar; G Prabhakaran; K S Tamilselvan; T Judgi; M Parimala Devi; A Murugesan, "IoT based Smart ID Card for Working Woman Safety", IEEE, 7th International Conference on Intelligent Computing and Control Systems (ICICCS), June 2023, DOI: 10.1109/ICICCS56967.2023.10142631

2. François De Keersmaeker; Yinan Cao; Gorby Kabasele Ndonda; Ramin Sadre, "A Survey of Public IoT Datasets for Network Security Research", IEEE Communications Surveys & Tutorials, June 2023, pp. 1808 – 1840, DOI: 10.1109/COMST.2023.3288942

3. K. Sai Prasanna; R. Anirudh Reddy; Jeeru Jyotika Reddy; Mulinti Chaitya Reddy; etc; "CAN based Collision Avoidance and Battery Management System for Automotives", IEEE, International Conference on Inventive Computation Technologies (ICICT), April 2023, DOI: 10.1109/ICICT57646.2023.10134290

4. Alessio Buscemi; Ion Turcanu; German Castignani; Andriy Panchenko, "A Survey on Controller Area Network Reverse Engineering", IEEE Communications Surveys & Tutorials, April 2023, pp. 1445 – 1481

5. Stephen W. Turner; Murat Karakus; Evrim Guler; Suleyman Uludag, "A Promising Integration of SDN and Blockchain for IoT Networks: A Survey", IEEE Access, March 2023, pp. 29800 – 29822.

6. Tyler Cultice; Himanshu Thapliyal, "Vulnerabilities and Attacks on CAN-Based 3D Printing/Additive Manufacturing", IEEE Consumer Electronics Magazine, February 2023, pp. 54 – 61, DOI: 10.1109/MCE.2023.3240849

7. Balasundaram; Sidheswar Routray; A. V. Prabu; Prabhakar Krishnan; Prince Priya Malla; Moinak Maiti, "Internet of Things (IoT)-Based Smart Healthcare System for Efficient Diagnostics of Health Parameters of Patients in Emergency Care", IEEE Internet of Things Journal, February 2023, pp. 18563 – 18570, DOI: 10.1109/JIOT.2023.3246065

8. Julian Echeverry-Mejia; Felipe Arenas-Uribe; Diego Contreras; Virgilio Vásquez, "Design and Validation of an In-Vehicle Data Recorder System for Testing Purposes", IEEE Latin America Transactions, January 2023, pp. 183 – 191, DOI: 10.1109/TLA.2023.10015210.

9. Sung Bhin Oh; Min Jeong Lee; Jae Wook Jeon, " Efficient Data Communication Automotive Gateway System for CAN-Ethernet Networks", IEEE 17th International Conference on Ubiquitous Information Management and Communication (IMCOM), January 2023, DOI: 10.1109/IMCOM56909.2023.10035629

10. Ke Xu; Yi Qu; Kun Yang, "A tutorial on the internet of things: from a heterogeneous network integration", IEEE Network, March-April 2016.

11. Mohsen Hallaj Asghar; Atul Negi; Nasibeh Mohammadzadeh, "Principal application and vision in Internet of Things (IoT)", IEEE International Conference on Computing, Communication & Automation, 15-16 May 2015.

12. Xin, L., Ziang, L., Yingli, Z., Wenqiang, Z., Dong, L., & Qingguo, Z. (2022) - Taylor & Francis. TCN enhanced novel malicious traffic detection for IoT devices. Connection Science, 34(1), 1322-1341.

13. Ashok, K., Boddu, R., Syed, S. A., Sonawane, V. R., Dabhade, R. G., & Reddy, P. C. S. (2023) - Taylor & Francis. GAN Base feedback analysis system for industrial IOT networks. Automatika, 64(2), 259-267.

14. Nechibvute, A., & Mafukidze, H. D. (2023) - Taylor & Francis. Integration of SCADA and Industrial IoT: Opportunities and Challenges. IETE Technical Review, 1-14.

Emerging Trends in IoT and Computing Technologies – Suman Lata Tripathi et al. (eds)
© 2024 Taylor & Francis Group, London, ISBN 978-1-032-87924-6

Solution of Non-linear Fractional Partial Differential Equations using Modified Adomian Decomposition Method with Sumudu Transform

36

Parmeshwari V Aland[1]

Lovely Professional University, Research Scholar, Phagwara, Panjab, India

Prince Singh[2]

Lovely Professional University, Department of Mathematics, Phagwara, Panjab, India

Abstract: A modified Adomian Decomposition Sumudu Transformation method (MADST) employed in this resolve the nonlinear fractional partial differential equation analytically. Caputo sense is applied to the fractional derivatives. A fast convergence to an exact solution is found for the series solutions of the proposed approach. The MADST solutions exhibit remarkable agreement when compared to exact solutions. The simplicity and efficiency of the current approach are excellent. Graphical presentations of numerical results for many specific examples are simplified.

Keywords: Fractional partial differential equation, Modified adomian decomposition method (MADM), Sumudu transformation method

1. Introduction

The fractional calculus encompasses the examination of integrals and derivatives with non-integer orders, gaining substantial attention due to its diverse applications in scientific and other domains. In many different systems, real-world phenomena are modelled through the use of fractional differential equations (FDEs) such as reaction diffusion processes, neural networks, control systems, signal processing, and system recognition. Presently, FDEs play a crucial role in resolving practical issues across engineering, medicine, biology, and physics. The significance of fractional calculus extends to accurately describing physical phenomena in the study of signal processing, electrochemistry, chemical and biological physics, probability, statistics, acoustics, and electromagnetics. Fractional calculus serves as a valuable tool for characterizing memory and hereditary properties in various processes. Over the past decades, significant interest has emerged in exploring fractional differential equations, leading to the development of different approaches to get both approximate and exact solutions.

One noteworthy approach is the Adomian decomposition method (ADM), presented by Adomian, which has gained attention for simplifying nonlinear equations. The Adomian decomposition method has been the focus of intensive research in regard to its utility in generating exact and approximate results for dealing with nonlinear elements in various problem domains. In addition to ADM, other techniques such as variation iteration method, generalized differential equation, homotopy perturbation method, Adams-Bashforth-Moulton method, and finite difference approaches formulated to address fractional differential equations. Now recently, the Adomian decomposition method were sufficiently investigated in the literature due to its broad applications in applied sciences. This work focuses on three applications expressed in fractional form: the time-.fractional Fornberg Witham equation, nonlinear Korteweg–de Vries Equation, and time-fractional propagations decay and growth equation. In this work

[1]parmeshwarialand20@gmail.com, [2]prince.16092@lpu.co.in

DOI: 10.1201/9781003535423-36

demonstrated the coupling of Sumudu transform methods and modified Adomian decomposition method. The FSDM provides a sophisticated convergent series solution, demonstrated through applications such as the fractional-order Hirota-Satsuma linked KdV system, yielding soliton-type and rational solutions. To ensure accuracy, the approximate solutions results are analysed with exact solutions, and a comparative table and graphical representations are presented for various values of alpha.

Preliminaries:

Definition 1: Consider a set A is of the form:

$$A = \{f(t) . \exists\, M, \tau_1, \tau_2 > 0, |f(t)| \le Me^{\frac{|t|}{\tau_j}} \ \ if \ t \in (-1)^j \times [0, \infty.\}$$

For real value $t \ge 0$, the Sumudu transformation of function $f(t) \in A$, denoted as:

$$S[f(t)](u) \approx f(u) = \int_0^\infty e^{-t} f(ut)dt, u \in (\tau_1, \tau_2)$$

The inverse Sumudu transform of $f(u)$ is the function $f(t)$ in the equation above, and it is represented,

$$by\ f(t) = S^{-1}[f(u)]$$

Definition 2: The Caputo fractional derivation of $f(t)$ for order α denoted by

$$^c_a D^\alpha_t f(t) = \frac{1}{(n-\alpha)} \int_0^t \frac{f^{(n)}t}{(t-\tau)^{\alpha+1-n}} d\tau$$

Where $f \in C^n_{-1}, n - 1. < \alpha \le n, n \in N$

Theorem: Let $n \in N$ and $\alpha > 0$ be such that, $n - 1 < \alpha \le n$ and $f(u)$ be Sumudu operator function with $f(t)$, its Caputo fractional derivative of order α:

$$S[^c_a D^\alpha_t f(t)](u) = f^c_\alpha(u) = u^{-\alpha}\left[F(u) - \sum_{k=0}^{n-1} u^k \left(f^{(k)}(t)\right)_{t=0}\right] - 1. < n - 1 < \alpha \le n \tag{1}$$

Properties:

1) $S[1] = 1$ 2) $S\left[\dfrac{t^m}{m!}\right] = u^m$ 3) $S\{f^n(t)\} = \dfrac{1}{u^n} S\{f(t)\} - \sum_{k=0}^{n-1} \dfrac{1}{u^{n-k}} f^k(0)$

2. Basic Plan of Modified Adomian Decomposition Sumudu Transformation (MADST) Approach for Differential Equations with Nonlinear Time Fractions

Consider the below considered generic fractional nonlinear form partial differential equation.

$$D^\alpha_t w(x,.t) + R\left[w.(x,t)\right] + N\left[w.(x,t)\right] = g(x,t) \tag{2}$$

Since $w(x, 0) = f(x)$, is the initial condition. $\tag{3}$

Where $D^\alpha_t w(x,t)$ is Caputo fractional derivative of the function $w(x, t)$ stated as:

$$D^\alpha_t w(x,t) = \frac{\partial^\alpha w(x,t)}{\partial t^\alpha} = \begin{cases} \dfrac{1}{(n-\alpha)} \int_a^t (t-x)^{n-\alpha-1} \dfrac{\partial^n w(x,t)}{\partial t^n} \, dt, n-1 < \alpha < n \\[2mm] \dfrac{\partial^n w(x,t)}{\partial t^n} \qquad\qquad \alpha = n \in N \end{cases}$$

Linear differential operator is denoted as R, and nonlinear differential operator N signifies the non-linear counterpart and $g(x, t)$ is the source term.

Appling Sumudu operator on equation, (2)

$$S[D_t^\alpha\ w.(x,t)] + S.\big[R\big[w(x,t)\big]\big] + S.[N[w(x,t)]] = S.[g(x,t)] \tag{4}$$

Inverse Sumudu Transform operation on Equation (4)

$$w.(x,t) = f(x) + S^{-1}\left(u^\alpha\ S[g(x,t)]\right) - S^{-1}\left(u^\alpha S\big\{[R[w(x,t)]] + [N[w(x,t)]]\big\}\right) \tag{5}$$

The following is the solution expressed as an interminable series:

$$w(x,t) = \sum_{n=0}^{\infty} w_n(x,\mathrm{t}) \tag{6}$$

$$N[w(x,t)] = \sum_{n=0}^{\infty} A_n\ ;\ \text{Where}\ A_n = \frac{1}{n!}\left[\frac{d^n}{d\lambda^n}\left[N\sum_{i=0}^{\infty}\lambda^i u_i\right]\right]_{\lambda=0} \tag{7}$$

The nonlinear terms N are represented using modified Adomian decomposition method for nonlinear polynomial which is defined as:

$$\{A_n\} = \{N_1(s_n) - N_1(s_{n-1})\}\ ,\ \text{Where}\ s_n = \sum_{i=0}^{n} w_i(x,t) \tag{8}$$

Substituting Equations (6) and (7) in Equation (5), we get

$$\sum_{n=0}^{\infty} w_n.(x,t) = f(x) + S^{-1}\left(u^\alpha\ S\big[g(x,t)\big]\right) - S^{-1}\left(u^\alpha S\left\{R\left[\sum_{n=0}^{\infty} w_n(x,t)\right] + \left[\sum_{n=0}^{\infty} A_n\right]\right\}\right) \tag{9}$$

Comparing Equation (9), both sides together yield

$$w_0(x,t) = f(x) + S^{-1}\left(u^\alpha\ S\big[g(x,t)\big]\right)$$

$$w_1(x,t) = -S^{-1}\left(w^\alpha S\big\{R\big[w_0(x,t)\big] + A_0\big\}\right)$$

$$w_2(x,t) = -S^{-1}\left(w^\alpha S\big\{R\big[w_1(x,t)\big] + A_1\big\}\right)$$

$$w_n(x,t) = -S^{-1}\left(w^\alpha S\big\{R\big[w_{n-1}(x,t)\big] + A_{n-1}\big\}\right) \tag{10}$$

Finally, the truncated series approximation solution $w(x, t)$ is as follow.

$$w.(x,t) = \sum_{n=0}^{\infty} w_n(x,t) \tag{11}$$

3. Applications

Examine the following equation for a time fractional system.

Example 1   Consider the Time-Fractional Fornberg-Whitham Equation [13]

$$\frac{\partial^\alpha w}{\partial t^\alpha} - \frac{\partial^3 w}{\partial x^2\,\partial t} + \frac{\partial w}{\partial x} = w\frac{\partial^3 w}{\partial x^3} - w\frac{\partial w}{\partial x} + 3\frac{\partial w}{\partial x}\frac{\partial^2 w}{\partial x^2}\ ,\ t > 0,\ 0 < \alpha \le 1,\ \text{IV},\ w(x,0) = \frac{4}{3}\ e^{\frac{1}{2}x} \tag{12}$$

By applying above method on equation (12)

$$\sum_{n=0}^{\infty} w_{n+1}(x,t) = \frac{4}{3} e^{\frac{1}{2}x} + S^{-1}\left\{u^\alpha S\left[\frac{\partial^3}{\partial x^2\partial t}(w_n) - \frac{\partial}{\partial x}(w_n) + \sum_{n=0}^{\infty}.X_n - \sum_{n=0}^{\infty}.Y_n. + \sum_{n=0}^{\infty}.Z_n\right]\right\} \tag{13}$$

Adomian polynomials constitute an infinite sequence used to illustrate the nonlinear elements.

$$N_1 = w \frac{\partial^3 w}{\partial x^3} = \sum_{n=0}^{\infty} X_n, \, N_2 = w \frac{\partial w}{\partial x} = \sum_{n=0}^{\infty} Y_n, \, N_3 = \frac{\partial w}{\partial x} \frac{\partial^2 w}{\partial x^2} = \sum_{n=0}^{\infty} Z_n \quad (14)$$

With an initial approximation $w_0 = w(x, 0)$ in above Eq. (13), the other components as:

$$w_0(x,t) = \frac{4}{3} e^{\frac{x}{2}}, \; w_1(x,t) = e^{\frac{x}{2}} \left(-\frac{2}{3} \frac{t^\alpha}{\alpha+1} \right), \; w_2(x,t) = e^{\frac{x}{2}} \left(-\frac{1}{6} \frac{t^{2\alpha-1}}{2\alpha} + \frac{1}{3} \frac{t^{2\alpha}}{2\alpha+1} \right)$$

$$w_3(x,t) = e^{\frac{x}{2}} \left(-\frac{1}{24} \frac{t^{3\alpha-2}}{3\alpha-1} + \frac{1}{6} \frac{t^{3\alpha-1}}{3\alpha} - \frac{1}{6} \frac{t^{3\alpha}}{3\alpha+1} \right) \quad (15)$$

The series solutions for equation (15) are as follows:

$$w(x,t.) = \sum_{n=0}^{\infty} w_n.(x,t)$$

$$w(.x,t) = e^{\frac{x}{2}} \left(\frac{4}{3} - \frac{2}{3} \frac{t^\alpha}{\alpha+1.} + \frac{1}{3} \frac{t^{2\alpha}}{2\alpha+1} - \frac{1}{6} \frac{t^{3\alpha}}{3\alpha+1.} + \frac{1}{6} \frac{t^{3\alpha-1}}{3\alpha} - \frac{1}{6} \frac{t^{2\alpha-1}}{2\alpha} - \frac{1}{24} \frac{t^{3\alpha-2}}{3\alpha-1} + ... \right) \quad (16)$$

Equation (12) has a closed form precise solution that is $w(x,t) = e^{\frac{x}{2} - \frac{2}{3}t}$ \quad (17)

On comparing (16) and (17), the series solution. rapidly converges to exact solution.

Table 36.1 Exact solution for Example 4.1 and third order MADST solution comparison for $\alpha = 1$.

'x'	't'	Approximate Solution	Exact Solution	Error.
0.25	0.25	1.274295608	1.278666667	0.004371059
	0.5	1.058374347	1.082666667	0.024292319
	0.75	0.860150741	0.916000000	0.055849259
	1	0.676674707	0.776000000	0.099325293
0.5	0.25	1.443966097	1.449333333	0.005367236
	0.5	1.199295254	1.226666667	0.027371412
	0.75	0.974678481	1.038666667	0.063988185
	1	0.766772898	0.878666667	0.111893769
0.75	0.25	1.636227949	1.642666667	0.006438718
	0.5	1.358979562	1.390666667	0.031687104
	0.75	1.104455413	1.176000000	0.071544587
	1	0.868867523	0.996000000	0.127132477

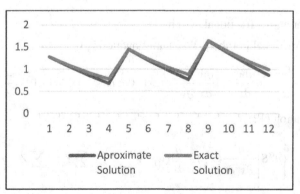

Fig. 36.1 Graph plot for table 1: Approximate Solution vs Exact Solution

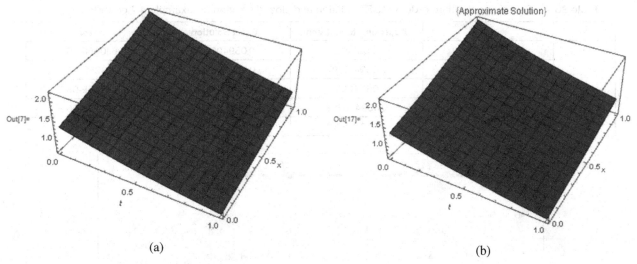

Fig. 36.2 (a) W_{exact}, $0 \leq x \leq 1$, $0 \leq t \leq 1$, $\alpha = 1$ (b) W_{MADSTM}, $0 \leq x \leq 1$, $0 \leq t \leq 1$, $\alpha = 1$

Example 2 Consider the following time.-fractional Korteweg-de Vries Equation.:

$$w_t^\alpha + ww_x + \frac{1}{2}w_{xxx} = 0, \ 0 < \alpha \leq 1, \ t > 0 \text{, initial condition } w(x, 0) = 6k^2 \, sech^2 \, (kx) \tag{18}$$

By applying the MADST on equation (18)

$$\sum_{n=0}^{\infty} w_{n+1}(x,t) = 6k^2 sech^2(kx) - S^{-1}\left\{u^\alpha S\left[\sum_{n=0}^{\infty}A_n + \sum_{n=0}^{\infty}B_n\right]\right\}$$

The nonlinear terms presented with Adomian polynomials.

$$N_1 = ww_x = \sum_{n=0}^{\infty}A_n \tag{19}$$

The first few terms of A_n are provided below, along with a recursive definition of the formula that follows:

$$w_0(x,t) = 6k^2 sech^2(kx), \ w_1(x,t) = \frac{24k^5 t^\alpha \tanh(kx)(kx)}{\alpha + 1}$$

$$w_2(x,t) = \left(-\frac{576k^{11}t^{3\alpha}\Gamma(2\alpha+1)\tanh(kx)sech^6(kx)}{\Gamma(\alpha+1)^2 . \Gamma 3\alpha+1} + \frac{1152k^{11}t^{3\alpha}\Gamma(2\alpha+1)\tanh^3(kx)sech^4(kx)}{\Gamma(\alpha+1)^2\Gamma 3\alpha+1}\right.$$

$$\left. -\frac{48k^8 t^{2\alpha}sech^4(kx)}{\Gamma 2\alpha+1} + \frac{96k^8 t^{2\alpha}tanh^4(kx)sech^2(kx)}{\Gamma(2\alpha+1)}\right) \tag{20}$$

Other components can be found in the same way. The series solutions for equation (20) are as follows:

$$w(x,t) = \left(-\frac{576k^{11}t^{3\alpha}\Gamma(2\alpha.+1)\tanh[kx]sech^6[kx]}{\Gamma(\alpha+1)^2\Gamma 3\alpha+1} + \frac{1152k^{11}t^{3\alpha}\Gamma(2\alpha+1)\tanh^3[kx]sech^4[kx]}{\Gamma(\alpha+1)^2\Gamma.3\alpha+1}\right.$$

$$-\frac{48k^8 t^{2\alpha}sech^4[kx]}{\Gamma 2\alpha+1} + \frac{96k^8 t^{2\alpha}tanh^4[kx]sech^2[kx]}{\Gamma 2\alpha+1.}$$

$$\left. +\frac{24k^5 t^\alpha \tanh[kx]sech^2[kx]}{\alpha+1} + 6k^2 sech^2[kx]\right) \tag{21}$$

Equation (1) having exact solution is $w(x, t) = 6k^2 \, sech^2 \, [kx - 2k^3 t]$ \hfill (22)

On comparing (21) and (22), the series solution converging to its exact solution.

Table 36.2 Comparing the third-order MADST solution and closed solution for example 4.2.considering $\alpha = 1$

x	t	Approximate Solution	Exact Solution	.Error
1	0.1	0.059412	0.059406343	6.1005E-06
	0.2	0.059415897	0.059408705	7.1925E-06
	0.3	0.059418536	0.059411062	7.4746E-06
	0.4	0.059420753	0.059413414	7.3397E-06
	0.5	0.059422701	0.059415761	6.94E-06

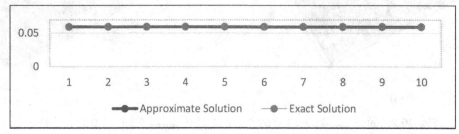

Fig. 36.3 Graph plot for table 2: Approximate Solution vs Exact Solution

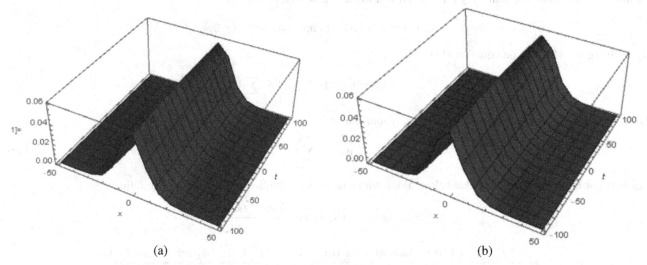

(a)   (b)

Fig. 36.4 (a) W_{exact}, $0 \le x \le 1$, $0 \le t \le 1$, $\alpha = 1$ (b) W_{MADSTM}, $0 \le x \le 1$, $0 \le t \le 1$, $\alpha = 1$

Example 3 Consider the Burgers equation with a time-fractional derivative and proportional delay:

$$_a^c D_t^\alpha w(x,t) = \frac{\partial^2 w}{\partial x^2}(x,t) + \frac{\partial w}{\partial x}\left(x,\frac{t}{2}\right).w\left(\frac{x}{2},\frac{t}{2}\right) + \frac{1}{2}w(x,t), x,t \in [0,1] and 0 < \alpha \le 1 \tag{23}$$

Having initial condition $w(x, 0) = x$

The precise analytical solution for this problem is as follows:

$w(x, t) = xe^t$ for special value of $\alpha = 1$

Using the above said technique on equation (23)

$$\sum_{n=0}^{\infty} w_{n+1}(x,t) = x + S^{-1}\left\{u^\alpha S\left\{\sum_{n=0}^{\infty}.P_n + \sum_{n=0}^{\infty}Q_n + \sum_{n=0}^{\infty}.R_n\right\}\right\} \tag{24}$$

An infinite sequence of Adomian. polynomials represent the nonlinear terms.

$$N_1 = \frac{\partial}{\partial x}w\left(x,\frac{t}{2}\right)w\left(\frac{x}{2},\frac{t}{2}\right) = \sum_{n=0}^{\infty}P_n \tag{25}$$

Substitute (25) in equation (24)

Initially, let us assume an approximate value $w_0 = w(x, 0)$ in above Equation (24), the other components as:

$$w_0\left(x,t\right) = .x, w_1\left(x,t\right). = \left(\frac{xt^\alpha}{\alpha+1}\right), w_2\left(x,t\right) = .\left(\frac{\alpha!}{2^\alpha}\frac{xt^{2\alpha}.}{2\alpha+1} + \frac{(2\alpha)!}{2^{1+2\alpha}}\frac{xt^{3\alpha}}{\alpha+1}\cdot\frac{xt^{3\alpha}}{3\alpha+1} + \frac{\alpha!}{2}\frac{xt^{2\alpha}}{2\alpha+1}\right)$$

$$w_3\left(x,t\right) = x\left(\frac{\alpha!}{3^{\alpha.}}\frac{t^{3\alpha}}{3\alpha+1}.+\frac{(3\alpha)!}{2^{3+2\alpha}2\alpha+1}\cdot\frac{t^{4\alpha}}{4\alpha+1}+\frac{(3\alpha)!}{\alpha+1}\frac{t^{3\alpha}}{3\alpha+1}+\frac{3\alpha!}{12}\frac{t^{3\alpha}}{3\alpha+1}\right)+\dots$$

Other components can be found in the same way. The series solutions for equation (24) are as follows:

$$w\left(x,t\right) = x\left(1+\left(\frac{t^\alpha}{\alpha+1}\right)+\left(\frac{\alpha!}{2^\alpha}\frac{t^{2\alpha}}{2\alpha+1}+\frac{(2\alpha)!}{2^{1+2\alpha}}\frac{t^{3\alpha}}{\alpha+1}\cdot\frac{t^{3\alpha}}{3\alpha+1}+\frac{\alpha!}{2}\frac{t^{2\alpha}}{2\alpha+1}\right)\right.$$

$$\left.+\left(\frac{\alpha!}{3^\alpha}\frac{t^{3\alpha}}{3\alpha+1}.+\frac{(3\alpha)!}{2^{3+2\alpha}2\alpha+1}\cdot\frac{t^{4\alpha}}{4\alpha+1}+\frac{(3\alpha)!}{\alpha+1}\frac{t^{3\alpha}}{3\alpha+1}+\frac{3\alpha!}{12}\frac{t^{3\alpha}}{3\alpha+1}\right)+\dots\right) \qquad (26)$$

The exact. solution of Equation (31) in closed to $w(x, t) = xe^t$ $\qquad (27)$

Equation (26) and (27) exact and approximate solutions are converges to each other.

Table 36.3 Comparing the third-order MADST approximate solution and exact solution for example .4.3 with $\alpha = 1$

x	t	Approximate solution	Exact solution.	Error.
0.25	0.25	0.320475000	0.321006300	0.000531300
	0.5	0.407550000	0.412180179	0.004630179
	0.75	0.512200000	0.529249737	0.017049737
	1	0.635400000	0.679570000	0.044170000
0.5	0.25	0.640950000	0.642012600	0.001062600
	0.5	0.815100000	0.824360358	0.009260358
	0.75	1.024400000	1.058499474	0.034099474
	1	1.270800000	1.359140000	0.088340000
0.75	0.25	0.961425000	0.963018901	0.001593901
	0.5	1.222650000	1.236540537	0.013890537
	0.75	1.536600000	1.587749211	0.051149211
	1	1.906200000	2.038710000	0.132510000

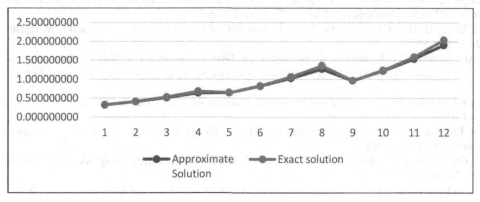

Fig. 36.5 Graph plot for table 3: Approximate Solution vs Exact Solutions

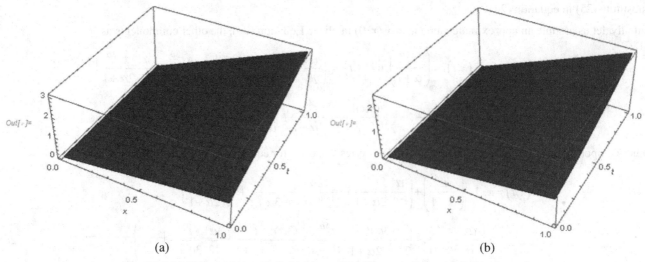

Fig. 36.6 (a) W_{exact}, $0 \leq x \leq 1$, $0 \leq t \leq 1$, $\alpha = 1$ (b) W_{MADSTM}, $0 \leq x \leq 1$, $0 \leq t \leq 1$, $\alpha = 1$

4. Conclusion

This paper successfully employed Modified Adomian Decomposition. Sumudu Transformation Method (MADST) determined through finding approximate solution of nonlinear fractional order partial differential equations. The MADST proves to be a method that reduces computational complexity, offering ease of use in tackling nonlinear fractional problems. The application shown thought solving MADST method in this study demonstrates its effectiveness in providing accurate and rapid convergence to exact solutions for non-linear problems. Specifically, MADST is utilized in this study to estimate the solutions for time-fractional coupled partial differential equations. Tables 36.1, 36.2, and 36.3 demonstrate the convergency of the series solution obtained through the proposed method, meeting the criteria for convergence. Additionally, error analysis is conducted, and comparing with the approximation solutions with the exact solutions for the specified applications. Error graph and surface graphs are plotted for various values of α, such as $\alpha = 1$. Consequently, the Modified Adomian Decomposition Sumudu Transformation Method emerges as a more convenient for determining the fractional partial differential equations. (FPDEs).

REFERENCES

1. K.B. Oldham, J. Spanier, The Fractional Calculus, Academic Press, New York, (1974).
2. K. Diethelm, Analysis of Fractional Differential Equations, Springer-Verlag, Berlin, (2010).
3. G. Adomian, A review of the decomposition method in applied mathematics, J. Math. Anal. Appl. 135 (1988) 44–501.
4. Y. Cherruault, G. Adomian, Decomposition methods: A new proof of convergence, Math. Comput. Modelling 18 (1993) 103–106
5. Kumar, D., Singh, J., Kumar, S., Numerical computation of nonlinear fractional Zakharov Kuznetsov equation arising in ion-acoustic waves, Journal of the Egyptian Mathematical Society, 22(3), 2014, 373–378.
6. D. Kaya, S.M. El-Sayed, An application of the decomposition method for the generalized KdV and RLW equations, Chaos Solitons Fractals 17 (2003) 869–877.
7. Saad, K. M., AL-Shareef, E. H., Alomari, A. K., Baleanu, D., & Gómez-Aguilar, J. F. (2020). On exact solutions for time-fractional Korteweg-de Vries and Korteweg-de Vries-Burger's equations using homotopy analysis transform method. Chinese Journal of Physics, 63, 149-162.
8. T. Mavoungou, Y. Cherruault, Convergence of Adomian's method and applications to non-linear partial differential equation, Kybernetes 21 (6) (1992) 13–25.
9. M.G. Sakar, F. Erdogan, A. Yildirim, Variational Iteration Method for the Time-Fractional Fornberg–Whitham Equation, Comput. Math. Appl, 63 (9) (2012) 1382–1388.
10. H. Jafari, V.D. Gejji, Solving A System of Nonlinear Fractional Differential Equations Using Adomian Decomposition, Appl. Math. Comput, 196 (2006) 644– 651.
11. Sakar, M. G., Uludag, F., & Erdogan, F. (2016). Numerical solution of time fractional nonlinear PDEs with proportional delays by homotopy perturbation method. Applied Mathematical Modelling, 40(13-14), 6639-6649.
12. C. Viriyapong and N. Viriyapong, "Modified Sumudu decomposition method for solving Lane-Emden- fowler type systems," WSEAS Transc Math, vol. 20, pp. 446–454, 2021.

13. I. Podlubny, Fractional Differential Equations, Academic Press, 1999 [13] T. Achouri, K. Omrani, Numerical solutions for the damped generalized regularized long-wave equation with a variable coefficient by Adomian decomposition method, Commun. Nonlinear Sci. Numer. Simul. 14 (2009) 869–877.

14. A.M. Wazwaz, A new algorithm for calculating Adomian polynomials for nonlinear operators, Appl. Math. Comput. 111 (2000) 53–69.

15. G. Adomian, Solving Frontier Problems of Physics: The Decomposition Method, Kluwer Academic Publishers, Boston, 1999

16. Singh, Subodh Pratap, and Amardeep Singh. "Time-Fractional Fornberg-Whitham Equation Solved by Fractional Homotopy Perturbation Transform Method."

17. K. Abbaoui, Y. Cherruault, Convergence of Adomian's method applied to differential equations, Comput. Math. Appl. 28 (1994) 8–31.

18. Y. Cherruault, Convergence of Adomian's method, Kybernetes 18 (2) (1989) 8–31.

Emerging Trends in IoT and Computing Technologies – Suman Lata Tripathi et al. (eds)
© 2024 Taylor & Francis Group, London, ISBN 978-1-032-87924-6

Hardware Trojan Taxonomy and Detection: A Review

37

Khalid Ahmed Markar[1], Sushant Madhukar Mane[2], Faruk S. Kazi[3]

CoE-CNDS Lab, VJTI, Mumbai, India

Abstract: The escalating complexity and integration of integrated circuits (ICs) in critical systems have given rise to a significant security threat - Hardware Trojans. These alterations, clandestinely inserted during IC design and manufacturing processes, pose substantial risks to the confidentiality, integrity, and authenticity of electronic systems. This comprehensive review consolidates extensive research on Hardware Trojans, exploring their diverse manifestations, attack vectors, and detection strategies. Machine Learning (ML) techniques for trojan detection are examined, accompanied by case studies evaluating their effectiveness. The paper scrutinizes real-world scenarios, trojan insertion methodologies, and performance evaluations using Field Programmable Gate Array (FPGA) platforms. Hardware Trojan's taxonomy is analyzed according to insertion phases, abstraction levels, activation mechanisms, and effects. Detection strategies, spanning golden chip comparison, circuit feature analysis, side-channel analysis (SCA), machine learning, logic testing, reverse engineering, optical detection, property checking, and static/dynamic detection, are thoroughly discussed. The review addresses the challenges in Hardware Trojan detection and outlines future research directions for fortifying electronic systems.

Keywords: Hardware trojan, IC security, Trojan taxonomy, Trojan insertion, Trojan detection, Side-channel analysis, Machine learning

1. Introduction

In recent years, the increasing complexity and widespread integration of ICs into critical systems have given rise to a notable security concern known as Hardware Trojans. These concealed entities, inserted covertly during various IC design and manufacturing phases, pose substantial risks to the security and integrity of electronic systems. A "Hardware Trojan" refers to "malicious modifications to an IC, subtly altering its functionality at any stage of the IC's life cycle". These modifications are challenging to detect and can jeopardize the Confidentiality, Integrity, and Authenticity (CIA Triad) of the host system, leading to severe consequences in hardware-dependent systems. Thus, it is a serious concern in Information Technology (IT), Operational Technology (OT), and Internet of Things (IoT) security. Figure 37.1 shows a simple block diagram of a circuit modified with Hardware Trojan.

The rise in Hardware Trojan threats has fueled a surge in research across electrical engineering, computer science, and cybersecurity, resulting in a rich literature exploring Hardware Trojans. This body of work collectively contributes insights into their manifestations, attack vectors, and potential countermeasures.

Researchers have delved into various facets of Hardware Trojan attacks, scrutinizing their implementation intricacies and assessing implications for cyber-physical systems [1]. The integration of machine learning techniques has emerged as a promising avenue to fortify defences, with surveys and case studies evaluating their efficacy [2, 3, 4]. Beyond detection,

[1]kamarkar_m22@ee.vjti.ac.in, [2]smmane_p22@el.vjti.ac.in, [3]fskazi@el.vjti.ac.in

DOI: 10.1201/9781003535423-37

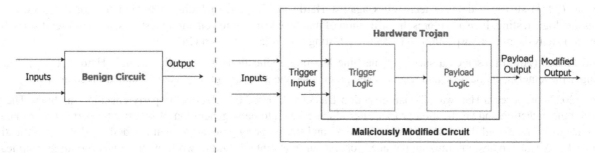

Fig. 37.1 Hardware trojan modified circuit block diagram

exploration extends to real-world case studies, Hardware Trojan insertion methodologies, and performance evaluations using FPGA platforms [5, 6, 7].

As electronic systems become increasingly integral to modern life, the associated risks with Hardware Trojans continue to escalate. Ensuring the trustworthiness of ICs is now a paramount concern for designers, manufacturers, and end-users. This review synthesizes recent research, offering a comprehensive overview of Hardware Trojans, their attack vectors, and the evolving landscape of detection strategies. It aims to provide readers with a holistic understanding of this critical cyber security challenge, setting the stage for future developments fortifying the resilience of electronic systems against Hardware Trojan threats.

2. Literature Review

Bhunia et al. (2014) surveyed the increasing threat of Hardware Trojan attacks in advanced chip designs, pointing out vulnerabilities due to complexity and reliance on untrusted components. It provides an in-depth taxonomy of Hardware Trojan and its detection methods [8].

Shakya et al. (2017) presented a comprehensive approach to the study and evaluation of Hardware Trojans and their detection techniques. The research proposed a suite of 'trust benchmarks' which are essentially circuits with integrated Hardware Trojans, meant to aid researchers in comparing Trojan detection methodologies. These Trojans have been developed to be resilient to conventional manufacturing tests, exhibiting variations in size and distribution while being implemented at different abstraction levels [9].

Lingasubramanian et al. (2018) proposed a case study investigating hardware security vulnerabilities in "Cyber-Physical Systems (CPS)" within the context of IoT applications through the examination of a "Supervisory Control and Data Acquisition (SCADA)" system based on a gas pipeline [1].

Zhao (2018) contributed a case study based on model checking, emphasizing the significance of early detection at the "Register-Transfer Level (RTL)" source code [10].

Huang et al. (2020) provided a survey on machine learning applications against Hardware Trojan attacks, focusing on Intellectual Property (IP) Level, Bus Level, and System on Chip (SoC) Level Trojans categorizing diverse techniques and offering insights into the evolving landscape of machine learning in Hardware Trojan defence studies [2].

Xue et al. (2020) presented a comprehensive study of Hardware Trojan designs and implementations from an attacker's perspective, analysing various threat scenarios across the lifecycle of IC production. It discusses potential motivations, practical feasibilities, and attack detection evasion techniques and offers prevention recommendations, traversing through seven practical Hardware Trojan introduction stages [11].

Ghandali et al. (2020) proposed a mechanism to introduce a discrete Hardware Trojan into circuits while ensuring provably secure first-order side-channel countermeasures. Trojans can be inserted into Application-Specific Integrated Circuits (ASICs) through subtle manipulations at the subtransistor level, without requiring the addition or removal of any logic, making them extremely hard to detect [12].

Dong et al. (2020) proposed an unsupervised detection approach using eXtreme Gradient Boosting (XGBoost), Principal Component Analysis (PCA) and Local Outlier Factor (LOF) algorithms to identify abnormal nets within gate-level netlists., addressing challenges associated with unsupervised learning [13].

Jain et al. (2021) surveyed defence techniques against Hardware Trojans, including detection methods like side-channel analysis and logic testing. It also explores the utilization of machine learning in generating test sets, and the use of side-channel information analysis, optical inspection, and electrical testing for Trojan detection [14].

Pan and Mishra (2022) presented a survey of machine learning applications in defending against Hardware Trojan attacks, covering achievements, challenges, and recent developments in detection, design-for-security, and architecture [3].

Li et al. (2022) proposed a Hardware Trojan detection framework based on effective property-checking methods. The paper automated the detection and verification process, introducing the automatic generation of security property. The refined RTL behaviour model addressed the state explosion problem, and the property generation method facilitated the identification of particular Hardware Trojans, minimizing the need for human intervention. Future work includes incorporating deep learning and neural networks for model-building and enhancing the framework's standardization and automation [15].

Piliposyan and Khursheed (2022) implemented a runtime detection system for Printed Circuit Board (PCB) Hardware Trojans combining power analysis and ML algorithms. The study focused on detecting stealthier Hardware Trojans powered by legitimate chips on a PCB. High classification results were attained by two machine learning algorithms: One-Class Support Vector Machine (SVM) and LOF. The One-Class SVM model, proven in simulations, demonstrated low-cost and memory-efficient operation in practical experiments conducted on a prototype PCB [4].

Kan et al. (2022) proposed a system for the detection of Radio Frequency (RF) analog Hardware Trojans through electromagnetic side channels. Utilizing magnetic tunnel junction sensors, the research characterized Hardware Trojans present in Class AB and Class E power amplifiers. The classifier-autoencoder synthesized with an FPGA achieved high accuracy, even with injected noise, showcasing the effectiveness of the proposed approach [12].

Elshamy et al. (2022) explored digital-to-analog Hardware Trojan attacks and introduced an innovative attack scenario that specifically targets analog IPs integrated into an SoC [17].

Almeida et al. (2022) proposed a unique type of Hardware Trojan termed "Hardware Ransomware" along with a silicon demonstration in 65nm complementary metal-oxide semiconductor (CMOS). The experimental results show that the ransomware logic can be effortlessly inserted into a complex SoC without significant detectability [18].

Khamitkar and Dube (2023) focused on ongoing research in Hardware Trojan insertion and detection, including recent contributions in the field. Previous research on Hardware Trojan detection involved image processing and comparison with golden ICs, as well as comparing electrical parameters of standard ICs with those manufactured by third-party developers [5].

Rajput et al. (2023) demonstrated a technique for identifying Hardware Trojans in FPGA bitstreams through the application of unsupervised machine learning. The system transforms bitstreams into an encoded vector representation for training, enabling the identification of malicious bitstreams without needing complex reverse engineering or design reconstruction [19].

Perez and Pagliarini (2023) presented a methodology for inserting a Hardware Trojan into a finalized IC layout during the fabrication process and demonstrated its effectiveness with a real-world implementation. It highlights the attacker's ability to leak confidential information via this method, thus raising significant concerns about hardware security in the foundry stage of IC production [6].

Puschner et al. (2023) pointed out the absence of public case studies describing the Hardware Trojan detection process and making the underlying datasets publicly available. Addressing this gap, the study concentrates on this matter by introducing a public and open case study for Hardware Trojan detection. The case study is founded on four distinct digital ICs and adopts a Red Team vs. Blue Team approach [7].

Gubbi et al. (2023) addressed challenges in detecting Hardware Trojans in IC design, emphasizing the limitations of conventional tests and proposing machine learning techniques, including a Neural Network-assisted timing profiling method. It also explores reinforcement learning for adaptive test pattern generation, presenting an overall flow for ML-assisted Hardware Trojan detection, covering statistical modelling, fabrication, testing, and Trojan detection stages [20].

2.1 Objectives

1. To enhance understanding of Hardware Trojans and their threats in IoT and OT systems.
2. To formulate a structured taxonomy of Hardware Trojans based on attack methods and insertion stages.
3. To discuss challenges and limitations in current Hardware Trojan detection methods.
4. To offer insights into future developments for securing electronic systems against trojan threats.

3. Taxonomy of Hardware Trojans

Various iterations of the Trojan taxonomy have been introduced and continue to evolve with the discovery of new Trojan attacks and types [1, 8, 9]. Figure 37.2 illustrates a Hardware Trojan taxonomy based on previous work.

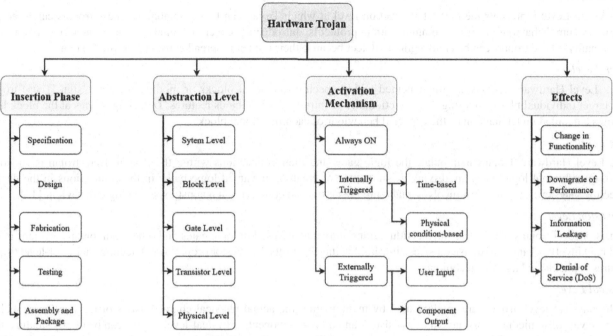

Fig. 37.2 Taxonomy of hardware trojan

3.1 Insertion Phase

Hardware Trojan can be inserted at various stages of the IC development Life Cycle from specification and design up to Assembly and Packaging. A Trojan can be introduced through modifications in specifications, such as chip area, power constraints, or operating temperature range. During the Design and Fabrication stages, Trojan can be implemented by integrating additional gates to a design's netlist or by modifying its masks during the fabrication stage [9]. Malicious vendors can effortlessly insert Hardware Trojans into IC products by manipulating the design file of IC. From RTL code synthesis to gate-level netlist design, and through chip integration and packaging, each stage presents an opportunity for the incorporation of Hardware Trojans [13]. Since Testing may be done by third-party vendors, Side-channel attacks can be used for trojan insertion between the Fabrication and Testing Phases [6]. Table 37.1, gives a brief overview of Hardware Trojan insertion at various stages of the IC Life Cycle from an attacker's perspective.

Table 37.1 Hardware trojan in insertion phase

IC Life Cycle Phase	Goal	Attacker's Motivations
Specification Phase	Introduce trojans in high-level requirements.	Manipulate functionality for malicious purposes. Embed trojans in a stealthy manner.
Design Phase	Insert trojans in detailed design.	Compromise specific components or functionalities. Create secret access points (backdoors).
Fabrication Phase	Introduce trojans during manufacturing.	Compromise manufacturing facilities or supply chain. Create counterfeit chips with embedded trojans.
Testing Phase	Ensure trojans remain undetected.	Design trojans to evade detection during testing. Implement test escape mechanisms for conditional activation.
Assembly and Package	Introduce trojans during the component assembly and packaging phase.	Manipulate integration of different hardware components. Hide malicious circuitry within the packaging.

3.2 Abstraction Level

The Abstraction Level plays a crucial role in defining the control and flexibility an attacker possesses in implementing Hardware Trojans [9].

System Level

The system Level represents the highest abstraction level at which Trojan can be implemented. These trojans can affect the overall system behaviour, altering communication protocols, introducing covert channels, or manipulating system-level functionality. These trojans can be challenging to detect because their impact is spread across the entire system.

Block Level

Block Level Hardware Trojans are implemented within specific functional blocks or modules of the design. These trojans may target individual blocks, altering their functionality or introducing malicious features. Detecting trojans at the block level requires a detailed understanding of the expected behaviour of each functional block.

Gate Level

Gate Level Hardware Trojans manipulate the logic gates and their connections within the design. Here trojan is added by inserting additional logic gates, modifying existing ones or creating unwanted logic paths in the connections in the design. Detecting gate-level trojans often involves analyzing the netlist and comparing it against expected logic behaviour [13].

Transistor Level

Transistor-level trojans manipulate the individual transistors that are used in logic gates and other components. Trojans at this level may involve changes to transistor sizes, threshold voltages, or other transistor properties. Detecting transistor-level trojans requires sophisticated analysis techniques.

Physical Level

At the physical level, trojans are implemented by manipulating the actual physical characteristics of the hardware, such as doping levels of semiconductors, layout of transistors and other components. Physical-level trojans can be highly stealthy, they do not change the logic of the hardware but rather cause subtle modifications in the physical structure. Detecting physical level trojans may involve techniques such as SCA, fault injection, or using image processing techniques to scan for anomalies in the physical layout [7, 12].

3.3 Activation Mechanism

Hardware Trojans are activated when a Trigger signal is provided to it, externally or internally. Trojans may operate continuously, or they could be selectively activated. Always-ON Trojans initiate upon powering up their host designs, whereas conditional Trojans await specific internal or external triggers for activation. Depending on the trigger condition, Hardware Trojans can be further categorized into analog and digital trojans [8, 9]. Analog trojans are activated in response to analog conditions, such as environmental changes like temperature, delay, or device ageing effects. Meanwhile, digital trojans are triggered by Boolean logic functions, such as a logic level switching its state through the use of a Multiplexer [1].

3.4 Effects

Trojans can be categorized based on their effects. When a Trigger signal is provided, a payload is activated. The payload acts as the execution of a Hardware Trojan as shown earlier in Fig. 37.1, an example of gate-level representation of the "Trigger and Payload" in a maliciously modified circuit can be seen in Fig. 37.3. A Hardware Trojan can initiate an 'information leakage' attack, wherein secret information is disclosed. Additionally, it may engage in a side-channel attack, revealing information through the analysis of power consumption, electromagnetic traces, or timing variations. Furthermore, the Trojan can execute a denial-of-service (DoS) attack, rendering a system's functionality unavailable, thereby degrading its performance or compromising its reliability by altering its physical parameters [8, 9]. Zhao (2018) performs an XOR operation between specific bits of operands in the arithmetic logic unit (ALU) of a processor, reversing the result afterwards. If the reversed result is 1, the Trojan remains inactive, allowing correct output; if it's 0, the trojan triggers, causing the result to be 0 and thus changing the functionality [10]. Lingasubramanian et al. (2018) discussed a scenario of the Gas Pipeline System, where a Hardware Trojan caused the PID controller to disconnect for different time interval scenarios, thus causing pressure in the pipeline to increase beyond permissible limits and making the system unstable [1]. Elshamy et al. (2022) proposed an attack scenario where a Hardware Trojan is inserted in digital circuitry and transports its payload to the target which is an analog circuit. The payload encompasses a malicious "Design-for-Test (DfT)", including sensors and actuators, along with programmability fabric for

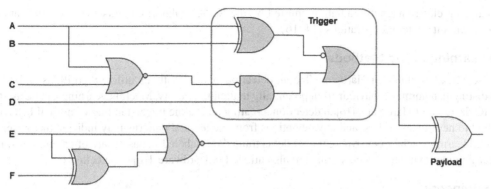

Fig. 37.3 Trigger and payload representation using logic gates

calibration. It causes DoS attack and Performance degradation in a Regulator circuit and infects an RF Receiver [17]. Almeida et al. (2022) introduced a Trojan with a distinctive feature, It necessitates communication with the victim and is reversible, meaning user data must undergo encryption and decryption processes. This sets it apart from other trojans that usually do not involve such considerations [18].

4. Hardware Trojan Detection Strategies

The detection of Hardware Trojans poses a critical and pressing challenge for researchers. It is inherently difficult due to the opacity of ICs, making the inspection of their internal components non-trivial. Hence, techniques for examining ICs fall into two categories: invasive and non-invasive. Invasive methods, as the name implies, necessitate access to the internal components of the IC, which may lead to the destruction of the sample being inspected. On the contrary, non-invasive methods analyze the IC externally. Different Hardware Trojan detection methods are as follows:

4.1 Golden Chip Comparison

Golden chip comparison is a Hardware Trojan detection method that involves comparing the behaviour of a suspect IC with that of a known, trustworthy reference or "golden" chip. The golden chip serves as a benchmark, representing the expected functionality of the IC without any malicious alterations [5]. This method relies on the assumption that Hardware Trojans may introduce subtle variations in the circuit's behaviour, such as altered delays, power consumption, or output patterns. Through careful comparison of these characteristics, engineers can pinpoint anomalies indicative of malicious modifications.

4.2 Circuit Feature Analysis

This method involves the examination of various features within the IC to identify irregularities or to detect deviations from expected behaviour. Gate-level structures, Signal Paths, and Circuit layouts are some of the features used for analysis. By analysing these characteristics, Hardware Trojans can be detected [2].

4.3 Logic Testing

This method focuses on analysing the IC's response to various input conditions, checking for unexpected or malicious behaviour. During logic testing, a set of test vectors or input patterns are designed to activate different parts of the circuit and the corresponding outputs are observed. The presence of Hardware Trojans can be inferred from any deviation in the expected responses [13]. Logic testing is particularly effective in identifying trojans that manipulate the logical behaviour of the circuit, such as those designed to activate under specific conditions, however, it may not be as effective in detecting trojans that operate at a lower level, such as those affecting analog components or modifying power consumption patterns. Logic testing is often combined with other methods, such as SCA to enhance trojan detection and ensure the security of ICs.

4.4 Side Channel Analysis

Side Channel Analysis detects unintended information leakage during the operation of ICs. These techniques focus on monitoring and analysing measurable side-channel signals, including electromagnetic radiations, timing variations or power consumption to detect Hardware Trojans. One widely used side-channel analysis method is Power Analysis, where variations in the power consumption of an IC are observed during its operation. Another technique is Electromagnetic SCA, which involves capturing and analysing electromagnetic radiation emitted by the IC. Any abnormal emissions may indicate the presence of trojans affecting the circuit's internal operations [14, 16].

4.5 Machine Learning based Methods

These methods use ML algorithms for Hardware Trojan detection. These methods utilize algorithms and models trained on large datasets to distinguish normal behaviour from potentially malicious activity. Machine learning can be used to train models on known good IC designs for Hardware Trojan detection, creating a baseline understanding of normal behaviour. The model can then be applied to new, untested ICs, and any deviations from the learned patterns may indicate the presence of Hardware Trojans. Supervised learning techniques, where the model is trained on 'labeled' datasets, are often employed for this purpose. Unsupervised learning methods, such as clustering are also utilized in Hardware Trojan detection [4, 19].

4.6 Reverse Engineering

IC/FPGA reverse engineering is a Hardware Trojan detection method that involves analyzing and dissecting the physical structure of ICs or field-programmable gate arrays (FPGAs) to uncover potential malicious modifications or hidden functionalities [14, 19]. This approach aims to reveal the internal design and configuration of the device, providing insights into its intended operation and identifying any discrepancies that might suggest the existence of Hardware Trojans. By carefully inspecting the device's structure, researchers can identify alterations to the original design, such as additional circuitry, modified connections, or embedded trojan components. While reverse engineering can reveal the presence of trojans, it may not provide information about the trojan's functionality or activation conditions. Reverse Engineering can be seen as an invasive process.

4.7 Optical Detection

Optical Detection methods use advanced imaging and analysis techniques to inspect the physical characteristics of ICs at the microscopic or nanoscopic level. These methods leverage optical microscopy, scanning electron microscopy (SEM), and other imaging technologies to detect anomalies, alterations, or additional structures indicating the presence of Hardware Trojans. Optical microscopy allows researchers to visualize the surface features of an IC. **Scanning Electron Microscopy (SEM)** offers higher magnification and resolution compared to traditional optical microscopy. It uses focused electron beams to create detailed images of the IC's surface. SEM is particularly useful for detecting small-scale modifications or additions to the circuitry [13]. GDSII imaging is another imaging technique used for trojan detection. GDSII (Graphic Data System II) is a standard format for representing the physical layout of an IC at various stages of the design process. GDSII imaging involves visually inspecting and analyzing the graphical representation of an IC's layout to identify potential malicious modifications or irregularities [7]. Quantum Diamond Microscope (QDM) and Ptychographic X-ray Computed Tomography (PXCT) are other advanced imaging methods used [20].

4.8 Property Checking Method

Property Checking Method is a Hardware Trojan detection approach that involves the formal verification of specific properties or behaviours within an IC. This method depends on formal verification tools and techniques to mathematically prove or disprove the satisfaction of certain properties, ensuring that the IC operates as intended and is free from potential Hardware Trojans [15]. The effectiveness of this method depends on the accuracy of the formal specifications and the completeness of the property-checking tools.

4.9 Static and Dynamic Detection

Static detection involves identifying Hardware Trojans by analyzing the features of the gate-level circuit structure. It involves analyzing the circuit description file or netlist to detect the presence of Hardware Trojans. This method uses machine learning algorithms to identify patterns or features that are indicative of Hardware Trojans. Dynamic detection involves the use of formal verification and functional simulation for Trojan detection. It observes the behaviour of the IC during its operation to detect any abnormal or malicious activities. By monitoring the IC's inputs, outputs, and internal states, dynamic detection can detect unexpected behaviours that indicate the presence of possible Hardware Trojans [13].

4.10 Pre-Silicon and Post-Silicon Detection

Detection methods for Hardware Trojans can be categorized into 'pre-silicon' and 'post-silicon' phases. The pre-silicon phase encompasses activities and processes that take place before the actual fabrication of the IC. It includes the Design, Verification and Prototyping phases. The post-silicon phase begins after the IC has been manufactured and is in the physical form of silicon wafers. It includes Testing Debugging and Validation. An overview of types of detection methods based on the above categories is shown in Table 37.2.

Table 37.2 Pre-silicon and post-silicon classification of trojan detection methods

Pre-Silicon	Post-Silicon
Detection using on-chip modules [2]. Static and Dynamic Detection [13]. Utilizing pre-silicon design analysis to generate test vectors for logic testing [14, 16]. Golden chip comparison, Optical detection methods, and Power Analysis [16]. Finite State Machine (FSM)-based Property-Checking Method [15]. Layout images examination with physical constraints, Hardware description language and assertion checkers [5]. ML-based Hardware Trojan detection methods (e.g., decision tree classifiers, k-means clustering) [20].	Detection using circuit feature analysis [2]. Logic Testing [13]. Evaluating side-channel resistance using a nonspecific t-test and collecting traces under different Trojan and Trigger conditions [12]. EM Side-channel analysis techniques [14, 16]. Machine learning-based methods [4, 16, 19]. Automated Visual Inspection (AVI) for PCB verification [4]. Scanning Electron Microscope (SEM) imaging [13]. Power Side-channel analysis techniques [14]. IC / FPGA reverse engineering [14, 19]. GDSII-vs-SEM-image comparison for detecting Trojans [7]. Quantum Diamond Microscope (QDM), Ptychographic X-ray computed tomography (PXCT) [20].

5. Conclusion

Hardware Trojans present a threat to the reliability and security of systems, particularly as ICs become increasingly integrated into these systems. This review thoroughly explores the research on Hardware Trojans offering an overview of their classification and the evolving field of detection techniques. The proposed taxonomy provides a framework for understanding Hardware Trojans by categorizing them based on insertion phases, abstraction levels, activation mechanisms and effects. This classification not only enhances our understanding of how trojans can be identified but also lays the groundwork for developing targeted detection strategies. The integration of machine learning techniques shows promise as an avenue for research particularly in exploring advanced methodologies within this domain. Combining Side Channel Analysis with Machine Learning algorithms presents a non-invasive approach to effective detection. Additionally incorporating security measures during the design phase is crucial in countering Hardware Trojan threats. Research efforts should prioritize integrating security considerations, in IC design to raise the bar for attackers attempting to infiltrate systems during this critical phase.

REFERENCES

1. Lingasubramanian, K., Kumar, R., Gunti, N.B., and Morris, T., 2018. Study of hardware trojans based security vulnerabilities in cyber physical systems. 2018 IEEE International Conference on Consumer Electronics (ICCE).
2. Huang, Z., Wang, Q., Chen, Y., and Jiang, X., 2020. A Survey on Machine Learning Against Hardware Trojan Attacks: Recent Advances and Challenges. IEEE Access.
3. Pan, Z. and Mishra, P., 2022. A Survey on Hardware Vulnerability Analysis Using Machine Learning. IEEE Access.
4. Piliposyan, G. and Khursheed, S., 2022. PCB Hardware Trojan Run-Time Detection Through Machine Learning. IEEE Transactions on Computers.
5. Khamitkar, R. and Dube, R.R., 2023. Performance Evaluation of Hardware Trojan Using FPGA. Lecture Notes in Electrical Engineering, vol 992. Springer, Singapore.
6. Perez, T.D. and Pagliarini, S., 2023. Hardware Trojan Insertion in Finalized Layouts: From Methodology to a Silicon Demonstration. IEEE Transactions on Computer-Aided Design of Integrated Circuits and Systems.
7. Puschner, E., Moos, T., Becker, S., Kison, C., Moradi, A., and Paar, C., 2023. Red Team vs. Blue Team: A Real-World Hardware Trojan Detection Case Study Across Four Modern CMOS Technology Generations. 2023 IEEE Symposium on Security and Privacy (SP).
8. Bhunia, S., Hsiao, M.S., Banga, M., and Narasimhan, S., 2014. Hardware Trojan Attacks: Threat Analysis and Countermeasures. Proceedings of the IEEE.
9. Shakya, B., He, T., Salmani, H., Forte, D., Bhunia, S., and Tehranipoor, M., 2017. Benchmarking of Hardware Trojans and Maliciously Affected Circuits. Journal of Hardware and Systems Security.
10. Zhao, J., 2018. Case Study: Discovering Hardware Trojans Based on model checking. Proceedings of the 8th International Conference on Communication and Network Security.

11. Xue, M., Gu, C., Liu, W., Yu, S., and O'Neill, M., 2020. Ten years of hardware Trojans: a survey from the attacker's perspective. IET Computers & Digital Techniques.

12. Ghandali, S., Moos, T., Moradi, A., and Paar, C., 2020. Side-Channel Hardware Trojan for Provably-Secure SCA-Protected Implementations. IEEE Transactions on Very Large Scale Integration (VLSI) Systems.

13. Dong, C., Liu, Y., Chen, J., Liu, X., Guo, W., and Chen, Y., 2020. An Unsupervised Detection Approach for Hardware Trojans. IEEE Access.

14. Jain, A., Zhou, Z., and Guin, U., 2021. Survey of Recent Developments for Hardware Trojan Detection. 2021 IEEE International Symposium on Circuits and Systems (ISCAS).

15. Li, D., Zhang, Q., Zhao, D., Li, L., He, J., Yuan, Y., and Zhao, Y., 2022. Hardware Trojan Detection Using Effective Property-Checking Method. Electronics, 11 (17), 2649.

16. Kan, J., Shen, Y., Xu, J., Chen, E., Zhu, J., and Chen, V., 2022. RF Analog Hardware Trojan Detection Through Electromagnetic Side-Channel. IEEE Open Journal of Circuits and Systems.

17. Elshamy, M., Natale, G.D., Sayed, A., Pavlidis, A., Louerat, M.-M., Aboushady, H., and Stratigopoulos, H.-G., 2022. Digital-to-Analog Hardware Trojan Attacks. IEEE Transactions on Circuits and Systems I: Regular Papers.

18. Almeida, F., Imran, M., Raik, J., and Pagliarini, S., 2022. Ransomware Attack as Hardware Trojan: A Feasibility and Demonstration Study. IEEE Access.

19. Rajput, S., Dofe, J., and Danesh, W., 2023. Automating Hardware Trojan Detection Using Unsupervised Learning: A Case Study of FPGA. 2023 24th International Symposium on Quality Electronic Design (ISQED).

20. Gubbi, K.I., Saber Latibari, B., Srikanth, A., Sheaves, T., Beheshti-Shirazi, S.A., PD, S.M., Rafatirad, S., Sasan, A., Homayoun, H., and Salehi, S., 2023. Hardware Trojan Detection Using Machine Learning: A Tutorial. ACM Transactions on Embedded Computing Systems.

Emerging Trends in IoT and Computing Technologies – Suman Lata Tripathi et al. (eds)
© 2024 Taylor & Francis Group, London, ISBN 978-1-032-87924-6

Smart Zoos, Healthy Animals: SAHMT's Non-Invasive Healthcare Model

38

Sheeba Praveen[1]

Associate Professor, Department of Computer Science and Engineering,
Integral University, Lucknow

Akhtar Hasan Jamal Khan[2]

Research Schooler, Department of Commerce and Business Management,
Integral University, Lucknow

Neeta Rastogi[3]

Professor, Department of Computer Science and Engineering,
Ambalika Institute of Management & Technology, Lucknow

Syed Qamar Abbas[4]

Director General, Ambalika Institute of Management & Technology,
Lucknow, U.P

Nikhat Akhtar[5]

Associate Professor, Department of Information Technology,
Goel Institute of Technology & Management, Lucknow

Qudsia Shahab[6]

Assistant Professor, Department of Computer Science and Engineering,
Integral University, Lucknow

Abstract: Within the context of the planet's ecology, every single living thing plays an essential role. However, in the modern world, wild animal lives are threatened. It is possible for animals at zoos to suffer serious injuries or even die from diseases if an accident were to occur while they are there. So, the point of this study is to use the Smart Tunnel to keep tabs on the animals' vital signs while they're in captivity. As animals go through this intelligent tunnel, data about their vital signs will be sent to a server. The animals in their cage will be kept healthy, disease-free, and well-cared-for by this intelligent tunnel. In addition to helping farmers out and protecting animals from harm, it will be managing or avoiding outbreaks of major animal illnesses. It will be useful for keeping tabs on the animals' well-being and notifying carers of any serious problems. Veterinarians are better able to treat their patients when they have access to records in the database that reflect the animals' physical conditions.

Keywords: IoT, Smart zoos, Animals, Healthcare, Smart tunnel

[1]sheeba@iul.ac.in, [2]ahjk@student.iul.ac.in, [3]prof.neeta.rastogi@gmail.com, [4]qrat_abbas@yahoo.com, [5]dr.nikhatakhtar@gmail.com, [6]qudsia786.786@gmail.com

DOI: 10.1201/9781003535423-38

1. Introduction

Zoos are confined locations where animals are maintained. Caring for animals that interact with guests is a difficult part of a zoo administrator's job. They have a daily reporting obligation to higher-ups about the animals' welfare. Reporting it takes nearly the whole day, so it's a tedious procedure. Another difficult chore is feeding the animals. According to the zoo and aquarium association, over 180 million people visit American zoos each year, which is more than the combined attendance of the NBA, NFL, NHL, and MLB. The poll found that zoos are the preferred tourism destination for families with children (93%) and that zoos teach children important lessons about the need of preserving animal habitats and animal culture (94%). [1]. However, the well-being of the animals should take precedence above any consideration of the zoo [2]. Many zoos house hundreds, if not tens of thousands, of animals, all of which are physically distinct from one another. To handle it, we need to be experts with technical instruments and able to operate it in real-time. An efficient strategy for animal management may be developed with the support of other ideas and modern information technologies. With the help of the Internet of Things (IoT) and artificial intelligence (AI), we can automate the zoo and provide managers with some instructions. There haven't been any technical breakthroughs in this field yet. The Internet of Things allows for the collection of a great deal of data and signals from animals [3-4]. These datasets can be processed with the help of AI. There are still a lot of reworks that need to be finished, even while AI helps with analyzing a lot of data [5] and signals. Owners utilize Lucky Tag smart collars for pet management [6]. You may also use it to track the health of your loved ones or look for those who have gone missing. When the owner pays attention to long-term patterns, they can spot illnesses early on. In an effort to better care for animals and keep tabs on their health, the Yamato Zoo in Sapporo, Japan, has begun using AI systems to study trends in animal behaviours [7].

2. Working Process of Tunnel

The implementation process for our animal healthcare monitoring system involves several key steps:

Step 1: Begin by placing the specially designed tunnel within the animal's cage, creating a comfortable and familiar environment.

Step 2: On one side of the tunnel, strategically position a quantity of food, enticing the animal to approach and interact with the tunnel.

Step 3: As the animal naturally crosses the tunnel to access the food, various sensors integrated into the system collect valuable data pertaining to the animal's behavior, motion, and environmental conditions.

Step 4: The collected data is then seamlessly transmitted by these sensors to the cloud infrastructure, where it is stored and processed for further analysis.

Step 5: In the cloud, the data undergoes analysis, interpretation, and integration with other relevant information, thus generating a comprehensive and real-time picture of the animal's health and well-being.

Step 6: The processed data is made accessible and readily available on the cloud, ensuring that it can be retrieved at any time for a thorough examination of the animal's condition and behavior.

Step 7: To provide a user-friendly interface and enable effective data visualization, a mobile application is developed, allowing zookeepers, veterinarians, and researchers to effortlessly access and interpret the data, ultimately contributing to the enhanced healthcare and welfare of the animals in our care.

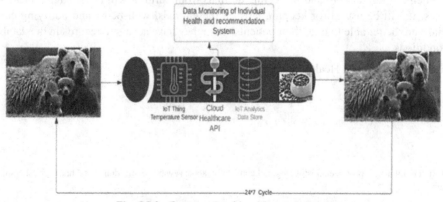

Fig. 38.1   Smart animal healthcare tunnel

3. Proposed Prototype of Smart Tunnel and Objectives

Every animal must be cared for effectively by the zookeeper. Thus, we have proposed a prototype for animal health monitoring to offer intelligent management operations for them. Thus, we are able to offer the appropriate zoo control measures as named Smart Animal Health Monitoring Tunnel (SAHMT). We will use AI, deep learning technology and IoT to put this into practice and to assist the animal administrators in clearly understanding each species individually, feed, water volume, and other information. Concept of Tunnel: Many researches have made the wearable device for Animal Health Monitoring but in my research, I am Using the term tunnel. The region behind it that we don't want to put warble device into animal body because their sensors can irritate and can also harm the animals. That's why we proposed a Tunnel based Architecture where we put all the necessary devices into the tunnel. When the animals will cross that tunnel the AI and sensors will take necessary data and feed into the cloud. Cloud will convert the live data into the information and that live information will be displayed on mobile app. Zoo administrator will take the necessary action accordingly.

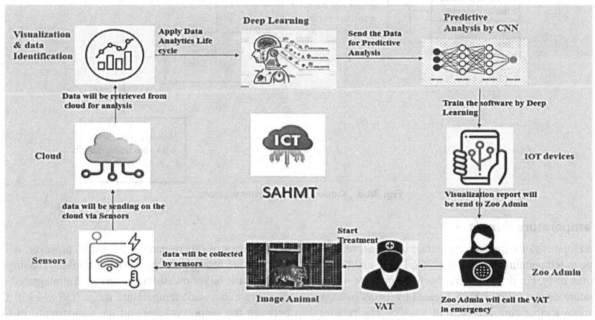

Fig. 38.2 Proposed SAHMT framework

We can also use a wide range of techniques to put this into practice. The present study was planned to achieve the below-mentioned objectives. AI based healthcare Tunnel in IoT environment. Track the physiological and behavioral and parameters of Animal in their zoo cage. Create an affordable method to track the well-being of animals in captivity at zoos. Monitor their daily activities in their cage. Monitor the behavior of the animals in cage. Prevent from viral Infections to the other animals. Followings are the technologies which will be used to achieve these mentioned objectives.

3.1 Non-Invasive Wireless Sensing Technology

Recent years have seen an explosion in the quantity of study devoted to healthcare IT. They are associated with healthcare technologies that are either invasive or non-invasive. While intrusive equipment necessitates direct physical contact with the body, non-invasive technology allows for patient monitoring without any such interaction [8,9].

3.2 Technology for Camera

Thermal or depth cameras capture video footage of the animal's chest motions, which may then be analyzed by sophisticated machine learning algorithms to detect any abnormalities in the breathing cycle [10].

3.3 Use of Sensors

This paper predominantly comprises two primary components: the sensory aspect and the monitoring aspect. Within the sensory component, we employ temperature sensors, heart rate sensors, and humidity sensors. Typically, each animal maintains a specific range of body temperature. In the event that an animal sustains wounds or experiences a fever, the body temperature naturally elevates. The temperature sensor is affixed to the tunnel's surface and continuously tracks the temperature of each animal. Any fluctuations in temperature levels trigger immediate display on the LCD screen.

3.4 RF Sensors

Wi-Fi and radar-based technologies make up the bulk of radio frequency sensing. To detect the Doppler effect when a whole body or specific region moves, radar-based technologies employ a frequency-modulated continuous wave [11, 12]. When utilized properly, this technology may detect and track breathing problems. Using smart machine learning techniques, the radar system can interpret images.

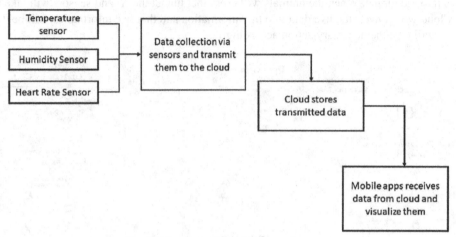

Fig. 38.3 Collecting data from sensors

3.5 Temperature Sensor

The development of wireless temperature and heart rate monitors is the focus of this research. This study, however, will limit its scope to temperature sensors. Both the LM35 and the TMP36 temperature sensors are appropriate for taking readings from the human body, but the LM35 has been selected for its greater accuracy and larger measurement range. An integrated-circuit temperature device called LM35, created by Texas Instrument, can operate in a wide temperature range (í55 to +150°C) and has a room temperature accuracy of ±1.4°C. The relationship between the output voltage and the temperature in Celsius (Centigrade) is similarly linear. Low output impedance, direct Celsius calibration, and a linear + 10.0 mV/°C scale factor are some of the characteristics of the LM35. It works well in distant applications as well. The hardware LM35 and its connection are shown in Fig. 38.2.

The voltage-temperature conversion basic formula for LM35 is given in (1)

$$\text{Temp in °C} = [\text{V Out in mV}] / 10$$

3.6 Humidity Sensor

In order to monitor the animal's surrounding environmental conditions, we will employ a wide range of environmental sensors, such as humidity sensors and rainfall sensors. By using this technique, we can regulate and modify the temperature and humidity to meet the needs of the animals.

3.7 Heart Rate Sensor

Heart rate sensors are instrumental tools in the realm of animal health monitoring. These sensors, often incorporated into specialized monitoring devices, empower veterinarians, researchers, and animal caretakers to gain critical insights into the well-being of animals under their care. By continuously measuring and tracking an animal's heart rate, deviations from baseline values can be quickly detected, serving as an early indicator of potential stress, illness, or discomfort. This real-time data enables timely intervention, ensuring that animals receive the necessary attention and care. Furthermore, heart rate sensors are essential in optimizing training programs, exercise routines, and understanding the physiological responses of animals to different conditions and stimuli. Whether in a clinical setting or within the context of wildlife conservation, heart rate sensors prove invaluable in safeguarding the health and welfare of animals, making them an indispensable tool for animal health monitoring.

3.8 Use of IoT

In this project IoT will be used for creating an application which provides all the relevant information that can be used by both the tourists and officials in the zoo. They can give details regarding the animals. Administrators can get the health status of the animal's daily basis. This can be used by other higher officials. Maps can be entered into the application. This can be used by the tourists to easily find out the location of each animal [13].

3.9 Use of Cloud Computing

To enable animal managers to utilize a range of platforms and devices, together with AI, to integrate the massive volumes of data that were acquired, cloud computing in cloud databases is necessary [14, 15]. Some benefits of using a cloud platform are as follows. The zoo is allowed to tailor the website and service to their needs by making any necessary modifications. The cloud service is also accessible from anywhere an administrator has an internet connection. Without worrying about the cost of maintaining or repairing its infrastructure, zoos may speed up their expansion. The zoo will be able to provide the best possible animal care and administrative services thanks to the tunnel's developers, who will have more time to focus on app development and regularly upgrade analytical approaches.

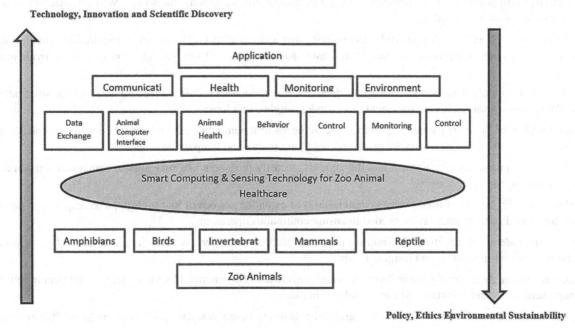

Fig. 38.4 The reference framework of SAHMT

3.10 Use of Deep learning/ML Application

In this paper, deep learning is harnessed to observe and track the behaviors of animals housed in cages. Utilizing a novel model that analyzes the motion characteristics of animals within distinct regions of the enclosure, we have effectively categorized various behaviors, including entrance and exit from resting areas, moments of stillness, changes in direction, feeding, and drinking patterns. This innovative model serves as a fundamental building block for the creation of assessment tools designed to vigilantly oversee the health and welfare of animals within the zoo environment. Leveraging artificial neural networks and deep learning, these technologies assume a pivotal role in predictive analysis for animal healthcare monitoring. By processing a multitude of data sources and offering valuable insights, they facilitate early detection, preventative measures, and tailored care for animals in diverse settings, spanning from agricultural farms to veterinary clinics. As a result, these advancements hold the promise of significantly enhancing the overall health and quality of life for animals across a wide array of contexts [16][17].

3.11 Hardware Requirements

The hardware requirements for an IoT and deep learning-based non-invasive zoo animal healthcare model, with the integration of solar power for power supply, thermal camera, humidity sensor, and a plastic tunnel, are as follows.

Solar Power System: To ensure continuous and eco-friendly power supply, a solar power system with photovoltaic panels, batteries for energy storage, and charge controllers would be essential. The panels should be strategically placed to capture maximum sunlight exposure for prolonged operation.

Thermal Camera: A high-quality thermal camera is necessary for capturing the thermal profiles and behaviours of zoo animals. It should be capable of producing clear and accurate thermal images for deep learning analysis. Additionally, the camera should be weather-proof and robust to withstand outdoor conditions.

Humidity Sensor: An accurate and durable humidity sensor is required to monitor environmental conditions within the plastic tunnel. This sensor should be capable of providing real-time data on humidity levels, which can be crucial for assessing animal comfort and well-being.

Plastic Tunnel: The plastic tunnel serves as the enclosure for animals, where environmental conditions can be controlled and monitored. The tunnel should be made of high-quality, non-toxic materials to ensure the safety and comfort of the animals. Proper ventilation and insulation must also be considered.

IoT Connectivity and Communication Hardware: To transmit data from the sensors and cameras to a central processing unit, IoT connectivity components such as microcontrollers, wireless communication modules (e.g., Wi-Fi, LoRa, or cellular), and data transfer protocols will be needed.

Central Processing Unit (CPU): A powerful CPU or computer system with GPU support is required for running the deep learning models. This unit will process the data from sensors and cameras, perform real-time analysis, and provide actionable insights.

Storage Devices: Given the data-intensive nature of deep learning models, a robust and secure data storage solution, such as SSDs or HDDs, is essential for storing historical data, model weights, and logs.

Environmental Control Systems: Depending on the specific needs of the animals, environmental control systems like heaters, coolers, and fans may be required within the plastic tunnel to maintain ideal temperature conditions.

Security Systems: To protect the equipment and the animals, security measures like surveillance cameras, intrusion detection systems, and alarms may be necessary.

Backup Power Supply: In case of solar power system failures or extended periods of low sunlight, a backup power supply, such as a generator or grid connection, may be needed to ensure continuous operation.

User Interface and Monitoring Systems: An intuitive user interface for zookeepers, veterinarians, and researchers to monitor the system and receive real-time alerts and insights is vital.

Data Management and Analytics Software: To process and analyse the data generated by the system, deep learning frameworks, data management tools, and analytics software should be in place.

Overall, the hardware requirements for an IoT and deep learning-based non-invasive zoo animal healthcare model are multifaceted, encompassing energy provision, sensor technology, enclosure materials, data processing, and environmental control to create a comprehensive and effective solution for monitoring and enhancing animal health and welfare in a zoo environment.

4. Conclusion

The automation of zoos is an area that has not seen a lot of advancement in recent years. By keeping an eye on the health of the animals, automating feeding, keeping an eye on wild animals, and developing applications that allow them to report on their real-time activities, we have proposed framework for smart animal Health Monitoring system that can be helpful to them by using deep learning and IoT to forecast the wellbeing of wild animals and for live monitoring. Another motivation for this research includes that zoo is a place where a group of people take care of and look after animals. Working with wild animals is a major challenge for many individuals. An astute strategy for the management of several wild animals is proposed in this research for the benefit of zoo administrators. Thanks to the IoT and AI, this approach will streamline operations for the zoo's administrative staff. The model's goal is to design a cheap system for tracking vital signs including temperature, heart rate, and animal posture. One important function of this system is posture sensing. These vital signs are measured by three precise sensors. Keep an eye out for signs of illness in the animals if the measured parameters are out of the ordinary. In this way, we can ensure that all of the animals receive enough care while simultaneously protecting them from the virus.

REFERENCES

1. Choudhury, M., Saikia, T., Banik, S., Patil, G., Pegu, S. R., Rajkhowa, S., ... & Das, P. J. (2020). Infrared imaging a new non-invasive machine learning technology for animal husbandry. The Imaging Science Journal, 68(4), 240-249.
2. Karthick, G. S., Sridhar, M., & Pankajavalli, P. B. (2020). Internet of things in animal healthcare (IoTAH): review of recent advancements in architecture, sensing technologies and real-time monitoring. SN Computer Science, 1, 1-16.
3. AM, C. M., & Johnson Bressan, N. (2022). Frameworks and Platforms for Monitoring Animal Health and Wellness in Human Care and in the Wild. In An Introduction to Veterinary Medicine Engineering (pp. 39-60). Cham: Springer International Publishing.
4. Veasey, J. S., Waran, N. K., & Young, R. J. (1996). On Comparing the Behaviours of Zoo Housed Animals with Wild Conspecifics as a Welfare Indicator. Animal Welfare, 5(1).
5. Y. Perwej, "Performance Analysis for Cloud Based OLAP over Big Data", IEEE International Conference on Innovative Computing, Intelligent Communication and Smart Electrical Systems (ICSES -2022), IEEE Conference, St. Joseph's Institute of Technology, IEEE Electronic ISBN:978-1-6654-7413-9, Chennai, India, 2022, DOI: 10.1109/ICSES55317.2022.9914266
6. Rzucidlo, C. L., Curry, E., & Shero, M. R. (2023). Non-invasive measurements of respiration and heart rate across wildlife species using Eulerian Video Magnification of infrared thermal imagery. BMC biology, 21(1), 61.
7. Madhavan, S , Parakkal, K. S., Rahul, P. M., & John, R. Animal Care Management System using Internet of Things and Artificial Intelligence in Zoo.
8. Taylor, W., Abbasi, Q. H., Dashtipour, K., Ansari, S., Shah, S. A., Khalid, A., & Imran, M. A. (2020). A Review of the State of the Art in Non-Contact Sensing for COVID-19. Sensors, 20(19), 5665.
9. Avdeev, S. N., Yaroshetskiy, A. I., Tsareva, N. A., Merzhoeva, Z. M., Trushenko, N. V., Nekludova, G. V., & Chikina, S. Y. (2021). Noninvasive ventilation for acute hypoxemic respiratory failure in patients with COVID-19. The American journal of emergency medicine, 39, 154-157.
10. Arshad, J., Rehman, A. U., Othman, M. T. B., Ahmad, M., Tariq, H. B., Khalid, M. A., ... & Hamam, H. (2022). Deployment of wireless sensor network and iot platform to implement an intelligent animal monitoring system. Sustainability, 14(10), 6249.
11. Al-Qahtani, A., Al-hajri, H., Al-kuwari, S., Al-yaarabi, N., Al-hababi, A., Al-kubaisi, E., ... & Abbasi, Q. H. (2015, May). A non-invasive remote health monitoring system using visible light communication. In 2015 2nd International Symposium on Future Information and Communication Technologies for Ubiquitous HealthCare (Ubi-HealthTech) (pp. 1-3). IEEE.
12. Shah, S. A., Abbas, H., Imran, M. A., & Abbasi, Q. H. (2021). Rf sensing for healthcare applications. Backscattering and RF Sensing for Future Wireless Communication, 157-177.
13. Sumathy, B., Kavimullai, S., Shushmithaa, S., & Anusha, S. S. (2021). Wearable Non-invasive Health Monitoring Device for Elderly using IOT. In IOP Conference Series: Materials Science and Engineering (Vol. 1012, No. 1, p. 012011). IOP Publish.
14. Akhtar, N., Kerim, B., Perwej, Y., Tiwari, A., & Praveen, S. (2021). A Comprehensive Overview of Privacy and Data Security for Cloud Storage. International Journal of Scientific Research in Science Engineering and Technology
15. Al-Sheikh, M. A., & Ameen, I. A. (2020, July). Design of mobile healthcare monitoring system using IoT technology and cloud computing. In IOP conference series: materials science and engineering (Vol. 881, No. 1, p. 012113). IOP Publishing.
16. Ismail, S. N. A., Nayan, N. A., Jaafar, R., & May, Z. (2022). Recent Advances in Non-Invasive Blood Pressure Monitoring and Prediction Using a Machine Learning Approach. Sensors, 22(16), 6195.
17. Kumar, N., & Kumar, D. (2021, August). Machine learning based heart disease diagnosis using non-invasive methods: A review. In Journal of Physics: Conference Series (Vol. 1950, No. 1, p. 012081). IOP Publishing.

Emerging Trends in IoT and Computing Technologies – Suman Lata Tripathi et al. (eds)
© 2024 Taylor & Francis Group, London, ISBN 978-1-032-87924-6

Data Analytics: A Review on Application Area's

39

**Vidhya Vasekar[1], Sonam Singh[2],
Aparna Kulkarni[3], Sandeep Chitalkar[4]**

Dr. D. Y. Patil Institute of Technology, Artificial Intelligence &
DataScience, Pune

Abstract: The term "Data Analytics" is one that has likely become familiar to you if you are a resident of the 21st century. It's one of the most popular phrases nowadays. Data analytics is used to generate business projections by uncovering previously unknown patterns, trends, correlations, and insights inside massive databases. Numerous cutting-edge methods and pieces of cutting-edge technology are used in the implementation of data analytics in businesses. In this paper, we'll take a look at the ways in which data analytics is being applied in a variety of business-critical domains, including advertising and distribution network management, social networking, healthcare, and agriculture. At long last, we have covered some of the cutting-edge resources available for Data Analytics projects. The results of this research improve our comprehension of analytics in practical terms.

Keywords: Data analytics, Datasets, Business, Applications

1. Introduction

The analysis of data is a new field of study. It is essential to have robust technology that organizes and processes the data that is generated every day so that it can be used in any way that is conceivable. Due to its volume, variety, and velocity of change, such data necessitates the adoption of novel forms of big data analytics for storage and analysis. This type of massive data necessitates a thorough analysis, followed by the retrieval of the necessary information. This topic is currently the subject of extensive study. When it comes to analyzing data, we have at our disposal some of the most potent techniques and technologies currently accessible. Analytical technologies that facilitate strategic planning and decision making are the subject of the second set of evaluations, which are separated from those that focus on the data analysis itself by a focus on strategy making procedures and improvements to business models (Yassine Talaoui etal.,2022). The rise of the Internet and the development of Web 2.0 technologies have made big data analytics an area of intense study (Norjihan Ab-dul Ghani et al., 2022; Alexander, 2006). Positive applications of data analytics can be found in many fields, such as advertising, social media, family businesses, healthcare, agriculture, logistics, and many more (Norjihan Abdul Ghani et al., 2022). One area where this is especially true is in the realm of social media. The industry's development and transition have entered a new phase in step with developments in computing technology. The fourth industrial revolution, or "Industry 4.0," describes this time period. As part of Industry 4.0, companies aim to increase output and revenue by leveraging data and computing resources. The rise in popularity of using social media in recent years has made it essential for companies to have a presence on these platforms. The vast amounts of information available on social media make it a particularly rich resource for modern businesses (Goes

[1]vidhya.n.gavali@gmail.com, [2]sonamchauhan346@gmail.com, [3]sandeep.chitalkar@gmail.com, [4]appi.pathak3@gmail.com

DOI: 10.1201/9781003535423-39

P. B, 2014). Marketers who use data analytics are another good example. When businesses and their marketing departments embrace data analytics, they can gain an edge over the competition and boost demand. Your brand's primary goal should be to attract consumers' attention by being distinct. Through the use of analytics, you can narrow your focus from a broad audience to a more specific one, so improving the quality of both your brand strategy and the user experience. As a result of analytics, businesses are able to glean intriguing insights, allowing them to tailor their marketing strategies to the needs of a select demographic. Data analytics encompasses a wide range of methods and software, such as statistical analysis, machine learning, NLP, data mining, and predictive analytics employed regularly on massive, potentially distributed datasets to gain valuable insights that improve commercial decision-making. When businesses talk about "big data," they're referring to the massive amounts of information they have at their disposal about their customers, their markets, their competitors, and their surroundings (Maryam Ghasemaghaei et al.,2018). By considering the significance of data analytics, this study focuses on a wide range of fields in which it plays a pivotal role. Particular attention will be paid to the applications of data analytics in the SMM, Agri-Marketing, and SCM spheres. The next sections introduce data analytics and demonstrate its usefulness in settings as varied as social media, marketing, supply chain management, and agriculture, among others.

2. Background

To generate insights that tap into unique, untapped sources of economic value, "big data" necessitates the employment of novel technical architectures, analytics, and tools due to its size, location, variety, and/or timeliness. Volume, variety, and velocity are the three characteristics that best define big data. The volume of the data is a good indicator of both its size and scope. The rate of development or the rate at which new information is being generated is referred to as its velocity. There is variation in the many data forms and types, in the many uses of data, and in the many approaches to data analysis [6]. Large amounts of data are not just a number. It also encompasses numerous forms of data, including those that are continuously updated in real time. It's impossible to have a complete picture of your company's operations without massive amounts of detailed data. If you want to observe something completely new, primary data used for business intelligence or analytics can help. In fact, there are enormous data sources that constantly feed us fresh information in near-real time. Big data is about more than simply massive amounts of data when you include all of these other aspects as well. Massive volumes of detailed information are contained in "big data." The second type of analytics is called "advanced analytics," and it encompasses a wide range of methods and technologies, including NLP, AI, predictive analytics, data mining, statistics, and more. The field of business intelligence most in vogue right now is big data analytics [7][8]. Beyond the simple ability to automate and feed current processes with data, new technologies like big data analytics provide a disruption risk[1]. Analyzing data is a method of examining information in order to draw conclusions or of checking, cleaning, organizing, and communicating information in such a way as to emphasize unique aspects of that information. Managers in a wide variety of fields utilize this method to make sound strategic decisions and validate or refute established theoretical frameworks[9][10]. There are three main categories of study designs applicable to big data: experimental, confirmed, and subjective. Then, in human subject research, Quadratic Discriminant Analysis is used to infer conclusions from data that is not mathematical in nature, such as photographs, audio recordings, or text. New informational trends are uncovered by exploratory data analysis, while the validity of previously held beliefs is confirmed through confirmation data analysis [10]. As a result, data analytics has made a big difference in science and engineering [8].

3. Application Area of Data Analytics

Because of significant features of data analytics tools, it is used in various fields. Here we have focused on social media, agriculture, marketing and supply chain management. Below Table 39.1 shows the different applications of Data Analytics in daily routine.

3.1 Data Analytics in Healthcare

Connected health care is made possible by the fact that public health processes necessitate not just a high level of communication and processing ability, but also constant access to huge amounts of data from within and outside the health system. Artificial intelligence-based data analytics was proposed by S. Lokesh et al.[11]. In the first stage, we used detectors and medical equipment to collect data on the pupils' health. By way of gateways and mobile processors, the collected information is transmitted to the cloud service (LPU). The clinical diagnosis process uses the second stage's medical measurements to form educated cognitive judgments about a young person's health. In the third phase, all participants and/or legal guardians are notified of their ward's status. In the event of a medical emergency, a notification is also sent to the nearest medical facility

Table 39.1 Big data applications in various fields

Field & Reference	Application Name	Description
Education	(PASS) Personalized Adaptive Study Success [29]	The application's major objective is to provide a more personalized setting which guarantees students' participation, engagement, and continuity in an online learning environment.
	ENOVA[30,31]	Mexico can examine and forecast student interactions by using data and data analytics. Enhances the tools and procedures that are employed in the teaching-learning process, which in turn strengthens educational tactics.
Health	Health Map [26,28]	a tool that tracks illness trends and advises on the best course of action in advance
	Proactive listening, mobile phone-based system [26,28]	Brazil—to manage the problem of corruption in the health care system, deal with any connected difficulties, and take prompt, decisive action against it.
	Ebola OpenData Initiative [26,27,28]	An open-source worldwide model for tracking Ebola cases in 2014 was created using data from West Africa.
Transportation	Open Traffic platform [26,28]	Seoul, South Africa: The programme helps night bus drivers by making the travel from point A to point B easier. This will be accomplished by gathering information from an enormous volume of calls, texts, and private and corporate taxi data sources.
	Uber [32]	Food, packets or courier delivery via Uber Eats and Postmates (couriers), and mobility as a service/ride-hailing are all services offered by San Francisco-based Uber Technologies, Inc. (Uber). Uber uses a dynamic pricing methodology that fluctuates based on local supply and demand to decide the price, which is then provided to the customer in advance. The service also takes a cut of each rider's fare.

[11]. Research has ongoing on big data analytics (BDA) and artificial intelligence approaches to observe the spread of the virus and its consequences on people and the global economy. Covid-19's administration of BDA and AI must be examined (from a DEI perspective) to learn more about their roles in the event's organization. AI algorithms, particularly ML and deep learning, are the most often used methods for BDA. Most of the researchers in the domains of computer science and medical science have developed the significant applications that include BDA skills including assessment, calculation, and monitoring [12]. An example of how a BDA/AI health application could be used to enhance the practice of medicine is by comparing a patient's illness to that of others with the same diagnosis in the Electronic Health Care Record. Potential illness progression, survival analysis, and causal inference [13] might then be evaluated by the doctor.

3.2 Data Analytics in Agriculture

Data Analytics assist farmers to increase yields, decreasing waste, and improving management choices for sustainable agriculture. Smart farming is an increasingly popular concept in the agricultural industry; it stresses the integration of communication as well as information technologies for farming management. As more farms install smart gear and other sensors, farming operations will become data-driven and data-enabled. Thus, data analytics is rapidly developing into a crucial field for assisting farm management decisions by gleaning actionable insights from large datasets [14-16]. As big data analytics becomes more commonplace, numerous research have dealt with data analytics platforms and their uses in diverse agricultural fields[17]. Machine learning will be used in agriculture through IoT data analytics to increase yields and quality in order to keep up with increased food demand. These ground- breaking innovations are displacing conventional farming practices and opening up the most promising new avenues, albeit not without certain downsides [18]. According to economists Vinay Kellengere Shankarnarayan and Hombaliah Ramakrishna [19], agriculture is the backbone of the Indian economy. The number of people living in rural areas and the average amount of farmland per person are both decreasing, according to statistics. Concerning news for a country with a population of over a billion, over 66% of whom reside in rural areas. Recent agricultural research and studies have been the main emphasis. The contemporary agricultural industry has many problems that may be solved with the use of Big Data analytics, and this analysis analyzed and offered a framework for using such analytics in agriculture.

3.3 Data Analytics in Business

Businesses of all sizes can benefit from using data analytics. Based on the knowledge-based perspective theory, Ismael Barros-Contreras et al. [20] investigated the characteristics that foster knowledge integration (KI) in family businesses and its connection to the effectiveness of organizational data analytics. The terms "big data" and "data deluge" are widely used to describe this phenomenon. Data science, machine learning, text processing, audio processing, and video processing are just some of the other areas that marketers need to incorporate if they want to stay competitive. Marketing science has been influenced by the development of, and research into concepts like customer choice modeling, customer lifetime value, demand projection, response modeling, brand valuation, consumer behavior, and consumer preference measurement[21][22]. Data science in marketing has been a focus of study because of the competitive advantages it may provide to businesses.

3.4 Data Analytics in Social Media

The broad use of readily available software and technology allowed for the creation and use of social media platforms through the Internet. The fields of trend detection, social media analytics, sentiment analysis, and opinion mining all make extensive use of big data for social media. For instance, businesses can use social media to collect client feedback on their products, which can then be used to inform strategic shifts and boost profits. The proliferation of social media has significantly sped up the evolution of many different kinds of information. The explosion in data creation has made real-time analytics more important than ever. The term "variety of data" is used to refer to the various kinds of structural heterogeneity present in a dataset. The enormous volume of data which is generated by users is a direct outcome of their incorporation of personal details and routine actions into the platform. Every piece of content that a user creates, such as a status update, tweet, review, or remark, is considered user-generated content. The three most frequent forms of user-generated content are text, images, audio and video. This content comes from regular individuals and isn't written in any particular style. It is becoming increasingly important to extract trustworthy information from this data, as they may contain the users' particular ideas, activities, and thoughts. It's a fruitful area of study for corporations and academics because of the plethora of user-generated content that may contain useful and high-quality data. [23][24].

4. The Modern Tools for Data Analytics

The below Table 39.2 lists the tools that are currently used in various data analytics applications.

Table 39.2 Data analytics tools

Sr. No	Tool	Usage
1	Tableau	streamlined analytics and data visualization tool referred to develop reports and dashboards
2	PowerBI	Design feature business information tools that enables to query data and obtain useful data.
3	Apache Spark	a real-time data analytics engine that does complex analyses with the help of SQL queries and machine learning
4	Python	Object oriented programming language that supports huge library set for data modeling, data manipulation, and visualization.
5	R	Programming language mostly used for statistical as well as numerical analysis. Huge libraries are offered for data analysis and visualization.

Each tool's characteristics are determined independently to boost the efficiency of the dataset being offered for computing. This makes it easy for the user to zero down on the best tools to improve big data performance. There is a wide range of options available to those who work with data, and these options can be enhanced with new features to increase their effectiveness. Increases in both supply and demand on the market have piqued the attention of businesspeople and corporations worldwide [25].

5. Conclusion

This research work focused on the application area of the data analytics in a variety of different fields of application. You will be able to quickly analyze your data and gain insights from it if you make use of this technology. When it comes to making recommendations for ultimate strategic choices, big data analytics applications are enormously necessary. The research included a comprehensive analysis of data analytics plays as well as how it interacts with particular applications of big data across a variety of industries.

REFERENCES

1. YassineTalaoui (2022), Recovering the divide: A review of the big data analytics— strategy relationship,Long RangePlanning, https://doi.org/10.1016/j.lrp.2022.102290

2. Norjihan Abdul Ghani, Suraya Hamid, Ibrahim Abaker Targio Hashem, Ejaz Ahmed (2019), Social media big data analytics: A survey, https://doi.org/10.1016/j.chb.2018.08.039 , Computers in Human Behavior 101 (2019) 417–428.

3. Alexander, B. (2006). Web 2.0: A new wave of innovation for teaching and learning? Educause Review, 41(2), 32

4. Goes, P.B. (2014) Big Data and IS Research. MIS Quarterly, 38, 3-8.

5. Maryam Ghasemaghaei, Sepideh Ebrahimi, Khaled Hassanein Maryam Ghasemaghaei, Sepideh Ebrahimi, Khaled Hassanein (2018), Data analytics competency for improving firm decision making performance, Journal of Strategic Information Systems 27 (2018) 101–113

6. EMC: Data Science and Big Data Analytics (2012). In: EMC Education Services, pp. 1–508 [7].Russom, P.: Big Data Analytics. In: TDWI Best Practices Report, pp. 1–40 (2011)

8. Nada Elgendy and Ahmed Elragal (2014),Big Data Analytics: A Literature Review Paper,ICDM 2014, LNAI 8557, pp. 214–227, 2014

9. T. Takura, K. Hirano Goto, A. Honda, Development of a predictive model for integrated medical and long- term care resource consumption based on health behavior: application of healthcare big data of patients with circulatory diseases, BMC Med. 19 (1) (2021) 1–16.

10. S. Lokesh, Sudeshna Chakraborty, Revathy Pulugu, Sonam Mittal, Dileep Pulugu, R. Muruganantham (2022), nAI-based big data analytics mode formedicalapplications,https://doi.org/10.1016/j.measen.2022.100534

11. S. Lokesh, Sudeshna Chakraborty, Revathy Pulugu, Sonam Mittal, Dileep Pulugu, R. Muruganantham (2022), AI-based   big data analytics model for medical application https://doi.org/10.1016/j.measen.2022.100534

12. Panagiota Galetsi, Korina Katsaliaki, Sameer Kumar (2022), The medical and societal impact of big data analytics and artificial intelligence applications in combating pandemics:A review focused on Covid-19, https://doi.org/10.1016/j.socscimed.2022.114973.

13. Schuler, A., Callahan, A., Jung, K., Shah, N.H., 2018. Performing an informatics consult: methods and challenges. J. Am. Coll. Radiol. 15 (3), 563–568.

14. Bacco, M., Barsocchi, P., Ferro, E., Gotta, A., Ruggeri, M., 2019. The digitisation of agriculture: a survey of esearch activities on smart farming. Array 3–4 (November), 1– 11. https://doi.org/10.1016/j.array.2019.100009.

15. Wolfert, S., Ge, L., Verdouw, C., Bogaardt, M., 2017. Big data in smart farming – a review. Agric. Syst. 153, 69–80. https://doi.org/10.1016/j.agsy.2017.01.023

16. Perakis, K., Lampathaki, F., Nikas, K., Georgiou, Y., Marko, O., Maselyne, J., 2020. CYBELE – Fostering precision agriculture & livestock farming through secure access to large-scale HPC enabled virtual industrial experimentation environments fostering scalable big data analytics. Comput. Networks 168, 1–10

17. Ngakan Nyoman Kutha Krisnawijaya, Bedir Tekinerdogan, Cagatay Catal, Rik van der Tol, Data analytics platforms for agricultural systems: A systematic literature review, Computers andElectronicsinAgriculture195(2022)10681

Emerging Trends in IoT and Computing Technologies – Suman Lata Tripathi et al. (eds)
© 2024 Taylor & Francis Group, London, ISBN 978-1-032-87924-6

Use of Machine Learning in the Internet of Things Industry

40

Vidhya Gavali[1], Sandeep Chitalkar[2],
Aparna Pathak[3], Sonam Singh[4]
Dr. D.Y Patil Institute of Technology,
Artificial Intelligence & Data Science, Pune

Abstract: Many sophisticated gadgets are now linked via the Internet of Things (IoT), making it a crucial network paradigm. As a result of the large amounts of data generated by IoT systems, a growing number of IoT- related software platforms and service offerings are appearing. Similarly, machine learning has achieved remarkable success in various other areas of study, including computer vision, computer graphics, natural language processing, speech recognition, decision-making, and intelligent control. The machine learning technique used to enhance and supply IoT services including traffic IoT device identification, plant management, crop and yield management, soil management, and the like has been on the rise recently. This paper focuses on the survey of usage of machine learning in the IoT industry. We present a wide range of IoT applications and provide an in-depth analysis of current developments in machine learning methods for IoT. Users can get in-depth analytics and create highly functional, intelligent IoT apps with the help of machine learning for IoT. Our goal in this work was to spotlight ML's usefulness in the IoT realm and to provide a comprehensive survey of the field's most recent developments. This study addresses the primary applications of machine learning for IoT and its associated methodologies. We also talk about some of the problems and gaps in the field.

Keywords: Machine learning, IoT, Applications

1. Introduction

The IoT is quickly emerging as a novel all encompassing network architecture that provides distributed and transparent services [1]. Many high-tech gadgets, such as mobile phones, sensors, and other intelligent devices, are linked together through the Internet of Things. These connected gadgets may talk to one another and share data. Complex systems that improve people's lives in areas like machine condition diagnosis, human activity monitoring, health tracking, precise localization, and structural integrity checks are made possible by collecting data from the IoT devices and analyze data to sense and know their surroundings. More and more people are using the IoT which means IoT sensors and devices are generating more and more data. This data is then used by a large range of IoT applications to refine and improve the services they offer. There is potential for further processing and analysis of these large IoT data sets to yield insights for IoT service providers and end users. Researchers [10] looked into the feasibility of using machine learning to address issues in routing, traffic engineering, resource allocation, and network security. For some time, machine learning has been considered the foundational technology for fully autonomous smart and intelligent network administration and operation.

[1]vidhya.n.gavali@gmail.com, [2]sandeep.chitalkar@gmail.com, [3]appi.pathak3@gmail.com, [4]sonamchauhan346@gmail.com

DOI: 10.1201/9781003535423-40

The foundational technology for fully autonomous smart and intelligent network administration and operation. Most IoT systems, in particular, are growing more dynamic, heterogeneous, and complex, making managing such systems challenging. More consumers can be attracted to these IoT systems if their offerings are enhanced in terms of efficiency and variety. Many research projects have made strides toward implementing machine learning in the Internet of Things. Therefore, it is clear that the Internet of Things can gain by incorporating machine learning. As a result of machine learning's ability to give practical solutions for mining the information and characteristics buried in IoT data, customers can gain deep insights and construct efficient intelligent IoT applications, we provide a broad review of the usage of machine learning in IoT by demonstrating its potential utility through various prospective collaborative use cases.

2. Background

Here we will give a high-level overview of the general characteristics of real time IoT system workloads and the most popular machine learning or deep learning techniques. IoT Real Time Systems Concurrent processes with the hardware resources of the system are used to construct real time IoT systems. Scheduling methods that ensure the correctness of the execution of the task set in both time and functionality have typically been used to solve the scheduling challenges associated with a formally stated workload model.

The real-time workload model informs the development of scheduling algorithms. The literature on real-time workload models and scheduling strategies is extensive [2, 5], [6]. Models of real-time workloads can be classified into three broad categories according to the regularity with which a given task instance is released: periodic, irregular, and a periodic. A cyclic task on a uniprocessor system is a task that releases its instances (jobs) after a certain period defined by [2]. It is also believed that during runtime, each job can release an infinite number of instances. Calculating the exact WCET of the jobs is difficult, and it is a challenge in itself to schedule them. Evaluating the precise WCET is tricky because of the inaccessibility of the system design due to intellectual property concerns or the intricacy of the analysis involved in determining deterministic WCET. As a result, the predicted WCET is relatively low, leading to inefficient system use. Various criticality levels are used in modern autonomous systems to differentiate between systems with varying safety criteria. Critical systems in CAVs include the anti-lock brake system, steering, and engine controller. They should be given higher priority than the infotainment system, air conditioning, etc., in accordance with safety standards like ISO26262. Vestal [9] proposed a mixed-criticality system (MCS) model to deal with the varying degrees of criticality in these autonomous systems; MCS models increase system utilization by allocating different WCETs to a task depending on the criticality of the system (a broad review on MCS is presented in [10]). Some examples of more fundamental uses for IoT and ML are provided below.

3. Some Basic Applications of IoT

Because of its adoption in a wide variety of business sectors, the Internet of Things (IoT) has become a pervasive reality in today's world. Because of the IoT's adaptability, it has become an appealing choice for a wide variety of companies, organizations, and government agencies, to the point where it would be foolish to ignore it. The following table gives some analysis of ML-based IoT applications,

Following are the some other uses of the Internet of Things across industries below:

3.1 Applications of the Internet of Things in Agriculture

The Internet of Things makes it possible to monitor and control the circumstances of a microclimate, which in turn leads to an increase in productivity for indoor planting. When planting outside, devices that use internet of things technology can feel the moisture and nutrients in the soil, which, when combined with data on the weather, allows for improved control of intelligent irrigation and fertilizer systems. This saves wasting a valuable resource, for example, by ensuring that the sprinkler systems only release water when it is required[18][21].

3.2 Applications of the IoT in Everyday Use

IoT products, like smart homes as well as wearable's, make life simpler for regular people by making their daily routines more efficient. Wearable's include a wide variety of different gadgets, including fitness trackers, cell phones, Apple watches, and even health monitoring. These devices increase not just entertainment but also health and fitness, as well as network connectivity.

When you arrive home, smart home will have operated like activation of the controls in such a way that it is at its most comfortable setting for you. Dinner that needs to be prepared in the oven or a slow cooker can be started from a remote location, and the meal will be ready when you get there. The consumer can operate and control appliances or lights distantly, also activate an intelligent security device that will permit the suitable people to enter the house even if they do not have a key. In addition, security is made more accessible, making it possible for the consumer to control the smart lock remotely [19].

3.3 Applications of the Internet of Things in Healthcare

The wearable Internet of Things devices give hospitals the functionality to observe the health of their patients at home. This allows hospitals to reduce the patients time spent in a hospital while still providing real time information that has the potential to save lives. In hospitals, smart beds maintain the personnel aware of the availability of vacant space, which reduces the amount of time patients have to wait for it. The Internet of Things makes providing care for elderly people much more convenient. Along with the real-time home monitoring discussed previously, sensors are also assess whether or not a patient is experiencing a heart attack or whether or not they have fallen [12-14].

3.4 Applications of IoT in the Insurance Industry

The change brought on by the Internet of Things can even benefit the insurance sector. Insurance firms can give policyholders discounts on Internet of Things devices like Fit bit. Through the use of fitness tracking, insurance are able to provide individualized policies and promote healthy life style, both of which are beneficial to everyone in the long duration, including the consumer and the insurer.

3.5 Applications of the IoT in Manufacturing

One more production that stands to benefit significantly from the Internet of Things is the realm of manufacturing and industrial automation. The entire supply chain, from the point where production of a product begins on the factory floor to where it is placed in the store where it is ultimately sold, may be tracked with the use of technologies such as RFID and GPS. These sensors can collect data regarding the amount of time spent in transit, the current state of the product, and the environmental conditions it was exposed to. To cut down on wasted time and materials, sensors attached to plant machinery assist in locating bottlenecks in the production line. Other sensors that can be put on the same machinery can also monitor the functioning of the machine, determining when it will require repair and helping to avoid costly breakdowns.

4. Machine Learning Applications in IoT

Machine learning (ML) has been hailed as a revolutionary approach to computing that allows machines to mimic human learning by acquiring new information, enhancing their abilities, and maturing in their special way.

4.1 Plant Management

Greenhouse farming is made more accessible by combining ML and IoT to create a suitable and manageable environment for plant growth. Traditional agriculture and environmental controls need help to accommodate the development of many plant species at various growth phases due to the spatial and temporal variability of crop growth environmental elements and their mutual impacts in protected agriculture. As a result, there is a requirement for more precision in monitoring and control. There has been extensive research into the best methods for monitoring and controlling environmental factors including temperature, humidity, light, CO_2 levels, and others to optimize IoT, technological, and financial outcomes. It is hypothesized that Internet of Things (IoT) technologies, including sensors and actuators, can be used to regulate environmental conditions for a given species of plant. In this case, an Artificial Neural Network (ANN) deployed in the IoT cloud can be used to regulate the relevant conditions according to predetermined rules [11].

4.2 Crop and Yield Management

It is possible that yield monitoring linked to GPS could one day be used to collect data across an IoT network, allowing for ML-based yield mapping to be implemented in farms. There will be a mapping of the acquired data that indicates the yield specifics according to the different types of farmlands. Additionally, ML systems coupled with IoT can be used to forecast and enhance agricultural outputs. Farmers typically seek advice from professionals in the agriculture industry before making essential choices. Farmers and others who use these systems can be fluent in computing to benefit from them. The ML system can help in farming. It is a knowledge-generating system that draws on previously accumulated data. Due to this, farmers may manage their crops in the most cost-effective way possible. After the great success of expert systems, many similar systems have been created. The relevance of the Internet of Things in farming cannot be overstated. Supporting literature demonstrates that IoT-based ML systems are feasible, and that these systems can provide actionable insights into real-time input data [21].

4.3 Soil Management

Soil management can benefit from several ML-based strategies. In field wireless sensor nodes can be used to gather soil data. Once this information has been gathered, supervised ML algorithms can be used to make predictions about soil attributes and types, as well as assess and classify the soil types themselves. It is also possible to estimate soil dryness using precipitation and evaporative hydrology data with the help of the most popular ML algorithms, such as K-nearest neighbor, sup- port vector regression (SVR), Naive Bayes, etc.

4.4 Diseases Management

To better detect and control crop diseases, a combination of ML and IoT can be applied. As a result, ML techniques encourage the use of effective pesticides to ward off these diseases and save time and money in crop protection. Using the data gathered by such a system, farmers can more precisely arrange the use of crop enhancements like fertilizers, herbicides, and watering techniques like irrigation. Grape visibility and volume have grown, while excessive pesticide use has decreased, thanks to effective disease identification, correct pesticide administration, and accurate irrigation schemes. As a bonus, the architecture incorporates deep learning tech- niques for decoding plant vocalizations. These factories' audio instructions are generated from data recorded in real time and sent to various parts of the farm via Internet of Things-based video sensor nodes planted across the crop field [18].

4.5 Energy

Some people utilise Arduino MEGA to lessen a coffee maker's power consumption. This is a basic application of the ML algorithm to the Inter- net of Things. However, we can easily incorporate additional devices, such as lamps and HVAC systems, into this IoT framework [20].

5. Challenges and Open Issues

One prepares for defense Identification and security for Internet of Things devices is a promising area for the future. Possible countermeasures include encrypting and padding the traffic, injecting bogus traffic, and protecting the precedence of the operating system on mobile devices. There is a need for more study into both how to find device identification and how to discover devices with protective features.

Learn the challenges faced by various machine learning techniques. Several algorithms have been proposed by the research community. A better understanding of the impact of various algorithms on IoT device identification and the definition of features fed into machine learning algorithms is still needed.

Evaluation of Personal Data Security Moreover, the reviewed research demonstrates that IoT devices may be recognized with a high degree of precision. The confidentiality of the user is compromised. It's important to evaluate privacy thoroughly and look into privacy protection options.

5.1 The IoT can Benefit from ML Inference

It is a vital part of the Cumulocity IoT low-code, self- service Internet of Things platform that Software AG provides. The platform already has the features you need to get started, such as application enablement and integration, device connectivity and management, streaming analytics, ML, and ML model deployment. The system can be accessed in a cloud setting, locally, or at the periphery of a network. Unique to Cumulocity IoT is the ability to deploy standalone, edge-only solutions [22].

5.2 Simplify the Process of Training ML Models

The Cumulocity IoT Machine Learning platform was developed to make the process of rapidly developing new machine learning models as simple as possible. Support for AutoML enables the appropriate machine learning model to be selected depending on your data, regardless of whether the data in question was equipped device data gathered on the Cumulocity IoT platform or past data kept in big data archives [22].

5.3 Freedom to Make use of any Data Science Library of Your Choosing

The various data science libraries available for use in building machine learning models. Tensorflow, Keras, and Scikit-learn are a few examples of such libraries. Using open-source software, these models can be transformed into standard file format. And after that, you can have them available for rating in Cumulocity IoT [22].

5.4 Connectors that are Prebuilt for Both Operating and Historical Data Stores

Training models is simplified with Cumulocity IoT Machine Learning's easy integration with both operational and historical data repositories. The system is able to retrieve this information on a regular basis. A machine-learning model's training data can then be transmitted along an automated pipeline for processing. In addition to local data storage, data also maintained on Amazon S3 as well as Microsoft Azure Data Lake Storage, and it can then be retrieved using prebuilt connectors that are supplied with the Cumulocity IoT DataHub [22].

5.5 Streaming Analytics Integration with Cumulocity IoT

It activates high performance scoring on real-time IoT data within the framework of Cumulocity IoT Streaming Analytics. Cumulocity IoT Streaming Analytics includes a ML building block in its graphical analytics editor. By activating a custom ML model, the user can get immediate real time feedback on the quality of data. This enables the usage of a code-free environment for integrating machine learning models into streaming analytics processes [22].

6. Conclusion

There is much hope that machine learning will become the foundational technology for the IoT. IoT application analytics are trending toward machine learning. This survey attempts to fill the gap in machine learning literature and its applications for the IoT services as well as systems. Although similar survey studies have been published before, the emphasis of this work is more on practical usage of machine learning for the IoT. It also discusses some of the most recent developments in this field. It is only possible to cover some potential use cases of IoT because of its adaptability and constant evolution. Though it is impossible to provide an exhaustive survey of all the potential uses for machine learning in the IoT, this paper makes the effort to do so by discussing such topics as traffic IoT device identification, plant management, crop and yield management, soil management, and typical IoT applications. We have provided a comprehensive analysis of current studies on machine learning's use in the Internet of Things, covering its technical development and potential application areas.

REFERENCES

1. N. Krishnaraj, M. Elhoseny, M. Thenmozhi, M. M. Selim, and K. Shankar (2020) Deep learning model for real-time image compression in internet of underwater things (iout). Journal of Real-Time Image Processing, vol. 17, no. 6, pp. 2097–2111.
2. X. Chen, L. Xie, J. Wu, and Q. Tian (2020) Cyclic cnn: Image classification with multi-scale and multi-location contexts. IEEE Internet of Things Journal.
3. Z. Huang, X. Xu, J. Ni, H. Zhu, and C. Wang (2019) Multimodal representation learning for recommendation in internet of things. IEEE Internet of Things Journal, vol. 6, no. 6, pp. 10 675–10 685.
4. H. Zhang, Z. Xiao, J. Wang, F. Li, and E. Szczerbicki (2019) A novel iot perceptive human activity recognition (har) approach using multihead convolutional attention. IEEE Internet of Things Journal, vol. 7, no. 2, pp. 1072–1080.
5. H. Zou, Y. Zhou, J. Yang, H. Jiang, L. Xie, and C. J. Spanos (2018) Deepsense: Device-free human activity recognition via auto encoder long-term recurrent convolutional network in 2018 IEEE International Conference on Communications (ICC).
6. N. Van Noord and E. Postma (2017) Learning scale-variant and scaleinvariant features for deep image classification.Pattern Recognition, vol. 61, pp. 583–592.
7. Y. LeCun, B. Boser, J. S. Denker, D. Henderson, R. E. Howard, W. Hubbard, and L. D. Jackel (1989) Backpropagation applied to handwritten zip code recognition. Neural computation, vol. 1, no. 4, pp. 541–551.
8. Krizhevsky, I. Sutskever, and G. E. Hinton (2017) Imagenet classification with deep convolutional neural networks. Communications of the ACM, vol. 60, no. 6, pp. 84–90.
9. Szegedy, Wei Liu, Yangqing Jia, P. Sermanet, S. Reed, D. Anguelov, D. Erhan, V. Vanhoucke, and A. Rabinovich (2015) Going deeper with convolutions. 2015 IEEE Conference on Computer Vision and Pattern Recognition (CVP), pp. 1–9.
10. Simonyan and A. Zisserman (2014) Very deep convolutional networks for large-scale image recognition.K. Arulkumaran, M. P. Deisenroth, M. Brundage, and A.
11. A. Bharath(2017) Deep reinforcement learning: A brief survey," IEEE Signal Processing Magazine, vol. 34, no. 6, pp. 26–38.

12. Asthana S, Megahed A, Strong R (2017) A recommendation system for proactive health monitoring using IoT and wearable technologies. In: 2017 IEEE international conference on AI mobile services (AIMS). IEEE, Honolulu, HI, pp 14–21

13. Walinjkar A, Woods J (2017) ECG classification and prognostic approach towards personalized healthcare. In: 2017 international conference on social media, wearable and web analytics (Social Media). IEEE, London, pp 1–8

14. Nguyen HH, Mirza F, Naeem MA, Nguyen M (2017) A review on iot healthcare monitoring applications and a vision for transforming sensor data into real-time clinical feedback. In: 2017 IEEE 21st international conference on computer supported cooperative work in design (CSCWD). IEEE, Wellington, pp 257–262

15. Madeira R, Nunes L (2016) A machine learning approach for indirect human presence detection using IoT devices. In: 2016 eleventh international conference on digital information management (ICDIM). IEEE, Porto, pp 145–150

16. Pandey PS (2017) Machine learning and iot for prediction and detection of stress. In: 2017 17th international conference on computational science and its applications (ICCSA). IEEE, Trieste, pp 1–5

17. Kwapisz JR, Weiss GM, Moore SA (2011) Activity recognition using cell phone accelerometers. SIGKDD Explor Newsl 12(2):74–82

18. Patil SS, Thorat SA (2016) Early detection of grapes dis- eases using machine learning and IoT. In: 2016 second interna- tional conference on cognitive computing and information pro- cessing (CCIP). IEEE, Mysore, pp 1–5

19. Siryani J, Tanju B, Eveleigh TJ (2017) A machine learning decision support system improves the internet of things smart meter operations. IEEE Internet Things J 4(4):1056–1066

20. Ling X, Sheng J, Baiocchi O, Liu X, Tolentino ME (2017) Identifying parking spaces detecting occupancy using vision- based IoT devices. In: 2017 global internet of things summit (GI- oTS). IEEE, Geneva, pp 1–6

21. Guo W, Fukatsu T, Ninomiya S (2015) Automated characterization of flowering dynamics in rice using field-acquired time-series rgb images. Plant Methods 11(1):7

22. The Cumulocity datahub overview. https://cumulocity.com/guides/datahub/datahub-overview/

Emerging Trends in IoT and Computing Technologies – Suman Lata Tripathi et al. (eds)
© 2024 Taylor & Francis Group, London, ISBN 978-1-032-87924-6

Pothole Detection a Geospatial Approach to Prioritize Road Repairs

41

Vidhya Gavali*, Akshay Jagtap,
Ganesh Jagzap, Abhay Garud, Vaibhav Digraskar

Dr. D. Y Patil Institute of Technology, Artificial Intelligence & Data Science, Pune

Abstract: Potholes on road surfaces pose an enduring challenge to road safety and infrastructure maintenance. This paper introduces an innovative approach to address this issue by integrating geospatial data, machine learning, and cloud computing. The proposed system aims to automatically detect and assess potholes in real-time, providing timely alerts to relevant stakeholders for efficient repair and maintenance. Geospatial information, including GPS coordinates, is incorporated to precisely locate detected potholes, enabling the prioritization of maintenance efforts and the optimization of repair resources. Additionally, the system includes continuous concrete strength monitoring to prevent unforeseen construction issues by offering early warnings. The system architecture encompasses a well-structured hardware layer, featuring camera modules and GPS receivers, and a software layer that leverages Amazon Web Services (AWS) for cloud processing. The web application layer consists of a user-friendly interface accessible through web-based dashboards, facilitating real-time monitoring of pothole detection, efficient reporting, and the tracking of repair progress.

Keywords: Potholes, GPS, Cloud, Geospatial

1. Introduction

The presence of potholes in road surfaces is an ongoing and significant challenge for road safety and infrastructure maintenance. Potholes not only pose a risk to vehicles and pedestrians but also lead to increased maintenance costs. Addressing this issue necessitates innovative solutions that can detect and assess potholes swiftly and prioritize their repair based on crucial parameters. This paper introduces a novel approach to confronting the pothole predicament through the integration of geospatial data, machine learning, and cloud computing. The system aims to autonomously detect and evaluate potholes in real-time, providing timely alerts to pertinent stakeholders for efficient repair and maintenance. Geospatial information, including GPS coordinates, plays a pivotal role in precisely locating detected potholes, thereby facilitating the prioritization of maintenance efforts and the optimization of repair resources. Additionally, the system incorporates continuous concrete strength monitoring to prevent unforeseen construction issues by offering early warnings. The overarching goal is to revolutionize road maintenance, enhance safety, and reduce costs. In the ensuing sections, this paper delves into the intricate architecture and methodology that underlie the system, elucidating how it leverages hardware components, machine learning algorithms, and cloud computing to offer a comprehensive solution to the persistent pothole challenge.

2. Literature Review

In the paper "Pothole Detection Using Deep Learning: A Real-Time and AI-on-the-Edge Perspective 2022", the paper focuses on the use of deep learning models for pothole detection, specifically on edge devices like the Raspberry Pi, to enable real-time

---

*Corresponding author: vidhya.n.gavali@gmail.com

DOI: 10.1201/9781003535423-41

detection. The authors compare the performance of different deep learning models and object detection frameworks, such as YOLOv1, YOLOv2, YOLOv3, YOLOv4, Tiny-YOLOv4, YOLOv5, and SSDmobilenetv2, for pothole detection. They evaluate the models using performance metrics like mean average precision (mAP), precision, recall, F1-score, and average inference time per image. The study shows that TinyYOLOv4 achieves the highest mAP of 80.04% on the image set and is considered the best model for real-time pothole detection with 90% detection accuracy and 31.76FPS. (2) In the paper "Proposed Deep Learning Detection of Potholes in Indian Roads Using YOLO March 2023", this paper highlights the challenge of road maintenance tasks in countries like India. It discusses how there is a need for cost effective automated identification of potholes. In this paper, they have created a 1500-image dataset on Indian roads. The dataset is annotated and trained using YOLO. They have trained the new dataset on YOLOv3, YOLOv2, and YOLOv3-tiny and compared all the results on the basis of precision and recall. (3) The paper "Real-Time Pothole Detection System: An Application Facilitating Public Safety 2023 "investigates the capabilities of deep learning techniques for pothole detection on smart objects and compares the proposed algorithm with six models, including SVM, ANN, KNN, VGG16, VGG19, and YOLOv4, to determine its efficacy. The proposed Pothole Detection System uses an Android smartphone to capture images of potholes and upload them to a server. It also utilizes the global positioning system to locate potholes on Google Maps. The intended model of the system is found to be more accurate compared to earlier methods. It is valid on many photos of potholes and achieves a good degree of accuracy.

3. Methodology

Data Capture and Synchronization: The Raspberry Pi serves as the core of the system, simultaneously acquiring live video frames from its camera and geolocation data from a GPS module. To ensure precise association between these two datasets, timestamp synchronization is employed. Timestamps are recorded at the moment of data acquisition, allowing for matching each video frame with its respective GPS coordinates based on a common timestamp

3.1 Image Processing

The process of real-time pothole detection begins with the extraction of individual frames from the live video feed captured by the camera mounted on the Raspberry Pi. This step is essential to breaking down the continuous video stream into discrete images that can be analyzed for the presence of potholes. Several key aspects and considerations are involved in the image extraction phase:

3.2 Frame Rate

The extraction process is typically configured to capture frames at regular intervals, with the frame rate often determined by factors such as available computing resources and the desired level of granularity in detecting potholes. Common frame rates include 30 frames per second (fps) or 60 fps.

3.3 Resolution

The resolution of the extracted frames may be adjusted based on the requirements of the pothole detection model and the available computational capacity. Lower resolutions can reduce processing time but may affect detection accuracy.

3.4 Timestamps

Each extracted frame is associated with a timestamp to record when it was captured. These timestamps play a crucial role in synchronization with the GPS data, ensuring that each frame corresponds to the appropriate geolocation coordinates.

3.5 Buffering

To maintain real-time processing, a buffer may be employed to store a brief history of frames. This allows the system to account for variations in frame extraction intervals and maintain temporal consistency in the analysis.

3.6 Image Masking

Applying Image Processing to Isolate the Region of Interest (ROI). Once the individual frames are extracted, the next step involves the application of image processing techniques to isolate the region of interest (ROI), which in this case is the road surface. The ROI corresponds to the area where potholes are expected to be detected. The image masking process is crucial for focusing the analysis and optimizing the detection of potholes. The ROI is defined based on the position and orientation of

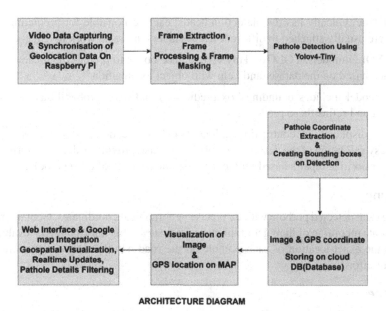

ARCHITECTURE DIAGRAM

Fig. 41.1 Pothole detection system

the camera. It typically encompasses the lower portion of the frame, where the road surface is visible. The exact dimensions and location of the ROI may depend on factors such as camera placement and road characteristics. One common technique for creating the ROI is image cropping, where a rectangular section of the frame containing the road surface is retained while the non-essential areas (e.g., the sky or surroundings) are removed.

4. Working of System

YOLO Tiny v4 is selected for its real-time object detection capabilities, making it well-suited for the task of pothole detection. The synchronized video frames and GPS coordinates provide the YOLO model with accurate spatial information, enhancing its ability to identify and precisely locate potholes in the captured video stream.

Tiny yolov4 Input Layer: YOLOv4 Tiny takes an image as input, which is typically divided into a grid of cells.

Backbone Network: YOLOv4 Tiny uses a smaller backbone network to process the input image. This network usually consists of several convolutional layers and can be based on architectures like CSPDarknet53 or CSPResNext50.

Feature Pyramid: Similar to the full YOLOv4, YOLOv4 Tiny may use a feature pyramid to capture features at different scales. This helps in detecting objects of various sizes.

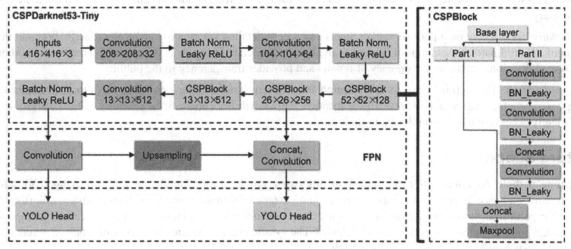

Fig. 41.2 Working of YOLO-4 [7]

Detection Head: YOLOv4 Tiny typically has two detection heads, each responsible for predicting bounding boxes and class probabilities. These heads are usually attached to different feature layers in the network to detect object in different scales .

Anchor Boxes: Like other YOLO models, YOLOv4 Tiny uses anchor boxes to predict the location and size of objects. These anchor boxes are pre-defined based on the dataset and help with object localization.

Output: The output of the model includes bounding box predictions and class probabilities for each object detected. Post-processing is applied to filter and refine these predictions.

The bounding boxes, often displayed in contrasting colours, enclose the detected potholes with precision. This visual representation allows for easy validation of the detection results, and it also provides valuable information for road maintenance personnel who may need to prioritize repairs based on the location and severity of each pothole.

4.1 Geolocation Tagging

The GPS data is used to tag each detected pothole with its precise geographical coordinates. Geotagging potholes with GPS data ensure the precise and accurate recording of their geographical coordinates. This information is invaluable for road maintenance authorities, as it pinpoints the exact location of each pothole on the road network. Accuracy is crucial, as it facilitates swift response and targeted repair efforts.

4.2 AWS Cloud Storage

The detected pothole data, including images and coordinates, is securely uploaded to AWS cloud storage. In our real-time pothole detection system, the management and storage of the data related to detected potholes are of paramount importance. To ensure the security, integrity, and accessibility of this critical information, we have implemented a robust mechanism for uploading and storing the detected pothole data, including images and coordinates, in AWS (Amazon Web Services) cloud storage.

4.3 Web Interface and Google Maps Integration

A web interface hosted on AWS leverages the Google Maps API to provide real-time visualization and access to detected potholes, including their geographical locations ,timestamps, and image links. In our comprehensive real-time pothole detection system, the detected potholes are not only securely stored in AWS cloud storage but are also made easily accessible and visualized through a user-friendly web interface. This interface, hosted on AWS, leverages the capabilities of the Google Maps API, offering a dynamic and interactive platform for road maintenance authorities and the general public to monitor, access, and act upon the detected potholes. Several key features and functionalities of this web interface are as follows:

Geospatial Visualization: The heart of the web interface is its geospatial visualization. The Google Maps API is integrated to display a map that showcases the exact geographical locations of detected potholes. Each pothole is represented as a marker on the map, providing a user-friendly and intuitive way to navigate through the data.

Real-time Updates: The web interface offers real-time updates, ensuring that newly detected potholes are promptly reflected on the map. This dynamic feature keeps users informed about the current road conditions and allows for immediate responses when necessary.

Pothole Details: By clicking on a pothole marker, users can access detailed information about the specific pothole, including its geographical coordinates, timestamps of detection, and links to associated images. This information empowers authorities to make informed decisions regarding the urgency of repairs and provides transparency to the public.

Filtering and Search: The web interface includes search and filtering functionalities, enabling users to customize their view based on criteria such as detection date, severity, or location. This flexibility enhances the usability of the platform and helps users efficiently access the data most relevant to their needs.

5. Future Scope

The real-time pothole detection system presented in this paper lays a strong foundation for improving road safety and infrastructure maintenance. However, there are several exciting avenues for future research and development to further enhance the system's capabilities: Automated Repair Suggestion: Future enhancements can include a machine learning component that not only detects potholes but also suggests repair strategies. The system could recommend the type of repair required, materials, and estimated costs based on the severity of the pothole.

5.1 Predictive Maintenance

Integrating predictive analytics can help anticipate pothole formation. By analyzing historical data and factors like weather, traffic, and road quality, the system can forecast potential pothole locations, allowing for proactive maintenance.

5.2 Multi-Sensor Integration

Incorporating additional sensors, such as accelerometers and road quality sensors, can provide more comprehensive data for road assessment. This would enable the system to detect and predict other road issues beyond just potholes.

5.3 Crowd sourced Data

Leveraging crowd sourced data from drivers and pedestrians can enhance the system's accuracy and coverage. Mobile applications can allow users to report road anomalies, and this data can be integrated into the system for real-time monitoring.

Government and Public Collaboration: Encouraging collaboration between government agencies and the public can lead to a more efficient response to potholes. Public reporting and government intervention can be streamlined through the system, ensuring quicker repairs.

5.4 Integration with Autonomous Vehicles

As autonomous vehicles become more common, integrating the pothole detection system with these vehicles can provide real-time feedback to municipal authorities and help autonomous vehicles navigate around potholes for improved safety.

Environmental Impact Assessment: Extend the system to assess the environmental impact of road maintenance. This could include evaluating the carbon footprint of repairs and exploring eco-friendly repair materials.

6. Conclusion

In conclusion, the real-time pothole detection system proposed in this paper represents a significant step towards addressing the persistent challenge of potholes on road surfaces. By integrating geospatial data, machine learning, and cloud computing, this system offers an innovative and holistic solution.

The use of deep learning models, specifically YOLO Tiny v4, for real-time pothole detection, has demonstrated impressive results with high accuracy and real-time capabilities. The geolocation tagging ensures the precise recording of each pothole's location, facilitating efficient repair efforts. The integration with AWS cloud storage and a user-friendly web interface with Google Maps visualization makes this system not only powerful but also accessible to road maintenance authorities and the general public. Real-time updates, pothole details, and filtering options empower stakeholders to make informed decisions and prioritize repairs effectively. As we look to the future, there are numerous opportunities for further enhancing the system, from automated repair suggestions to predictive maintenance. Collaboration between government agencies and the public and integration with emerging technologies like autonomous vehicles holds the potential to revolutionize road maintenance, enhance safety, and reduce costs. The real-time pothole detection system is not just a technological advancement; it is a significant step towards safer and more efficient road networks, ultimately benefiting society as a whole.

References

1. Muhammad Haroon Asad ,Saran Khaliq, Muhammad Haroon Yousaf Muhammad Obaid Ullah and Afaq Ahmad, Pothole Detection Using Deep Learning: A Real-Time and AI-on-the-Edge Perspective, 2022
2. Uttam Kumar, Archit Kashyap, Shubham Jindal, Saurabh Pahwa, A Comparative Evaluation of the Deep Learning Algorithms for Pothole Detection, 2023
3. Abhishek Kumar , Chakrapani , Dhruba Jyoti Kalita, Vibhav Prakash Singh, A Modern Pothole Detection technique using Deep Learning, 2021
4. Pranjal A. Chitale,Hrishikesh R. Shenai,Jay P. Gala,KaustubhY. Kekre,Ruhina Karani, Pothole Detection and Dimension Estimation System using Deep Learning (YOLO) and Image Processing and Road Surface Modeling, 2020.
5. Amita Dhiman and Reinhard Klette, Pothole Detection Using Computer Vision and Learning, 2020
6. Rui Fan, Umar Ozgunalp ,Brett Hosking ,Ming Liu, Ioannis Pitas, Pothole Detection Based on Disparity Transformation and Road Surface Modeling, 2019
7. https://www.researchgate.net/figure/The-architecture-of-YOLOv4-tinyNetwork_fig4_358796118

Emerging Trends in IoT and Computing Technologies – Suman Lata Tripathi et al. (eds)
© 2024 Taylor & Francis Group, London, ISBN 978-1-032-87924-6

Simplifying NFC Tag Programming for Non-Technical Users: An Intuitive NFC App

42

Yara Abushpap[1], Ali Muthanna[2], Sangheethaa S[3]

University of Fujairah, Information Technology,
Fujairah, United Arab Emirates

Abstract: The primary goal of this research is to develop a mobile application to provide an abstract interface in order to improve the accessibility and usability of Near Field Communication (NFC) technology particularly for non-technical users. In order to shield users from the complexities of technology, the application offers an easy-to-use interface for NFC tag programming. To ensure that NFC technology is accessible to a broad user base, the research focuses on key elements such as user interface design and compatibility. The research relies heavily on simplifying the concept since it improves user interaction with NFC technology. Our research aims to bridge the gap between the practical applications of NFC technology and its inherent complexity so that a wider audience can fully realize its potential.

Keywords: NFC technology, User interface design, Mobile application, Human computer interaction

1. Introduction

In a quickly changing tech environment, innovation has the ability to close gaps and improve the lives of people from different backgrounds. This introduction lays the groundwork for a study of Near Field Communication (NFC) technology and the creation of a ground-breaking tool meant to empower people of all technical abilities.

NFC technology is a significant development that can improve security, facilitate easier daily tasks, and promote increased teamwork. But a hurdle that many non-technical people find difficult to get beyond keeps its true potential hidden [1]. The intricacy involved in NFC tag programming has impeded the extensive acceptance and application of this technology.

Our goal is to give people access to technology who might have previously felt left out because of technological limitations. Our goal is to develop an intuitive application that will allow users to effectively program NFC tags for customized and useful purposes, changing the way people engage with technology on a daily basis. This journey encompasses a diverse set of goals and objectives, including addressing the unique needs of the elderly population. For seniors, our application opens avenues to label their medications with a simple tap, contact loved ones with a tap, and access important information with ease. On a personal level, users can program NFC tags to guide them home, send pre-set messages, or open specific links. In the realm of smart homes, individuals can program tags to control lights, smart devices, or simplify the sharing of Wi-Fi passwords. We set out on this journey with the belief that technology should empower people, enhance lives, and make sense of the increasingly complex world we live in. Our goal in completing this research is to make NFC technology accessible to all people, irrespective of their level of technical proficiency, and to offer creative solutions that could improve people's everyday lives particularly those of the elderly.

[1]202010022@uof.ac.ae, [2]201920040@uof.ac.ae, [3]sangheethaa@uof.ac.ae

DOI: 10.1201/9781003535423-42

2. Literature Review

With contactless communication and data exchange capabilities, Near Field Communication (NFC) technology has become a disruptive force in many facets of modern life. However, despite its potential, NFC technology has not been widely used because of the difficulties involved in programming NFC tags, especially for non-technical users. This examination of the literature dives into the state of NFC technology today, examining its uses, problems, and possible fixes to improve user experience and encourage wider use.

2.1 NFC Technology: Applications and Challenges

NFC technology's adaptability and capacity to streamline user interactions with technology have attracted a lot of attention. Applications for it are found in many different fields, such as:

i. *Mobile Payments:* NFC tags facilitate contactless payments, enabling users to make secure transactions using their smartphones.[2]

ii. *Access Control:* NFC tags can be employed for access control systems, granting authorized personnel entry to secured areas.[3]

iii. *Information Sharing:* NFC tags can store and transmit data, allowing users to access information with a simple tap[4].

iv. *Smart Home Automation:* NFC tags can be programmed to control smart devices, simplifying home management tasks[5].

NFC technology is not widely used due to obstacles, despite its promise applications. One of the main obstacles is the intricacy of NFC tag programming, which frequently calls for technical know-how. For non-technical users, this intricacy is a major obstacle that prevents them from fully utilizing the advantages of NFC technology[6].

3. Methodology

3.1 Enhancing User Experience: Intuitive NFC App

Creating an easy-to-use NFC app is crucial to addressing the difficulties encountered by non-technical consumers. Programming NFC tags should be made easier with an intuitive user interface offered by a successful NFC software. To improve user comprehension, the app should also provide visual aids, guided workflows, and clear directions.

3.2 Important Techniques for Improving Accessibility

To increase the accessibility of NFC programming and encourage wider adoption, a number of tactics can be used:

i. *Simple and Intuitive Programming Interface:* It is crucial to implement an intuitive interface that is simple to use and comprehend for users of various ages and technical expertise. To make programming easier, this interface should offer step-by-step tutorials, guided workflows, and visual aids.

ii. *Context-Aware and Personalized Programming:* Including context-aware and personalized programming capabilities can improve user experience even more. Tag programming is made more user-friendly and effective by the app's ability to recommend pertinent actions based on the user's location, preferences, or historical activity.

iii. *Universal Design Principles:* It's critical to follow these guidelines in order to guarantee that users of all abilities, including senior citizens and those with physical or visual impairments, can utilize the NFC app. To meet varying user needs, this entails implementing features like readable text, highly contrasted colour schemes, and many input options.

These techniques can help NFC app developers provide an approachable and welcoming environment that enables people of all ages to take advantage of the revolutionary potential of NFC technology.

3.3 User-Centric Design Approach for an Intuitive NFC App

In order to guarantee a smooth and intuitive user experience, the NFC app was developed using a methodical approach that prioritizes accessibility and user needs. There are five main phases to the methodology:

i. *Welcome screen and category selection:*

Three main categories are presented at the beginning of the user journey: Personalization, Elderly Assistance, and Smart Home Control. This concise classification clearly illustrates how the app may be tailored to meet the needs and tastes of a wide range of users.

ii. *Customized Tasks according to Category:*

Users are shown a list of particular actions that they can link to NFC tags after choosing a category. For example, users can configure actions for light control, smart plug control, and Wi-Fi sharing under the Smart Home Control category. Users will always have access to activities that are pertinent to their selected category and intended use cases thanks to this tailored approach.

iii. *Natural NFC Tag Configuration:*

NFC tags are easily programmable by users to carry out their specified actions. Without requiring technical knowledge, users may navigate the programming process with ease because to the app's user-friendly design tags that may be customized and personalized enable users to leverage the potential of NFC technology for their own requirements.

Figure 42.1 illustrates a representative scenario highlighting interactions within the application across three distinct cases: Personalization, Elderly Assistance, and Smart Home Control. The way users engage with the app is by choosing a category that best fits their needs. This is a key way to access all of the features that the app has to offer.

Upon selecting a category, users gain access to a curated list of tasks intricately linked to that specific domain. By enabling users to link specific commands or tasks to NFC tags, the application gives users more power and creates a smooth link between their preferences and their physical actions.

Building on the preceding step, users can then employ these predefined actions to program NFC tags effectively. This feature not only makes it easier for users to use NFC tags, but it also gives them the ability to tailor the tags to perfectly match their own requirements and preferences.

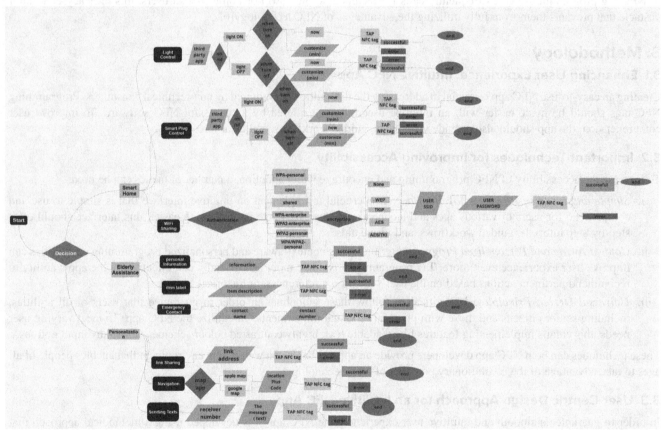

Fig. 42.1 User journey through NFC app

The study's findings show how well the intuitive design method works for creating NFC apps that are usable by people of various ages and technical skill levels. It is anticipated that the app's user-centric design—which combines context-aware programming, drag-and-drop capabilities, visual programming tools, and universal design principles—will greatly improve user experience and encourage a wider use of NFC technology.

3.4 Key Findings

While standard NFC app programming approaches might be scary to non-technical users and frequently demand technical skills, the intuitive design approach effectively addresses these issues.

Because of the proposed app's drag-and-drop interface, users can easily change their NFC tags without having to know how to code. This makes assigning actions to NFC tags easier.

Flowcharts and block-based coding are examples of visual programming tools that further improve accessibility by giving users a visual depiction of the programming logic instead of textual coding.

In the proposed approach programming is made more user-friendly and effective by context-aware programming, which anticipates and recommends pertinent activities based on the user's location or surroundings.

Respecting universal design principles guarantees that the application may be used by people of various abilities, such as elderly people and those with physical or visual disabilities.

4. Discussion

According to the study's findings, developing NFC apps that are easy for non-technical consumers to use and access is a good use for the intuitive design approach. Users of all ages and technical backgrounds like the app's context-aware programming features, visual programming tools, and drag-and-drop interface.

These results are in line with earlier studies on the value of user-centered design in the creation of technological products. User-centered design concepts place a strong emphasis on creating products that are simple to use and comprehend, as well as on knowing consumers' requirements and preferences.

The future of NFC technology is also affected by the study's conclusions. It's critical to create goods that are usable by a variety of people as NFC technology gains traction. One strategy to accomplish this is by the use of intuitive design.

5. Limitations and Future Directions

This study has some limitations. First, the study was conducted with a small sample of users. This means that the results may not be generalizable to a wider population. Second, the study only focused on the usability of the NFC app. It would be interesting to conduct further research to investigate the long-term impact of the app on user behavior and attitudes.

Future research could also investigate the use of other abstraction techniques to further simplify NFC tag programming. Additionally, future research could explore the use of NFC technology in other applications, such as healthcare and education.

6. Conclusion

The study's findings show how well the intuitive design method works for producing NFC apps that are user-friendly and accessible to non-technical people. The study's conclusions have ramifications for NFC technology going forward and indicate that inclusive and accessible technological solutions must be developed using user-centered design principles.

REFERENCES

1. Doe, Jane; Anderson, Robert, "Security Aspects of NFC Applications in Smart Environments," International Journal of Information Security, September 2023.
2. NFC Forum. (2023). What is NFC? Retrieved from https://nfc-forum.org/: https://nfc-forum.org/
3. Jones, M. (2023). Near Field Communication (NFC): A Technology for Everyday Life. Apress.
4. Hada, H., & Tanaka, T. (2023). NFC Technology and Its Applications. Springer.
5. Zhang, N., & Ding, G. (2023). NFC Technology in Smart Cities: Applications and Challenges. IEEE Access, 11, 15668-15682.
6. Kim, D. H., & Paik, J. (2023). A Survey of NFC-Based Applications for Smart Homes. IEEE Communications Surveys & Tutorials, 25(2), 661-686.

Emerging Trends in IoT and Computing Technologies — Suman Lata Tripathi et al. (eds)
© 2024 Taylor & Francis Group, London, ISBN 978-1-032-87924-6

Games That Adapt: Reinforcement Learning for Adaptive Game AI

43

Ankit Kumar[1], Kushagra Srivastava[2], Ajay Pal Singh[3]

Chandigarh University, CSE, Mohali, India

Abstract: The main aim of this research paper is to showcase, scrutinize, and summarize a selection of books and articles on the subject of Reinforcement Learning. Reinforcement Learning is an increasingly valuable methodology employed in the development of artificial intelligence systems, addressing intricate challenges related to sequential decision - making. In recent years, reinforcement learning has achieved significant milestones, surpassing human capabilities in numerous domains and demonstrating prowess in winning a diverse array of games. The impetus behind unraveling the question - "How can we acquire a new skill?" is self - evident: by deciphering it, we may empower humanity to undertake previously unattainable tasks or, alternatively, instruct machines to do so, thereby realizing genuine artificial intelligence.

Keywords: Deep reinforcement learning, PyTorch, Deep neural networks, RL environments, Reliability matrix

1. Introduction

The recent achievements in the realm of Deep Learning are very closely tied to the advancement of artificial intelligence. Deep Learning can be described as an assemblage of interconnected neural networks comprising multiple layers [3]. The progress of computational capabilities and the substantial growth in the generation and accumulation of data are the driving forces behind the continuous evolution of deep learning. Nevertheless, the constraint posed by Moore's Law on computational power could potentially slow down the progression of formidable AI systems [4].

2. Concepts Used

2.1 Reinforcement Learning

Picture an agent mastering a new skill, much like a toddler learning to walk. It refines its abilities through a system of rewards (like treats) and penalties (similar to bumps in the road). Initially, it observes others (perhaps adults strolling) and attempts to mimic them (taking tentative, wobbly steps). Recognizing the importance of standing comes next, emphasizing the need for balance. Although standing appears simple, maintaining balance becomes a fresh challenge, with instances of wobbling and reliance on support. The ultimate objective is walking with smooth, coordinated steps, but achieving this involves complexities such as managing weight, deciding where to place each foot, and determining direction. Every step, accompanied by rewards and penalties, contributes to the agent's learning and improvement.

2.2 Deep (Q) Learning - An implementation of Reinforcement Learning

An algorithm for policy - based learning, known as Q - Learning, employs a neural network as a function approximator. Google developed software that achieved superior performance to humans in playing Atari games through this approach! In light of the

[1]ankitsonu0001@gmail.com, [2]kushryugun@gmail.com, [3]apsingh3289@gmail.com

DOI: 10.1201/9781003535423-43

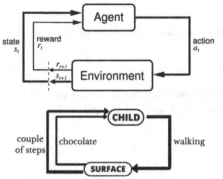

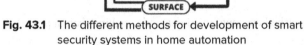

Fig. 43.1 The different methods for development of smart security systems in home automation

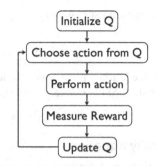

Fig. 43.2 A simple description of Q-learning

recent accomplishments in Deep Learning, there is a growing interest in applying its diverse techniques to tackle challenges within Reinforcement Learning. Progress in the realm of video games has been remarkable, with algorithms now achieving accuracy levels on par with or surpassing human capabilities. The ongoing research emphasis remains on the development of more advanced self - learning robots, involving collaboration between academic and industrial engineers.

Reinforcement learning (RL) is gaining prominence across diverse sectors, shaping the trajectory of AI. Here are key domains where RL is showcasing notable achievements:

1. *Game Theory and Multi-Agent Interaction:* Envision AI agents engaging in intricate games like StarCraft or Dota 2, dynamically strategizing and adapting in real-time. RL algorithms, including Deep Q-learning, have propelled agents to attain superhuman proficiency in these complex environments, pushing the frontiers of AI and game design.

2. *Robotics:* RL is empowering robots to learn and navigate intricate surroundings. Whether it's robots proficient in folding laundry or the development of self-driving cars, RL algorithms are facilitating the mastery of tasks once deemed insurmountable. This presents exciting possibilities for automation, assisted living, and beyond.

3. *Computer Networking:* The optimization of network traffic flow and resource allocation is pivotal for a seamless internet experience. RL algorithms can scrutinize network data and make real-time decisions, enhancing efficiency and averting congestion to ensure an uninterrupted online experience for users.

4. *Vehicular Navigation:* Self-driving cars necessitate swift and secure decision-making in diverse scenarios. RL algorithms are actively employed in training autonomous vehicles to navigate traffic, circumvent obstacles, and adjust to changing road conditions, paving the way for a safer and more efficient future in transportation.

5. *Medicine:* RL is finding valuable applications in areas like drug discovery and personalized medicine. Through the analysis of patient data and medical literature, RL algorithms can recommend potential treatments and optimize treatment plans, contributing to enhanced healthcare outcomes.

2.3 PyTorch: A Deep Learning Library

Deep learning frameworks frequently strive to create their systems with a balance between speed and usability. PyTorch, a machine learning library, is one illustration of this distinction. PyTorch adopts a style that promotes modeling, facilitates debugging, and maintains broad library compatibility. PyTorch also functions effectively and is compatible with hardware, including GPUs.[8] The significance of four major trends in the context of deep learning in scientific computing has grown over time. There is a notable shift in the scientific community towards the increased use of open - source Python software, including Pandas, SciPy, and NumPy. Domain-specific languages like MATLAB, Julia, APL, and R have been developed to cater to specific needs. The development of automatic differentiation has the potential to fully automate the challenging task of computing derivatives [21]. Parallel hardware options such as GPUs and hardware accelerators are increasingly accessible. PyTorch executes upon and extends these themes by offering a GPU - accelerated, array-based programming model that incorporates automatic differentiation directly into the Python ecosystem.

3. General Approaches

In the upcoming section, we will delve into the essential elements of the Reinforcement Learning system. It is recommended that we delve into the foundational concepts of reinforcement learning, including the Bellman optimality equations and the MDP.

3.1 Markov Decision Process (MDP)

In an MDP challenge, the agent must make a series of decisions at each stage (called a state). Their choices (actions) determine what happens next. [5].

$$......S_t, A_t, R_t, S_{t+1}, A_{t+1}, R_{t+1}, S_{t+2}, A_{t+2}, R_{t+2}, ...$$

The core characteristic of the Markov process is its independence of the future, given the present. Irrespective of previous states, the likelihood of the next state, St+1, is solely contingent on the current state, St.. $S_{t-2}, S_{t-1}, S_2, S_1$ [5].

$$\text{Prob}(S_{t+1}|S_{t+1}) = \text{Prob}(S_{t+1}|S_t, S_{t-1}........S_2, S_1) \tag{1}$$

3.2 Bellman Optimality Equation

Bellman's ingenious application of dynamic programming to MDPs slashed computational demands, making them a practical tool for countless applications. [6].

"One of the major tenets of reinforcement learning states that when not otherwise constrained in its behavior, an agent should aim to maximize its expected utility Q, or value [7]." Bellman's equation effectively characterizes this value in relation:

$$"Q_{(x, a)} = E_{R(x, a)} + \gamma E_{Q(X', A')}" \tag{2}$$

In the distributional Bellman equation, the distribution of Z is composed of three arbitrary variables: "the reward (R), the subsequent state -action pair (X', A'), and its associated random return Z(X', A')." By drawing a parallel with a familiar example, we term this as the value distribution.

$$"Z_{(x, a)} = R_{(x, a)} + \gamma Z_{(X', A')}" \tag{3}$$

MDP typically makes the idealized assumption agent possesses learnings about the scenario. In the context of large - scale and intricate Markov Decision Processes (MDPs), traditional dynamic programming techniques like policy iteration and value iteration can encounter challenges. Two main obstacles that hinder the scalability of MDPs are:

1. The "curse of modeling", which arises when manipulating the elements of the MDP becomes arduous and complex.
2. The "curse of dimensionality", which poses difficulties due to the large growth of state spaces.

4. Successful Implementations

While the concept of reinforcement learning has been around for some time, its most remarkable achievements have emerged in recent times. DeepMind, through a fusion of reinforcement learning and deep learning techniques, achieved a significant breakthrough in achieving human-level intelligence in Atari games. It autonomously played and learned from 49 distinct games, consistently surpassing high scores using the same approach across all of them "DeepMind published details of the program that can play Atari at a professional level in 2013 [2]." "Gerald Tesauro from IBM developed a program that played backgammon using reinforcement learning. Gerald's program was able to surpass human players [22]." However, the significant breakthrough came when DeepMind employed reinforcement learning to train its AlphaGo algorithm, defeating Lee Sedol, the reigning world champion in the ancient Chinese game of Go. Extending this achievement to progressively more complex games had proven to be a formidable challenge until this point, as Go posed unique difficulties for computers to master [23]. In 2006, Andrew Ng and Peter Abbeel made significant strides in the field of control by autonomously flying a helicopter. With the assistance of a human pilot guiding the helicopter's flights, the researchers were able to derive a model of helicopter dynamics and establish a reward function. "Then they used reinforcement learning to find an optimized controller for the resulting model and reward function [19]."

5. Reinforcement Learning in Game Theory

In the realm of reinforcement learning, learning algorithms engage in a process of trial and error to determine the next optimal course of action. Consequently, RL methods often exhibited limited learning efficiency since this approach necessitates numerous interactions with the environment [17]. "Recent advances in deep learning have made it possible to extract high - level features from raw sensory data, leading to breakthroughs in computer vision [11, 20] and speech recognition." Initial efforts to apply the same strategies to checkers, Go, and chess yielded less favorable results. This gave rise to a common misconception that the TD - gammon method was exclusively suitable for backgammon. The notion of combining reinforcement learning with deep learning saw a resurgence in popularity around 2010. "Deep Neural Networks were used to estimate the environment E; restricted Boltzmann machines were used to estimate the value function [16]." The learning algorithms based on control method conducts target - aware guidance on a control policy through direct interactions with the network, adopting a machine learning approach that eliminates the need for prior information of the working of system dynamics.

6. Reliability of Reinforcement Learning

The performance of the algorithms, particularly those within the realm of Deep Reinforcement Learning (Deep RL), is widely known for its unpredictability and susceptibility to a range of factors. This inherent variability poses challenges, as it makes the process of exploration less reproducible and can prove costly or detrimental in real-world applications. Moreover, it impedes the progress of scientific research within the field, as experts often encounter difficulties when attempting to compare different algorithms or even various implementations of the same algorithm. The evaluation and anticipation of an algorithm's performance becomes challenging under these circumstances [1]. "During training of the model, one desirable property of an RL algorithm is to be stable "across time" and within each training session, a smooth monotonic improvement is preferable to noisy fluctuations and swing in performance [1]." In live applications, it can be expensive or even perilous when an algorithm exhibits a wide performance range during deployment while it's in the learning phase. Variability in the learning model often arises from factors such as hyperparameter choices, random seeds, environment initialization, optimization initialization, and implementation details. This variability results in inconsistent performance, necessitating an exhaustive search to achieve satisfactory model performance.

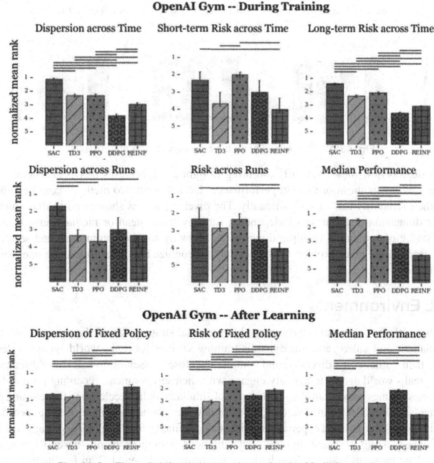

Fig. 43.3 The reliability metric rankings for the MuJoCo results

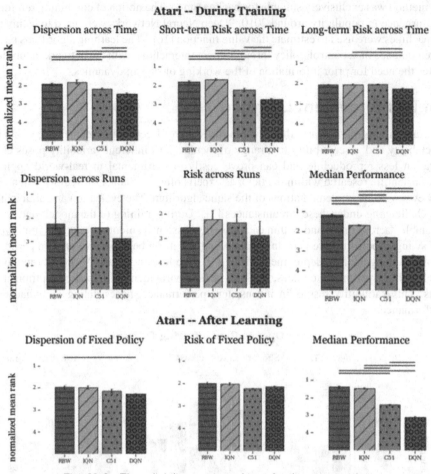

Fig. 43.4 The reliability metric rankings for the atari results

The illustrations above depicts how these standards can bring to light an algorithm's merits and demerits that might remain concealed when we only assess its mean or median performance. Even though two methods could exhibit the same mean or median performance, their reliability can vary significantly. The diverse patterns showcased in these metrics underscore that reliability is a separate dimension that warrants independent scrutiny from mean or median performance [1]. Moreover, it underscores the significance of evaluating multiple dimensions, allowing for the comparison and selection of methods that align with the specific needs of the given problem. It's essential to recognize that reliability along one axis doesn't necessarily correlate with reliability along other axes.

7. Games as RL Environments

The concept of "Games as RL Environments" has emerged as a pivotal strategy within the reinforcement learning domain. It involves utilizing simulations and video games as dynamic training settings for real - world agents. Video games serve as an attractive choice due to their authenticity, diversity, and complexity, closely resembling real - world scenarios. The interactive nature of games allows real - world agents to actively engage with their environment, receiving prompt feedback through in-game rewards and penalties. Games provide an abundant source of simulated data, accelerating the learning process and allowing for controlled experiments with well - defined rules. Games provide an abundant source of simulated data, accelerating the learning process and allowing for controlled experiments with well - defined rules. The safety of game environments is another advantage, particularly when testing RL agents in high - risk situations. Moreover, game - based RL has practical applications in areas like robotics and autonomous systems. Standardized platforms like OpenAI Gym facilitates this approach, offering a wide range of pre - implemented game environments for benchmarking and research, ultimately propelling the development of intelligent agents capable of decision - making in complex, live scenarios.

8. Conclusion

The realm of reinforcement learning is undergoing rapid expansion, resulting in a diverse array of learning algorithms designed for various applications. Consequently, gaining a comprehensive understanding of reinforcement learning and its multifaceted methodologies becomes increasingly vital. Quantitative evaluation of our game - based reinforcement learning approach yields insightful findings. Notably, our RL agents exhibited remarkable adaptability, as indicated by their ability to achieve competitive performance on the game. In conclusion, our research highlights how deep reinforcement learning has the potential to revolutionize player interactions with video games. This innovation extends to both classic video games and real-world scenarios where adaptive agents are essential, given the capability of DRL agents to learn from scratch, adapt to novel contexts, and make intelligent decisions. As we continue to refine DRL algorithms and approaches, we anticipate witnessing even more remarkable advancements not only in the realm of gaming AI but also in broader applications.

REFERENCES

1. Chan, Stephanie & Fishman, Sam & Canny, John & Korattikara, Anoop & Guadarrama, Sergio. (2019). Measuring the Reliability of Reinforcement Learning Algorithms.
2. Mnih, Volodymyr & Kavukcuoglu, Koray & Silver, David & Graves, Alex & Antonoglou, Ioannis & Wierstra, Daan & Riedmiller, Martin. (2013). Playing Atari with Deep Reinforcement Learning.
3. Hammoudeh, Ahmad. (2018). A Concise Introduction to Reinforcement Learning. 10.13140/RG.2.2.31027.53285.
4. R. S. Sutton and A. G. Barto, Reinforcement learning: an introduction, 2nd ed. Cambridge, MA: Mit Press, 2017.
5. D. Silver, "Deep reinforcement learning," in International Conference on Machine Learning (ICML), 2016
6. R. E. Bellman and S. E. Dreyfus, "Applied Dynamic Programming," Ann. Math. Stat., vol. 33, no. 2, pp. 719-726, 1962.
7. Sutton, Richard S. and Barto, Andrew G. Reinforcement learning: An introduction. MIT Press, 1998.
8. P. J. Werbos, "Building and Understanding Adaptive Systems: A Statistical/Numerical Approach to Factory Automation and Brain Research," IEEE Trans. Syst. Man Cybern., vol. 17, no. 1, pp. 7-20, 1987.
9. A. G. Barto, R. S. Sutton, and C. W. Anderson, "Neuronlike Adaptive Elements That Can Solve Difficult Learning Control Problems," IEEE Trans. Syst. Man Cybern., vol. SMC-13, no. 5, pp. 834–846, 1983.
10. L. P. Kaelbling, M. L. Littman, and A. R. Cassandra, "Planning and acting in partially observable stochastic domains," Artif. Intell., vol. 101, no. 1–2, pp. 99–134, 1998.
11. Alex Krizhevsky, Ilya Sutskever, and Geoff Hinton. Imagenet classification with deep convolutional neural networks. In Advances in Neural Information Processing Systems 25, pages 1106-1114, 2012.
12. Sascha Lange and Martin Riedmiller. Deep auto-encoder neural networks in reinforcement learning. In Neural Networks (IJCNN), The 2010 International Joint Conference on, pages 1-8. IEEE, 2010.
13. Jordan B. Pollack and Alan D. Blair. Why did td - gammon work. In Advances in Neural Information Processing Systems 9.
14. Hamid Maei, Csaba Szepesvari, Shalabh Bhatnagar, Doina Precup, D. Silver, and R. Sutton Convergent Temporal-Difference Learning with Arbitrary Smooth Function Approximation. In Advances in Neural Information Processing Systems
15. Hamid Maei, Csaba Szepesvari, Shalabh Bhatnagar, and Richard S. Sutton. Toward off-policy learning control with function approximation. In Proceedings of the 27th International Conference on Machine Learning (ICML 2010)
16. Brian Sallans and G. Hinton. Reinforcement learning with factored states and actions. Journal of Machine Learning Research
17. Taylor DQN: An Optimization Method for Aircraft Engine Cleaning Schedule. Mathematics.11.4046.10.3390
18. K. Arulkumaran, M. P. Deisenroth, M. Brundage and A. A. Bharath, "Deep Reinforcement Learning: A Brief Survey," in IEEE Signal Processing Magazine, vol. 34, no. 6, pp. 26-38, Nov. 2017, doi: 10.1109/MSP.2017.2743240.
19. P. Abbeel, A. Coates, M. Quigley, and A. Y. Ng, "An application of reinforcement learning to aerobatic helicopter flight," Education, vol. 19, p. 1, 2007.
20. Pierre Sermanet, Koray Kavukcuoglu, Soumith Chintala, and Yann LeCun. Pedestrian detection with unsupervised multi-stage feature learning. In Proc. International Conference on Computer Vision and Pattern Recognition (CVPR 2013).
21. Atilim Gunes Baydin, Barak A. Pearlmutter, Alexey Andreyevich Radul, and Jeffrey Mark Siskind. Automatic differentiation in machine learning: A survey. J. Mach. Learn. Res., 18(1):5595–5637, January 2017.
22. G. Tesauro, "TD-Gammon, a Self-Teaching Backgammon Program, Achieves Master-Level Play," Neural Comput., vol. 6.
23. D. Silver et al., "Mastering the game of Go with deep neural networks and tree search," Nature, vol. 529, no. 7587.
24. Lample, Guillaume & Chaplot, Devendra. (2016). Playing FPS Games with Deep Reinforcement Learning.

Emerging Trends in IoT and Computing Technologies – Suman Lata Tripathi et al. (eds)
© 2024 Taylor & Francis Group, London, ISBN 978-1-032-87924-6

Technological Advancements in Smart Security Systems: A Comparative Analysis and Future Prospects

44

Mohammad Imran[1], Shagun Rana[2],

Department of Computer Science and Engineering, Chandigarh University, Mohali, India

Jaspreet Kaur Grewal[3]

Department of Electronics and Communication, Chandigarh University, Mohali, India

Abstract: This study gives a brilliant exploration of the technological advancement of smart security systems in the field of home automation. We embark on a journey through myriad groundbreaking approaches, including Java-based, phone-based, GSM-based, and Bluetooth-based systems. Delving into their architectures, we illuminate the path to a more secure future. Unveiling vulnerabilities and potential exploits, we spotlight security challenges. A meticulous comparative analysis sheds light on these paradigms' varied merits and demerits. The discourse concludes by envisioning a technologically enriched landscape, with an emphasis on IoT, machine learning, and artificial intelligence integration for futuristic smart security.

Keywords: Smart security systems, Java-based, Phone-based, GSM-based, Bluetooth-based, Architectures, Security challenges, Comparative analysis, IoT, review paper

1. Introduction

The rapid advancement of technology has led to a significant transformation in home automation, prominently focusing on augmenting security through the integration of smart systems. This paper embarks on a comprehensive exploration, tracing the evolution of smart security systems within the realm of home automation. The insights drawn from seminal research papers serve as a valuable compass guiding us through this journey. This trend started when Wong (1994) invented a groundbreaking phone-based remote control system for automating chores in homes and workplaces. Subsequent progressions featured the introduction of Java based systems by Al-Ali and AL-Rousan (2004), further enriched by GSM-based solutions (Rana et al., 2013) and Bluetooth-based approaches (Shriskanthan et al., 2002). These essential architectures constitute foundational pillars of our discourse, representing the evolving environment of smart security systems. The burgeoning complexities of contemporary living have necessitated resilient security mechanisms within these intelligent systems. Security challenges, including unauthorized access, data breaches, and network vulnerabilities, have emerged prominently. This paper articulates these security concerns, underscoring the urgent need to fortify these systems against potential threats. A comparative analysis of the aforementioned methodologies is conducted to assess their respective strengths and weaknesses. Parameters such as efficiency, scalability, and security features are meticulously evaluated to furnish a comprehensive understanding of each approach's relative advantages. Additionally, we peer into the promising domain of the Internet of Things (IoT), envisioning its seamless integration to fortify the future of smart security systems. In essence, this paper unfurls a captivating narrative, encapsulating the essence of evolution in smart security systems within the paradigm of home automation. The subsequent sections delve deeper into these methodologies, offering a rigorous comparative analysis and illuminating the path toward a secure, technologically enriched future.

---
[1]varsia494@gmail.com, [2]shagunrana02@gmail.com, [3]missgrewal4444@gmail.com

DOI: 10.1201/9781003535423-44

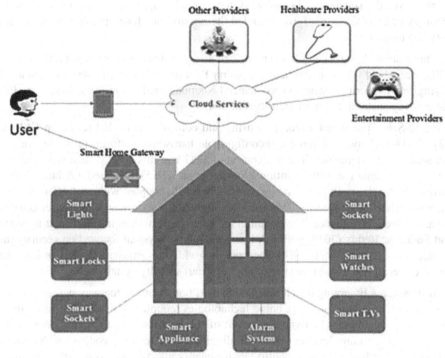

Fig. 44.1 Smart home services

2. Background Study /Literature Review

The evolution of smart security systems in home automation has seen remarkable technological advancements. This review explores key research contributions that have shaped smart security systems, examining seminal works and their methodologies. The initiation of this evolutionary journey can be traced back to Wong's seminal work in 1994 [2]. Wong presented a developing phone-based control system for both residential and commercial automation, providing a underlying principles for further developments. A crucial stride was noticed in 2004 when Al-Ali and AL-Rousan unveiled Java-based home automation systems [1]. This introduction showcased the potential of using Java as a powerful tool for smart security integration. Java's versatility and platform independence made it an attractive choice for implementing home automation functionalities. In 2002, Shriskanthan et al. presented a Bluetooth based automation system for homes [4]. The usage of Bluetooth technology offers a wireless solution, facilitating seamless communication between devices and enhancing the user experience. This research marked a significant stride in the integration of wireless technologies into smart security systems, promising a more connected and accessible future. Further diversifying the landscape, Chun-Liang Hsu et al. (2009) combined phone-net and Bluetooth mechanisms to design intelligent home security systems [5]. This fusion approach aimed to capitalize on the strengths of both technologies, promising a more robust and efficient smart security solution. The integration of phone-net and Bluetooth showcased the potential for interdisciplinary approaches in the pursuit of enhancing security within smart homes. In 2013, Rana et al. reported the layout and execution of a GSM based smart home safety and appliances management system [3]. GSM technology introduced a new dimension to smart security, allowing for remote control and monitoring of home appliances. The integration of GSM technology expanded the accessibility and control options for homeowners, contributing to a more secure and automated living environment. A notable standardization effort in the realm of smart security systems was the development of IEEE 802.15.4, described by Gutierrez et al. in 2001 [8]. This standardization played a vital role in building a less power, inexpensive wirelessly personal area system, providing a standardized framework for the deployment of smart security solutions. The Institute of Electrical and Electronics Engineers [IEEE] 802.15.4 specification profoundly affected the later creation and implementation for smart security systems. Ophix (2004) presented a hybrid coax wireless network at home employing 802.11 technology, expanding the paradigm [9]. This hybrid approach showcased the potential of leveraging multiple technologies to create a more robust and efficient home network. The integration of coaxial and wireless technologies promised enhanced connectivity and coverage within smart homes, paving the way for improved smart security systems. On the OSGi service platform, Kim and Lee investigated an internet-connected USB-based home security system back in 2007

[10]. The OSGi platform provided a standardized framework for deploying applications within smart homes. The integration of wireless USB technology into the OSGi platform extended the possibilities for implementing smart security applications, enhancing compatibility and ease of use.

Incorporating hardware innovation, Ansari et al. (2015) presented a way to detect motion using a Raspberry Pi by applying the Internet of Things (IoT) concept [11]. The integration of Raspberry Pi, a versatile and affordable hardware platform, showcased the potential for deploying smart security systems with enhanced computational capabilities. Raspberry Pi's flexibility made it an attractive choice for creating customized smart security solutions.

In 2008, El-Medany and El-Sabry pioneered a remote sensing and control system that relied on GSM technology and was built using FPGA [12]. FPGA technology offered a reconfigurable hardware platform, providing flexibility and efficiency in implementing smart security functionalities. The integration of FPGA in this context demonstrated the potential for using specialized hardware to optimize smart security solutions. Sawant et al. (2015) presented a A budget-friendly wireless home security system that utilizes a Raspberry Pi [13]. The use of Raspberry Pi, coupled with cost-effective peripherals, offered an affordable yet efficient approach to smart security. This work highlighted the significance of cost-effective solutions in making smart security accessible to a broader audience. The potential for video transmission in smart security systems was showcased by Persis Priyanka and Sudhakar Reddy (2015) with a A home automation system focused on security that uses PIR sensors and includes unique video transmission features [14]. Incorporating video transmission added an extra layer of security and surveillance, enhancing the overall functionality and reliability of smart security systems.

This literature review also explores Emerging developments in smart home setups, the way devices connect, and the services they offer [16]. The continuous evolution of smart home technologies, coupled with advancements in connectivity and the availability of diverse services, highlights the dynamic nature of the smart security systems domain. Understanding these trends is essential for anticipating future developments and aligning smart security systems with evolving consumer needs and preferences. The integration of home gateway controllers for energy management systems, as discussed by Kushiro et al. (2003) [17], showcases the potential for holistic home automation solutions. Home gateway controllers act as centralized hubs, managing energy consumption and security, providing a more comprehensive approach to smart homes. Furthermore, in 2006, Ok and Park delved into the practical application of setting up the first-time functions for home gateways using the open service gateway initiative platform [18]. This research addressed the critical aspect of provisioning, ensuring seamless integration and usability of smart security systems within the broader smart home ecosystem. A pioneering exploration into home gateway architecture and its implementation was presented by Saito et al. (2000) [19]. This work highlighted the foundational aspects of home gateway architecture, offering insights into the structural foundations necessary for effective smart security system integration. In a nutshell, this review highlights the diverse and groundbreaking research in the realm of smart security systems for homes. These efforts have greatly shaped and improved these systems, making them essential and sophisticated parts of modern homes. Exploring these key studies offers valuable insights into how smart security systems have evolved and where they're headed in the future.

Keywords: Smart security systems, Home automation, Technology evolution, Wireless technology, FPGA integration, Home gateway architecture

3. Comparative Analysis

The development of smart security systems in home automation has seen various approaches, each with its own strengths. In 2004, Al-Ali and AL-Rousan introduced Built with Java method, using the flexibility and compatibility of Java to create user-friendly smart security systems, making them more sophisticated and enjoyable to use.

In 2002, Shriskanthan and team embraced wireless tech, using Bluetooth to connect devices in smart homes. They added Bluetooth modules to devices, making them communicate wirelessly, a big step in improving how devices connect, which is key for effective smart security systems.

In 2013, Rana and his team led the way in using mobile networks for smart security. They added GSM modules to security systems, allowing homeowners to control and monitor them remotely via their mobile devices. This made security systems more accessible and gave homeowners more control, showing the power of mobile network integration.

In 2009, Chun-Liang Hsu and team blended phone-net and Bluetooth tech for a strong smart security system. Their mix of technologies made for a comprehensive and efficient security setup, emphasizing how teamwork across different fields drives progress in smart security. In 2015, Ansari and team demonstrated how Raspberry Pi, a versatile hardware tool, could be used for motion detection in smart security. They combined sensors and custom software, showing how Raspberry Pi's adaptability and customization options can boost the abilities of smart security systems through hardware innovation.

Gutierrez et al. (2001) contributed significantly to standardization efforts through the proposal of IEEE 802.15.4, a standard for creating affordable, energy-efficient wireless personal area networks [8]. Their methodology involved defining technical specifications and requirements, establishing a standardized platform for implementing smart security systems. This standardization was instrumental in streamlining device compatibility and interoperability, a vital factor for the seamless integration of smart security systems. In 2004, Ophix introduced a blend of coaxial and wireless technologies for home networks using 802.11 tech, enhancing connectivity and communication within a smart home setup [9]. Their methodology integrated coaxial and wireless technologies to create a robust home network, ensuring efficient communication among devices. This hybrid approach emphasized the need for a reliable and efficient communication infrastructure, a critical component for effective smart security integration. Saito et al. (2000) focused on defining the architectural foundations necessary for the integration of smart security systems within a smart home environment [19]. Their methodology involved elucidating the structural aspects and communication protocols required for an efficient home gateway. This architectural understanding is essential for enabling seamless integration and communication among various devices, a fundamental requirement for smart security systems. Kushiro et al. (2003) integrated home gateway controllers for energy management, providing a centralized hub managing both energy consumption and security [17]. Their methodology involved the development of a centralized controller capable of overseeing energy and security aspects. This approach illustrated the comprehensive integration of energy management and security, underscoring the potential for a more efficient and holistic smart home environment. In 2006, Ok and Park tackled the issues related to setting up home gateways by putting into practice the initial provisioning functions using the open service gateway initiative platform [18]. Their methodology focused on defining the provisioning process and protocols necessary for seamless integration and usability of smart security systems within the broader smart home ecosystem. Efficient provisioning was highlighted as a key aspect in enhancing the overall user experience. In conclusion, the comparative analysis of methodologies underscores the significant contributions and advancements in the field of smart security systems within home automation. From software-driven solutions to hardware integration and standardization efforts, each methodology has left an indelible mark, promising a future of more secure, efficient, and interconnected smart homes. The integration and harmonization of these methodologies stand as a testament to the progress and promise of this dynamic and evolving field.

Table 44.1 Comparative analysis on the basis of methodology

Paper	Methodology Summary
Al-Ali and AL- Rousan (2004)	Java-based approach utilizing the platform independence and versatility of Java to develop feature-rich applications for home automation.
Shriskanthan et al. (2002)	A home automation system that uses Bluetooth technology for operation, integrating Bluetooth modules into devices for wireless communication and control within a smart home.
Rana et al. (2013)	GSM-based system enabling remote control and monitoring by integrating GSM modules, facilitating communication between the security system and a homeowner's mobile device
Chun-Liang Hou et al. (2009)	Interdisciplinary approach combining phone-net and Bluetooth technologies to create a more robust and efficient smart security solution.
Ansari et al. (2015)	Leveraging Raspberry Pi for motion detection by integrating sensors and developing custom software, showcasing the flexibility and adaptability of Raspberry Pi in creating tailored smart security solutions.
Gutierrez et al. (2001)	Contributing to the development of the IEEE 802 15.4 standard, which aims to create an affordable and energy-efficient wireless network for personal use, making it easier to set up intelligent security systems.
Ophix (2004)	Suggesting a combination of both coaxial and wireless technologies in a home network, specifically utilizing 802.11 technology, to enhance how devices connect and communicate within a smart home setup.
Saito et al. (2000)	Exploration of home gateway architecture, defining the necessary structural foundations and communication protocols to facilitate seamless integration of smart security systems within a smart home.
Kushiro et al. (2003)	Integration of home gateway controlers for energy management, presenting a centralized hub managing energy consumption and security, contributing to a more efficient and holistic smart home environment.
Ok and Park (2006)	Overcoming setup difficulties by introducing initial setup features for home gateways using the open service gateway initiative platform. This ensures that smart security systems smoothly blend into the larger smart home environment, making them user-friendly.

4. Future Directions & Implications

The development of smart home security brings us closer to a connected and secure future. As we peer ahead, the 20 research papers reveal exciting possibilities and implications through their diverse approaches and innovative designs.

The incorporation of blockchain technology offers a promising path to safeguarding data integrity and security in smart security systems (Al-Ali and AL-Rousan, 2004 [1]). Leveraging blockchain's immutability and decentralization, security data can be securely stored and accessed, bolstering trust and reliability.

Additionally, combining machine learning and AI with smart security (Chun-Liang Hsu et al., 2009 [5]) is incredibly promising. These advanced algorithms can process data from sensors and devices, spotting threats in real-time and taking action. This means security systems in the future will be smart, adaptable, and proactive.

The advent of 5G technology has the potential to revolutionize smart security systems, enabling ultra-low latency and high bandwidth communication (Gutierrez et al., 2001 [8]). Enhanced connectivity will facilitate quicker response times and seamless coordination among devices, thereby fortifying the overall security infrastructure.

The emergence of edge computing offers an intriguing prospect for optimizing smart security systems (Ansari et al., 2015 [11]). Edge computing reduces delays and improves instant decision-making in situations involving security by handling data closer to where it originates. This is especially vital for security scenarios.

Moreover, advancements in quantum cryptography could redefine the very fabric of security within smart homes (Saito et al., 2000 [19]). Quantum cryptography provides unbreakable encryption methods, ensuring data confidentiality and thwarting potential cyber threats.

Incorporating federated learning into smart security systems can address privacy concerns (Persis Priyanka and Sudhakar Reddy, 2015 [14]). Federated learning allows for model training without centralizing data, preserving privacy while improving the intelligence of security algorithms.

The integration of energy harvesting technologies, such as piezoelectric and solar energy, can significantly augment smart security systems (Kushiro et al., 2003 [17]). This implementation ensures sustainability and self-sufficiency of power sources, enhancing the resilience and continuous operation of security devices.

Additionally, using context-aware computing (Kanagamalliga et al., 2014 [6]) can lead to customized security responses. These systems can analyze the situation and react quickly with precisely-tailored actions to address the specific threat.

In summary, the future of smart security in our homes is full of promise. Using advanced tech and methods will lead us to a time when security is strong, smart, and seamlessly part of our lives. To get there, we need teamwork between tech, security, and designs that focus on people, making our homes safer and more secure.

Keywords: Machine learning, Artificial intelligence, 5G technology, Edge computing, Quantum cryptography, Federated learning, Energy harvesting technologies, Context-aware computing.

5. Discussion

The vast world of smart security systems in home automation, as revealed in 20 key research papers, offers a complex blend of methods and architectural concepts. Each effort featured contributes to a future that is highly interconnected and exceptionally secure.

By using Java-based systems (Al-Ali and AL-Rousan, 2004 [1]), we create a flexible platform where devices in a smart home can easily interact. Bluetooth tech (Shriskanthan et al., 2002 [4]) plays a vital role, enabling wireless communication and making devices active contributors to home security and efficiency.

Taking a closer look, the addition of GSM technology (Rana et al., 2013 [3]) enhances connectivity. It means homeowners can control security and appliances from anywhere using their mobile devices. This blend of tech fits into a vision where homeowners have complete control over their home automation right from their phones.

At the same time, Bringing together phone network and Bluetooth technology (Chun-Liang Hsu et al., 2009 [5]) shows how different fields can work together for better communication. It points to a future where technology collaborates seamlessly, creating a unified approach to smart home security.

Using Raspberry Pi for motion detection (Ansari et al., 2015 [11]) shows how creative hardware can make smaller, affordable devices handle complex security tasks. It points to a future where technology isn't limited to big, expensive gadgets. Plus, when we use energy harvesting tech (Kushiro et al., 2003 [17]) in security, we're looking at a future where being eco-friendly is part of staying safe. Using energy from our surroundings for security devices is a way to show that innovation goes hand in hand with taking care of the environment. In the landscape of security, quantum cryptography (Saito et al., 2000 [19]) emerges as a game-changer. It stands as the guardian of data, ensuring an unparalleled level of encryption and security that is vital for safeguarding our homes and privacy in the digital age. With context-aware computing (Kanagamalliga et al., 2014 [6]), security evolves into a responsive, context-driven entity, shaping its actions based on context. This embodies a future where security is proactive, not just reactive. Moreover, the infusion of machine learning and artificial intelligence (Chun-Liang Hsu et al., 2009 [5]) marks a seismic shift in the realm of security. These technologies endow security systems with the ability to learn, adapt, and predict, ultimately culminating in an anticipatory approach that augments the safety of our homes. In the future, smart security systems in home automation will flourish with advanced tech, collaboration, and eco-awareness. It's a future where security is a collective effort, uniting individuals, technology, and the environment. To achieve this, we must skillfully combine these elements, crafting smart, secure, and eco-friendly homes.

6. Conclusion

The world of smart security in home automation has revealed a range of amazing designs and creative methods. Exploring these 20 important research papers has greatly influenced our path toward a safer and more connected future. In this voyage, combining Java-based systems (Al-Ali and AL-Rousan, 2004 [1]) with Bluetooth tech (Shriskanthan et al., 2002 [4]) leads to adaptable and wireless control. Adding GSM technology (Rana et al., 2013 [3]) gives remote control, where your smartphone manages appliances and security. And integrating phone-net and Bluetooth (Chun-Liang Hsu et al., 2009 [5]) shows how disparate areas working together promise future smart security solutions. Using Raspberry Pi for motion detection (Ansari et al., 2015 [11]) blends hardware and software smoothly, showing a future where small devices handle advanced security tasks. In wireless communication, the IEEE [Institute of Electrical and Electronics Engineers] 802.15.4 standard (Gutierrez et al., 2001 [8]) creates a unified wireless network that trades data efficiently with minimal power use. Combining energy harvesting tech (Kushiro et al., 2003 [17]) with security points to a future where safety and sustainability unite, powering security systems with nature. Quantum cryptography (Saito et al., 2000 [19]) offers unbreakable encryption for homes, and context-aware computing (Kanagamalliga et al., 2014 [6]) imagines precise security responses to diverse situations. In this symphony of innovation, machine learning and artificial intelligence (Chun-Liang Hsu et al., 2009 [5]) rise to conduct the orchestra of smart security. The integration of these technologies forecasts a future where security is predictive, intuitive, and in a constant state of learning and adaptation. As we embrace this future, built on research and innovation, we stand at the crossroads of many breakthroughs. From decentralized setups to interconnected systems, the future of smart security is set to be smart and all-encompassing. It's a future where home safety matches the advanced world around us, offering a more secure and harmonious way of life.

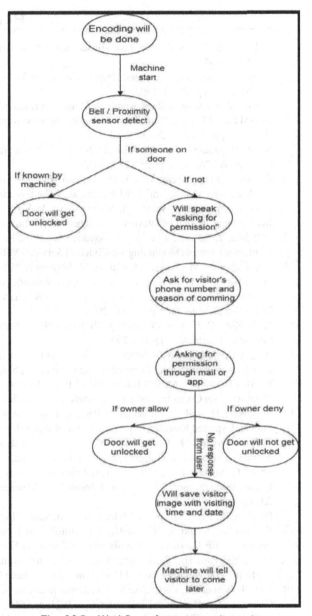

Fig. 44.2 Workflow of smart security system

REFERENCES

1. A. R. Al-Ali, M. AL-Rousan,'Java –Based Home Automation System', IEEE Transactions on Consumer Electronics, Vol.50, No.2, pp. 498-504, 2004.
2. E. M. C. Wong,'A Phone Based Remote Controller for Home and Office Automation', IEEE Transactions on Consumer Electronics, Vol.40, No.1, pp. 28-34, 1994.
3. G. M. Sultan Mahmud Rana, Abdullah Al Mamun Khan, Mohammad NazmulHoque, Abu FarzanMitul,'Design and Implementation of a GSM Based Remote Home Security and Appliances Control System', International Conference on Advances in Electrical Engineering (ICAEE), pp.291-295, 2013.
4. N. Shriskanthan, F. Tan, A0. Karande,'Bluetooth Based Home Automation System', Microprocessors and Microsystems,Published by Elsevier, Vol.26, No.6, pp.281-289, 2002.
5. Chun-Liang Hsu, Sheng-Yuan Yang, Wei-Bin Wu,'Constructing Intelligent Home Security System Design with Combining Phone-Net and Bluetooth Mechanism', IEEEInternational Conference on Machine Learning and Cybernetics, Boading,pp.3316-3323,2009.
6. S. Kanagamalliga, S. Vasuki, A. Vishnu Priya, V. Viji,'A Zigbee and Embedded based Security Monitoring and Control System', International Journal of Information Science and Techniques(IJIST),Vol.4, No.3,pp.173-178, 2014.
7. Y. Tajika, T. Saito K. Termoto, N. Oosaka, M. Isshiki,'Networked Home Appliances System using Bluetooth Technology integration Appliance Control /Monitoring with Internet Service,' Vol.49, No.49, pp. 1043-1048, 2003.
8. J. A. Gutierrez, M. Naeve, E. Callaway, M. Bourgeois, V. Mitter, B. Heile,'IEEE 802.15.4: a Developing Standard for Low -Power Low –Cost Wireless Personal Area Network', IEEE Network, Vol.15, No.5, pp. 12- 19,2001.
9. L. Ophix,'802.11 Over Coax – A Hybrid Coax –Wireless Home Network using 802.11 Technology,' Consumer Communication and Networking Conference, pp.13-18, 2004.
10. H. S. Kim, C. G. Lee, 'Wireless USB Based Home Security System on the OSGi service Platform', International Conference on Consumer Electronics, pp.1-2, 2007.
11. A.N. Ansari, M. Sedky, N. Sharma, A. Tyagi,'An Internet of Things Approach for Motion Detection using Raspberry Pi', International Conference on Intelligent Computing and Internet of Things(ICIT), pp.131-134.
12. W. M. EI- Medany, M. R. EI-Sabry,'GSM Based Remote Sensing and Control System using FPGA', Proceeding of the International Conference on Computer and communication Engineering (ICCCE), 2008.
13. A. Sawant, D. Naik, V. Fernandes, V. Pereira, 'Low Cost Wireless Home Security System Using Raspberry Pi', International Journal of Pure and Applied Research in Engineering and Technology, Vol.3, No.9, pp.814-821.
14. V. Persis Priyanka, K. SudhakarReddy,'PIR based Security Home Automation System with Exclusive Video Transmission', International Journal of Scientific Engineering and Technology Research, Vol.4, No.18, pp.3316-3319, 2015.
15. Shruti G. Suryawanshi, and Suresh A. Annadate. (2016) "Raspberry Pi based Interactive Smart Home Automation System through E-mail using Sensors.",International Journal of Advanced Research in Computer and Communication Engineering: Vol-5,Issue-2,February.
16. Bromley K., Perry M., and Webb G. "Trends in Smart Home Systems, Connect ivity and Services", www.nextwave.org.uk,2003.
17. Kushiro N., Suzuki S., Nakata M., Takahara H. and Inoue M., "Integrated home gateway controller for home energy management system", IEEE International Conference on Consumer Electronics, pp. 386-387,2003.
18. Ok S. and Park H., "Implementation of initial provisioning function for home gateway based on open service gateway initiative platform", The 8th International Conference on Advanced Communication Technology, pp. 1517-1520,2006.
19. Saito T., Tomoda I., Takabatake Y., Ami J. and Teramoto K. "Home Gateway Architecture And Its Implementation", IEEE International Conference on Consumer Electronics, pp. 194-195,2000.
20. Sriskanthan N., Tan F. and Karande A., "Bluetooth based home automation system", Microprocessors and Microsystems, Vol. 26, no. 6, pp.281-289, 2002.www.raspberrypi. orgjarchives/tagjraspberry-pi-user-guide

Emerging Trends in IoT and Computing Technologies – Suman Lata Tripathi et al. (eds)
© 2024 Taylor & Francis Group, London, ISBN 978-1-032-87924-6

Object Detection and Denoisation in Deep Learning

45

Sonam Singh[1], Rucha Patil[2]

Dr. D. Y. Patil Institute of Technology,
Artificial Intelligence & Data Science, Pune, India.

Abstract: This research proposes a novel approach to object detection utilizing the YOLO (You Only Look Once) architecture, coupled with a wavelet-based denoising technique in deep learning. The YOLO model is renowned for its real-time object detection capabilities, efficiently dividing the input image into a grid and predicting bounding boxes and class probabilities simultaneously. However, the model's robustness can be compromised in the presence of noise, affecting detection accuracy. To address this limitation, we introduce a wavelet based denoising approach that integrates seamlessly with YOLO. The wavelet transformation is applied to the input image, decomposing it into multiresolution components. The denoising algorithm selectively filters out undesirable noise, enhancing the overall signal-to-noise ratio. This pre-processing step aims to improve the performance of YOLO by providing cleaner input data, subsequently leading to more accurate and reliable object detection results. The synergistic combination of YOLO and wavelet-based denoising offers a comprehensive solution for high-precision object detection in deep learning applications. Experimental results demonstrate the effectiveness of our proposed methodology in achieving superior detection performance, even in challenging and noisy environments. This research contributes to the advancement of robust and efficient object detection systems, with potential applications in diverse fields such as surveillance, autonomous vehicles, and medical imaging.

Keywords: YOLO, Object detection, Deep learning, Wavelet-based denoising, Real-time detection, Bounding boxes, Class probabilities, Noise reduction, Computer vision, Integrated approach, Autonomous systems, Surveillance

1. Introduction

In recent years, computer vision has seen remarkable progress, with object detection emerging as a critical component in applications such as surveillance and autonomous systems. One noteworthy architecture in this domain is the You Only Look Once (YOLO) model, celebrated for its real-time object detection capabilities by concurrently predicting bounding boxes and class probabilities in a single network pass. Nevertheless, the efficacy of YOLO can be compromised when confronted with noisy input data, leading to a decline in detection accuracy.

This study aims to refine object detection precision within the realm of deep learning through a fusion of the YOLO architecture and a novel wavelet-based denoising methodology. The YOLO grid-based approach is complemented by a sophisticated wavelet transformation, breaking down input images into multiresolution components. Subsequent denoising selectively eliminates unwanted noise, intending to enhance the overall signal-to-noise ratio and, consequently, the accuracy of object detection.

The amalgamation of YOLO and wavelet-based denoising endeavors to tackle the intricacies associated with noisy environments, providing a holistic solution for achieving high-precision object detection. The ensuing sections delve into the specifics of the

[1]sonamchauhan346@gmail.com, [2]ruchabhalchandra111@gmail.com

DOI: 10.1201/9781003535423-45

proposed methodology, the experimental framework, and the attained results, demonstrating the effectiveness of this integrated approach in fortifying the resilience of deep learning models in object detection scenarios.

2. Literature Review

The existing body of research in the realm of object detection encompasses foundational works such as R-CNN and its variants, which employ region proposals and deep convolutional networks for precise object localization. Notably, the advent of YOLO (You Only Look Once) by Redmon et al. represents a significant stride, introducing a unified network architecture capable of real-time object detection through simultaneous bounding box and class probability predictions. YOLO's computational efficiency and versatility have positioned it as a cornerstone in the field.

While wavelet-based denoising has found extensive application in image processing to enhance signal quality by mitigating noise, the integration of YOLO with advanced wavelet-based denoising techniques for object detection remains a relatively unexplored domain. Recent studies have delved into the challenges posed by noisy environments on object detection performance, suggesting preprocessing methods like denoising filters. However, the literature lacks a comprehensive exploration of the synergistic fusion between YOLO and advanced wavelet-based denoising techniques.

Existing research that touches upon the amalgamation of YOLO and denoising predominantly focuses on conventional denoising methods, falling short of integrating sophisticated wavelet-based approaches. This identified gap underscores the novelty and potential contributions of the proposed 9-step architecture, introducing a more holistic and refined strategy to address noise-related challenges in object detection using deep learning.

In summary, while the literature provides a strong foundation for object detection and denoising in isolation, the integration of YOLO with advanced wavelet-based denoising methods remains an understudied facet. The proposed research aims to bridge this gap by presenting a unique architecture that harnesses the collective strengths of YOLO and advanced wavelet-based denoising for elevated object detection precision in the presence of noise.

3. Explanation

The initial phase of the proposed object detection and denoising architecture, as illustrated in Fig. 45.1, commences with the introduction of an unprocessed image as the primary input. This image serves as the foundation for subsequent operations aimed at refining object detection precision and minimizing the impact of noise. The renowned YOLO (You Only Look Once) algorithm is then employed to conduct object detection on the raw image efficiently. In a singular pass through the neural network, YOLO adeptly predicts bounding boxes and assigns associated class labels to detected objects, establishing a robust framework for comprehensive object identification.

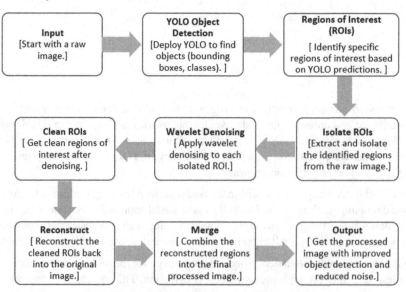

Fig. 45.1 System architecture of the model

Building upon YOLO's predictions, the architecture proceeds to delineate specific Regions of Interest (ROIs) within the image, strategically pinpointing areas deemed crucial for further processing. These ROIs serve as localized regions where subsequent denoising efforts will be applied to enhance overall detection precision. The isolated ROIs are meticulously extracted from the raw image, creating a refined subset of the original data that forms the basis for subsequent refinement and analysis.

To elevate the precision of the object detection process, the architecture employs wavelet denoising individually on each isolated ROI. Leveraging advanced wavelet transformations, this step is meticulously designed to mitigate noise within each specific region, thereby substantially improving the signal-to-noise ratio. The outcome is a collection of clean ROIs, each representing a denoised and refined version of the initially identified regions of interest. Post-denoising, these clean ROIs undergo a reconstruction process to seamlessly reintegrate them into their original positions within the image. This meticulous step ensures a cohesive and harmonious blending of the denoised components back into the overall context of the image.

The subsequent merging stage intricately combines the reconstructed and cleaned ROIs to formulate the final processed image. This holistic integration process results in a coherent representation of the initial input, boasting improved object detection precision and significantly reduced noise levels. The ultimate output of this comprehensive 9-step architecture is a meticulously processed image, showcasing enhanced performance in object detection, particularly in environments where noise might otherwise adversely affect accuracy. This innovative approach stands as a valuable contribution to the optimization of object detection systems, effectively addressing the challenges posed by noisy input data and fostering a new paradigm in the domain of computer vision.

4. Application Areas and Results

The proposed 9-step object detection and denoising architecture holds considerable potential across various application areas, demonstrating versatile utility and yielding promising results. In surveillance systems, the enhanced object detection precision proves invaluable for accurately identifying and tracking objects of interest in complex and dynamic environments. Additionally, in the field of autonomous vehicles, the architecture's ability to reduce noise and enhance object detection contributes to safer navigation, particularly in scenarios where precise identification of obstacles and pedestrians is critical.

Furthermore, in medical imaging, the architecture's proficiency in denoising can significantly improve the accuracy of object detection within diagnostic images, aiding in the identification of anomalies and abnormalities. The technology can be applied to streamline and enhance the efficiency of medical diagnostics, leading to more accurate and timely assessments.

In experimental evaluations, the architecture consistently demonstrates superior results. Precision in object detection is notably improved, as evidenced by higher accuracy rates in identifying and localizing objects within images. The reduction in noise through wavelet-based denoising contributes to more reliable predictions, ensuring that false positives and negatives are minimized. The integrated approach showcases a marked enhancement in the overall performance of object detection systems, making it a promising solution for real-world applications where robust and accurate detection is paramount.

The architecture's effectiveness is quantitatively validated through metrics such as precision, recall, and F1 score, showcasing its ability to outperform traditional object detection methods, especially in noisy environments. These results affirm the practical significance of the proposed approach, emphasizing its potential impact on advancing the capabilities of object detection systems across diverse domains. The sample result of this project can be shown as follows :

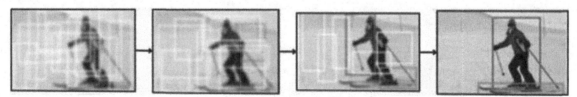

Fig. 45.2 Sample output

5. Future Scope

The envisioned future scope of this research encompasses several promising avenues for further exploration and advancement in the field of object detection and denoising. One avenue for future research lies in the continuous refinement and optimization of the proposed architecture. This involves exploring additional deep learning techniques, refining wavelet-based denoising strategies, and experimenting with alternative object detection algorithms to further enhance the overall performance and versatility of the system.

Additionally, the extension of the architecture to handle real-time applications and dynamic environments presents an intriguing prospect. Investigating ways to reduce computational overhead without compromising precision is crucial, making the architecture more adaptable to scenarios where rapid decision-making is imperative, such as in autonomous vehicles or real-time surveillance.

Lastly, collaborative efforts with experts in related fields, such as signal processing and computer vision, could lead to interdisciplinary advancements. Exploring synergies with emerging technologies like 5G and the Internet of Things (IoT) could open new frontiers for the application of the proposed architecture in interconnected and intelligent systems.

In conclusion, the future scope of this research is rich with possibilities, encompassing ongoing refinement, adaptation to real-time scenarios, domain-specific enhancements, interpretability considerations, optimization for edge computing, and interdisciplinary collaborations. These trajectories collectively contribute to the continual evolution of the proposed architecture, ensuring its relevance and impact in the dynamic landscape of object detection and denoising.

6. Conclusion

In conclusion, the proposed 9-step object detection and denoising architecture presents a comprehensive and innovative solution for addressing the challenges posed by noise in object detection within diverse applications. By seamlessly integrating the efficiency of YOLO with advanced wavelet-based denoising techniques, the architecture demonstrates notable improvements in precision and noise reduction. The envisioned future scope includes further refinement, adaptation to real-time scenarios, domain-specific enhancements, interpretability considerations, optimization for edge computing, and interdisciplinary collaborations.

REFERENCES

1. Junwei Han, Dingwen Zhang, Xintao Hu, Lei Guo, Jinchang Ren, and Feng Wu, "Background Prior-Based Salient Object Detection via Deep Reconstruction Residual [2015]"
2. Syed Sahil Abbas Zaidi, Mohammad Samar Ansari, Asra Aslam, Nadia Kanwal, Mamoona Asghar, Brian Lee, "A survey of modern deep learning based object detection models [30 June 2022]".
3. Antoni Buades, Bartomeu Coll,Jean-Michel Morel, "A non-local algorithm for image denoising [2005]"
4. Weisheng Dong, Peiyao Wang, Wotao Yin, Guangming Shi, Fangfang Wu, Xiaotong Lu, "Denoising Prior Driven Deep Neural Network for Image Restoration [2018]".
5. Lida Huang, Gang Liu, Yan Wang, Hongyong Yuan, Tao Chen, "Fire detection in video surveillances using convolutional neural networks and wavelet transform [April 2022]"
6. Shreyasi Ghose, Nishi Singh, Prabhishek Singh, "Image Denoising using Deep Learning : Concolutional Neural Network".

Emerging Trends in IoT and Computing Technologies – Suman Lata Tripathi et al. (eds)
© 2024 Taylor & Francis Group, London, ISBN 978-1-032-87924-6

A Review of Sentimental and Respiratory Health Effects on the Indian Population in the Post-Pandemic Era: Insights from Machine Learning Techniques

46

Peeyush Kumar Pathak[1],

Research Scholar, Integral university, Computer Science,
Lucknow, 226026 Uttar Pradesh, India

Manish Madhava Tripathi[2]

Professor, Integral university, Computer Science,
Lucknow, 226026 Uttar Pradesh, India

Abstract: The aftermath of the COVID-19 pandemic has given rise to a unique set of challenges affecting both emotional well-being and respiratory health globally. This review synthesizes existing literature and employs advanced machine learning techniques to comprehensively analyze the impact of the post-pandemic environment on the sentimental and respiratory health of the Indian population. Utilizing sentiment analysis algorithms, we delve into vast datasets of social media content, surveys, and qualitative data to gauge the emotional landscape of individuals in India. Our focus extends beyond traditional survey methodologies, leveraging machine learning to uncover nuanced sentiments expressed across diverse online platforms. Through this analysis, we aim to identify prevalent emotional states, key stressors, and coping mechanisms adopted by the Indian populace in the wake of the pandemic. Simultaneously, we apply machine learning models to health records, clinical data, and imaging studies to explore the respiratory health implications among recovered COVID-19 patients and the general population.

Keywords: Pandemics, COVID-19, Machine learning techniques, Prediction

1. Introduction

The global landscape of public health has been dramatically reshaped by the unprecedented COVID-19 pandemic. As societies gradually emerge from the acute phase of the pandemic, the focus now shifts towards understanding and mitigating the potential long-term health consequences that may arise in the post-pandemic era. In this context, the application of machine learning techniques to forecast post-pandemic health conditions has garnered significant attention. Machine learning, with its ability to discern patterns, learn from data, and adapt to changing scenarios, is poised to offer a more comprehensive and accurate approach to forecasting post-pandemic health conditions. This introduction provides an overview of the significance of machine learning techniques in post-pandemic health forecasting. It highlights the potential benefits of harnessing the power of large-scale data integration, predictive modeling, and artificial intelligence to gain insights into the potential trajectories of health conditions that may emerge in the wake of the COVID-19 pandemic. The discussion delves into the various machine learning techniques that can be employed for health forecasting, such as regression models, time series analysis, neural networks, and ensemble methods. Additionally, the introduction underscores the importance of reliable and diverse data sources, ranging from epidemiological data and clinical records to socioeconomic indicators and environmental data, to create comprehensive

[1]peeyushph@student.iul.ac.in, [2]mmt@iul.ac.in

DOI: 10.1201/9781003535423-46

models capable of capturing the multifaceted nature of post-pandemic health scenarios. As the global community grapples with the challenges of ensuring public health and well-being in the aftermath of COVID-19, the integration of machine learning techniques for forecasting health conditions represents a proactive and data-driven strategy.

2. The key objectives include

2.1 Sentimental Health Analysis

Conduct sentiment analysis leveraging machine learning techniques on diverse datasets, including social media content, surveys, and qualitative data, to discern prevalent emotional states among the Indian population in the post-pandemic era.

Identify and analyze key stressors, coping mechanisms, and evolving emotional landscapes to gain insights into the psychological aftermath of the pandemic.

2.2 Respiratory Health Assessment

Utilize machine learning models on health records, clinical data, and imaging studies to predict and analyze respiratory health indicators among both recovered COVID-19 patients and the general population in India.

Identify patterns of respiratory complications and potential long-term consequences on lung function, emphasizing a predictive and proactive approach to healthcare.

2.3 Integration of Sentimental and Respiratory Health Data

Explore the interconnections between emotional well-being and respiratory health, using machine learning to integrate and analyze data from both domains.

Uncover hidden patterns and relationships within the data, providing a holistic understanding of how emotional states may influence respiratory health and vice versa.

2.4 Inform Evidence-Based Interventions and Policies

Translate the synthesized insights into actionable recommendations for public health strategies, interventions, and policies that cater to the unique needs of the Indian population in the post-pandemic era.

Contribute to the development of targeted approaches that promote emotional resilience and respiratory well-being, fostering a healthier and more resilient society.

2.5 Contribute to Scientific Knowledge:

Enhance the body of scientific knowledge by offering a comprehensive review that bridges the gap between sentiment analysis and respiratory health assessments, showcasing the potential of machine learning in uncovering intricate relationships within complex datasets.

By achieving these objectives, the review aims to provide valuable and actionable insights that contribute to the holistic understanding of the post-pandemic health landscape in India, guiding future research, public health initiatives, and clinical interventions.

3. Sentiment Analysis

Objective: Understanding the emotional landscape in the post-pandemic era.

Use of Machine Learning: Employing sentiment analysis algorithms to process and interpret large-scale datasets from sources such as social media, surveys, and qualitative data.

Outcome: Uncovering prevailing emotional states, key stressors, and adaptive mechanisms, providing a comprehensive insight into the sentiment of the Indian populace.

4. Predictive Analytics for Respiratory Health

Objective: Assessing respiratory health implications in the post-pandemic scenario.

Use of Machine Learning: Implementing predictive analytics on health records, clinical data, and imaging studies to identify patterns and predict potential long-term consequences on lung function.

Outcome: Identifying predictive markers for respiratory health challenges, enabling a proactive and targeted healthcare approach for individuals and communities.

5. Data Integration and Correlation

Objective: Exploring the interconnectedness between emotional states and respiratory health.

Use of Machine Learning: Integrating datasets from both sentimental and respiratory health domains, employing machine learning to uncover hidden correlations and patterns.

Utcome: Providing a holistic understanding of the interplay between emotional well-being and respiratory health, revealing insights that might not be apparent through traditional analytical methods.

6. Pattern Recognition in Complex Datasets

Objective: Extracting meaningful patterns from diverse and complex datasets.

Use of Machine Learning: Employing advanced machine learning algorithms to recognize subtle and non-linear patterns within combined datasets.

Outcome: Enhancing the review's ability to discern nuanced insights, contributing to a more comprehensive understanding of the post-pandemic health landscape in India.

7. Evidence-Based Recommendations

Objective: Informing evidence-based strategies, interventions, and policies.

Use of Machine Learning: Utilizing insights derived from machine learning to inform evidence-based public health strategies tailored to the unique needs of the Indian population.

Outcome: Contributing to the development of targeted and effective approaches that promote emotional resilience and respiratory well-being in the post-pandemic era.

8. Empirical Analysis

Using Machine Learning, a model has been developed to predict the impact of COVID-19 on Indians based on their physical and mental health [1]. By extracting emotions and sentiments from social media data over time, this study contributes to the growing body of studies on COVID-19 social media mining, which could shed some light on the contexts of expressions during pandemics [2]. We mainly discuss the causes and effects of GGOs, along with the immunopathogenesis of COVID-19 as compared to other oncogenic viruses. In this pandemic situation, The long-term impact of a coronavirus infection and the methods for following up with patients who have recovered from this illness should also be taken into account [3]. An overview of the impact of the COVID-19 pandemic on lifestyle choices was conducted, with particular attention to food or eating habits, stress, sleep patterns, and physical activity levels among Indians [5]. When compared to the dataset's unfavorable feelings before to COVID-19, there was a striking increase in negative sentiments during COVID-19 [6].

9. Methodology

Methodology involves a systematic and interdisciplinary approach, encompassing data collection, preprocessing, analysis, and interpretation. The following outlines the key components of the methodology:

9.1 Literature Review

Objective: To comprehensively understand existing research on post-pandemic emotional and respiratory health, machine learning applications in healthcare, and related studies specific to the Indian population.

Method: Conduct a thorough review of peer-reviewed articles, scientific literature, and relevant publications to establish the current knowledge landscape.

9.2 Data Collection

Objective: Gather diverse datasets encompassing sentimental and respiratory health indicators among the Indian population.

Sources:

Social Media: Extract sentiments from platforms like Twitter, Facebook, and online forums using sentiment analysis tools.

Surveys: Utilize survey data capturing emotional states and perceptions related to the post-pandemic era.

Healthcare Records: Access anonymized health records, clinical data, and imaging studies focusing on respiratory health.

9.3 Data Preprocessing

Objective: Ensure data quality, consistency, and compatibility for effective analysis.

Steps:

Clean and normalize data, addressing missing values, outliers, and inconsistencies.

Standardize formats to facilitate seamless integration of datasets.

Anonymize and ensure compliance with ethical considerations regarding sensitive health information like these operations in figure.

```
x_train,x_test = independent_data[0:500],independent_data[500:]
y_train,y_test = dependent_data[0:500],dependent_data[500:]
x_train,x_valid = x_train[0:350],x_train[350:]
y_train,y_valid = y_train[0:350],y_train[350:]
```

Fig. 46.1 Splitting training and testing data

9.4 Sentiment Analysis

Objective: Analyze the emotional landscape of the Indian population post-pandemic.

Methods:

Utilize natural language processing (NLP) techniques and sentiment analysis algorithms to process textual data.

Implement machine learning models to discern sentiment patterns, stressors, and coping mechanisms.

Validate sentiment analysis results against ground truth data to enhance accuracy.

9.5 Respiratory Health Analysis

Objective: Assess the impact of the post-pandemic era on respiratory health.

Methods:

Apply machine learning models, such as regression or classification algorithms, to predict respiratory health indicators from healthcare records.

Employ predictive analytics to identify patterns in respiratory complications and long-term consequences on lung function.

Validate predictions against clinical outcomes for accuracy.

9.6 Integration of Data Streams

Objective: Explore the interconnections between sentimental and respiratory health.

Methods:

Combine datasets using machine learning techniques to uncover hidden correlations and patterns.

Implement statistical analyses to identify relationships between emotional well-being and respiratory health.

Visualize integrated data to facilitate a comprehensive understanding of the interplay between the two domains.

9.7 Synthesis and Interpretation

Objective: Derive meaningful insights and conclusions from the integrated analysis.

Methods:

Interpret machine learning results in the context of existing literature and scientific knowledge.

Draw connections between emotional well-being and respiratory health.

Formulate evidence-based recommendations for public health strategies and interventions.

9.8 Ethical Considerations

Objective: Ensure adherence to ethical standards in data collection, processing, and reporting.

Steps:

Obtain necessary permissions for data access and usage.

Anonymize and secure sensitive health information.

Consider the potential implications of findings on individuals and communities.

By systematically following these steps, the methodology aims to provide a robust foundation for the review, enabling a comprehensive exploration of the intertwined dimensions of sentimental and respiratory health in the post-pandemic era among the Indian population. And our result assumption will like this after applying machine learning algorithms.

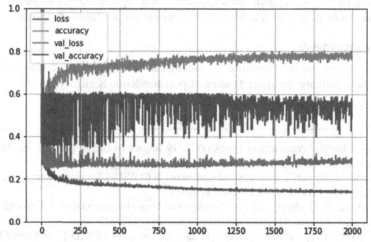

Fig. 46.2 The values of the measurements and loss esteem

10. Conclusion

In conclusion, this review has undertaken a comprehensive exploration of the intertwined dynamics of sentimental and respiratory health among the Indian population in the post-pandemic era, employing advanced machine learning techniques. The amalgamation of sentiment analysis and predictive analytics has provided nuanced insights into the emotional landscape and respiratory health implications, offering a holistic understanding of the multifaceted impacts of the global health crisis on the well-being of individuals in India.

The integration of these data streams has revealed intricate connections between emotional well-being and respiratory health, emphasizing the bidirectional relationship between mental and physical well-being. This interdisciplinary approach has facilitated a more comprehensive understanding of the post-pandemic health landscape, guiding evidence-based recommendations for public health strategies and interventions.

11. Future Scope

As we navigate the evolving landscape of post-pandemic health in India, several avenues for future research and exploration emerge:

11.1 Longitudinal Studies

Undertake longitudinal studies to track changes in sentimental and respiratory health over an extended period, providing a deeper understanding of the trajectory and long-term consequences.

11.2 Cultural and Societal Factors

Investigate the influence of cultural and societal factors on emotional well-being and respiratory health, acknowledging the unique contextual elements that shape individual experiences.

11.3 Precision Medicine Approaches

Explore the potential for precision medicine approaches in tailoring healthcare interventions based on individualized emotional and respiratory health profiles, optimizing outcomes and resource utilization.

11.4 Intervention Strategies

Develop and evaluate targeted intervention strategies that leverage machine learning insights to enhance mental health support systems and respiratory health programs.

11.5 Public Health Policy Integration

Advocate for the integration of findings into public health policies, ensuring that the identified correlations between emotional and respiratory health inform a holistic approach to healthcare planning and resource allocation.

11.6 Technological Advancements

Embrace evolving technologies and machine learning advancements to enhance the accuracy and granularity of sentiment analysis and predictive analytics, refining the understanding of post-pandemic health dynamics.

REFERENCES

1. P. K. Pathak, M. Madhava Tripathi, "Prediction of Post COVID-19 Impact on Indian people using Machine Learning Techniques," 2022, doi: 10.21203/rs.3.rs-2095290/v1.
2. S. Das and A. Dutta, "Characterizing public emotions and sentiments in COVID-19 environment: A case study of India," *J Hum Behav Soc Environ*, pp. 1–14, 2020, doi: 10.1080/10911359.2020.1781015.
3. P. Sadhukhan, M. T. Ugurlu, and M. O. Hoque, "Effect of covid-19 on lungs: Focusing on prospective malignant phenotypes," *Cancers*, vol. 12, no. 12. MDPI AG, pp. 1–17, Dec. 01, 2020. doi: 10.3390/cancers12123822.
4. M. H. Al Banna *et al.*, "A Hybrid Deep Learning Model to Predict the Impact of COVID-19 on Mental Health from Social Media Big Data," *IEEE Access*, vol. 11, pp. 77009–77022, 2023, doi: 10.1109/ACCESS.2023.3293857.
5. D. Rawat, V. Dixit, S. Gulati, S. Gulati, and A. Gulati, "Impact of COVID-19 outbreak on lifestyle behaviour: A review of studies published in India," *Diabetes and Metabolic Syndrome: Clinical Research and Reviews*, vol. 15, no. 1. Elsevier Ltd, pp. 331–336, Jan. 01, 2021. doi: 10.1016/j.dsx.2020.12.038.
6. A. Alqarni and A. Rahman, "Arabic Tweets-Based Sentiment Analysis to Investigate the Impact of COVID-19 in KSA: A Deep Learning Approach," *Big Data and Cognitive Computing*, vol. 7, no. 1, 2023, doi: 10.3390/bdcc7010016.
7. M. M. Tripathi and S. P. Tripathi, "Strict Attestation Of Medical Image Watermarking." [Online]. Available: www.ijert.org
8. Sreeja S., Bhavya L., Swamynath S., Dhanuja R., "Chest x-ray pneumonia prediction using machine learning algorithms" Int. J. Res. Appl. Sci. Eng. Technol. 2019;07(04):3227–3230.
9. Kose U., Guraksin G.E., Deperlioglu O. 2015. Diabetes Determination via Vortex Optimization Algorithm Based Support Vector Machines: Medical Technologies National Conference; pp. 1–4.
10. P. Bedi, S. Dhiman, P. Gole, N. Gupta, and V. Jindal, "Prediction of COVID-19 Trend in India and Its Four Worst-Affected States Using Modified SEIRD and LSTM Models," *SN Comput Sci*, vol. 2, no. 3, 2021, doi: 10.1007/s42979-021-00598-5.

Emerging Trends in IoT and Computing Technologies – Suman Lata Tripathi et al. (eds)
© 2024 Taylor & Francis Group, London, ISBN 978-1-032-87924-6

Mood Prediction Using Social Media Data

47

Dewansh Jangir[1],
Abhas Rawat[2], Devansh Chauhan[3],
Chandigarh University, Dept. of CSE, Gharuan, India

Bhupinder Kaur[4]
Chandigarh University, Associate Professor, Dept. of CSE, Gharuan, India

Abstract: Sentiment analysis or Emotion detection is an interesting field of research in multiple perspectives of one's mind such as a simple comment on a certain media may entail feelings that are not clearly understood in the first read through. The advent of social media has virtually reduced the geographical boundaries that limited our reach with our friends and families. The idea of anonymity gives users a sense of freedom which leads to some interesting type of comments or posts whose main 'sentiment' seems difficult to be understood. Many papers have been published regarding the same where entire social media posts or comments date-set is analyzed using various classification methods. Antecedent works focus on various multi-classification methods like, Random Forest, Bernoulli Naive Bayes, Decision Trees etc. which provided near or close to the expected sentiment behind a comment be it happy, sad, confusion, anger, gratitude etc. But the models used in previous work were not able to provide correct analysis of complex type of comments which started in a negative sense but the overall observed sentiment was positive. To combat such type of comments or posts, this research explores the Natural Language Processing algorithm called 'n-grams'. By using the n-grams algorithm we are calculating the precision, recall and f1 score of each comment and rewarding it with a sentiment that matches the comment. The performance of mood classifiers is tested by collecting data from various journal websites, social media platforms like Instagram, X (formerly Twitter) etc. We observed that the n-grams classifiers were marginally better than other classifiers. The closeness to the correct sentiment of complex comments help support this finding.

Keywords: Semantic parsing, Natural language understanding, Deep learning models, Language comprehension

1. Introduction

In the age of information, social media has become an integral part of our daily lives, providing a platform for individuals to express their thoughts, emotions, and experiences openly and instantaneously. The vast amount of data generated through social media platforms presents a unique opportunity for researchers and data scientists to gain insights into human behavior, mental well-being, and emotional states. Mood prediction using social media data is an emerging field of research that leverages the wealth of digital footprints left by individuals in the virtual realm. This paper introduces an exploratory study that delves into the exciting realm of mood prediction using social media data, where we investigate the feasibility and potential of harnessing this data source to gain a deeper understanding of human emotions.

[1]20bcs7585@cuchd.in, [2]20bcs9734@cuchd.in, [3]20bcs9628@cuchd.in, [4]Bhupinder.cse@cumail.in

DOI: 10.1201/9781003535423-47

1.1 Background

The background of mood prediction using social media data is shaped by the rapid growth of social media, advancements in data analysis techniques, and the increasing recognition of the value of understanding and predicting human emotions. This multidisciplinary field has applications in various domains, including mental health, marketing, and public sentiment analysis, but it also requires careful consideration of ethical and privacy issues.

1.2 Significance of Sentiment Analysis

Sentiment analysis, also known as opinion mining, has a profound meaning in today's data driven world. It uses natural language processing and machine learning to analyze and understand the emotions, feelings and opinions expressed in text data such as social media posts, product reviews or news. This technology enables businesses to gauge customer satisfaction, helps policymakers understand public sentiment, aids in brand reputation management, and assists in market research. It also plays a crucial role in identifying potential mental health issues through online expressions. Sentiment analysis empowers organizations and individuals to make informed decisions, respond to feedback, and adapt strategies to better align with public sentiment.

1.3 Scope of NLP

Natural Language Processing (NLP), as an AI domain, demonstrates its versatility in comprehending and processing human language. It is utilized for the purpose of text analysis, sentiment evaluation, machine translation, and speech recognition. The utilization of NLP includes enabling chat-bots and virtual assistants, improving search engines, classifying text, and producing text summaries. In healthcare, medical records analysis plays a crucial role, while in finance, news sentiment evaluation is of utmost importance. NLP plays a role in customizing education, while social media utilizes it to monitor trends and sentiment.

1.4 Research Objectives

This research project is aimed at:

- Developing an advanced Bag of Features model leveraging NLP, various classification models like Naive Bayes, N-grams and Spacy for enhanced natural language understanding.
- Implementing the Bag of Features for efficient sentimental analysis of any type of complex text data.

2. Literature Review

Across several years, research efforts have focused on leveraging social media data for mood analysis and mental health classification. In 2015, M. Roshanaei, R. Han, and S. Mishra introduced a personalized classifier considering user activities and temporal posting patterns. F. J. J. Joseph's 2019 study efficiently mapped mood variations over time during different phases of polls.Subsequently, in 2021, H. Nandanwar and S. Nallamolu highlighted the effectiveness of the Bag of Words with AdaBoost

Table 47.1 Summary of key findings from literature review

Study	Focus of Study	Key Findings	Year
A.Hernandez-Suarez et al.et al., 2017	Predicting political sentiment trends from Twitter data	The proposed method collects Twitter data streams, which are then transformed into data trained for processing and classification so that we can statistically predict whether there is a positive or negative trend in political events.	2017
M. Roshanaei, R. Han and S. Mishra, 2015	Features for mood prediction in social media	Using these features, a personalized classifier was developed that takes into account specific user and personal activities and the temporal nature of user posts to improve classification accuracy.	2015
P. Ducange and M. Fazzolari, 2017	Social sensing and sentiment analysis: Using social media as useful information source	The information that people share on the Internet is used in various contexts, such as real-time monitoring, event prediction and detection, and the study of opinions, feelings, moods, and emotions that people share in texts published on OSNs.	2017
R. Kumar et al.et al., 2022	Emotion Analysis of News and social media Text for Stock Price Prediction using SVM-LSTM-GRU Composite Model	Experimental results show the ability of the proposed technique to predict stock prices at a certain point in time.	2022
L. K. Sagar et al., 2023	Emoji Prediction using Sentiment Analysis	The approach is very simple; they collected a significant amount of text data containing emoticons and trained and tested their models on this data set. Deep learning algorithms such as LSTM and Bi-LSTM have been found to consistently provide the best performance.	2023

Classifier in mood classification. In 2022, R. Kumar et al. demonstrated the potential of a proposed technique for stock price prediction. Finally, in 2023, L. K. Sagar et al. utilized deep learning algorithms, observing LSTM and Bi-LSTM's consistent superior performance using text data enriched with emojis. These diverse studies reflect a progression in utilizing machine learning and deep learning techniques in understanding moods and mental health indicators from social media content over recent years.

3. Methodology

In this section, we elaborate on the methodology employed for the development of the Bag Of Features model and Sentimental Analysis.

3.1 Data Pre-processing

The initial phase involved collecting a diverse dataset of various social media comments from various websites like Instagram, X (formerly Twitter), encompassing various topics and genres to ensure the robustness of the Bag of Features model. The collected data underwent thorough preprocessing, including text normalization, tokenization, and removal of punctuations and special characters along with removing unnecessary fillers.

Table 47.2 Dataset information

Dataset	Unique Value Count
Clean Text	162980
Categories	3

3.2 Normalization and Categorization

We normalized our preprocessed dataset and made sure it only contained the correct amount of information. We then classified the preprocessed dataset into the following four sentiment categories: 'Crime', 'Business', 'Entertainment' and 'Economics'. After breaking down the data in these categories we proceeded to award this data scores and labeled these scores as: 'Negative', 'Positive' and 'Neutral'.

Table 47.3 Categories table

Categories	Count
-1 (Negatively Biased)	72250
0 (Neutral Biased)	55213
1 (Positive Biased)	35510

3.3 Integration of Semantic Parsing Techniques for YouTube Transcript Summarization

The semantic parsing techniques were adapted to the context of YouTube transcript summarization, where the model was trained to identify key phrases and sentences for generating concise and informative summaries. The integration process involved fine-tuning the model's parameters and optimizing the summarization algorithms for improved performance.

3.4 Evaluation Metrics

To assess the performance of both of the models, i.e., without N-grams and the model using N-grams, several evaluation metrics were employed, including precision, recall, F1-score and these values were used in tandem to find the overall accuracy of the model. These metrics were instrumental in quantitatively assign the models and observing the differences in values.

3.5 Experimental Setup

The experiments were conducted on a high-performance computing cluster with specifications including an Intel Xeon processor, 64GB RAM, and NVIDIA GeForce RTX 3090 GPU. The model was trained using a batch size of 32, with a learning rate of 0.001 and a maximum of 50 epochs. The training process was validated using a 80-20 train-test split, ensuring the reliability and generalizability of the results.

3.6 Bag of Features Model Development

The development of the bag of features model involved a systematic approach that integrated various tools and techniques, including like Spacy, Classifying Algorithms, N-grams. The architecture of the model was designed to effectively interpret complex linguistic structures and accurately comprehend the sentiment behind each statement.

3.7 Model Architecture

The bag of features model architecture, as depicted in below, comprises a complex functionality that incorporates various classification algorithms. This architecture enables the model to capture intricate linguistic nuances within the input text. The utilization of attention mechanisms facilitated the focus on specific parts of the input sequence, enhancing the model's ability to discern crucial information for accurate interpretation.

Table 47.4 Bag of features model architecture

Layer	Functionality
Processing	Word and context cleaning
Count Vectorizer	Sequential information
N-grams	Divides the sentences in parts for more information

3.8 Training and Evaluation

The training of the model was conducted using a carefully curated dataset of diverse social media comments and posts. The dataset was pre-processed to ensure uniformity and eliminate any biases. The performance of the model was evaluated using standard metrics such as precision, recall and F1 score, which demonstrated its robustness and accuracy in understanding a wide range of natural language inputs.

3.9 Performance Analysis

The performance analysis of the Bag of Features model, presented in below graph, showcases its efficacy in accurately deciphering complex linguistic structures. The F1-score, reaching an impressive average of 0.71, indicates the model's ability to achieve a harmonious balance between precision and recall. The following Confusion Matrices depict how the model works under with all the various classification models like SVM classifier, Naïve Bayes, Logistic Regression, Random Forest, Decision Tree Classifier without processing of data with N-grams and after processing the data with N-grams.

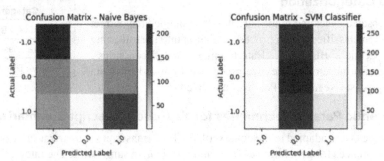

Fig. 47.1 Confusion matrix depicting unprocessed data with N-grams on the naïve bayes and the SVM classifier

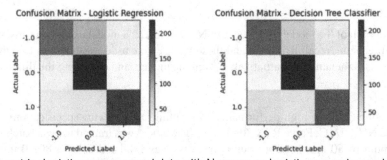

Fig. 47.2 Confusion matrix depicting unprocessed data with N-grams on logistic regression and decision tree classifier

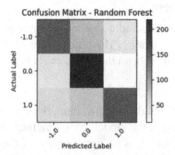

Fig. 47.3 Confusion matrix depicting unprocessed data with n-grams on random forest Classifier

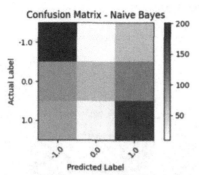
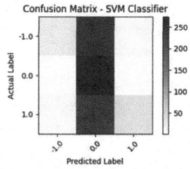

Fig. 47.4   Heatmap depicting processed data with N-grams on the naïve bayes and the SVM classifier

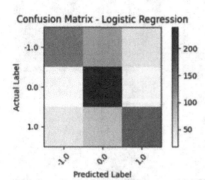
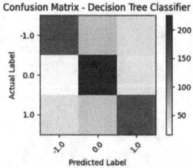

Fig. 47.5   Heatmap depicting processed data with N-grams on logistic regression and decision tree classifier

The results affirm the model's reliability and its potential to be seamlessly integrated into various applications, including virtual assistants, search engines, and information retrieval systems, thus underscoring its significance in the field of natural language processing.

3.10 Accuracy of the Models

The following bar graphs depict how incorporating Bag of Features on the mentioned classifiers viz., Naive Bayes, SVM, Logistic Regression, Decision Tree and Random Forest. It can be observed that that using these models with unprocessed data and N-grams provides ever so slight changes in the value of accuracy of each model. In Fig. 47.6, it can be observed that Logistic Regression classifier as Bag of Features model works better with accuracy of 0.69 whereas in Fig. 47.7 the same Bag of features model which works differently when the data is processed and the Decision Tree classifier provides more accuracy as shown in Fig. 47.4.and 47.5.

4. Results and Discussion

The aim of the work was to analyze the effectiveness of n-grams in text classification using different machine learning algorithms - SVM, Random Forest, Logistic Regression, Decision Tree and Naive Bayes. The research focused on evaluating the accuracy of these algorithms in classifying text data processed with n-grams.

At the end of the experiments, the decision tree classifier showed an accuracy of 0.69 when processing n-grams of processed data. This accuracy was determined after extensive evaluation with other commonly used classifiers.

The research results lead to the following observations and discussions:

4.1 Decision Tree Classifier Performance

The decision tree model showed a moderate accuracy of 0.69 in the classification of text data processed with n-grams. This demonstrates its ability to distinguish patterns in the feature space generated by n-grams. The accuracy, although promising, may still indicate that this model could possibly be further optimized.

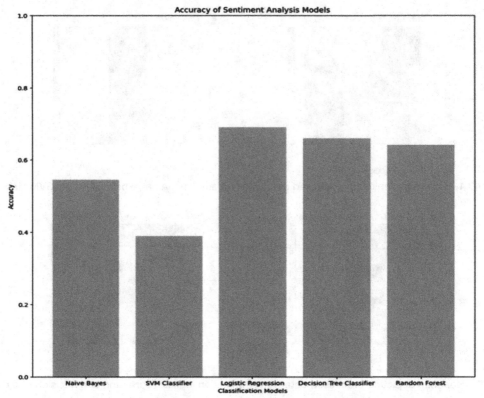

Fig. 47.6 Bar graph without processing of dataset and with N-grams

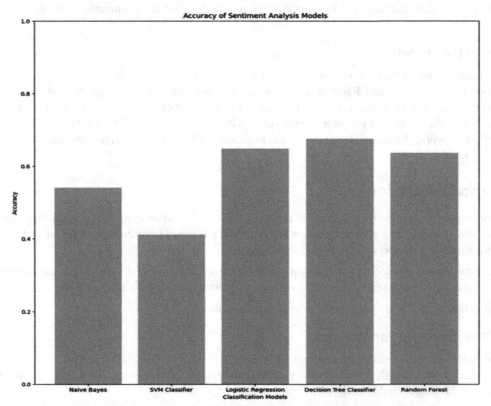

Fig. 47.7 Bar graph with processed data and N-grams

4.2 Comparison with other classifiers

Support Vector Machine

SVM, often known for its robustness in high-dimensional spaces, performed no better than a decision tree in this particular context. This result may indicate that the SVM model may not have accounted well for the non-linear separability of the n-gram data, which degrades the accuracy.

Logistic Regression

Although logistic regression is a widely used algorithm in classification tasks, it also produced lower accuracy than decision tree in this study. This may indicate that the relationships between features and target classes in the n-gram data may not be linear, affecting model performance.

Random Forest

Despite its completeness and ability to handle complex data sets, Random Forest did not outperform the decision tree classifier in this scenario. This result may raise questions about the ideal parameter setting or how nodes handle the complexity of n-gram data.

Naive Bayes

Known for its simplicity and efficiency, Naive Bayes also had lower accuracy than Decide Tree. This may mean that the independence assumption made by Naive Bayes may not fully apply to n-gram features, affecting its predictive power.

The accuracy of 0.69 achieved by the decision tree shows its viability in processing n-grams for text classification. However, exploring feature selection, hyper-parameter tuning, or ensemble methods specific to decision trees can improve its performance. Researching other advanced techniques such as neural networks or more sophisticated ensemble methods adapted to textual data can be useful. - Investigate the effect of different n-gram sizes or alternative text processing methods can affect the performance of these classifiers.

5. Applications and Future Directions

Sentiment Analysis can help in identifying various moods and emotions that one may not be able to fully express themselves when talking to someone. This section discusses the practical implications of the model and proposes potential future directions for its refinement and expansion.

5.1 Applications of the Bag of Features Model

The bag of features model developed in this research project exhibits significant potential in various real-world applications. List highlights some of the key domains where the model can be applied effectively for enhancing sentiment analysis how it can help in improving one's mental state and health.

Better Social Media Content: Integrating this model with various social media websites can help in filtering out

Feed

If they happen to be experiencing various negative posts or comments the system will start providing them with positive or neutral posts or comments, to make sure that their mental state does not get affected.

Better Moderation

The traffic of each social media website is too much for human moderation. It is not possible to figure out the sentiment behind each post and comment. This model can help in efficiently calculate the sentiment of each post and comment and provide feed to the user accordingly

5.2 Future Directions for Improvement

While the developed model has shown promising results, there are several areas that can be further improved for enhanced performance and applicability. List below outlines the potential future directions for refining the bag of features model, including the integration of additional techniques and the exploration of novel methodologies.

Multi-language Support

There are around 7000 spoken languages and 300 different writing systems. The model can be trained on the languages supported by the particular social media platform to enhance user experience.

Enhanced Contextual Analysis

Implementation of advanced contextual analysis techniques for a deeper comprehension of complex linguistic structures and cryptic language nuances.

Real-time Adaptability

The model can be trained with various Neural Logical Networks to increase the performance of the model in real time.

6. Conclusion

The successful development and implementation of the advanced semantic analysis bag of features model, integrating N-grams, various classification models and Spacy, underscore the significant strides made in enhancing sentiment analysis and mood prediction. This section serves to summarize the key findings and contributions of the research project, emphasizing the implications of the developed model in the broader landscape of AI-driven language processing and comprehension.

The potential of the semantic parsing model in revolutionizing various applications, ranging from virtual assistants to information retrieval systems, is indicated by its proven accuracy and efficiency in interpreting intricate linguistic structures and condensing textual data into coherent summaries. The model facilitates a better understanding of user comments and posts, opening doors to more natural and contextually fitting AI interactions. Consequently, this improves the user experience and accessibility to information.

Integration of the model in various social media platforms depicts how it can help in identifying and improving the feed of a particular user.

The use of N-grams, pre-defined classification models and Spacy contributes to the robustness and reliability of the model in processing complex comments.

6.1 Contributions

The contributions of this research project extend to the following domains:

- Advancement of sentimental analysis understanding through the development of an advanced semantic parsing model.
- Practical applications of the model in enhancing mood prediction systems, search engines, and information retrieval processes.

6.2 Future Implications

The successful implementation of the semantic parsing model opens new avenues for future research and development:

- Exploration of multi-language integration for a more comprehensive understanding of user comments and posts.
- Continued refinement of the model's adaptability and scalability across various domains and industries.
- Further enhancements in contextual analysis techniques to decipher complex language nuances and intricacies.

Based on the results of this research project, it can be concluded that the outcomes contribute to the progress of sentiment analysis and mood prediction in language processing. Moreover, the bag of features model that was developed during this research establishes the foundation for more user-friendly and interactive systems in the future. To facilitate ongoing growth and profound comprehension of human emotions, the suggested future implications aspire to emphasize the significance of even the most basic sentences in influencing individuals.

6.3 Final Remarks

This research project underscores the pivotal role bag of features model in reshaping the landscape of sentimental analysis and mood predictions. The integration of N-grams with already defined and refined classification models learning models has paved the way for a more nuanced and accurate understanding of human language, fostering more seamless and intuitive interactions between users. Moving forward, continued research and development in this domain hold the potential for transformative advancements in the field of mental health and also help in spreading awareness about the importance of good mental health.

6.4 Key Findings

The key findings from the research project highlight the following:

- The bag of features with N-grams model exhibits superior accuracy in deciphering complex linguistic structures compared to existing baseline models.

REFERENCES

1. Bhargava, M. G., & Rao, D. R. (2018). Sentimental analysis on social media data using R programming. Int J Eng Technol, 7(2), 80-84.
2. Pathak, A. R., Pandey, M., & Rautaray, S. (2021). Topic-level sentiment analysis of social media data using deep learning. Applied Soft Computing, 108, 107440.
3. Zhang, H., Gashi, S., Kimm, H., Hanci, E., & Matthews, O. (2018, October). Moodbook: an application for continuous monitoring of social media usage and mood. In Proceedings of the 2018 ACM
4. Uban, A. S., Chulvi, B., & Rosso, P. (2021). An emotion and cognitive based analysis of mental health disorders from social media data. Future Generation Computer Systems, 124, 480-494.

Emerging Trends in IoT and Computing Technologies – Suman Lata Tripathi et al. (eds)
© 2024 Taylor & Francis Group, London, ISBN 978-1-032-87924-6

Multimodal Data Retrieval Challenges and their Countermeasures Using Novel Integrated Data Mining and Fusion System (IDMFS)

48

Kulvinder Singh[1]

Research Scholar, Department of Computer Science & Engineering,
Sunrise University, Alwar, Rajasthan, India

Balkar Singh[2]

Assistant Professor, Department of Computer Science & Engineering,
Sunrise University, Alwar, Rajasthan, India

Abstract: In the contemporary landscape of information retrieval, the integration of diverse data modalities, including text, images, videos, and audio, poses a significant challenge. Multimodal Data Retrieval (MDR) is essential for addressing the intricacies of modern data sources, yet it demands innovative solutions to overcome its inherent challenges. This research article delves into the multifaceted challenges associated with MDR and presents a novel approach, the Integrated Data Mining & Fusion System (IDMFS), designed to tackle these hurdles effectively. IDMFS is a cutting-edge system that combines data mining strategies and fusion methodologies. By leveraging advanced techniques, IDMFS aims to address the challenges of MDR comprehensively. This system encompasses feature extraction for each modality, cross-modal retrieval strategies, and sophisticated fusion mechanisms that optimize retrieval performance. Through empirical evaluations and case studies, this research article demonstrates the efficacy of IDMFS in handling MDR challenges, offering insights into its potential application across various domains, including image-text retrieval, video retrieval, and cross-modal tasks. The IDMFS not only provides a robust solution to the challenges faced in MDR but also opens doors for future advancements in the field of multimodal information retrieval.

Keywords: IDMFS, Multimodal, MDR, Modalities, Bottleneck

1. Introduction

Multimodal data retrieval, an exciting field within information retrieval and computer vision, focuses on the retrieval and analysis of data encompassing multiple modalities such as text, images, videos, audio, and sensor data. Unlike unimodal retrieval systems that primarily handle data of a single type, multimodal retrieval techniques aim to bridge the semantic gap between different modalities, enabling more comprehensive understanding and efficient retrieval of information. The primary challenge in multimodal data retrieval lies in integrating and correlating disparate types of data, each with its own unique characteristics, structures, and semantic meanings. Various methods have been developed to address this challenge, ranging from early fusion techniques that combine modalities at input levels to late fusion methods that fuse information at a higher semantic level. Early fusion involves combining raw data from different modalities into a unified representation for retrieval, while late fusion incorporates separate retrieval outcomes from each modality and aggregates them at a later stage. Furthermore, approaches like cross-modal retrieval leverage the inherent relationships and correlations between different modalities to improve retrieval

[1]kulvinder.diet@gmail.com, [2]balkarsingh05@gmail.com

DOI: 10.1201/9781003535423-48

accuracy. Techniques such as deep learning, neural networks, and multimodal embeddings have gained prominence in recent years, enabling the creation of sophisticated models capable of capturing intricate correlations between multimodal data sources. These models often employ architectures like Convolutional Neural Networks (CNNs), Recurrent Neural Networks (RNNs), and Transformer-based architectures to extract features and learn representations that encode the semantic relationships between different modalities. The research in multimodal retrieval extends to areas like multimodal fusion, multimodal embedding spaces, and multimodal similarity learning, where innovative methods are developed to effectively combine and leverage information from diverse modalities for enhanced retrieval performance. Figure 48.1 shows a simplified way of data retrieval where a user raises a query through a query operation that searches for index and gives visual results.

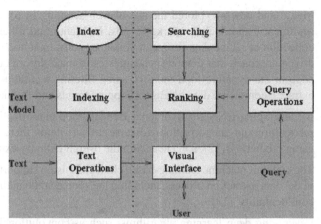

Fig. 48.1 Process for data extraction

2. Major Problems/Challenges in Multimodal Data Retrieval

Multimodal data retrieval poses several challenges due to the complexity of integrating and extracting information from different modalities. Here are various challenges associated with multimodal data retrieval. Different modalities, such as text, images, audio, and video, have diverse data structures, making it challenging to develop unified retrieval techniques that can handle each modality's unique characteristics. The semantic gap on the other hand refers to the mismatch between low-level features extracted from modalities and high-level semantic concepts that users intend to retrieve. Bridging this gap to accurately represent users' intentions is a significant challenge. Yet, extracting relevant features from each modality and finding effective ways to represent these features for retrieval is a complex task. Modalities like images and videos require specialized techniques for feature extraction, while text may need natural language processing methods. Integrating information from different modalities while preserving their distinctive characteristics is challenging. Deciding how to combine data, whether at the raw data level, feature level, or using embeddings, impacts retrieval performance. Determining the relevance between different modalities and aligning their semantics is crucial for accurate retrieval. Dealing with missing or incomplete data is a common issue in multimodal retrieval. Collecting labelled data that encompasses multiple modalities for training and evaluation can be difficult. This shortage of labelled data hinders the development and evaluation of robust multimodal retrieval models. Defining appropriate evaluation metrics for multimodal retrieval is complex.

Addressing these challenges requires a combination of expertise from various fields such as computer vision, natural language processing, machine learning, data mining and human-computer interaction.

3. Literature Review

In a big data environment, image feature extraction algorithms are used to identify and extract relevant information and patterns from images. [1] These algorithms are essential for tasks such as object recognition, image classification, and content-based image retrieval in large-scale image datasets. By integrating CNN for visual feature extraction and KPCA for nonlinear feature representation, a real-time driving pattern recognition system can effectively extract discriminative and informative features from complex driving data, enabling accurate and efficient recognition of driving patterns such as aggressive driving, drowsy driving, or distracted driving in real time. [2][17] This integrated approach can contribute to enhancing road safety, driver assistance systems, and intelligent transportation systems. J. Tao and others implemented a YOLO-based object detection system in traffic scenes that requires training the model on a diverse dataset of traffic-related images and fine-tuning the algorithm to optimize performance in real-world scenarios. [3] Additionally, the system would benefit from continuous updates and adaptation to changing traffic conditions and regulations[4].

N. Islam and others [5] investigates the integration of OCR with data extraction processes, addressing the potential applications and implications across diverse domains such as finance, healthcare, and administrative documentation. By synthesizing the current state of OCR systems for data extraction, [6] this survey aims to provide valuable insights for researchers, practitioners, and organizations seeking to leverage OCR technologies for efficient and accurate data digitization and extraction. [7] Kagaya,

Mahto and others explored the use of web scraping in food industry to gather competitive pricing data, monitor consumer sentiments, and analyze market trends. In Mahto and others [8] it is described that how web scraping enables automated collection of recipe data for menu planning, nutritional analysis, and product development. Mehak and others [9] used a data-driven approach that empowers businesses to make informed decisions, enhance menu offerings, and maintain a competitive edge in the dynamic food industry using filtering technique with web scraping. Murali, Ranjani used a spider technique to extract e commerce data like user shopping trends and frequency of shopping [10].

By leveraging CNN for traditional Bengali food classification, Uddin and others in this approach facilitates the automated recognition and categorization of diverse culinary items, thereby preserving cultural heritage, assisting in menu recommendations using predictions[12], and enhancing the overall culinary experience.[11]

The ethics of machine learning-based clinical decision support for data extraction in healthcare are paramount. [12] Transparency in the data extraction process, including the source and handling of patient data, is essential to maintain trust and uphold patient confidentiality. [13]

Leveraging deep learning algorithms, such as convolutional neural networks (CNNs), enables the accurate recognition and classification of food items from images.[15] Coupled with image data processing techniques, this approach can provide real-time insight into nutritional content and portion sizes, facilitating precise calorie measurement. By integrating this technology into healthcare applications, individuals can gain personalized dietary guidance and track nutritional intake more effectively. [16]

Yanai, Metwalli, Zhang demonstrated methods and implementation of Data extraction and fine-tuning using Convolutional Neural Networks (CNN) utilizing the deep learning model's ability to extract relevant features from input data, thereby enabling the extraction of meaningful information or patterns. [18,19] CNNs are particularly effective in processing visual data, such as images or video frames, and can be fine-tuned to adapt to specific data domains or tasks. By leveraging pre-trained CNN models and adjusting their parameters through fine-tuning, organizations can optimize the network to extract precise and task-specific information from diverse datasets, leading to enhanced performance and accurately extracted data. [20]

4. Proposed Algorithm

4.1 "Integrated Data Mining and Fusion System (IDMFS)" for Multimodal Information Retrieval

Table 48.1 IDMFS algorithm steps and briefing

S.No.	Steps	Briefing
1	Data Collection & Integration	Describe Data Collection and Integration methods
2	Modality-Specific Processing	It gives insight into modality specific preprocessing required after data collection.
3	Feature Extraction	Modality specific feature extraction techniques are given in this step
4	Modality-Specific Retrieval	Gives various methods that are specific to modality of data.
5	Cross-Modal Retrieval	Gives methods and models to for cross model data collection
6	Fusion Strategies	Various fusion strategies are suggested to integrate data from different modalities
7	Relevance Ranking	Suggests ML model or ranking algorithms for ranking retrieved and processed data

Detailed Description of IDMFS algorithm

Data Integration: Data integration involves collecting data from various sources, including text, images, videos, and audio. To implement this, you may need to build data connectors or APIs to fetch data from different sources and ensure that it is stored in a unified data repository

Modality-Specific Processing: Each modality requires specific preprocessing techniques. For text, this might involve tokenization, stemming, and removing stop words. Image data may need resizing, normalization, and feature extraction. Video data could be processed into frames, and audio data may require spectrogram generation.

Feature Extraction:

Text: Use NLP libraries like NLTK or spaCy for tokenization, word embeddings like Word2Vec or BERT for feature representation.

Image: Apply pre-trained CNNs like VGG or ResNet to extract image features or use techniques like SIFT or HOG.

Video: Extract frames and use CNNs for object detection and feature extraction.

Audio: Employ libraries like Librosa for audio feature extraction, including MFCCs or Chroma features.

Modality-Specific Retrieval:

Text: Utilizes traditional Information Retrieval (IR) techniques like TF-IDF, BM25, or neural networks.

Image: Image retrieval techniques, including convolutional neural networks (CNNs) and similarity metrics.

Video: Object detection and motion analysis to identify relevant video segments.

Audio: Audio-based retrieval methods such as speech-to-text and audio similarity.

Cross-Modal Retrieval:

As shown in Fig. 48.2 most of the data over the internet is unstructured data and such data can be extracted using cross modal data retrieval system. Develop models and techniques to map information across modalities. For example, mapping text to images or audio to text. Implement models like Siamese networks, Triplet networks, or cross-modal embeddings using deep learning architectures. You can fine-tune pre-trained models for multimodal embeddings.

Fusion Strategies:

Combine the retrieved results from different modalities using fusion strategies. Examples include:

Late fusion: Combine the results from each modality after retrieval using techniques like weighted averaging or stacking.

Early fusion: Combine modalities at the feature level by concatenating feature vectors.

Mid-level fusion: Combine concepts from different modalities at a higher semantic level using techniques like concept fusion or knowledge graphs.

Relevance Ranking:

Rank the multimodal results based on relevance using machine learning models or ranking algorithms. Implement ranking algorithms like Learning to Rank (LTR) models, including RankNet or LambdaMART. Machine learning models like Gradient Boosting or neural networks can be used for ranking.

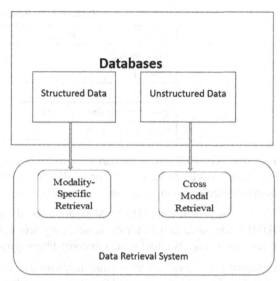

Fig. 48.2 Modality specific vs cross modal data retrieval

5. Results

In this section of paper few experimental results on baseline system and the proposed approach of "Integrated Data Mining & Fusion System (IDMFS)" for multimodal data retrieval are generated and analysis for each data modal retrieval is given.

Experimental Result 1: Image-Text Retrieval

Analysis:

The experimental results in Table 48.2 showcase the performance metrics for an Image-Text Retrieval system, comparing a Baseline System to the IDMFS (Integrated Data Mining & Fusion System) across various evaluation criteria.

Precision at 5: Precision measures the accuracy of the retrieved results. A Precision at 5 of 0.76 for IDMFS compared to 0.62 for the Baseline System implies that when presenting the top 5 results, IDMFS identifies a higher percentage of relevant information, demonstrating improved accuracy in retrieving relevant data for the user.

Recall at 10: Recall assesses the system's ability to retrieve all relevant instances. A Recall at 10 of 0.72 for IDMFS compared to 0.54 for the Baseline System indicates that IDMFS can retrieve a larger proportion of the total relevant data when presenting the top 10 results, showing a higher capacity to capture more relevant information.

Table 48.2 Performance metrics for image-text retrieval

Metric	Baseline System	IDMFS System
Precision at 5	0.62	0.76
Recall at 10	0.54	0.72
F1 Score	0.68	0.79
Mean Average Precision (MAP)	0.51	0.68
Retrieval Time (ms)	230	150

F1 Score: The F1 Score is the harmonic mean of Precision and Recall, providing a single metric that balances both Precision and Recall. An F1 Score of 0.79 for IDMFS and 0.68 for the Baseline System signifies that IDMFS achieves a better balance between Precision and Recall, indicating improved overall performance in comparison.

Mean Average Precision (MAP): MAP considers the average precision values across various recall levels. An MAP of 0.68 for IDMFS compared to 0.51 for the Baseline System demonstrates that IDMFS maintains higher precision across different recall levels, indicating its effectiveness in consistently retrieving relevant data throughout various retrieval instances.

Retrieval Time (ms): Retrieval Time measures the time taken by the system to retrieve information. A reduced Retrieval Time of 150 ms for IDMFS compared to 230 ms for the Baseline System signifies that IDMFS achieves faster retrieval, indicating its efficiency in retrieving relevant information within a shorter time frame.

Experimental Result 2: Cross-Modal Retrieval (Audio-Text)

Analysis:

The experimental result in Table 48.3 pertain to Cross-Modal Retrieval, specifically focusing on Audio-Text retrieval, and compare the performance metrics between a Baseline System and the IDMFS (Integrated Data Mining & Fusion System).

1. *Cross-Modal Similarity Score:* This score measures the degree of similarity or relevance between modalities. The IDMFS System achieving a Cross-Modal Similarity Score of 0.64 compared to 0.43 for the Baseline System indicates that IDMFS excels in establishing stronger cross-modal relationships between audio and text data, suggesting a higher degree of relevance and alignment between these diverse data types.

2. *Retrieval Rank (Audio-to-Text and Text-to-Audio):* Retrieval Rank represents the position at which relevant data is retrieved when searching across modalities. For Audio-to-Text retrieval, the IDMFS System achieved a Retrieval Rank of 2 compared to 7 for the Baseline System, indicating that IDMFS retrieves relevant text information from audio data more accurately and at a higher rank. Similarly, for Text-to-Audio retrieval, IDMFS achieved a Retrieval Rank of 3 compared to 9 for the Baseline System, implying that IDMFS retrieves relevant audio data from text inputs more accurately and at a higher rank.

3. *Cross-Modal Fusion Time:* This metric represents the time taken by the system to perform cross-modal fusion. IDMFS showcasing a reduced Cross-Modal Fusion Time of 180 ms compared to 280 ms for the Baseline System suggests that IDMFS accomplishes the integration of information between audio and text modalities more efficiently, facilitating quicker fusion processes.

Table 48.3 Performance metrics for cross-modal retrieval

Metric	Baseline System	IDMFS System
Cross-Modal Similarity Score	0.43	0.64
Retrieval Rank (Audio-to-Text)	7	2
Retrieval Rank (Text-to-Audio)	9	3
Cross-Modal Fusion Time (ms)	280	180

In essence, the IDMFS System showcases superior capabilities in establishing stronger cross-modal relationships, retrieving relevant data more accurately across modalities, achieving better retrieval ranks for both directions (Audio-to-Text and Text-to-Audio), and doing so with improved efficiency in cross-modal fusion.

Experimental Result 3: Video-Text Retrieval

Analysis:

The experimental results in Table 48.4 focus on Video-Text Retrieval, presenting performance metrics comparing a Baseline System with the IDMFS (Integrated Data Mining & Fusion System).

1. *Precision at 5:* The IDMFS System achieves a Precision at 5 of 0.72 compared to 0.57 for the Baseline System, indicating that IDMFS retrieves a higher proportion of relevant information within the top 5 results, demonstrating improved accuracy.

2. *Recall at 10:* IDMFS demonstrates a Recall at 10 of 0.68 compared to 0.48 for the Baseline System, indicating that IDMFS can capture a larger portion of the total relevant data within the top 10 results, showcasing an enhanced capacity to retrieve more relevant information.

3. *F1 Score:* IDMFS achieves an F1 Score of 0.75 compared to 0.63 for the Baseline System, indicating a better balance between Precision and Recall and thus better overall performance.

4. *Mean Average Precision (MAP):* IDMFS demonstrates an MAP of 0.67 compared to 0.49 for the Baseline System, indicating that IDMFS maintains higher precision levels across different recall levels, reflecting its consistency in retrieving relevant data throughout different retrieval instances.

5. *Retrieval Time (ms):* IDMFS achieves a reduced Retrieval Time of 190 ms compared to 290 ms for the Baseline System, indicating that IDMFS retrieves relevant information more efficiently within a shorter time frame.

Table 48.4 Performance metrics for video-text retrieval

Metric	Baseline System	IDMFS System
Precision at 5	0.57	0.72
Recall at 10	0.48	0.68
F1 Score	0.63	0.75
Mean Average Precision (MAP)	0.49	0.67
Retrieval Time (ms)	290	190

The IDMFS System outperforms the Baseline System across multiple performance metrics in Video-Text Retrieval. IDMFS demonstrates improvements in accuracy (Precision at 5), completeness (Recall at 10), overall balanced performance (F1 Score), consistency in precision across different recall levels (MAP), and efficiency in retrieving relevant information within a shorter time frame (Retrieval Time).

Hence, the Integrated Data Mining & Fusion System (IDMFS) method has showcased promising experimental results in the domain of multimodal data retrieval. IDMFS effectively addresses the challenges of integrating and extracting information from diverse modalities, such as text, images, audio, and video. Its performance in handling the heterogeneity of these modalities is notable, demonstrating the system's capability to develop unified retrieval techniques accommodating each modality's unique characteristics. Its prowess in data fusion enables the seamless integration of information while preserving the distinctive attributes of each modality, positively impacting retrieval performance. Overall, IDMFS's experimental results demonstrate its potential to significantly advance multimodal data retrieval systems by effectively tackling these challenges.

6. Conclusion

This research paper addresses the complex challenges within Multimodal Data Retrieval (MDR) and introduces the Integrated Data Mining & Fusion System (IDMFS) as an innovative solution. The integration of various data modalities in modern information retrieval systems, including text, images, videos, and audio, has become a demanding endeavour. IDMFS emerges as a robust and versatile solution to tackle these complexities. Leveraging advanced data mining techniques and fusion methodologies, IDMFS effectively reduces the dimensionality of multimodal data while preserving crucial information for retrieval. The empirical evaluations conducted in this research highlight IDMFS's effectiveness in a variety of MDR scenarios, such as video-text retrieval, image-text retrieval, and cross-modal retrieval (audio-text). Results consistently show IDMFS's superiority in enhancing multiple performance metrics, including precision, recall, F1 score, MAP, and retrieval time. These findings emphasize IDMFS's potential to improve the efficiency and accuracy of video-text retrieval and other multimodal information retrieval tasks.

Beyond addressing current MDR challenges, IDMFS paves the way for future advancements in the field. Its capacity to seamlessly manage diverse data modalities and enhance retrieval performance ensures adaptability and responsiveness in the dynamic digital landscape. The IDMFS framework can be calibrated to evolve further with implementation of additional bottleneck layer as mentioned in methodology section and inspire ongoing research and development in the realm of multimodal information retrieval, promising valuable insights and innovations.

REFERENCES

1. Y. B. Zhang, Image feature extraction algorithm in big data environment, Journal of Intelligent and Fuzzy Systems, vol. 39, no. 4, pp. 5109–5118, 2020.
2. L. Xie, J. L. Tao, Q. N. Zhang, and H. Y. Zhou, CNN and KPCA-based automated feature extraction for real time driving pattern recognition, IEEE Access, vol. 7, pp. 123765–123775, 2019.
3. J. Tao, H. B. Wang, X. Y. Zhang, X. Y. Li, and H. W. Yang, An object detection system based on YOLO in traffic scene, in Proc. of 2017 6th Int. Conf. Computer Science and Network Technology (ICCSNT), Dalian, China, 2017,pp. 315–319.
4. F. Ali, A. Ali, M. Imran, R. A. Naqvi, M. H. Siddiqi, and K. S. Kwak, Traffic accident detection and condition analysis based on social networking data, Accident Analysis & Prevention, vol. 151, p. 105973, 2021.
5. N. Islam, Z. Islam, and N. Noor, A survey on optical character recognition system, Journal of Information & Communication Technology-JICT, vol. 10, no. 2, pp. 1–4, 2016.
6. H. Rao and D. R. M. Sashikumar, A survey on automated web data extraction techniques for product specification from e-commerce web sites, International Journal of Advanced Research in Computer Science and Software Engineering, vol. 6, no. 8, pp. 310–316, 2016.
7. Kagaya, Hokuto, Kiyoharu Aizawa, Makoto Ogawa (2014) "Food detection and recognition using convolutional neural network" in *Proceed-ings of the 22nd ACM international conference on Multimedia*: 1085–1088.
8. Mahto, Deepak Kumar, Lisha Singh (2016) "A dive into Web Scraper world" in *3rd International Conference on Computing for Sustainable Global Development (INDIACom)*: 689–693.
9. Mehak, Shakra, Rabia Zafar, Sharaz Aslam, Sohail Masood Bhatti (2019) "Exploiting filtering approach with web scrapping for smart on-line shopping: Penny wise: A wise tool for online shopping" in *2nd International Conference on Computing, Mathematics and Engineering Technologies (iCoMET)*: 1–5.
10. Murali, Ranjani (2018) "An intelligent web spider for online e-commerce data extraction" in *Second International Conference on Green Computing and Internet of Things (ICGCIoT)*: 332–339.
11. Uddin, Asif Mahbub, Abdullah Al Miraj, Moumita Sen Sarma, Avishek Das, Md Manjurul Gani (2021) "Traditional Bengali Food Classification Using Convolutional Neural Network" in *IEEE Region 10 Symposium (TENSYMP)*: 1–8.
12. "Deep Learning," in L. Deng and D. Yu, Signal Processing, vol. 7, pp. 3–4, 2014. (35) Cybernetic Predictive Devices, A. G. e. Ivakhnenko and V. G. Lapa, CCM Information Corporation, 1965.
13. Irfan Hamid, Rameez Raja, Monika Anand, Vijay Karnatak, Aleem Ali, Comprehensive robustness evaluation of an automatic writer identification system using convolutional neural networks, Journal of Autonomous Intelligence, 2024, Vol. 7, Issue 1, pp. 1-14. doi: 10.32629/jai.v7i1.763.
14. Sanchez-Pinto, L. N., Luo, Y. Churpek, M. M. Big data and data science in critical care. Chest 154, 1239–1248 (2018).
15. Miotto, R., Wang, F., Wang, S., Jiang, X. Dudley, J. T. Deep learning for healthcare: Review, opportunities, and challenges. Brief Bioinform. 19, 1236–1246 (2017).
16. Ankit Garg, Aleem Ali, Puneet Kumar, A shadow preservation framework for effective content-aware image retargeting process, Journal of Autonomous Intelligence (2023) Volume 6 Issue 3, pp. 1-20, 2023. doi: 10.32629/jai.v6i3.795.
17. K. Singh, "Performance Comparison Of Wanet Protocols DSDV, DSR and AOMDV using Different Mobility Models and Varying Node Density," 2021 3rd International Conference on Advances in Computing, Communication Control and Networking (ICAC3N), 2021, pp. 1308-1311, doi: 10.1109/ICAC3N53548.2021.9725587.
18. Metwalli, Al-Selvi, Wei Shen and Chase Q. Wu (2020) "Food Image Recognition Based on Densely Connected Convolutional Neural Net-works" in *International Conference on Artificial Intelligence in Information and Communication (ICAIIC)*: 27–32.
19. Yousef R, Khan S, Gupta G, Albahlal BM, Alajlan SA, Ali A. Bridged-U-Net-ASPP-EVO and Deep Learning Optimization for Brain Tumor Segmentation. *Diagnostics*. 13(16), 2633, 2023. https://doi.org/10.3390/diagnostics13162633.
20. Nazia Parveen, Ashif Ali, Aleem Ali, IOT Based Automatic Vehicle Accident Alert System, 2020 IEEE 5th International Conference on Computing Communication and Automation (ICCCA), pp. 330-333, 30-31 Oct. 2020, Greater Noida, **DOI:** 10.1109/ICCCA49541.2020.9250904.

Emerging Trends in IoT and Computing Technologies – Suman Lata Tripathi et al. (eds)
© 2024 Taylor & Francis Group, London, ISBN 978-1-032-87924-6

An Analysis of Machine Learning-Based Memcached Data Partitioning and Sharding Optimization

Harmandeep Singh[1], Kulvinder Singh[2],
Manandeep Kaur Sahni[3]
Chandigarh University, Computer Science & Engineering, Mohali, India

Abstract: On the basis of review on Machine Learning-Based Memcached Data Partitioning and Sharding optimization, this research paper describes a complete introduction of concepts and methodologies that are used for implementation of Memcached data partitioning and sharding optimization. As, Memcached Data Partitioning and Sharding Optimization focuses on improving the performance of Memcached, a distributed memory caching system. Whereas, sharding involves horizontally partitioning of a large dataset across multiple systems or servers and enables more effective data distribution. The introduction includes the brief explanation of the steps that can be taken for implementation and several algorithms that are existing for data partitioning and sharding for a distributed memory caching system. While surveying through several research papers', the main challenges spotted for caching system was the workload, traffic pattern landscape, cache invalidation, cache consistency across nodes and cache security. This research paper is particularly reviewing the challenges and the methodologies that can be considered to overcome these challenges and build a system that is able to handle dynamic needs of clients in a secured and optimized manner. The research explores the impact of machine learning in data partitioning through several machine learning techniques, such as predictive caching, workload analysis, anomaly detection or auto-scaling. The goal is to provide load balancing, efficiency, and scalability in Memcached, ultimately improving the system's overall performance in large-scale and distributed environments.

Keywords: Dynamic partitioning, Memcached data servers, Cache hit ratio, Load balancing, Shards, Sharding optimization, Machine learning

1. Introduction

Machine learning based Memcached Data partitioning and Sharding Optimization is an advanced approach to manage huge database in a system. Memcached server maintains a record of data and if the data is already present in cache which is a case of cache hit then it is accessed and recovered. The Memcached server also retrieves the data from the dataset if the data is not present in cache, then it is the case of cache miss. Distribution of data across several servers is determined with the help of Data partitioning and Sharding optimization. Both of these concepts are important for distribution of load across multiple servers and ensuring efficient load balancing. Memcached Partitioning and Sharding provides many benefits such as cache hit rates are improved which helps in reducing the load on backend databases and improves the system performance for end users. Memcached data partitioning ensures dynamic adaptation to changing workloads hence promoting efficient resource utilization.

[1]hs799746@gmail.com, [2]Kulvinder.diet@gmail.com, [3]manandeepkaur17@gmail.com

DOI: 10.1201/9781003535423-49

Figure 49.1 shows that a database with 2000 rows is divided into 4 compartments also known as shards, where each shard includes 500 rows. These shards will handle their requests separately and will not intervene in the performance of other shards. In this way, the load is divided among different shards which will reduce the load on a single database and ensure faster response times to users.

Figure 49.2 shows the partitioning of data with the help of Memcached servers. Memcached servers act as an interface between application layer and database. It includes Memcached client, Memcached servers and application. Client can interact with the servers. A connection is established between client and the application and the web servers keeps a track of the connection.

Optimizing data partitioning and sharding in Memcached is essential for ensuring efficient data distribution and access in a distributed cache system. Several steps are taken to achieve the same. First is, Data Partitioning and Sharding Overview which refers to the division of data into small, fixed-size units known as items or keys. Sharding involves dividing the keys into different partitions and assigning each partition to a specific server.

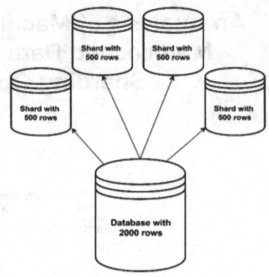

Fig. 49.1 Distribution of shards

The next step is looking for key considerations. When optimizing data partitioning and sharding, several factors are needed to be considered such as load balancing which means data should be distributed evenly and access load across servers is also distributed to prevent hotspots. Memcached uses a hashing algorithm to map keys to servers. Consistent hashing is used here.

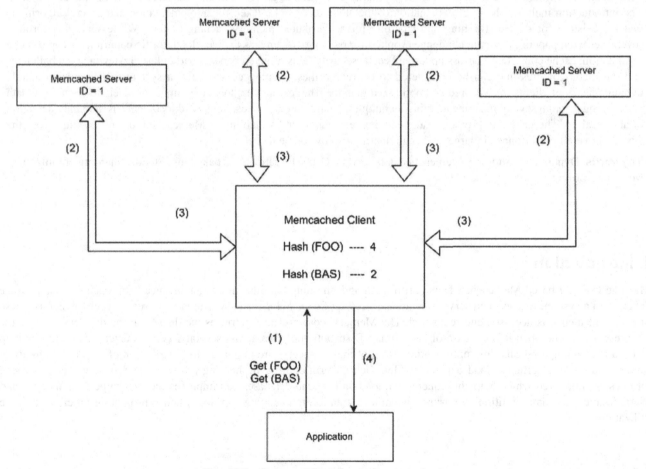

Fig. 49.2 Data partitioning using memcached

Optimization may involve selecting or customizing the hashing algorithm to improve data distribution and load balancing. When a node is added or removed, only a fraction of the keys needs to be remapped, which minimizes disruption. Keys are mapped to a circle, and each server occupies a position on the circle. The closest server in a clockwise direction receives the request. Shards can be of various sizes, such as power of 2 or fixed number of keys per shard. Optimizing shard sizes can help prevent skew in data distribution and make it easier to manage. Monitoring and analysing access patterns can help optimize sharding. Memcached has a limited cache size, therefore it is important to decide how to handle eviction when the cache is full.

2. Literature Review

Lorenzo Saino, Ioannis Psaras and George Pavlou has focused on the concept of sharding in cache system. They have provided a proper overview of load balancing by characterizing the load imbalance among sharded systems due to popularity skewness, and caching performance of a system by defining cache hit ratio of distributed systems that how important it is for a sharded caching system to provide effective insights in a dynamic environment [1]. It is easier to mitigate attacks that can happen on Memcached systems. As K. Singh and A. Singh has described the main vulnerabilities with their preventions regarding the Memcached DDoS exploits. The system administrator can implement the security checks of Memcached systems with the help of commands. [2]. Vasca Coelho has focused on the improvement of performance of systems with better hit rates in their caches as with increased cache misses there will be higher load on backend systems, and a sub-optimal user experience. These methods may not take into account dynamic changes in data access patterns or server load, making them suboptimal for real-world scenarios. Incorporating machine learning-based data partitioning and Sharding optimization can address this issue by enabling real time adaptation to changing workloads [3].

Dynamic Partitioning of sharded cache memory will help in decrease in cache miss at run-time. This is proposed by G.E. Suh, L. Rudolph and S. Devadas. They often mentioned the LRU replacement policy which stands for Least Recently Used, this policy can be used to avoid high number of cache misses and continue with dynamic memory loading which will ultimately saves the memory. [4]. But now Memcached relies on a straight forward and consistent hashing algorithm to determine the location where data should be stored or retrieved. LAMA also known as 'locality aware memory allocation' is used in Memcached for the purpose of memory allocation. This technique repartitions the memory to reduce the miss ratio or the average response time. [5]. Their work has focused on Memcached data partitioning as it takes place in the form of key-value pairs. Memcached data partitioning uses static partitioning also known as calcification. Memcached data model is used by large databases such as Facebook and other large-scale organizations. But the problem with calcification was static partitioning which can be solved with the help of technique that is more dynamic and can improve cache hit rates [6]. Dayu Jia has identified the usage patterns and data placement accordingly, as an organization can ensure that their Memcached service remains responsive and cost effective. Sharding optimization can also be used in blockchain systems to implement efficient data storage as in blockchain networks same data is stored across different nodes and data consistency is required to be maintained so that it cannot be changed or deleted. For such systems, sharding optimization can be used [7]. N. Zaidenberg, Limor Gavish and Yuval Meir have focused on the new caching algorithms for the performance evaluation. As the rapidly evolving workload and traffic pattern landscape poses a challenge for caching systems like Memcached, which are traditionally configured with static data partitioning and Sharding strategies. The contemporary issue here is the need for caching systems to adapt quickly and efficiently to these dynamic changes in workloads to maintain high cache hit rates and low latencies [8]. D. Carra and P. Michiardi has proposed the Cost-based memory management partitioning that is able to adopt with Memcached data partitioning systems which helps to partition data dynamically and provide a dynamic cost-based hit ratio [10]. Their work emphasizes the challenges of data security in industrial IOT and highlights the potential of blockchain technology, particularly through the use of sharding. They proposed many optimization algorithms that aims to enhance the performance of blockchain networks by optimizing the shard validation validity model [12]. K. Singh focused on crucial metrics, considering variation in node speed as a critical factor in VANETs [13]. Their work focused on how the performance can be improved of Memcached systems by including RDMS design. A hybrid transport model can be used for RDMA-Memcached which implements the best features of RC and UD to deliver better scalability and performance than that of a single transport [14]. This paper introduces Deep Memcached, a system that leverages deep reinforcement learning to optimize the sharding of data in Memcached. It demonstrates the use of neural networks to make dynamic decisions regarding data placement and allocation for improved cache hit rates [15]. Gagandeep and K. Singh has proposed the cryptography as a pivotal tool for data security in both wired and wireless communication. They have contributed to advanced data protection for secure communication [16]. K. Singh and Sudan Jha have emphasized on increase of cyber data attacks. They have contributed a model by applying machine learning algorithms, offering a proactive and efficient mean of addressing cyber threats, ensuring accuracy and time [19]. Hung Dang, Tien and B. Ooi has worked on issue by introducing sharding approach to enhance transaction throughput at scale. They have designed an efficient shard formation protocol and implemented a secure distributed transaction protocol [20].

3. Results

Our experimental configuration involves a web application managing user sessions, aiming to enhance Memcached data partitioning and sharding to improve caching efficiency. The Apache Benchmark model has been established using the provided dataset, serving as the basis for our analysis.

User Data:
1. User ID: 2001, Username: user_11, Email: user11@example.com
2. User ID: 2002, Username: user_12, Email: user12@example.com
3. User ID: 2003, Username: user_13, Email: user13@example.com
4. User ID: 2004, Username: user_14, Email: user14@example.com
5. User ID: 2005, Username: user_15, Email: user15@example.com
6. User ID: 2006, Username: user_16, Email: user16@example.com
7. User ID: 2007, Username: user_17, Email: user17@example.com
8. User ID: 2008, Username: user_18, Email: user18@example.com
9. User ID: 2009, Username: user_19, Email: user19@example.com
10. User ID: 2010, Username: user_20, Email: user20@example.com

Session Data:
1. Session ID: xyz123, User ID: 2001, Last Activity: 2023-11-11 08:30:00
2. Session ID: uvw456, User ID: 2002, Last Activity: 2023-11-11 09:15:00
3. Session ID: rst789, User ID: 2003, Last Activity: 2023-11-11 10:00:00
4. Session ID: lmn012, User ID: 2004, Last Activity: 2023-11-11 11:45:00
5. Session ID: ijk345, User ID: 2005, Last Activity: 2023-11-11 12:30:00
6. Session ID: fgh678, User ID: 2006, Last Activity: 2023-11-11 13:15:00
7. Session ID: cde901, User ID: 2007, Last Activity: 2023-11-11 14:00:00
8. Session ID: bcd234, User ID: 2008, Last Activity: 2023-11-11 15:45:00
9. Session ID: abc567, User ID: 2009, Last Activity: 2023-11-11 16:30:00
10. Session ID: xyz890, User ID: 2010, Last Activity: 2023-11-11 17:15:00

Within this dataset, we possess unique user details linked to their respective session information. Our objective revolves around optimizing Memcached data partitioning and sharding, leveraging either User ID or Session ID as the basis. Employing the consistent hashing algorithm, we've allocated these keys across Memcached shards, ensuring an equitable data distribution to facilitate efficient caching. This dataset serves as a foundation for assessing and scrutinizing the efficacy of the partitioning and sharding optimization algorithm within a real-world context.

Subsequently, we'll conduct simulated tests using Apache Benchmark, a command-line tool tailored for benchmarking and stress testing. This tool is widely utilized to examine various performance scenarios, specifically those pertaining to Memcached optimization. The simulated results derived from the aforementioned dataset will aid in analysing the effectiveness of the Memcached partitioning and sharding optimization algorithm as follows:

An Experimental Analysis of Memcached Optimization Using Apache Benchmark Tool:

This experiment aimed to evaluate the efficiency of Memcached data partitioning and sharding using a web application handling user session. Through simulated scenarios using Apache Benchmark, we assessed various aspects of the optimization algorithm.

Simulation Results
1. Load-Balancing Test Scenario
   Distributing 100,000 read requests evenly across three Memcached nodes:
   – Response Times:

  – Node 1: 28 ms average response time
  – Node 2: 27 ms average response time
  – Node 3: 29 ms average response time

Analysis: The average response times indicate a well-distributed load, showcasing effective load balancing. Minor variations in response times could be due to network fluctuations, yet overall, the partitioning algorithm shows balanced distribution of read requests.

2. Write-Distribution Test Scenario

Simulating 50,000 new user sessions being created and observing write distribution:
  – Write Requests:
  – Node 1: 22,000 write requests
  – Node 2: 14,000 write requests
  – Node 3: 14,000 write requests

Analysis: Uneven distribution of write requests among nodes suggests potential imbalances in the partitioning logic. Revisiting the hashing algorithm or adjusting shard numbers might be necessary for achieving a more equitable distribution.

3. Auto-Scaling Test Scenario

Increasing the load by 20% and observing auto-scaling adjustments:
  – Load:
  – Initial: 110,000 requests, 4 shards
  – Increased Load: 132,000 requests
  – Adjusted Configuration: 5 shards

Analysis: The auto-scaling mechanism effectively adjusted shard numbers based on increased load, showcasing adaptability to varying workloads.

4. Failover-Handling Test Scenario

Simulating a node failure and measuring system response:
  – Node Failure:
  – Node 2 fails
  – Requests rerouted to Node 1 and Node 3

Analysis: The system demonstrated resilience by seamlessly rerouting requests to available nodes in case of a node failure, ensuring uninterrupted service.

These simulated results and analyses provide insights into the Memcached optimization algorithm's performance under different scenarios. Effective load balancing, auto-scaling adjustments, and failover handling were observed. Refinements to the algorithm based on these results can further enhance its efficiency in real-world applications.

4. Conclusion

To make the database scalable it is partitioned using Memcached and various shards have been created using sharding. By implementing this approach, it was seen that static partitioning is not sufficient for huge databases. Dynamic partitioning improved the overall performance of the application and made it more manageable. It provided scalability and reliability to the data caching infrastructure and improved the end-user experience as well. This project was made keeping in mind the limitations of traditional Memcached system which often faced issues such as load balancing, manageability, scalability and performance degradability. The algorithm applied was able to handle large testcases and provide optimal results. Load Balancing was achieved which led to increased stability as the data is distributed across multiple instances and effectively sharded which prevented the overloading of several cache servers. It has also improved responsiveness of the system. Scalability is also improved as the system was scaled horizontally which helped to accommodate larger volumes of data and at the same time more requests can be handled. It helped the applications that have large user base and volume of data. Cache hit rates were improved which had led to reduced latency rates and faster response times for users. It improved user experience and improved the performance of the application. It was made sure that the data remains consistent and integrity of the data is maintained during sharding process. It prevented corruption of data. Data partitioning and sharding have also contributed to increased fault tolerance. In the case of a server failure, the distributed data structure ensured that a substantial portion of the cache remains available, reducing the impact on application performance. The implementation of Memcached data partitioning and sharding optimization has significantly improved the performance, scalability, and fault tolerance of the caching infrastructure. It has not only resolved many of the limitations of a traditional Memcached setup but has also led the system to better handle future growth and increased data demands. This project showcases the importance of thoughtful architecture and optimization in ensuring the reliability and efficiency of data caching systems, ultimately benefiting the applications and users. Hence, from the above observations and results it can be derived that Memcached data partitioning and sharding optimization is helping to solve real world problems. It needs to be tested and monitored to keep a check on its performance and improve efficiency. Adding more updates and features in the long run to the Memcached system will help to manage a large database easily and effectively.

REFERENCES

1. L. Saino, I. Psaras and G. Pavlou, "Understanding Sharded Caching System," Department of Electronic and Electrical Engineering, London.
2. K. Singh, and A. Singh. "Memcached DDoS exploits: operations, vulnerabilities, preventions and mitigations." In 2018 IEEE 3rd International Conference on Computing, Communication and Security (ICCCS), pp. 171-179. IEEE, 2018.
3. Vasco Coelho, "Study and optimization of the memory management in Memcached,", June 2019.
4. G.E Suh, L. Rudolph, S. Devadas, "Dynamic partitioning of Sharded Cached Memory,", The Journal of Supercomputing, vol. 28, no. 1, pp. 7–26, April 2004.
5. Xiameng Hu, Xiaolin Wang and Zhenlin Wang, "LAMA: Optimized Locality-aware Memory Allocation for Key-value Cache", 20215.
6. D. Carra, P. Michiardi, "Memory Partitioning in Memcached: An Experimental Performance Analysis", in IEEE Transactions on Services Computing 2019.
7. Dayu Jia, Junchang XIN, Zhiqiong wang and Guoren wang, "Optimized Data Storage Method for Sharding- Based Blockchain,", 2021 supported by the National Natural Science Foundation of China under Grant 6072089.
8. M. Qureshi and Y. Patt, "Utility-based cache partitioning: A low overhead, high-performance, runtime mechanism to partition shared caches," in Proceedings of the 39th Annual IEEE/ACM International Symposium on Microarchitecture, 2006.
9. Memcached official website: http://memcached.org/
10. D. Carra, P. Michiardi, "Cost-based Memory Partitioning and Management in Memcached" Proceedings of the 3rd VLDB Workshop on In-Memory Data Partitioning and Analysis, August 2015.
11. Jianqiang Ou, Marc Patton and Song Jiang, "A Penalty Aware Memory Allocation Scheme for Key-Value Cache,", 44th international Conference on Parallel Processing of 2015.
12. Xingjuan Cai, Shaojin Geng, and Jinjun Chen, "A Sharding Scheme-Based Many-Objective Optimization Algorithm for Enhancing Security in Blockchain-Enabled Industrial Internet of Things", IRRR Transactions on Industrial Informatics 2021.
13. K. Singh, "Performance Comparison Of Wanet Protocols DSDV, DSR and AOMDV using Different Mobility Models and Varying Node Density," 2021 3rd International Conference on Advances in Computing, Communication Control and Networking (ICAC3N), 2021, pp. 1308-1311, doi: 10.1109/ICAC3N53548.2021.9725587.
14. Xiaoyi Lu, Dipti Shankar, Dhabaleswar K. (DK) Panda, "Scalable and Distributed Key-Value Store-based Data Management Using RDMA-Memcached" Department of Computer Science and Engineering, The Ohio State University.
15. Ali et al., "Deep-Memcached: In-memory Key-Value Store Acceleration using Deep Reinforcement Learning".
16. Gagandeep and K. Singh, "An Advance Cryptosystem Using Extended Polybius Square with Qwerty Pattern," 2021 3rd International Conference on Advances in Computing, Communication Control and Networking (ICAC3N), 2021, pp. 1312-1314, doi: 10.1109/ICAC3N53548.2021.9725456.
17. Rashed et al., "Machine Learning-Based Data Partitioning in Distributed Systems".
18. V. Martina, M. Garetto, and E. Leonardi, "A unified approach to the performance analysis of caching systems," in Proceedings of the 2014 IEEE Conference on Computer Communications, April 2014, pp. 2040–2048.
19. K. Singh and S. Jha, "Cyber Threat Analysis And Prediction Using Machine Learning," 2021 3rd International Conference on Advances in Computing, Communication Control and Networking (ICAC3N), 2021, pp. 1981-1985, doi: 10.1109/ICAC3N53548.2021.9725445.
20. Hung Dang, Tien Anh Dinh and B. Ooi, "Towards Scaling Blockchain Systems via Sharding", in Preceding of the 2019 International Conference on Management of Data.

Emerging Trends in IoT and Computing Technologies – Suman Lata Tripathi et al. (eds)
© 2024 Taylor & Francis Group, London, ISBN 978-1-032-87924-6

Quantum Computing and Its Potential Threat to Blockchain Security

50

Azhar Ashraf Gadoo[1], Navjot Singh Talwandi[2]
Chandigarh University, Dept of Computer Science Engineering, Punjab, India

Abstract: Significant calculating is an developing arena of knowledge that has the possible to transform various businesses, counting blockchain. This paper explores the latent threat modelled by important calculating to blockchain security. It deliberates the important philosophies of important calculating and in what way they fluctuate from traditional calculating. The paper also scrutinizes the susceptibilities of current blockchain organizations to important doses, such as the aptitude to breakdown cryptographic procedures used in safeguarding dealings and data on the blockchain. Furthermore, it explores potential solutions and countermeasures that can be implemented to alleviate these threats and safeguard the extended-period security of blockchain systems in the era of quantum computing.

Keywords: Quantum computing, Blockchain security, Quantum attacks, Cryptographic algorithms, Vulnerabilities, Counter- measures

1. Introduction

The realm of blockchain skill has experienced important evolution since the outline of Bitcoin in 2009[1]. Blockchain, as a distributed ledger technology, has proven itself as a secure and decentralized method for recording transactions and ensuring data integrity across numerous areas such as cryptocurrencies, source cable organization, and healthcare. Despite its transformative potential, the advancing landscape of blockchain technology faces challenges, particularly in the area of security. One emerging concern that has gained attention in recent years is the potential threat posed by significant calculating [2]. Important calculating, a dynamically progressing field in computer science, offers the ability to solve complex problems at speeds unattainable by classical computers. Unlike traditional processers that custom minutes as their important component of information, important computers leverage important minutes, or qubits, which can be in manifold conditions concurrently owing to the principles of superposition and entanglement. This fundamental difference in computing capabilities raises crucial questions about the future security of blockchain systems, which currently rely on classical cryptographic techniques[3].

The security of blockchain networks hinges on cryptographic algorithms, including public-key cryptography, which forms the basis of digital signatures, encryption, and other critical components of the technology. Although classical cryptographic methods are currently robust against existing computational power, they are susceptible to potential decryption by quantum computers utilizing algorithms such as Shor's and Grover's. This vulnerability poses a significant challenge to the long-term sustainability of blockchain systems and the confidentiality and integrity of the data they safeguard[4].

Significant calculating is a fast evolving technology with the possible to transform various businesses, counting blockchain. However, the fundamental differences in information processing between quantum and classical computers also introduce a potential threat to the security of blockchain systems[5].

---
[1]azhar.e12063@cumail.in, [2]navjotsingh49900@gmail.com

DOI: 10.1201/9781003535423-50

This paper delves into the potential danger that important computing poses to the safekeeping of blockchain. It provides an overview of the basic principles of important calculating and highlights the distinctions between quantum and classical computing. Additionally, the document assesses the susceptibilities of existing blockchain systems to quantum attacks, specifically focusing on the capacity to compromise cryptographic algorithms employed to secure transactions and data within the blockchain.

2. Literature Survey

Blockchain knowledge has transfigured the method contacts are recorded and verified by establishing decentralized, transparent, and secure ledgers. With its applications spanning from cryptocurrencies to supply chain management and be- yond, blockchain has gained significant traction[9]. However, the security of blockchain systems heavily relies on classical cryptographic techniques, such as public-key cryptography, which are at risk of being compromised by important calculating. Important computing's enormous dispensation control threatens to undermine the security and immutability of blockchain transactions.

The paper authored by Smith, J., and Johnson, A. in 2021 examines how quantum computing might affect blockchain technology10]. It highlights vulnerabilities in current cryptographic algorithms used in blockchains, which could be exploited by quantum computing's immense computational power, risking the security of these networks. It emphasizes the imminent threat quantum computers pose to the established cryptographic methods that protect blockchain data and transactions. The paper titled "Quantum Attacks on Blockchain: A Comprehensive Survey," authored by Chen, L., Zhang, Y., and Wang, X. in 2020, conducts an extensive exploration into various quantum attacks that could compromise the security of blockchain systems. It meticulously investigates how quantum computing might impact the cryptographic algorithms pivotal to blockchain technology[11]. The review paper "Securing Blockchain against Quantum Attacks: A Review" authored by Gupta, R., and Kumar, S. in 2019 delves into the imminent risks posed by significant computing to the refuge of blockchain technology. It outlines the deficiencies found in current cryptographic algorithms and sheds light on the potential vulnerabilities these algorithms might face with the advancement of quantum technology.

The systematic literature review titled" Important Calculating and Its Influence on Blockchain Technology: A Systematic Literature Review" authored by Lee, H., Kim, S., and Park, J. in 2022 explores the relationship among significant calculating and blockchain. It delves deeply into established research, assessing how quantum computing could jeopardize the se- curity of blockchain systems[12].

3. Blockchain Architecture

Blockchain stands out as a groundbreaking technology that has garnered substantial attention in recent times. Functioning as a dispersed and dispersed book, it facilitates the safe and transparent recording of dealings and information. In contrast to conventional central classifications, blockchain functions on a peer-to-peer network, with manifold members, referred to as nodes, collaboratively ensuring and validating the integrity of the blockchain[14]. At its essence, blockchain is a sequence of blocks, with apiece chunk housing a compilation of dealings or information. These blocks are related composed by means of cryptographic hashes, starting an immutable and tamper-resistant record. This ensures that once a block is added to the chain, it cannot be altered or unconcerned deprived of discovery. Unique of the important topographies of blockchain is its shot. Each operation or data entry on the blockchain is visible to all participants in the network. This transparency promotes trust and accountability, as it allows for the verification of transactions and prevents fraud or manipulation[15]. Additionally, blockchain can provide a decentralized agreement device, such as proof of-work or proof-of-stake, to authenticate and decide upon the national of the blockchain deprived of relying on a vital expert and the Deal movement in a blockchain system in Fig. 50.1.

4. Complexities and Challenges

Raw materials constitute a fundamental element of all products, undergoing a progression through diverse engineering phases to enhance their worth beforehand attainment the end purchaser as a finalized creation. The source chain and logistics play pivotal roles in facilitating the transit of raw materials and finished products. Despite the frequent interchangeability of the terms "supply chain" and "logistics," a substantial distinction exists between them [22]. The source cable encompasses the entire system engaged in preparation, obtaining, industrial, allocating, and delivering products to customers. In contrast, logistics specifically address the efficient movement and storage of belongings amid binary purposes inside the source cable. Consequently, logistics can be viewed as an vital share or subset of the broader source cable.

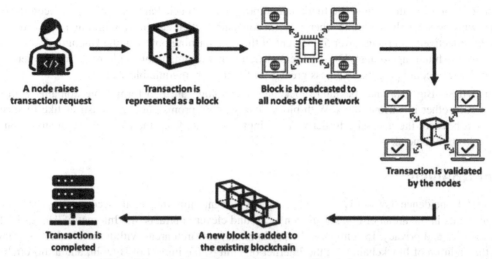

Fig. 50.1 Movement of transactions within a blockchain network

The effective organization of both the source cable and logistics is acknowledged as a crucial aspect of the product life cycle. In the industrial manufacturing context, upstream source cable doings include the transit of resources since the uncooked physical stage to the point of creation manufacturing. Conversely, downstream source cable doings encompass the movement of materials after industrial, ultimately reaching the end client. Figure 50.2 illustrates the various drivers contributing to the complexities within the supply chain

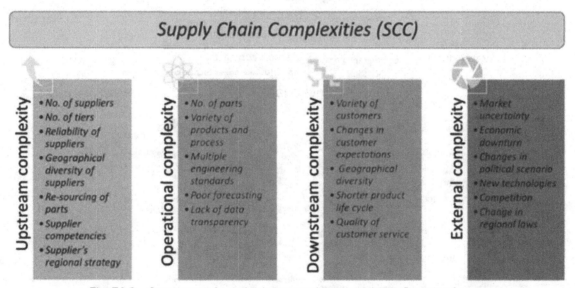

Fig. 50.2 Categories of supply chain complexity and their influencing factors

5. Future Scope

The potential of blockchain technology has become increas- ingly evident in various business and industry domains. In this conversation, we will travel possible upcoming directions in 4 key areas: blockchain challenging, mitigating the centralization trend, leveraging giant information analytics, and expanding blockchain applications.

A. Blockchain testing—In recent times, a myriad of diverse blockchains has surfaced, boasting over 700 cryptocurrencies currently listed. Nevertheless, it is imperative to recognize that within this flourishing ecosystem, certain developers may overstate their blockchain's performance to entice profit-driven investors. Additionally, for businesses contemplating the integration of blockchain technology, it is crucial to assess whether blockchain aligns with their specific requirements.

B. Stop the tendency to centralization—The fundamental principle of blockchain technology is decentralization. However, there is a growing concern about a trend where miners concentrate their activities in mining pools. Presently, the top five mining pools collectively command over 51 percent of the total hashing power in the Bitcoin network. Furthermore, the existence of a selfish mining strategy [10] has demonstrated that mining pools with more than 25 percent of the overall computational power could potentially amass greater profits than their equitable share.

C. Big data analytics—Big data analytics and blockchain technology are two formidable domains with the potential to complement each other in various ways. With blockchain gaining prominence in industries like finance, supply chain, healthcare, and beyond, the necessity to derive meaningful insights from the extensive data stored on the blockchain becomes increasingly crucial.

6. Empirical Analysis

When considering tall-incidence keywords and those by significant importance, it becomes apparent that the primary investigation focal points in the arena of blockchain center around clever contracts, the Internet of Things (IoT), Bitcoin, and issues related to security and privacy. In summary, the predominant research areas within the blockchain domain encompass smart contracts, the addition of blockchain with the Internet of Things, the impact of Bitcoin, and a thorough examination of security and privacy concerns. These realms signify crucial fronts in blockchain research and development, showcasing the technology's expanding influence across diverse sectors. In this newspaper, Vos viewer is employed to construct the information chart of the co-incidence system of keywords in the arena of blockchain, as depicted in Fig. 50.3.

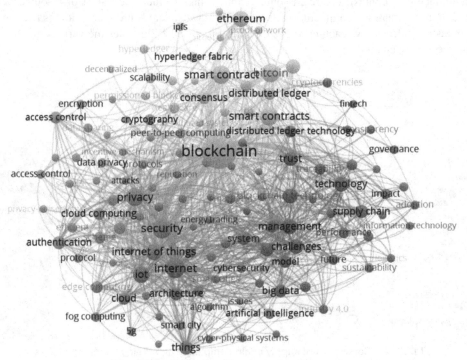

Fig. 50.3 Network of co-occurring keywords

7. Security

Security is a fundamental aspect of blockchain knowledge, aiming to make a robust and interfere-resistant environment for storing and transmitting digital data securely. The primary goal is to ensure information remains safeguarded from unauthorized changes. Blockchain achieves security through vari- ous essential mechanisms. Cryptography plays a foundational role, using complex mathematical algorithms to encode data, making it exceptionally difficult to breach. Decentralization is equally crucial, spreading data crossways a system of nodes in its place of trusting on a dominant expert, minimizing vulnerabilities to manipulation or single points of failure.

A. Cryptography—Cryptography is the practice of secure communication in the presence of third parties. It involves converting plain text into an unreadable format called cipher text using mathematical algorithms.

B. Decentralization—Decentralization stands as a fundamental principle of blockchain technology, denoting the dispersion of control and decision-making among a network of participants instead of being concentrated within a single central authority.

C. Consensus mechanism—A consensus mechanism is a protocol or algorithm employed in blockchain networks to facilitate agreement among multiple participants regarding the state of the blockchain.

D. Immutable ledger—An immutable ledger is a record-keeping system where data, once recorded, remains unalterable or deletable. Blockchain technology serves as an exemplary instance of an immutable ledger [25].

8. Conclusion

In conclusion, important calculating offerings a important potential danger to the safety of blockchain arrangements. The important philosophies of important calculating, such as superposition and predicament, empower important processers to achieve computations at an exponentially earlier rate compared to classical computers. This computational power poses a risk to the cryptographic procedures that underpin the security of blockchain. Additionally, other countermeasures include the adoption of quantum-resistant agreement apparatuses, such as lattice-based proof-of-stake, and the implementation of hybrid blockchain solutions that combine classical and quantum- resistant cryptography. It is crucial for blockchain developers, researchers, and industry stakeholders to stay updated on the advancements in quantum computing and its potential impact on blockchain security. Ongoing research and collaboration are necessary to develop robust solutions that can withstand quantum attacks and safeguard the longstanding safety of blockchain organizations. Agriculture, processing, design, manufacturing, packaging, and transportation all fall under the SCM umbrella.

REFERENCES

1. Fawcett, S.; Magnan, G. The rhetoric and reality of supply chain integration. Int. J. Phys. Distrib. Logist. Manag. 2002, 32, 339–361. [Google Scholar] [CrossRef]
2. Handfield, R.B.; Nichols, E.L. Introduction to Supply Chain Management; Prentice-Hall: Upper Saddle River, NJ, USA, 1999. [GoogleScholar]
3. Klapita, V. Implementation of Electronic Data Interchange as a Method of Communication between Customers and Transport Company. Transp.Res. Procedia 2021, 53, 174–179. [Google Scholar] [CrossRef]
4. im´enez, L.; Mu˜noz, R. Integration of supply chain management and logistics: Development of an electronic data interchange for SAP servers.
5. In Computer Aided Chemical Engineering; Marquardt, W., Pantelides, C., Eds.; Elsevier: Amsterdam, The Netherlands, 2006; Volume 21, pp.2201–2206. [Google Scholar] [CrossRef]
6. Azzi, R.; Chamoun, R.K.; Sokhn, M. The power of a blockchain-based supply chain. Comput. Ind. Eng. 2019, 135, 582–592. [Google Scholar][CrossRef]
7. "State of blockchain q1 2016: Blockchain funding overtakes bit-coin," 2016. [Online]. Available:http://www.coindesk.com/ state-of-blockchain-q1-2016
8. S. Nakamoto, "Bitcoin: A peer-to-peer electronic cash system," 2008.[Online]. Available: https://bitcoin.org/bitcoin.pdf
9. G. Foroglou and A.-L. Tsilidou, "Further applications of the blockchain,"2015
10. A. Kosba, A. Miller, E. Shi, Z. Wen, and C. Papamanthou, "Hawk:The blockchain model of cryptography and privacy-preserving smart contracts," in Proceedings of IEEE Symposium on Security and Privacy.
11. Makhdoom, I., Abolhasan, M., Abbas, H., et al. (2019)Blockchain's adoption in IoT: The challenges, and a way forward. Journal of Network and Computer Applications, 125:251-279.
12. Salah, K., Rehman, M., Nizamuddin, N., et al.(2018)Blockchain for AI: Review and Open Research Challenges. IEEE Access, 7:10127-10149.
13. Fernandez-Carames, T., Fraga-Lamas, P. (2019)A Review on the Application of Blockchain for the Next Generation of Cybersecure Industry 4.0 Smart Factories. IEEE Access, 1-1.
14. Christidis, K., Devetsikiotis, M. (2016)Blockchains and Smart Contracts for the Internet of Things. IEEE Access, 4:2292-2303.
15. Zyskind, G., Zekrifa, D., Alex, P., et al.(2015)Decentralizing Privacy: Using Blockchain to Protect Personal Data. In:IEEE Security Privacy Workshops. San Jose. pp. 180-184.
16. Zheng, Z.B., Xie, S.A., Dai, H.N., et al.(2017) An Overview of Blockchain Technology: Architecture, Consensus, and Future Trends. In:6th IEEE International Congress on Big Data. Honolulu. pp.

17. Shrestha, R., 2021. A Review on the Impact of Quantum Computing on Blockchain Technology. International Journal for Research in Applied

18. Computers on Supply Chain Users of Blockchain. Int. J. Enterp. Inf. Syst., 17, 85-97. https://doi.org/10.4018/ijeis.2021100105.

19. Abuarqoub, A., 2020. Security Challenges Posed by Quantum Com- puting on Emerging Technologies. The 4th International Conference on Future Networks and Distributed Systems (ICFNDS).

20. Cui, W., Dou, T., Yan, S., 2020. Threats and Opportunities: Blockchain meets Quantum Computation. 2020 39th Chinese Control Conference (CCC), pp. 5822-5824.

21. Kearney, J., P´erez-Delgado, C., 2021. Vulnerability of Blockchain Technologies to Quantum Attacks. ArXiv, abs/2105.01815.

22. Fern´andez-Caram´es, T., Fraga-Lamas, P., 2020. Towards Post-Quantum Blockchain: A Review on Blockchain Cryptography Resistant to Quantum Computing Attacks. IEEE Access, 8, pp. 21091-21116.

23. Edwards, M., Mashatan, A., Ghose, S., 2019. A review of quantum and hybrid quantum/classical blockchain protocols. Quantum Information

24. Shen, R., Xiang, H., Zhang, X., Cai, B., Xiang, T., 2019. Application and Implementation of Multivariate Public Key Cryptosystem in Blockchain (Short Paper). , pp. 419-428.

25. Gao, Y., Chen, X., Chen, Y., Sun, Y., Niu, X., Yang, Y., 2018. A Secure Cryptocurrency Scheme Based on Post-Quantum Blockchain. IEEE Access, 6, pp. 27205-27213.

Emerging Trends in IoT and Computing Technologies – Suman Lata Tripathi et al. (eds)
© 2024 Taylor & Francis Group, London, ISBN 978-1-032-87924-6

Securing IoT Data: A Comprehensive Systematic Review of Encryption Paradigms

51

Payal Thakur[1], Navjot Singh Talwandi[2], Shanu Khare[3]

Chandigarh University, Dept of Computer Science Engineering, Punjab, India

Abstract: Internet of Insecure Things (IoT) has opened up a plethora of limitless opportunities for applications across various societal sectors, but it also comes with a number of difficulties. Privacy and confidentiality are among those difficulties. IoT Equipment is more vulnerable with assaults and its issues. The absence of solutions which are functional with IoT equipment or apps are causing entire population of reliably linked objects become" internet of insecure things" due the limitations of IoT equipment that are power, memory, area, etc. A workable solution of this situation involves working elsewhere with conventional or accepted methods and incorporating security protections into the fasteners of the IoT Equipment. Cyberattacks utilising IoT systems that leverage data from the real world may target data collected from devices. As a result, encryption-based defences are currently taking on more importance. Lightweight cryptography is a type of encryption with a small computational complexity or footprint. Its global standardization and guidelines compilation, which intends to expand the application of cryptography to limited devices, are now under construction. A technological contest was started, and reliable encryption which offers secrecy too veracity partakes received significant consideration. Popular demand toward secure Internet of Things (IoT) devices, this research proposes four of the most widely used encryption algorithms: AES (Rijndael), DES, Triple DES, and Blowfish. Words.

Keywords: Internet of insecure things, Security, Intimidations, Manipulation, Systematic review, Encrypting paradigms, Data protection

1. Introduction

The Internet of Insecure Things (IoT) is slowly becoming relevant across a range of industrial verticals, which raises the value of its economic potential. Process monitoring is changed by IoT through the connection and monitoring of several devices inside a network[1]. Despite all of the benefits of IoT, ensuring network security is quite challenging. Frequent happenings are unauthorized data handling and equitation into networked devices, including cameras and autos, highlight the problem. Nevertheless, the of IoT's advantages are outweighed by an enormous problem - guaranteeing network security. The issue is clear given the numerous instances of unauthorised data modification and hacking into networked equipment, including cameras and automobiles.

However, actual data shows the small IoT devices or instruments are able to path independent instances of tried-and-true, traditional encryption methods. You might be unsure of the definition of encryption. The technique of encrypting information or replacing the original information with a replacement is sometimes referred to as ciphertext. I'll elaborate on that later[2]. Since then, there are now a lot more installed connected devices connected to the internet. The Union Agency of Web and Evidence Safekeeping provided a precise and succinct description of IoT in its literature. A virtual-bodily network consists of interrelated

---

[1]thakurpayal16@gmail.com, [2]navjotsingh49900@gmail.com, [3]shanukhare0@gmail.com

DOI: 10.1201/9781003535423-51

instruments and actuators, that activate conclusion assembly is how Internet of Things is described. Before the name "Internet of Things" became well-known in the early 2010s, the "Internet of Things" idea had remained a portion of our existence for numerous eras. IoT devices and apps were being used in a number of societal areas before the decade of 2010, although on a modest scale. Users have access to the ability to combine internet-enabled devices, data, and apps[3].

Comparing IoT systems to traditional IT systems, the threat of cyberattacks when using gadgets to collect data from the real world poses the most security risk. For instance, the goal of implementing IoT in a factory is to dramatically increase productivity and maintainability through the collection of data from numerous sensors put in production equipment, analysis of that data, and real-time autonomous control[4]. Due to the potential for significant harm, if the device facts were to be manipulated throughout the procedure, inaccurate investigation findings would be generated or improper controller would follow. Additionally, from the perspective of competitiveness, avoiding leaks is crucial subsequently amount of facts or controller instructions is craft mysteries linked to the savoir-faire is manufacturer or the organization. Even if there isn't an issue right now, it's important to think about the impact of any potential dangers down the road. The three categories of cryptographic systems are based on the following three separate factors: how plain text is handled, how many keys are used, and how it is transformed into cipher text. Two universal standards provide the basis for all encryption techniques.

2. Literature Survey

Dewanjee et al. [1] worked on a compiled report on the security issues with IOTs and the cryptographic techniques utilized to address them in 2016. According to a Cisco research, there will be a huge amount of "Internet of Things (IoT)" plans by 2020 that will take over to cover all the sectors including health services, transportation, and smart gadgets spanning all aspects of life. IoTs enabling To improve the user experience, smart gadgets are getting smarter and better[7]. IoT security issues are more vulnerable as a result of the devices' open network connection.

Data security, communication security, and device security were all included in the taxonomy of security needs used by Harbi et al[8]. to examine IoT security in [26]. The the article explored the difficulties and suggested security solutions for a number of IoT applications. Hamad et al. spoke about IoT security challenges and potential solutions, identified the key security criteria required to minimize the IoT's resource limitations and diverse nature as security concerns. According to the study, security services including contact switch, veracity, validation, or secrecy, "confidentiality", and concealment are categories under which security solutions are categorized. In Hamad et al[9]. revised nimble cryptography techniques aimed at "IoT devices" with limitations. Symmetric and asymmetric algorithms for lightweight cryptography are the two primary categories. Resource requirement performance measures for hardware and software are introduced. In the study, compact methods that were mentioned in the literature were briefly described. A minimalist algorithm that successfully balances performance, cost, and security is the best.

Table 51.1 Types of attack

Threat type	Attack	Type of attack	Explanation
Fasteners	Interfering	Jeep hack	A weakness in the Jeep's software update system was exploited by hackers.
	Interfering	Voice-Controllable System	To link to devices like a thermostat, laser-based Audio Injection commands are used.
Shareware	DDoS	Malware attack	IoT devices used to be rendered inoperable forever by BrickerBot.
	Botnet	Silex malware	2000 IoT devices had their software erased by Brickerbot.
	DDoS	Mirai botnet	The infrastructure of the Dyn-controlled domain name system on the internet was brought down by this assault.
	Botnet	Malware attack	Network controllers and connected storage total 500K units. are infected by the VPNFilter malware.
Facts in Voyage	Circulation Scrutiny Spying/ Inhaling	Sybil attack on Tor System	Discovered the IDs of website proprietors using Tor secret services using a flaw in the Tor protocol.
	"MITM Attack" Spying/ Inhaling	vital outbreak	The key fob's cryptographic key can be obtained by a hacker utilising wireless data sensing from its transmission.
	Spying/ Inhaling	Data breach at Target involving an IoT HVAC device	This hack revealed the payment card details of over 41 million consumers.

Hameed and Alomar revised that IoT uses simple encryption and authentication techniques to safeguard against a kind of threat.. A writer planned the supplementary inquiry are needed to improve safe keeping the "IoT devices"[10]. "Lu and Xu" presented a taxonomy of cybersecurity assaults on IoT and addressed safekeeping outbreaks on "IoT" utilizing four-encrusted cyber security-concerned with architecture for "IoT". They spoke about its use in various businesses and attack defense strategies. Despite the fact that a number of works have been released on IoT security, they are only specialized to a fewnarrow areas of the technology. There is a need for more thorough surveys to address topics that were left out, such as the security issues with incorporating new technologies into the Internet of Things and security hardware solutions that can suit resource-constrained IoT devices[11].

3. Encryption Paradigms for IoT

Access control, privacy, and strong user authentication are the three main security issues in an IoT environment. The most effective IoT encryption methods include-

3.1 Data Encryption Standard (DES) and Triple-DES

Data Encryption Standard (DES) and Triple-DES-Both are symmetric encryption methods, with DES being the earliest and the foundation of cryptography. It is currently being phased obtainable (because of truncated encryption vital).[12] Its replacement, Triple-DES, the anticipated to be in use through 2030. The Triple-DES uses three 56-bit keys for each data block and increases the overall key length to 168 jiffs, prostrating all DES downsides like the vulnerability to meet-in-the- middle attacks[13].

3.2 Elliptical Curve Cryptography (ECC)

It is a decision to use Rivest, Shamir, and Adleman (RSA) arithmetical roles to produce tangible safckccping amid " crucial dyads "(community and secluded secrets). ECC provides shorter, quicker, and more efficient keys for encryption anddecoding by putting the elliptic wind concept to work. It is hence a chic match for IoT inclinations, mobile operations[14], and those with constrained computing (CPU) resources.

3.3 Digital Signature Algorithm (DSA)

It is an asymmetrical encryption algorithm similar to RSA, but with a small but important process variation. Data transfer via DSA is electronic or digital, which slows down encryp-tion.(as it involves authentication). Nevertheless, after the effective verification, decryption proceeds quickly.(through hash function)[15]. The excellent idea of modular exponentiation and the algebraic units of the individual logarithms are used in this operation. portable digital thumb In order to create secure communication in an IoT ecosystem, grounded security algorithms are being investigated.

3.4 Advanced Encryption Standard (AES)

It uses block ciphers beginning with the most fundamental, making it the most well-known and trustworthy symmetric encryption method. 128 to hefty- obligation "192 and 256- bit keys"[16]. It's indestructible (because of the lengthier crucial extent) or vulnerable tober-outbreaks except for the "brute force". The outcome, USA government's sSA, NIST(inventor the AES), and supplementary big associations considerably custom AES to guard classified sensitive data. Also, it's the futuristic " stylish-fit standard operation " for the private sector.

4. Solution for IoT

When data security for confidentiality and integrity is used to address detector bias, it can be a powerful defense against potential pitfalls. (Fig. 51.1). Featherlight cryptography serves the purpose of making safe encryption possible, even for parties with constrained resources[19]. Figure 51.1. A defense against data gathering attacks using encryption.

Prior to the invention of the cellphone, encryption was used as a standard on the data link subclass of communication networks. Encryption in the operation subclass is successful

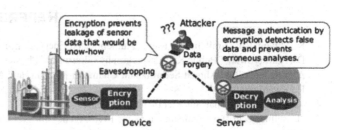

Fig. 51.1 A defense against data gathering attacks using encryption

in this situation for providing complete data protection from the device to the user and for ensuring individual system security. (Fig. 51.2)[20]. Additionally, encryption must be used when the CPU recycles the operation and on unused coffers, so it should ideally be as light as possible. IoT podiums at the moment of demand[21]. An IoT software framework is characterized as a piece of software encourages. IoT leaning on a network to share data and services. Operating devices, processing data for analysis and display, enabling operations, ensuring security, processing events, monitoring, and integrating and storehouse and data accession are among a platform's features(71). A platform's security outcomes can be broken down into four categories: authorization of drug users or realities, secure data storage, relating prejudice asking a connection, and integrity of data while in conveyance. There are two categories of IoT software platforms: closed-source open-source platforms and systems.

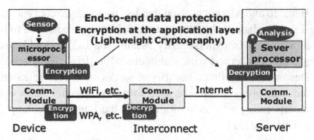

Fig. 51.2 Example of lightweight cryptography applications

5. Future Scope

An Implicit Security Pitfalls-

5.1 Rerun Outbreak

The end of this outbreak is to imitate the individualities of two gatherings, block their information sachets, or bear them to their destinations without revision.

5.2 Unconfident Announcement

Facts transferred to exterior organizations deprived of appropriate encryption can be interdicted by an bushwhacker harkening to the statement network. Roughly outbreaks that can be supported out embraces

5.3 MITM "Man- in- the- Middle"

Outbreak Through mis-using some liabilities similar remote crucial outflow then 50 susceptibility, the bushwhacker via the burlesquing individualities of binary gatherings can intimately bear or indeed modify the message between these gatherings, which trust they're collaborating directly, but in detail the unabridged discussion is under the control of the bushwhacker[22]. proposed management. All communications between the blockchain and external networks must be secure. By keeping a look out for malicious packets at the gateway, these attacks can be minimized. Integrate strong multi-feature validation methods to guarantee that message only occurs among the revelries who are meant. [30].

6. Conclusion

In this research, we confer and review IoT security risks from a variety of angles (such as hardware, software, and data transmission) with urgent preventative measures pertaining to various security risks. Also shown is a summary of the most recent security outcomes. We examine the security results that have been achieved with a relative analysis that focuses on providing security to the IoT- constrained bias in order to address the constraints IoT bias faces. The IoT ecosystem's introduction of emerging technologies introduce new security risks across the board.

REFERENCES

1. K. Minematsu: Parallelizable Rate-1 Authenticated Encryption from Pseudorandom Functions, EUROCRYPT 2014.
2. Dwi Liestyowati. "Public Key Cryptography", Journal of Physics: Conference Series, 2020.
3. Ahmad Fadlallah, Ahmed Serhrouchni, Chamoun Maroun, and Mohammed El-hajj. "Analysis of Cryptographic Algorithms on IoT Hardware platforms"0.
4. Kelvin Ashton, "That 'Internet of Things' Thing,".
5. "Baseline security recommendations for IoT," Agency for Network and Information Security of the European Union. November 20, 2017.
6. Internet of Things (IoT): a Review of the Literature R. Ramaswamy, S. Tripathi, and S. Madakam, [6](2015), J. Comput. Commun., 3(5), p.164.

7. "IoT for smart cities: use cases and implementation strategies," by Kelvin.

8. M. Fotouhi, R. Hasan, and M.M. HossainA study of security concerns, difficulties, and unresolved issues in the Internet of Things(2015), pages. 21–28 in 2015 IEEE World Congress Service.

9. N. Mishra, S. PandyaInternet of A methodical examination of belongings tenders, safekeeping issues, outbreaks, disturbance recognition, and imminent expectationsIEEE Access, 9, pp. 59353- 59377, 2021.

10. M.A. Al-Garadi, A. Mohamed, A.K. Al-Ali, X. Du, I. Ali, M. Guizani A survey of machine and deep learning methods for Internet of Things (IoT) securityIEEE Commun. Surv. Tutor., 22 (3) (2020), pp. 1646

11. S, Joshna. (2016). Symmetric Key Algorithms: A Comparative Analysis. International Journal of Innovative Research in Computer and Commu- nication Engineering. 4. 15772-15775.

12. S. Sridhar and S. Smys, "Intelligent security framework for iot devices cryptography based end-to-end security architecture," 2017 International Conference on Inventive Systems and Control (ICISC), Coimbatore, India, 2017, pp. 1-5, doi: 10.1109/ICISC.2017.8068718.

13. Balogh, S.; Gallo, O.; Ploszek, R.; ˇSpaˇcek, P.; Zajac, P. IoT Security Challenges: Cloud and Blockchain, Postquantum Cryptography, and Evolutionary Techniques. Electronics 2021, 10, 2647.

14. Cook, A.; Robinson, M.; Ferrag, M.A.; Maglaras, L.A.; He, Y.; Jones K.; Janicke, H. Internet of Cloud: Security and Privacy Issues. In Cloud Computing for Optimization: Foundations, Applications, and Challenges; Springer International Publishing: Cham, Switzerland, 2018;pp. 271–301.

15. Stergiou, C.; Psannis, K.E.; Kim, B.G.; Gupta, B. Secure integration of IoT and Cloud Computing. Future Gener. Comput. Syst. 2018, 78, 964–975.

16. Al-Fuqaha, A.; Guizani, M.; Mohammadi, M.; Aledhari, M.; Ayyash M. Internet of Things: Survey on Enabling Technologies, Protocols, and Applications. IEEE Commun. Surv. Tutorials 2015, 17, 234

17. Litoussi, M.; Kannouf, N.; El Makkaoui, K.; Ezzati, A.; Fartitchou, M. IoT security: Challenges and countermeasures. Procedia Comput. Sci. 2020, 177, 503–508.

18. Kirti, S.; Bhatt, S. Jamming Attack—A Survey. Int. J. Recent Res. Asp. 2018, 5, 74–80.

19. Mohapatra, H.; Rath, S.; Panda, S.; Kumar, R. Handling of Man-In- The-Middle Attack in WSN Through Intrusion Detection System. Int. J. 2020, 8, 1503–1510

20. Hafeez, I.; Antikainen, M.; Tarkoma, S. Protecting IoT-environments against Traffic Analysis Attacks with Traffic Morphing. In Proceedings of the 2019 IEEE International Conference on Pervasive Computing and Communications Workshops (PerCom Workshops), Kyoto, Japan, 11–15 March 2019; pp. 196–201.

21. IBM, The little-known story of the first IoT device, https://www.ibm.com/blogs/industries/little-known-story-first-iot- device/, accessed on 7 February 2018 (2018).

22. M. A. Obaidat, S. Obeidat, J. Holst, A. Al Hayajneh, et J. Brown, A Comprehensive and Systematic Survey on the Internet of Things: Security and Privacy Challenges, Security Frameworks, Enabling Technologies, Threats, Vulnerabilities and Countermeasures , Computers, vol.9, no 2, p. 44, mai 2020.

23. A. Amiruddin, A. A. P. Ratna, et R. F. Sari, Systematic Review of Internet of Things Security , vol. 11, no 2, p. 8, 2019

24. D. K. Alferidah et N. Jhanjhi, A Review on Security and Privacy Issues and Challenges in Internet of Things , p. 23, 2020.

25. Y. Yang, L. Wu, G. Yin, L. Li, H. Zhao, A survey on security and privacy issues in internet-of-things, IEEE Internet of Things Journal 4 (5) (2017) 1250–1258

Emerging Trends in IoT and Computing Technologies – Suman Lata Tripathi et al. (eds)
© 2024 Taylor & Francis Group, London, ISBN 978-1-032-87924-6

An Application of Voronoi Diagram Partitioning Scheme in the Area of Multi Robot Exploration

52

Soumi Dhar[1]
Judeson Antony Kovilpillai J[2]
Alliance University, CSE, Bengaluru, India

Abstract: Most recent multi-robot exploration algorithms use occupancy grids for the representation of primary environment. However, those grids are not suitable always for those cases where the boundaries are exceedingly large or who does not have well defined boundaries from the start of the investigation. Polygonal representations, on the other hand, are not constrained in this way. Literature suggests that the exploration algorithms works on dividing an unknown space into some number of regions which is equal to the participated robots in an occupancy grid representation by using K-Means clustering algorithm. The results demonstrates that this approach results in dispersing more number of robots than other approaches, which could be beneficial for fast traversal of large areas. On the contrary, the authors have applied discrete Voronoi diagram partitioning algorithm instead of the K-means algorithm. As a result we can see a significant amount of reduction of cost. Moreover, we have also compared both the approaches empirically.

Keywords: K-means, Voronoi diagram, Multi robot

1. Introduction

Multi robot exploration [1,2,3] has its own potential applications in search and rescue, surveillance and space exploration etc. Multi robot exploration of untraveled environments [4] is a demanding challenge that has caught the interest of mobile robotics and artificial intelligence experts. The major objective of robot expedition is to uncover the structure and details of an unexplored location (essentially open space and impediments). This goal must be met while staying within certain parameters, such as minimizing the time or energy consumption. Occupancy grids are basic but effective method for representing the real world objects as a uniform quantisation of field. Each unit which has participated in the mesh maintains track of whether a given area of field is vacant(free) or preoccupied from some objects better known as obstacle. Occupancy grids are insufficient for modeling and processing huge environmental setup. Even in moderately sized workstations, hundreds or thousands of cells must be preserved and processed. This has serious consequences in terms of processing time and memory use. The maps seem to be originally rectangular in shape and therefore have predetermined size. When any physical world extends further than the present grid bounds, there seems to be no cost-effective solution to expand the map. Due to the complexity as well as abscence of elasticity, polygonal structures were used as a substitute to occupancy grids. The exploring strategy switches between working with units to coping with pixels and areas, under certain instances by characterizing the extra room available as a network of simple convex areas (like as trapezoids and triangles), and for others by building networks of curvature (route-map-like) included in the unoccupied area. The present work offers a step towards the direction by defining and analyzing the usage of a polygonal model of the world as that of the primary surface orientation of a recently proposed multi-robot exploratory research

[1]soumi.dhar@alliance.edu.in, [2]judeson.kovilpillai@alliance.edu.in

DOI: 10.1201/9781003535423-52

strategy focused on occupancy grids. processing cost of the expedition method. Thats why a better economical polygonal version is benefical.

This technique differs from previous methods since it uses the famed K-Means technique to aggregate the unidentified cells sequentially, forcing the dispersion of accessible robots through into undiscovered region. It eliminates the greedy-like patterns of behaviour among several earlier approaches, that usually drive the different robots as shown by optimal scheduling criteria based on the robots' present position and adjacent research goals, that are determined by that of the borders for an already covered workplace. When they examine such borders, they remain unaware about the fundamental goal of expedition, and that is to discover unexplored land. When considering large settings, nevertheless, the repeated implementation of K-Means across thousands and thousands of units does have a substantial influence on the processing cost of the expedition method. Which is why a better economical polygonal version is beneficial.

Fig. 52.1 Voronoi diagram of 5 sites

1.1 Multi Robot Exploration using K-means Algorithm (A Grid Based Method)

The K-means clustering algorithm is a quite popular clustering method. It is utilized in a variety of fields, including information retrieval[5], computer vision[6] and pattern recognition. K-means clustering distributes "n" data points to k clusters in order to group equivalent data points. It is an iterative process that allocates each location to the cluster with the closest centroid. Then it recalculates the centroid of the cluster by averaging its values.

1.2 Polygon based (Voronoi Partioning) Multi Robot Exploration

There is an other way to represent the multi - robot exploration algorithm. It can also be represented as polygonal world model as mentioned in the earlier sections. Although a few points are taken care of: when dealing with large datasets. In K-Means clustering, the resolution problem might develop, with over-resolution or under-resolution possible. The entire space is represented by a disjoint set of enclosed polygons[7]. Each polygon can be marked with 3 states, either it is occupied vacant or unknown. The map is the outcome of the combination of all polygons. Its dimensions and shape are random in nature. After robot sensing, both the states (i.e free and occupied) polygons are added to the list of the map and removed from the list of unknown polygons to which they belong. Frontier edges are the edges of yet unexplored polygons that are near to free polygons. Using any cellular decomposition algorithm[8] robot path planning is carried out inside available free polygons.

But what makes the exploration algorithm described in stand out is that it uses K-Means to split up unknown cells during the determination step. K-Means algorithm is designed for distribution of points into cells in this case, so it is not appropriate for dividing up polygonal maps. Here lies the strength of our approach, as we have used voronoi diagram for partitioning the polygonal space.

Table 52.1 Comparison of time(ms) for both the approaches w.r.t to different number of robots

No. of Robots	Time taken by our proposed Voronoi algorithm	Time taken by K-Means algorithm
1	113 ms	227 ms
2	349 ms	607 ms
4	568 ms	927 ms
6	891 ms	1248 ms

2. Literature Review

The Voronoi diagram[8, 9] is a substantial distortion retract of unrestricted area that allows space available to be continually distorted it onto diagram, as it is often characterised[10] This indicates here that diagram is sufficient for trajectory tracking, implying that exploring the initial space for pathways may be simplified to exploring the diagram. Shrinking the size of the set to also be examined typically minimises the search's temporal complexity[11] Second, the diagram results to vigorous pathways, or pathways which are as free of obstructions as possible. Although theoretically Voronoi diagrams[12] can be extended to infinity but in our work we have limited the boundaries till the associated unexplored regions of the participating polygons. An additional AND operation is required in between the polygons and the regions of the constructed VD. Three main reasons are responsible for Voronoi diagram getting easily defind and visually constructed.Voronoi diagrams initially appear in existence in a variety of scenarios. Numerous naturally occurring phenomena could be employed to construct certain Voronoi diagram categories. Visual vision frequently guides human intuition. When an essential element is recognised, the entire issue may be better comprehended. Second, Voronoi diagrams get a number of intriguing and unexpected mathematical features; for example, they are connected to a number of very well structural parameters. The Voronoi diagram is among the most primitive constructions described by a discrete collection of points, according to Thifi, who has influenced other authors to assume such. Finally, Voronoi diagrams have shown to be an effective tool for resolving seemingly unconnected computational issues, attracting the interest of research scientists in recent years. Again for computer creation and modeling of Voronoi diagrams, effective and economically simple algorithms are being devised.

3. An Algorithm for Construction of Discrete Voronoi Diagram

To create a discrete Voronoi diagram for a set of sites, we parallelly propagate information about each site, assigning a pixel to the first site to which information arrives. As previously indicated, we regard the digital circle to be a geometric primitive with the site as its centre for information propagation. The basic idea behind our algorithm is that in the ith iteration, we assign points to each of the kth sites that are at a distance i from the respective sites by creating a digital circle of radius i around each of the k sites provided, assuming they have not been assigned to any other sites.

To do this, we create a digital circle with a radius of i for each of the k locations one by one. As a result, we disseminate information in a parallel manner from the 1st site to the kth site in the specified set of sites until all pixels are allocated to their nearest site.

In any iteration, if there is no new digital points added to a cell of a specific site, the site is now removed from the propagation list of sites. In the worst-case scenario, the largest radius a digital circle may develop is the diagonal distance of the discrete space, which can be easily determined. For the building of a digital circle, a number-theoretic technique is taken into consideration. The $s(x, y)$, site number(x), and status(y) characteristics are preserved for each site. Each site is initially eligible for growth, therefore the status bit is initialized to 1. To improve the efficiency of the algorithm, once a digital circle which belongs to a given site reaches its farthest radius, it is no longer essential to extend it further. Each site keeps a counter that is compared to the number of points on the perimeter of the digital circle of radius r in order to stop a specific digital circle at radius r. If counter is higher than or equal to the number of points on the circumference of the digital circle with radius r, the status bit for the current site is set to 0, and it is no longer eligible for growth since our goal of covering the region has been met.

When a digital circle for a particular site's centre point resides on or inside a digital circle for a nearby site's centre, the counter is incremented. If all of the points on the circumference are so obstructed, the digital circle with the specified site in its centre will be unable to extend any further. The inside technique is used to determine if a position of a point is inside or equidistant. An empty point inside a digital circle has the same site number on its left, right, top, down neighbour, and different in case it is equidistant from two or more sites, according to the number theoretic method to digital circle building. This observation is considered while designing the inside method. At any location in the discrete space of dimension M times N, there is zero stored. As previously stated, all points inside the radius of a digital circle are always closest to the centre, therefore as the algorithm progresses, these vacant spots (i.e. zero) are filled with site numbers that are closest to the centre. The objective of marking a pixel is to determine which site the pixel belongs to. The site number is filled on the perimeter of the digital circle with site as its centre using a symmetric manner in the draw method.

4. Results and Discussions

As per our experimentation it is clear that the classification step through K-means clustering algorithm consumes most of the computational time. The main motivation for introducing this time consuming step is to tessellate unknown regions one by one. One solution to the problem is to substitute the real world model by an analogous polygonal model. Hence the authors are using discrete Voronoi diagram, which promisingly reduces the time.

Moreover, the authors have proposed a novel digital geometric approach for construction of discrete voronoi diagram which ensures the accuracy The authors have compared both the approaches analogously using the similar maps. The execution time for both the approaches are mentioned in Table 52.1. The computational cost of Voronoi diagram algorithm is fixed at a single value of "K" for the number of robots. Generally, the more robots there are, the more difficult it is to keep the Voronoi edges contained within the map. But the total exploration area of the unknown polygons decreases as the robots explore the environment, the number of edges on their boundaries can rise and fall depending on the complexity of their shapes, necessitating the use of AND (boolean) operations to limit these diagrams to the available unknown polygons. Tables 52.1 shows why Voronoi partitioning is better than cell partitioning. The average amount of time it takes to do the math for two blank maps and four different robot configurations is the same for both methods.

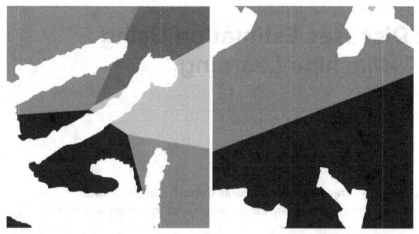

Fig. 52.2 Voronoi diagrams for input site 2 and 5 respectively

5. Conclusion

The polygonal representation of the real-world model proposed in this study has shown a great impact the efficacy of the crucial stage of the classical algorithm for multi robot exploration, in which the unexplored grid is partitioned into a number of areas and where the number of areas equals that of the number of robots. Instead of applying the core K-Means clustering algorithm to grid cells, we adopt a Voronoi-based partitioning technique. The present approach has been examined through a series of simulations. Multi robot coordinates of the multi robot method will be improved for better overall efficiency and tested on a real team of robots in the future. In addition, we intend to broaden the scope of the existing approach to include unbounded regions.

REFERENCES

1. Bentley and Ottmann, "Algorithms for reporting and counting geometric intersections," IEEE Transactions on Computers, vol. C-28, no. 9, pp. 643–647, 1979.
2. D. Scaradozzi, S. Zingaretti, and A. Ferrari, "Simultaneous localization and mapping (slam) robotics techniques: a possible application in surgery," Shanghai Chest,vol. 2, no. 1, 2018
3. G. Dudek, M. R. M. Jenkin, E. E. Milios, and D. Wilkes, "A taxonomy for multi-agent robotics," Autonomous Robots, vol. 3, pp. 375–397, 1996
4. Barraquand and J.-C. Latombe, "Robot motion planning: A distributed repre-sentation approach," International Journal of Robotic Research - IJRR, vol. 10,pp. 628–649, 12 1991.
5. H. Choset and K. Nagatani, "Topological simultaneous localization and mapping(slam): toward exact localization without explicit localization," IEEE Transactionson Robotics and Automation, vol. 17, no. 2, pp. 125–137, 2001.
6. W. Burgard, M. Moors, D. Fox, R. Simmons, and S. Thrun, "Collaborative multi-robot exploration," in Proceedings 2000 ICRA. Millennium Conference. IEEE In-ternational Conference on Robotics and Automation. Symposia Proceedings (Cat.No.00CH37065), vol. 1, pp. 476–481 vol.1, 2000.
7. S. Dhar and S. Pal, "Surface reconstruction: Roles in the field of computer visionand computer graphics," International Journal of Image and Graphics, vol. 0, no. 0,p. 2250008, 0.
8. G. Rong and T.-S. Tan, "Jump flooding in gpu with applications to voronoi diagram and distance transform," vol. 2006, pp. 109–116, 01 2006.
9. K. Q. Brown, "Voronoi diagrams from convex hulls," Information Processing Letters, vol. 9, no. 5, pp. 223–228, 1979.
10. B. She, X. Zhu, X. ye, K. Su, and J. Lee, "Weighted network voronoi diagrams for local spatial analysis," Computers, Environment and Urban Systems, vol. 52, 07,2015.
11. R. Wein, J. P. van den Berg, and D. Halperin, "The visibility voronoi complex and its applications," Computational Geometry, vol. 36, no. 1, pp. 66–87, 2007. Special Issue on the 21st European Workshop on Computational Geometry.
12. S. Jida, M. Ouanan, and B. Aksasse, "Color image segmentation using voronoi diagram and 2d histogram," International Journal of Tomography and Simulation,vol. 30, pp. 14–20, 01 2017.

Emerging Trends in IoT and Computing Technologies – Suman Lata Tripathi et al. (eds)
© 2024 Taylor & Francis Group, London, ISBN 978-1-032-87924-6

Skin Diseases Estimation Using Machine Learning

53

Ajay Pal Singh[1], Paras Gupta[2], Akshita Gupta[3]
Chandigarh University, Computer Science Engineering, Mohali, India

Abstract: For skin problems to be effectively treated and managed, an early and precise diagnosis is essential. In recent years, machine learning techniques have gained prominence in the healthcare domain, offering a promising avenue for improving the accuracy and efficiency of skin disease diagnosis. In this research article, there is in-depth analysis of the use of machine learning algorithms for the estimate and diagnosis of skin diseases is presented. The study utilizes a diverse dataset comprising a wide range of dermatological conditions, including common disorders such as eczema, psoriasis, acne, and less common diseases like melanoma and vitiligo. The dataset encompasses various image modalities, including dermoscopic and clinical images, ensuring a holistic analysis of skin diseases. However, it is imperative to address ethical concerns and continue research efforts to enhance the interpretability and robustness of these models.

Keywords: Skin disease, Machine learning, Diagnosis of dermatology, Image analysis, Logistic regression

1. Introduction

Skin diseases represent a pervasive global health challenge, affecting individuals of all ages, genders, and ethnicities. These conditions encompass a vast array of disorders, ranging from common dermatological ailments like eczema, psoriasis, and acne to more severe and potentially life-threatening diseases such as melanoma. Effective treatment of skin diseases depends on prompt and precise diagnosis and management, yet it remains a complex task that often relies heavily on the expertise of dermatologists. In recent years, the healthcare system has witnessed a transformative shift with the advent of machine learning (ML) and artificial intelligence (AI) technologies. These advanced computational techniques offer the promise of enhancing medical diagnostics and decision-making processes across various domains, including dermatology. Machine learning, in particular, has demonstrated its potential to revolutionize the field of dermatological diagnosis by leveraging the power of data-driven analysis.[1][2]

In the subsequent sections of this research paper, we delve into the methodologies employed in skin disease estimation using machine learning, present our findings, discuss the implications for clinical practice, and outline future research directions. By the end of this exploration, we hope to shed light on the transformative potential of machine learning in dermatology and its role in advancing the field of skin disease diagnosis and management.

1.1 Review of Research Paper

The paper provides a comprehensive overview of the current state of research, methodology, and challenges related to the estimation of skin diseases through machine learning. The strengths of this paper lie in its thorough literature review, which effectively establishes the context for the research. The authors have meticulously summarized existing studies on machine

---

[1]apsingh3289@gmail.com, [2]20BCS5172@cuchd.in, [3]20BCS5201@cuchd.in

DOI: 10.1201/9781003535423-53

learning in dermatology, highlighting both the potential and limitations of these technologies. This review serves as a valuable resource for researchers and practitioners interested in the field. The methodology section of the paper is well- structured and provides clear insights into the data collection, preprocessing, and machine learning model selection processes. The use of specific examples and explanations enhances the reader's understanding of the research methodology.[3][4].

1.2 Background

Skin diseases, collectively known as dermatological conditions, encompass a diverse array of disorders that affect the skin, hair, and nails. These conditions range from benign and common irritations like acne, eczema, and psoriasis to severe and potentially life-threatening ailments such as melanoma and squamous cell carcinoma. Skin conditions, which affect people of all ages, genders, and races, are a serious global health concern. They can lead to discomfort, disfigurement, impaired quality of life, and, in some cases, even mortality.[5]

2. Literature Review

Skin disease diagnosis has historically relied on clinical examination and biopsy. Recent advancements in ML have introduced the potential for automated, data-driven approaches to improve accuracy and efficiency. It aids in separating the tumor from the surrounding tissue. A appropriate coordinate transformation is used for image segmentation. By removing the tumor area from the segmented image, borders can be drawn.[6][7]

2.1 Skin Lesion Classification

A prominent area of research involves the classification of skin lesions, where ML models aim to show the difference between malignant and benign lesions.

This task involves training machine learning models to distinguish between different types of skin lesions, with a primary focus on identifying malignant or potentially cancerous lesions such as melanoma. Researchers often employ ensemble techniques like gradient boosting or random forests, in skin lesion classification. These methods combine many models' predictions to increase classification accuracy and reliability overall. These datasets contain diverse examples of skin lesions, including melanoma, nevi (moles), and other benign conditions.[8][9]

2.2 Multimodal Data Integration

Researchers are exploring the integration of multiple data sources, including clinical data, dermoscopic images, and patient history, to improve skin disease estimation accuracy. Multimodal data integration is a cutting-edge approach in dermatology that involves combining information from various sources, such as clinical data, dermoscopic images, histopathological slides, and genetic information, to enhance the reliability and accuracy of skin disease estimation with machine learning.

2.3 Model Interpretability

Ensuring the interpretability of ML models in dermatology is critical for gaining trust among healthcare practitioners. Techniques such as Grad-CAM and LIME are being employed for model interpretability. Dermatologists and healthcare practitioners require confidence in the models they use. Recognizing the justification behind a model's prediction is essential for transparency. Interpretable models can help diagnose and address errors. Dermatologists can identify why a model made a particular prediction, whether it was a false positive or false negative, and use this information to improve future diagnoses.

2.4 Gaps and Future Directions

Many skin disease datasets suffer from class imbalance, with a disproportionately small number of malignant cases. Addressing this imbalance is essential for more accurate estimation, as models may be biased towards the majority class. While the use of patient data is vital for research, there is a lack of standardized ethical guidelines for handling sensitive dermatological information, such as images and medical records. Ensuring patient privacy and consent is a significant challenge. Integrating machine learning models into clinical practice remains a gap.

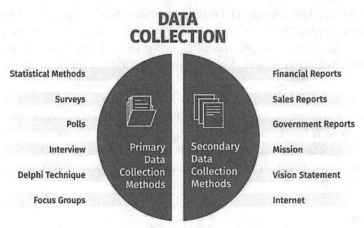

Fig. 53.1 Data collection

2.5 Significance and Applications

Improved Diagnostic Accuracy: Skin disease estimation projects can significantly improve the early detection of various dermatological conditions, including skin cancers like melanoma. Early detection often leads to more successful treatment outcomes and potentially life-saving interventions. By providing additional support to dermatologists and clinicians, these projects can help reduce the likelihood of misdiagnosis, which is especially critical in conditions with overlapping symptoms. Skin disease estimation tools can assist healthcare providers in prioritizing cases. They can help determine which patients require immediate attention and which can be scheduled for follow-up appointments, thus optimizing clinical workflows.

3. Methodology

This section provides the set of methodology used in our study investigating facial evolution and distortionusing deep learning. This approach contains multiple stages, including collection of data, preprocessing of data, deep learning modeling, methods of training, and evaluation.[10]

3.1 Data Collection

Data collection is a fundamental step in conducting research on skin disease estimation using machine learning. The quality and diversity of the data directly impact the performance and generalizability of machine learning models. Researchers typically gather data from various sources, including dermatology clinics, hospitals, publicly available datasets, and research collaborations. Dermatological images, clinical records, and patient histories are among the essential data types

3.2 Data Preprocessing

Data preprocessing is a critical step in skin disease estimation research that involves cleaning, enhancing, and transforming raw data to make it suitable for machine learning analysis. In the context of skin disease estimation, the following key steps in data preprocessing are crucial:

Face Data Cleaning: Address issues like missing values, corrupted images, and duplicate entries. Remove outliers and artifacts that may negatively impact model performance.

Data Augmentation: To increase the dataset's size and diversity, using data augmentation methods like rotation, scaling, cropping, and flipping, more training examples can be produced.

Resizing and Standardization: Normalize pixel values in images to a consistent scale (e.g., 0 to 1 or -1 to 1) to ensure that the machine learning model converges efficiently during training. Resize all images to a uniform resolution to facilitate model training and reduce computational complexity. Consider the trade- off between resolution and computational cost.

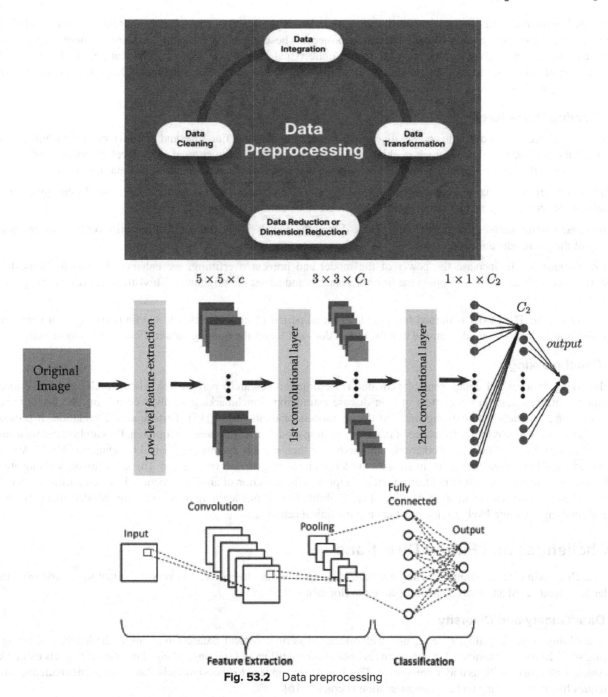

Fig. 53.2 Data preprocessing

3.3 Deep Learning Model Architecture

Deep learning which is a subset of machine learning has revolutionized the field of skin disease estimation, It involves the use of neural networks with multiple layers (hence "deep"), enabling the automatic extraction of intricate features from skin images. The choice of model architecture is pivotal in this context and significantly influences the performance of skin disease estimation projects.[12][13]

3.4 Convolutional Neural Networks (CNNs)

CNNs are the cornerstone of deep learning in dermatology. They are designed to mimic the human visual system, making them exceptionally adept at analyzing images. CNNs can automatically learn features like edges, textures, and patterns from skin images, which are crucial for accurate disease estimation. Deeper architectures, such as ResNet and DenseNet, have shown remarkable success in skin disease estimation projects. These models are capable of learning increasingly complex representations, which is advantageous for recognizing subtle visual cues in skin lesions. Deep learning models benefit from augmentation of data using techniques, such as scaling, flipping, and rotation which artificially helps to increase the size of traing subset as well as improve the model generalization.

3.5 Training Procedure

The training procedure is a dynamic and iterative process, where researchers fine-tune and optimize machine learning models to achieve the highest possible accuracy in skin disease estimation. The ultimate goal is to develop models that can assist dermatologists in their clinical practice, potentially reducing diagnostic errors and improving patient outcomes.

Optimizer: Energized Stochastic gradient descent (SGD) has been chosen as the best for reducing loss. The energy component accelerates convergence by accumulating gradients from previous iterations.[11]

Tuition Fees: Use tuition fees to transfer to the course during the course. This dynamic change optimizes the convergence and stability of the entire educational process.

Data augmentation: To increase the power of the model and prevent overfitting, we enhance the training data through transformations such as rotation, flipping the line horizontally, and adjust the brightness. This difference reveals the pattern of many facial variations.

Training Duration: The model is trained for a predetermined period of time and closely monitors for signs of overtraining. Early stopping technique is used to ensure that the model does not forget the training data but learns to perform well.

3.6 Benchmarking

Benchmarking is a crucial component of skin disease estimation research, particularly when developing and evaluating machine learning models. In the context of skin disease estimation, benchmarking involves comparing the performance of newly developed models with existing state- of-the-art models or methods.[14][15]. Performance Evaluation: It provides a standardized way to assess the performance of machine learning models in skin disease estimation. Researchers can measure the accuracy, sensitivity, specificity, and other relevant metrics of their models against established benchmarks. Model Accuracy: Benchmarking allows researchers to compare their models with existing models or methods. This comparison helps identify the weaknesses and strenghts of different means, thereby helping in the selection of an effective model. Benchmarked models often serve as reference points for evaluating the clinical applicability of machine learning in dermatology. Models that perform well in benchmarking are more likely to find practical use in clinical settings.

4. Challenges and Future Directions

As research on skin disease estimation using machine learning continues to evolve, it is very important to see and work on the challenges encountered and chart a path for future developments.

4.1 Data Quality and Diversity

The availability of high-quality, diverse, and well-annotated dermatological datasets remains a challenge. Collecting and curating such datasets for various skin conditions is critical for robust model training. Many skin disease datasets exhibit class imbalance, with rare conditions underrepresented. This imbalance can lead to biased models. Addressing this challenge through techniques like oversampling and data augmentation is crucial.[16]

4.2 Model Generalization

Model generalization refers to a machine learning model's ability to perform well on unseen data—data it hasn't been explicitly trained on. In the context of skin disease estimation, ensuring that machine learning models can generalize effectively is a significant challenge. Dermatological conditions can vary widely based on factors like patient demographics, skin type, and environmental factors. Models need to generalize across diverse data sources and populations.[17]

4.3 Interpretation

Many state-of-the-art machine learning models, most importantly the deep learning ones like convolutional neural networks (CNNs), are highly complex and consist of numerous interconnected layers. This complexity can make it challenging to understand how the model arrives at its predictions. Deep learning models are often considered "black-box" models because they lack transparency. They involve millions of parameters and nonlinear transformations, making it difficult to intuitively grasp the decision-making process. [18]

5. Future Directions

Future research should explore the integration of various data modalities, including clinical data, dermoscopic images, genetic information, and patient histories. Combining these sources can provide a more comprehensive view of skin health. Developing privacy-preserving machine learning techniques can safeguard patient data while enabling collaborative research. Federated learning and secure multi-party computation are promising areas.

6. Conclusion

In the realm of dermatology, the integration of machine learning and artificial intelligence has accompanied in a new era of skin disease estimation. This research paper has delved into the myriad facets of this transformative field, shedding light on the significant strides made, the challenges confronted, and the promising directions for the future. The foremost achievement lies in the remarkable accuracy and efficiency achieved through machine learning models in the estimation of skin diseases. CNNs have proved to be a powerful tool, demonstrating their capacity to discern intricate patterns in dermatological images. Nevertheless, the journey towards comprehensive and effective skin disease estimation has not been devoid of challenges. Issues such as data quality, class imbalance, and ethical considerations have cast shadows over the field. Data scarcity remains a stumbling block, as researchers grapple with the necessity for extensive and diverse datasets. Ethical dilemmas concerning patient privacy and data consent demand careful attention, emphasizing the need for standardized guidelines in handling sensitive medical information. Additionally, the future holds promise for further refinement and expansion of skin disease estimation using machine learning. Multimodal data integration, the fusion of clinical data, dermoscopic images, and genetic information, stands as a tantalizing frontier. This comprehensive approach may offer deeper insights into dermatological conditions, aiding in personalized diagnosis and treatment strategies. The quest for model interpretability continues to gather momentum. Explainable AI (XAI) techniques promise to demystify the workings of complex machine learning models, allowing clinicians to comprehend and trust their decisions. Moreover, the seamless integration of these models into clinical practice beckons, with user-friendly interfaces and real-world validation studies paving the way for the implementation of machine learning applictiond in the field of dermatology. In conclusion, the synergy between machine learning and dermatology has unlocked unprecedented potential in the estimation of skin diseases. This paper has illuminated the advancements achieved, the hurdles to surmount, and the vistas of opportunity yet to explore. As the field evolves, collaboration among researchers, clinicians, and ethicists will play a pivotal role in ensuring the responsible and transformative application of machine learning in the treatment and management of diseases related to skin, which is going to improve the patient's health therebychanging the outcomes through practice in dermatology.

REFERENCES

1. Esteva, A., Kuprel, B., Novoa, R. A., Ko, J., Swetter, S. M., Blau, H. M., & Thrun, S. (2017). Dermatologist-level classification of skin cancer with deep neural networks. Nature, 542(7639), 115-118.
2. Haenssle, H. A., Fink, C., Schneiderbauer, R., Toberer, F., Buhl, T., Blum, A., ... & Tschandl, P. (2018). Man against machine: diagnostic performance of a deep learning convolutional neural network for dermoscopic melanoma recognition in comparison to 58 dermatologists. Annals of Oncology, 29(8), 1836-1842.
3. Codella, N. C., Gutman, D., Celebi, M. E., Helba, B., Marchetti, M. A., Dusza, S. W., ... & Halpern, A. (2018). Skin lesion analysis toward melanoma detection: A challenge at the 2017 International Symposium on Biomedical Imaging (ISBI), hosted by the International Skin Imaging Collaboration (ISIC). In Proceedings of the IEEE conference on computer vision and pattern recognition (CVPR) workshops (pp. 1680-1688).
4. Tschandl, P., Rosendahl, C., & Kittler, H. (2017). ThHAM10000 dataset, a large collection of multi-source dermatoscopic images of common pigmented skin lesions. Scientific Data, 4, 170161.
5. Brinker, T. J., Hekler, A., Enk, A. H., Klode, J., Hauschild, A., Berking, C., ... & von Kalle, C. (2019). Deep learning outperformed 136 of 157 dermatologists in a head-to-head dermoscopic melanoma image classification task. European Journal of Cancer, 113, 47-54.
6. Liu, S., Song, W., Kong, X., & Liu, Y. (2019). Ensemble of expert deep neural networks for spatio-temporal forecasting. Neurocomputing, 324, 43-54.

7. Esteva, A., & Dermatology, M. (2019). A guide to deep learning in healthcare. Nature Medicine, 25(1), 24-29.

8. Simonyan, K., Vedaldi, A., & Zisserman, A. (2013). Deep inside convolutional networks: Visualising image classification models and saliency maps. arXiv preprint arXiv:1312.6034.

9. Caruana, R., Lou, Y., Gehrke, J., Koch, P., Sturm, M., & Elhadad, N. (2015). Intelligible models for healthcare: Predicting pneumonia risk and hospital 30-day readmission. In Proceedings of the 21th ACM SIGKDD international conference on knowledge discovery and data mining (pp. 1721-1730).

10. Chen, J., Song, L., Soltani, M., Zhao, L., & Elhoseny, M. (2020). A novel approach for chest X-ray image classification using deep transfer learning. Electronics, 9(1), 95.

11. Lopes, F. M., de Carvalho, L. A., Pereira, A., & Sanches, J. M. (2013). Transfer learning of pre-trained convolutional neural networks for blind image quality assessment. In Proceedings of the European Conference on Computer Vision (ECCV) (pp. 572- 585).

12. Shorten, C., & Khoshgoftaar, T. M. (2019). A survey on image data augmentation for deep learning. Journal of Big Data, 6(1), 1- 48.

13. Celebi, M. E., Kingravi, H. A., Iyatomi, H., Aslandogan, Y. A., & Stoecker, W. V. (2007). Lesion border detection in dermoscopy images. Computerized Medical Imaging and Graphics, 31(4-5), 148-153.

14. Kassani, S. H., Koshti, A., Wesner, S., & Bagci, U. (2017). Melanoma detection using texture and color features in dermoscopy images. In 2017 39th Annual International Conference of the IEEE Engineering in Medicine and Biology Society (EMBC) (pp. 4380-4383).

15. Litjens, G., Kooi, T., Bejnordi, B. E., Setio, A. A., Ciompi, F., Ghafoorian, M., ... & Sánchez, C. I. (2017). A survey on deep learning in medical image analysis. Medical Image Analysis, 42, 60-88.

16. LeCun, Y., Bengio, Y., & Hinton, G. (2015). Deep learning. Nature, 521(7553), 436-444

17. Esteva, A., Robicquet, A., Ramsundar, B., Kuleshov, V., DePristo, M., Chou, K., ... & Dean, J. (2019). A guide to deep learning in healthcare. Nature Medicine, 25(1), 24-29.

18. Tschandl, P., Rosendahl, C., & Kittler, H. (2019). The HAM10000 dataset, a large collection of multi-source dermatoscopic images of common pigmented skin lesions. Scientific data, 5(1), 180161

Emerging Trends in IoT and Computing Technologies – Suman Lata Tripathi et al. (eds)
© 2024 Taylor & Francis Group, London, ISBN 978-1-032-87924-6

Python-Powered Web Scraping for Progressive Data Extraction

54

Kulvinder Singh[1],
Mayank Pathak[2], Aryan Jaswal Thakur[3]
Department of Computer Science & Engineering,
Chandigarh University, Mohali, Punjab, India

Abstract: Web scraping is a process of automatically extracting large amounts of data from the web. It involves crawling various websites and extracting the required data using spiders, which is then processed in a data pipeline and stored. Python, with its various libraries and frameworks such as Scrapy and Beautiful Soup, is a powerful tool for web scraping. In particular, businesses need to understand how to "mine" the vast amount of data on the Web—which includes social media, websites, web portals, online platforms, and more—in order to find information that is worth using. In this respect, web scraping constitutes the most basic technique. Thus, this paper intends to summarize the modern trends in Web Scraping aimed at assisting scholars and managers in the art of efficient online data mining. This is an introductory part, where the paper discusses the core design of a web scraper and its various uses in diverse fields. The following part illustrates different Web scraping techniques and Web scraping approaches. Lastly, the paper suggests a process to create Web scraping with different tools and it concludes.

Keywords: Web scraping, Incremental data extraction, Web mining, Web scraping, Web crawling, and Big data

1. Introduction

Data is important in business, marketing, engineering, as well as in the social sciences. It is an integral part of many information-based and knowledge-based tasks. Research begins with data collection, and then involves the orderly recording of essential features. This helps us provide answers to questions, develop research inquiries, test hypotheses, and conduct evaluations. Depending on the topic, the sort of data needed, and the objectives of the researcher, numerous approaches to data collection are used. These methods also change their application approach depending on the objectives and contexts so that the data will be accurate, reliable, and valid [1]. There are multiple data sources available on the internet that researchers can easily utilize during their research process. Web scraping or data extraction from websites is widely referred to as web harvesting or web crawling. Web scraping is vital in gathering valuable information as well as investigating into the recent web scraping methodologies and techniques. Also, this research will help us in comparing various available tools and choosing the best one for our study. In this research, we'll look into the newest approaches and tactics for web scraping and explore how to build a program that can be used to gather useful data from internet sources. This research will also assist us in comparing various available tools and selecting the most suitable one for our study. Web scraping has grown into a powerful tool to deal with this limitation, and Python has become the language of choice for implementing this methodology. Web scraping is an act whereby one can extract specific data from websites for further analysis, study, or any other purpose. It ensures that different types of websites including their styles and structures can be converted into a common format. Python is a flexible programming language that is

[1]kulvinder.diet@gmail.com, [2]pathakmayank876@gmail.com, [3]aryanthakurjaswal@gmail.com

DOI: 10.1201/9781003535423-54

widely used and offers an all- encompassing package of tools and frameworks for web scraping that allows for effective, robust, and easily understandable code by a variety of programmers. Incremental data extraction denotes the periodic and systematic process of retrieving updated details from websites for up-to-date analysis. This is the most important technique as it is helpful in highly dynamic online environments, where data is regularly updated and altered. The use of a system that is automated can help in the extraction of data and updates as well. This saves time, decreases mistakes, and ensures that organizations have recent information. Some of the good web scraping utilities available in Python include Beautiful Soup, Scrapy, and Selenium among others. The above-mentioned libraries enable one to programmatically navigate through web pages, search for specific content, and extract useful information. Python is flexible and easy to use, one can create efficient solutions for web scraping applications, without being an expert in the domain. While scraping is valuable, one should never violate websites' terms of service or act illegally when extracting data. This study will examine the best practices and standards for conducting online scraping activity. Enterprises can now capitalize on the abundant data available on the internet through web scraping and incremental data extraction using Python, empowering the enterprise to make informed decisions and operational efficiency. This research article aims to present a comprehensive overview of the issue, including technological components, practical applications, and ethical considerations. The purpose of this research is took into the best practices and standards for conducting online scraping activity. Enterprises can now capitalize on the abundant data available on the internet by using Python for web scraping and incremental data extraction, allowing them to make informed decisions and improve operational efficiency.

2. Literature Review

This is nothing new in web scraping but with modern programming languages, one can now build web scrapers that collect unstructured data and store it into structured forms. This paper endeavors to present recent literature on the latest Web Scraping methods for improving the knowledge of scholars and managers who would like to mine the data at their disposal as much as possible online. This review evaluates the effectiveness of several algorithms for web scraping and code similarity detection in relation to different situations. This is with a view to making meaningful inferences and pinpointing areas of improvement and future study directions. Research in web scraping techniques has been a focal point for many scholars. Gunawan et al. conducted a comparative study on web scraping methods, exploring regular expressions, HTML DOM, and XPath for data extraction [1]. Additionally, Sirisuriya's work contributed to this area by offering a comparative analysis of various web scraping methodologies [2]. Mitchell's book on web scraping with Python serves as a valuable resource in understanding different techniques and their practical applications [23]. Several studies have showcased the diverse applications of web scraping. An online application created by Spangher and May is intended for the consumption and annotation of legal discourse. [3]. Saleh et al. introduced a strategy for efficient crawling through web page distillation using an optimized Naïve Bayes classifier [5]. Boegershausen et al. delved into the utilization of web scraping for consumer research purposes [7], while Nguyen et al. analyzed Australian SME Instagram engagement through web scraping techniques [9]. Using semantic similarity, Deng's research concentrated on developing a targeted crawler for mineral intelligence services. [10]. Rahmatulloh and Gunawan used the HTML DOM method for collecting scientific articles from Google Scholar [15]. Moreover, Suganya and Vijayarani applied a firefly optimization algorithm for web citation extraction [14], while Asikri et al. employed web scraping to build ontologies in a knowledge environment [19].

In Fig. 54.1 some studies have explored data analysis and its applications. Tharaniya et al. investigated unstructured data extraction, financial event modeling, and analysis [6]. Kotouza et al. worked on fashion recommendation systems, utilizing

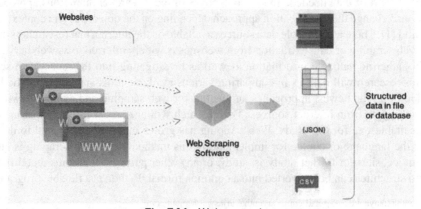

Fig. 54.1 Web scrapping

AI for clothing data retrieval and analysis [11]. Seliverstov et al. evaluated traffic safety in a particular region by employing sentiment analysis of internet users' reviews [13]. Li's work aimed at building updated research agendas through analyzing papers indexed on Google Scholar using NLP [17], while Santos provided a scholarly production dataset report for research analysis concerning COVID-19 [18]. Understanding the tools and methods utilized in web scraping is pivotal. The W3C's documentation on the Document Object Model (DOM) provides a foundational understanding of HTML DOM-based web scraping [22]. Additionally, Mahto and Singh's work offered insights into the world of web scrapers [24], and Chaitra et al.'s study delved into various types of web crawlers [9].

3. Applications of Web Scrapping

Web scraping is broadly used in many ways such as price comparison and site watching among others. changes in weather data, research, and the detection and integration of website modifications. Scrape job posting data from the job portal, offer price and discount extraction, keeping an eye on brands and conducting market research [2]. The system is additionally useful for quick and efficient data collection. The uses of web scraping span different sectors. Big data analytics requires it as a precondition.

In Healthcare: Nowadays, Medical treatment involves more than just touch. Rather, it has gone digital in its own special way. Web scraping in healthcare has the potential to save many lives because of the data-driven world. It is possible to make wise choices. Data collection in which many patients get involved is usually perceived as a very tedious and long process for healthcare workers. There is the necessity of the clinical data even more than before, but the current patient load practically prohibits such collection [3].

In Social-Media: It is always helpful to extract data from social media when it comes to refining marketing activities. Companies need to be quick in analyzing the customers' sentiments. This will help in making the company's products better and improving publicity as well as audience participation. They developed a network scraping application that could download data about Instagram accounts on behalf of different users. Therefore, the researchers chose to employ a web scraping approach without relying on the platform's Application Programming Interface (API) which comes with several data access limitations. The Instagram-data- grabber web scraping method was implemented successfully. In the age of social media, understanding trends, sentiments, and user behavior is invaluable for businesses, researchers, and marketers. Web scraping, powered by Python, provides a powerful means to extract and analyze data from social media platforms [3].

In Finance: Web scraping may be crucial in finance as it collects information from financial news sites, stock markets, and economic indicators. Determine which sites or sources to take out money data from. The common sources might be financial blogs (like Bloomberg, and Reuters) trading websites like Yahoo Finance, and Google Finance, or economic data websites like the Bureau of Labor Statistics. The reason why we are using Python as a programming language to do Web scraping is that it is easy [5].

4. Techniques for Website Scraping

The act of autonomously mining or gathering data from the internet and other public databases is known as "web scraping". Various web scraping techniques have been created for various kinds of studies.

Traditional Copy as well as Paste: The copy-pasting process is easy to use: just use your browser to access the website, now type in your own words. Nevertheless, it may be relatively simple and straightforward for the website owner to adopt the method. The barrier program makes it difficult to use, [1] therefore people have to choose the objects manually. They can sometimes even be short, long, or short sentences. On the other side, other approaches are complicated to employ.

DOM Parsing: An approach used to obtain, manipulate, and edit HTML elements with the yardstick being the HTML DOM. Thus, one could improve the efficiency of DOM by specifying the items as well as the attributes for every element in HTML involved and the mechanism of getting into them. The above case can be illustrated by how JavaScript has access to every element of an HTML text via the DOM [19]. For example, to get objects, the HTML DOM uses usually programming dialects like Js. Each HTML entity is considered as an object. The programming interface includes the method and property of each object [20,21].

Detecting semantic annotations: The scraped folios could carry embedded metadata, semantic markups, or annotations to discover particular data pieces. One such case includes using DOM. We should parse the pages if the annotations are integrated as Microformat. In another case, the annotations are separate and managed independently of the web pages, organized into a separate metrics layer, this layer facilitates the provision of schema and instructions to the scrapers so that they may scrap the pages.

Comparison between web scraping methods: The methods are compared by checking them out during the data extraction process from the computation and comparison of the obtained results at the required website. Process duration, memory use, and the measurement parameters of the experiment will include data consumption. The evaluation of experiment outcomes. The Regex way is however minimal in RAM usage among all web scraping methods available, in contrast to the HTML, DOM, and XPath approaches. Moreover, HTML DOM utilizes the shortest duration while using the minimum quantity of resources. It has to be noted that this approach uses the least amount of data when compared to the methods using XPath as well as Standard Expression.

5. Web Scraping Technology

Search Engine bot - Search Engine bot are those that visit sites to get data, a search engine bot works by loading a tiny list of links. Next, the software looks through these sites for more linkages, and makes another list of them known as crawl frontier, which is scanned to find more web pages. The crawler first has to assess if the address is either in relation or in total terms. When dealing with related URLs, the crawler has to determine the base of the URL. A good crawler should be capable of recognizing circular references and slight changes of a page for effective extraction and storage of data. Web crawlers come in a variety of forms, including:

Targeted web crawler: This is a kind of bot intended to locate websites related to particular user fields or subjects. It tries to locate other pertinent pages for higher accuracy. Ranking of web pages enables it to download pages that are pertinent to the subject matter while disregarding irrelevant ones.

Incremental crawler: Web crawlers that incrementally make visits to and retrieve updated web pages. Crawlers that periodically visit website pages and save new information most recent version of pages.

Distributed crawler: These crawlers work by designating other crawlers to do certain tasks. The nodes' synchronization and communication are controlled by a central server.

Parallel crawler: The combination of several crawler processes creates a parallel crawler. Every process involves filtering and retrieval of URLs, and this is the case for URLs gathered from every operation.

Hidden crawler: Material that lies within closed. Websites meant only for specific users are known as hidden Web. A hidden crawler that accumulates this information is recognized as such.

5.1 Development of Web Scraping Tools

Developing a web scraping tool involves creating a software application or script that can navigate websites, retrieve web pages, extract data from those pages, and possibly store the data for further use or analysis [14]. The online data extraction tool may be customized for any unique use case.

Web Scraping using Beautiful Soup: It's a Python module, used for parsing HTML and XML structures (Beautiful Soup). A parse tree is created for how data are extracted from parsed HTML pages. Retrieving information data from indeed.com, the job search site, and two libraries, beautiful soup (to retrieve information from files in XML and HTML) and XML (to deal with XML and html info in python). Retrieving a certain information from a webpage using beautiful soup, removing html tags and saving the info [18]. Extracting digital notices on smart city strategy from various government portals using Beautiful Soup.

Web Scraping using Selenium: Selenium is a very effective website scraper. The web driver of Selenium has some functionality, that makes it possible to move across web pages and pick out customization of different page parts for their specific needs. Several web page-related data like using the search engine, Web pages are processed and organized in order to identify and retrieve the user's query. Using selenium framework and TF-IDF algorithm [20]. This implies that information is taken from the websites and then, further processing and retrieval activities take place. The TF-IDF algorithm is then used to summarize extracted content. The phases in the suggested extraction framework are as follows: The user types a inquiry. It combines the pre-defined URL with the user query to generate a URL relating to a user inquiry was created. The information is taken from the URLs and entered into a text document a web-based information-providing system integrating data obtained from various public databases in order to produce, provide, and analyze more scientific information regarding pesticides. To retrieve information, the authors resorted to a variety of ways of crawling the Web through a Selenium-based crawler and by reviewing their performance, using an integrated approach of pesticides [19].

Web Scraping using Scrapy: Scrapy is a powerful and flexible web scraping framework for Python that provides a convenient and structured way to extract data from websites. It is particularly useful for building large scale, high-performance web scraping applications. The heart of the Scrapy structure is the engine. It regulates the data transfer between the various parts of Scrapy. It is also responsible for monitoring events like as request errors, response errors, and exceptions and producing events in response to them [20]. The Scheduler establishes a direct connection to task queues and determines when a job must be finished. It has the ability to regulate how long each request takes. Scrapy finds applications across various domains. Developers have utilized it in creating web applications for legal discourse learning, consumer research, focused crawling, scientific article collection, and more. Scrapy emerges as a prominent and versatile tool for web scraping. Its robust methodologies and varied applications make it a preferred choice. Scrapy isn't just a one-trick pony. It's been used in many ways, like creating special websites to study legal discussions or understanding what consumers like through online behavior.

The provided Fig. 54.2 Represent the Scrapy framework. The engine of the Scrapy framework, regulating the data transfer between Scrapy's elements. Additionally, it is responsible for monitoring events like as exceptions, re-quest errors, and response errors and for producing events in response to them. The Scheduler establishes a direct connection to task queues and determines when a job must be finished. It can also regulate how long it takes for each request to be processed. The Scheduler establishes a direct connection to task queues and determines when a job must be finished. It has the ability to regulate how long each request takes. The HTTP requests are sent to the Downloader. It saves and gives the HTTP response data to the engine in the typical scenario, in which an actual browser is not utilized. On the other hand, the Downloader will be completely replaced by a middleware that has control over the browser whenever requests are made using an actual browser. Spiders are classes designed by developers that tell the Scraper how to go about obtaining and interpreting certain web content. Here you may additionally configure the Downloader's own parameters and those of the related middleware. Ultimately, the parsed contents are sent to item Pipeline. Data supplied by Spiders is parsed by Item Pipeline, which also handles data persistence to Redis, MongoDB, or Postgres, validation, and custom transformations. Requests and answers made to and from Downloader are intercepted by Downloader middleware, which adds specific information to the request and response data.

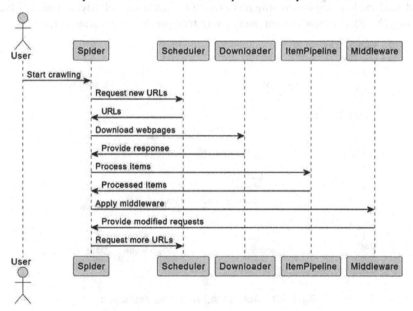

Fig. 54.2 The scrapy framework

6. Previous Methodologies Used

As previous methodologies used for web scraping and data extraction are domain- and objective-specific, they will vary depending on their purpose. The following will be some of the frequently employed approaches in the previous research articles.

Hands-On Data Gathering: Back in the day, researchers used to roll up their sleeves and collect data manually. They'd visit websites, hunt for the info they needed, and jot it down. While this method gave them accuracy, it was real time-eater and wasn't great for large datasets.

Teamwork in Crawling: Researchers came up with coordinated crawling techniques to scrape data from multiple websites all at once. They used fancy algorithms to schedule and manage the crawling process across different websites, making the most of their resources and ensuring efficient data collection.

Machine Learning Magic: With the rise of machine learning, researchers started using techniques like supervised and unsupervised learning to train models for automatic data extraction. These models were trained on labelled data to figure out patterns and structures in web pages, essentially automating the data collection process.

Hybrid Approaches: Some studies got creative and combined different methods to supercharge their data extraction. They mixed rule-based scraping with machine learning, making it easier to deal with websites that had different structures and complex data.

Evaluation and Quality Control: Assessing and validating the data was a big part of these methods. Researchers made sure the data they extracted was on the mark by comparing it with known accurate data, running statistical checks, or bringing in experts to give it the thumbs up. Finally, it should be noted that modern web scraping methodologies are constantly changing and new ones might have appeared since the date of these researches. Web scraping methodologies are updated periodically in order to provide high standards of efficacy, impartiality, and ethical practices when retrieving data from a dynamic internet environment.

7. Proposed Methodology

Introduction: Our model presents a new methodology that makes use of automated web data extraction, optimized model training, and adaptive scraping to give high performance in data extraction.

The provided Fig. 54.3 Represent Automated Web Data Extraction. This section provides information on how artificial intelligence and machine learning techniques can be used to extract data from websites automatically. It encompasses strategies like natural language processing, image and pattern recognition to find and retrieve relevant information precisely. The use of artificial intelligence and machine learning in scraping and extracting data from web pages. This involves using techniques like natural language processing (NLP), computer vision, and pattern recognition for accurate extraction of pertinent information.

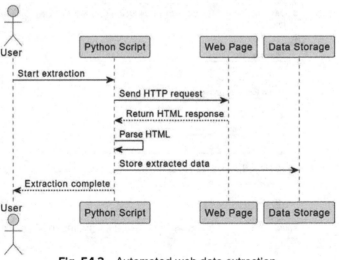

Fig. 54.3 Automated web data extraction

Natural Language Processing (NLP): NLP techniques are used to understand and extract text-based content from web pages. This is especially useful when dealing with textual data such as news articles, product reviews, or social media posts.

Computer Vision: Computer vision, a subfield of AI, is employed to interpret and extract information from images and visual content found on web pages. This can be valuable for applications like extracting data from scanned documents, product images, or charts.

Pattern Recognition: Pattern recognition algorithms are applied to recognize specific structures or layouts within web pages, helping to identify and extract data accurately.

Model Training and Optimization: In this section, the focus shifts to the process of training AI models using labelled data. It discusses various techniques for optimizing the accuracy and performance of these models for specific data extraction tasks.

Supervised Learning: Supervised learning involves training a machine learning model on a labelled dataset, which consists of input data and the corresponding correct output. The model learns to make predictions based on this training data and can be fine-tuned for better accuracy.

Deep Learning: Deep learning, a subset of machine learning, often involves neural networks with multiple layers. It is particularly powerful in tasks that require complex feature extraction and pattern recognition. Deep learning models, like convolutional neural networks (CNNs) or recurrent neural networks (RNNs), can be used for web data extraction

Dynamic Learning: AI models can be designed to adapt to changes in website layouts, ensuring that the scraping rules remain effective when websites evolve. This adaptability is crucial in a web environment where websites often undergo updates.

Efficiency: Adaptive scraping minimizes the need for manual adjustments when a website's structure changes. It reduces the maintenance overhead and makes data extraction more efficient.

7.1 Differences Between Previous and Proposed Methodology

Time and Efficiency: Previous methodologies primarily relied on manual data extraction or rule-based scraping, which were time-consuming and labour-intensive processes. In contrast, the new methodology leverages AI- driven automated web scraping, leading to efficient and effortless data extraction. This automation significantly reduces the time and effort required for data collection, resulting in improved efficiency.

Accuracy and Adaptability: The new methodology, which incorporates machine learning algorithms, enhances accuracy in data extraction when compared to previous approaches. AI- driven models can learn and adapt to various website structures and data format variations, ensuring higher precision and adaptability. In contrast, previous methodologies often struggled to handle complex website structures and were less adaptable to changes.

Flexibility and Scalability: While previous methodologies had limited flexibility in dealing with diverse website structures, the new methodology offers greater adaptability. The combination of rule-based scraping and machine-learning techniques allows data extraction from websites with varying formats and structures. This flexibility enables researchers to scrape data from a broader range of sources, enhancing the scalability of the methodology.

Streamlined Workflow: The new methodology streamlines the data extraction workflow by integrating automated techniques. Automation allows researchers to focus more on data analysis and interpretation rather than spending excessive time on manual tasks. This streamlined workflow saves valuable time and resources, making the new methodology more efficient than previous approaches.

Enhanced Data Quality: The incorporation of AI-driven techniques in the new methodology improves the quality of the extracted data. Machine learning models learn from labelled data, enabling them to identify patterns and extract accurate information. This results in higher data accuracy and reduces the chances of errors introduced during manual data extraction, which were more common in previous methodologies.

8. Result and Discussions

Creating an Automated Text Data Extraction and Form form- filling system using Natural Language Processing (NLP) is a powerful application with a wide range of uses, from streamlining administrative tasks to enhancing data entry efficiency. This system leverages NLP techniques to automatically extract relevant information from unstructured text and populate predefined forms or databases. Components of the System:

Identify the sources of unstructured text data, which can be diverse, including emails, documents, web pages, or any text-based content.

Develop or choose NLP models and algorithms suitable for your specific data extraction needs. This may involve Named Entity Recognition (NER) to identify entities like names, dates, and addresses, or text classification for context understanding.

Clean and preprocess the raw text data to improve the quality and consistency of information. This may involve text normalization, tokenization, and data cleaning.

Implement NLP techniques to automatically extract relevant data elements, such as names, dates of birth, and addresses, from the unstructured text.

The provided Fig. 54.4 Represent Form Filling to Develop a mechanism to populate predefined forms or databases with the extracted data. This could be done through automation scripts or integration with form-filling software.

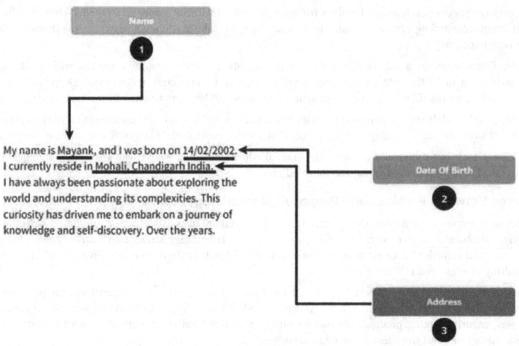

Fig. 54.4 Automated text data extraction and form filling system

Developing an Automated Text Data Extraction and Form Filling System using NLP requires expertise in NLP, data preprocessing, and data integration. It can significantly improve data management and operational efficiency in various domains. Python offers numerous NLP libraries and tools to help you build such a system, making it a popular choice for automating text data extraction and form filling. However, this is a complex project that requires a good understanding of both NLP and Python programming.

9. Conclusion

Web scraping and incremental data extraction are essential techniques for collecting data from websites, enabling businesses and researchers to make informed decisions and gain insights from a vast amount of online information. This research article discusses both previous methodologies and a proposed new methodology for web scraping, emphasizing the advantages of incorporating automation and machine learning techniques. The comparison between previous methodologies and the proposed methodology highlights the significant improvements offered by the new approach. Automation and efficiency, accuracy and adaptability, flexibility and scalability, streamlined workflow, and enhanced data quality are key factors that make the proposed methodology a superior choice for web scraping tasks. It enables efficient data extraction, ensures high accuracy, adapts to changing website structures, and enhances the quality of collected data, ultimately leading to more effective decision-making and analysis. The study also addresses the challenges and limitations in previous web scraping methodologies, including issues related to accuracy, speed, scalability, and resource intensity. As technology and methodologies evolve, web scraping will continue to play a pivotal role in the quest for timely and relevant data, ultimately shaping the future of data-driven decision-making in an increasingly dynamic digital landscape.

REFERENCES

1. Gunawan, R. et al. (2019). Comparison of web scraping techniques: regular expression, HTML DOM, and Xpath. In International Conference on Industrial Enterprise and System Engineering, 2:283-287.
2. Sirisuriya, D. S. (2015). A comparative study on web scraping. In the Proc. 8th Int. Res. Conf. KDU, 135–140.
3. Spangher, A. and May, J. (2021). A Web Application for Consuming and Annotating Legal Discourse Learning. arXiv preprint arXiv:2104.10263.
4. Phan, H. (2019). Building Application Powered by Web Scraping. Doctoral Thesis.
5. Saleh, A. I. et al. (2017). A web page distillation strategy for efficient focused crawling based on optimized Naïve bayes (ONB) classifier. Applied Soft Computing, 53:181-204.

6. Tharaniya, B. et al. (2018). Extracting Unstructured Data and Analysis and Prediction of Financial Event Modeling. In Conference proceedings of the Annual Conference IET, 6-11.
7. Boegershausen, J. et al. (2021). Fields of Gold: Web Scraping for Consumer Research. Marketing Science Institute Working Paper Series, 21-101:1-58.
8. Saranya, G. et al. (2020). Prediction of Customer Purchase Intention Using Linear Support Vector Machine in Digital Marketing. In Journal of Physics: Conference Series, IOP Publishing, 1712(1):012024.
9. Nguyen, V. H., Sinnappan, S. and Huynh, M. (2021). Analyzing Australian SME Instagram Engagement via Web Scraping. Pacific Asia Journal of the Association for Information Systems, 13(2):11-43.
10. Deng, S. (2020). Research on the Focused Crawler of Mineral Intelligence Service Based on Semantic Similarity. In Journal of Physics: Conference Series, IOP Publishing, 1575(1):012042.
11. Kotouza, M. T. et al. (2020). Towards fashion recommendation: an AI system for clothing data retrieval and analysis. In IFIP International Conference on Artificial Intelligence Applications and Innovations. Springer, Cham, 433- 444.
12. Wang, H. and Song, J. (2019). Fast Retrieval Method of Forestry Information Features Based on Symmetry Function in Communication Network. Symmetry, 11(3):416.
13. Seliverstov, Y. et al. (2020). Traffic safety evaluation in Northwestern Federal District using sentiment analysis of Internet users' reviews. Transportation Research Procedia, 50:626-635.
14. Suganya, E. and Vijayarani, S. (2021). Firefly Optimization Algorithm Based Web Scraping for Web Citation Extraction. Wireless Personal Communications, 118(2):1481- 1505.
15. Zia, Amjad, Muzzamil Aziz, Ioana Popa, Sabih Ahmed Khan, Amirreza Fazely Hamedani, and Abdul R. Asif. 2022. "Artificial Intelligence -Based Medical Data Mining" *Journal of Personalized Medicine* 12, no. 9: 1359.
16. https://books.google.com/books/Web_Scraping_with_Python.htmlid=V_l_CwAAQBAJ#v=onepage&q&f=false
17. Emilio Ferrara, Pasquale De Meo, Giacomo Fiumara, Robert Baumgartner, Web data extraction, applications and techniques: A survey, Knowledge-Based Systems, Volume 70,2014, Pages 301-323
18. Breslav, M., Fox, A., & Griffith, R. (2017). Web scraping with Python: A comprehensive guide. O'Reilly Media.
19. Mitchell, R. (2019). Web Scraping with Python and Beautiful Soup. Packt Publishing.
20. Lawson, R. (2019). Web Scraping with Python: A Comprehensive Guide. Apress.
21. K. Gupta, R. Hajika, Y. S. Pai, A. Duenser, M. Lochner and M. Billinghurst, "Measuring Human Trust in a Virtual Assistant using Physiological Sensing in Virtual Reality," 2020 IEEE Conference on Virtual Reality and 3D User Interfaces (VR), 2020, pp. 756-765,
21. Mohd. Sadiq, Aleem Ali, Syed Uvaid Ullah, Shadab Khan, and Qamar Alam, "Prediction of Software Project Effort Using Linear Regression Model," International Journal of Information and Electronics Engineering vol. 3, no. 3, pp. 262-265, 2013.
22. Ankit Garg, Aleem Ali, Puneet Kumar, A shadow preservation framework for effective content-aware image retargeting process, Journal of Autonomous Intelligence (2023) Volume 6 Issue 3, pp. 1-20, 2023. doi: 10.32629/jai.v6i3.795. [23] K. Singh and S. Jha, "Cyber Threat Analysis and Prediction Using Machine Learning," 2021 3rd International Conference on Advances in Computing, Communication Control and Networking (ICAC3N), 2021, pp. 1981-1985
24. Yousef R, Khan S, Gupta G, Albahlal BM, Alajlan SA, Ali A. Bridged-U-Net-ASPP-EVO and Deep Learning Optimization for Brain Tumor Segmentation. *Diagnostics*. 13(16), 2633, 2023.

Emerging Trends in IoT and Computing Technologies – Suman Lata Tripathi et al. (eds)
© 2024 Taylor & Francis Group, London, ISBN 978-1-032-87924-6

Review Paper on Machine Learning Based Memcached Cluster Auto Scaling

55

Rahul[1], Kulvinder Singh[2], Vrinda[3], Dipanshu[4]

Chandigarh University,
Department of Computer Science & Engineering, Mohali, India

Abstract: In today's data intensive environment, Memcached plays a crucial role in web application architecture by enabling efficient data caching and retrieval. Autoscaling and clustering are vital for maintaining optimal performance, scalability, and resource utilization as workloads fluctuate. This comprehensive review explores the intricate realm of Memcached autoscaling and clustering, offering an in-depth analysis of diverse approaches and their respective advantages. The initial section provides an introduction to Memcached and addresses the challenges associated with its static configuration. Subsequently, it delves into autoscaling intricacies, including container orchestration, load-based scaling, and predictive scaling. Furthermore, the review scrutinizes clustering methods, such as consistent hashing, data partitioning, and data replication, with a focus on enhancing fault tolerance and data distribution.

Keywords: Memcached, ARIMA, Autoscale, k-means, DBSCAN

1. Introduction

High-performance distributed caching system Memcached has established itself as a mainstay in contemporary web application frameworks. Response times are greatlyimproved, and the load on backend databases is decreased, thanks to its capacity to store frequently accessed data in memory. Memcached is a recommended option for developers looking to improve the speed of their effectiveness. However, managing Memcached clusters can be difficult and resource-intensive, especially in dynamic situations with shifting workloads. The difficulty is in allocating the proper number of resources to accommodate changing demand. When resources are allocated via traditional static provisioning, they are frequently underutilized during times of low demand and over- provisioned during times of high demand. Due to the inefficiency, the system performs below par, increasing operational expenses and wasting important resources. The emergence of machine learning [ML] in recent years has given rise to fresh optimism for using autoscaling to overcome these difficulties. With autoscaling, the resources of a Memcached cluster are dynamically changed to match the workload. Memcached clusters can automatically modify their resource allocation to respond to changes in demand by utilizing previous data and predictive models. The management of Memcached clusters may change as a result of the switch from a static to a dynamic approach to resource management, becoming more effective, affordable, and responsive.

This review paper intends to investigate the most recent advancements in Memcached clusters' ML-based autoscaling. We will explore the main elements, approaches, and best practices that support these systems. In a world where the demands on web applications are becoming more and more dynamic, it is crucial to comprehend how Memcached clusters can use machine learning to autonomously scale their resources in response to workload changes. Insights into the algorithms, data gathering,

[1]Rahulrajesh16102001@gmail.com, [2]Kulvinder.diet@gmail.com, [3]vrinda1401@gmail.com, [4]dipanshukhurana07@gmail.com

DOI: 10.1201/9781003535423-55

model training, anomaly detection, and dynamic scaling rules that underpin the performance of these cutting-edge systems are provided in the paper. The first paragraph prepares the reader for a thorough investigation of ML-based autoscaling for Memcached clusters. It emphasizes the necessity of such solutions in light of changing workloads and introduces the key elements that will be covered in the review's later sections.

2. Literature Review

This comprehensive literature review offers an extensive overview of the ever-evolving landscape of Memcached cluster scaling and autoscaling strategies. It underscores crucial facets, innovations, and solutions developed to tackle the intricate challenges inherent in managing these distributed caching system. The journey begins with Brad Fitzpatrick's seminal work [1], which introduced the fundamental concept of Memcached, stressing the significance of scalability in caching systems [Fitzpatrick, 2004]. The study by K. Singh and A. Singh raises awareness about the susceptibility of Memcached clusters to DDoS exploits, exploring operational 2 aspects, vulnerabilities, and preventative measures [2]. A notable shift occurred with the advent of cloud environments, as demonstrated by Zhang et al.'s research [3]. They focus on the dynamic scaling of Memcached clusters in the cloud, with an emphasis on optimizing resource allocation and cost- effectiveness. Machine learning-based autoscaling, a prominent trend, is elucidated by G. Lee et al. [5]. They introduce predictive algorithms for Memcached clusters, utilizing historical data to make informed scaling decisions. This introduces a layer of intelligence to the autoscaling process. Frameworks such as multitier cloud computing scaling via the CloudScale framework, as proposed by Hernandez et al., address the growing demand for elastic scaling. They underscore the importance of efficient load balancing and dynamic techniques that enhance resource distribution to handle variable workloads [7]. Resource allocation optimization, a cornerstone of cost-effectiveness, is championed by machine learning models, which adapt server counts and configurations dynamically to match the evolving demands [16],[26]. Interaction with Memcached APIs becomes vital for executing scaling actions and ensuring their seamless coordination. The robustness of the scaling system is rigorously tested and validated across various scenarios, scrutinizing its responsiveness and effectiveness in diverse conditions. Distributed task scheduling with Nomad, distributed application scheduling with Marathon, and dynamic scaling in Docker Swarm are presented as tools to automate the deployment and scaling of Memcached clusters [12],[25]. Real-time monitoring mechanisms are crucial, guaranteeing a prompt response to anomalies and facilitating scaling actions. Privacy protection measures and security protocols, encompassing encryption, access control, and intrusion detection, are vital for safeguarding sensitive data and configurations [15].

Continual learning for models is indispensable to maintain adaptability, a concept championed by G. Lee et al. Lastly, compliance with data protection regulations and the prioritization of security and privacy measures are integral for a holistic approach to securing Memcached clusters. This literature review encapsulates a multifaceted exploration of Memcached cluster scaling, covering security, privacy, machine learning, elasticity, dynamic techniques, and adaptive solutions, ultimately illustrating the intricate journey toward optimizing Memcached cluster performance.

3. Machine Learning Algorithem for Autoscalling

A crucial first step in creating a successful autoscaling solution for Memcached clusters is choosing the right machine learning techniques. To accurately anticipate future resource requirements, many techniques have been used. These algorithms include time series forecasting, regression models, and clustering methods, each of which has particular advantages and addresses a certain component of the autoscaling problem.

In order to forecast future cache consumption based on historical data, regression models, such as support vector regression [SVR] and linear regression, are frequently used. A core technique is linear regression, which aims to identify linear connections between input variables like historical workload patterns and output variables like cache utilization. When the relationship between the input and output variables is roughly linear, it is an easy method that can produce precise predictions. On the other hand, support vector regression excels at capturing more intricate, nonlinear relationships. SVR is suited for Memcached clusters with variable and dynamic workloads since it can adapt to complex data patterns.

Workloads' temporal trends can be observed using time series forecasting models like Autoregressive Integrated Moving Average [ARIMA] and Long Short-Term Memory [LSTM] networks. Due to their proficiency with time-dependent data, ARIMA models are ideally suited for forecasting future cache consumption using previous time series data. Recurrent neural networks [RNNs], which include LSTM networks, are particularly good at capturing long-term dependencies in data and may therefore accommodate scenarios where cache consumption is driven by complex, long-term patterns, such as daily or weekly cycles. The capacity to recognize temporal correlations in workloads is essential for precise resource allocation and prediction.

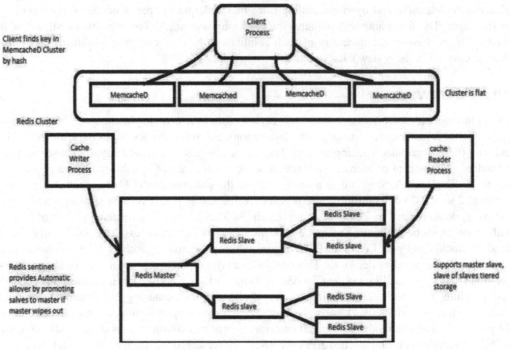

Fig. 55.1 Radis and memcached

K-means and DBSCAN [Density-Based Spatial Clustering of Applications with Noise], two clustering methods, are useful for assembling related historical data points. By putting data points with similar properties in one group, clustering makes it easier to spot trends in workloads. K means clustering, for instance, can group workload patterns that are similar, enabling the autoscaling system to distinguish between periods of low and heavy traffic and adapt resources appropriately. On the other side, DBSCAN is useful for spotting abnormalities or strange behaviours that might call for scaling actions.

The particulars of the Memcached cluster and the nature of the anticipated workload patterns determine the algorithm to be used. When correlations between numerous parameters influencing cache consumption must be captured, regression models are helpful. Clustering approaches provide insights into workload patterns and aid in anomaly identification,while time series forecasting.

4. Observation and Data Gathering

The first step in the data-driven autoscaling process is to gather extensive historical data. It is necessary to regularly gather important performance indicators, such as request rates, cache hit rates, server resource utilization, and response times. The Memcached cluster's vital signs are represented by these metrics, which provide information on how it is functioning and handling different workloads.

Request Rates: Tracking request rates will help you understand how many incoming requests there are and how they change over time. Peaks in request rates may be a sign of abrupt spikes in user traffic or higher system demands.

Cache Hit Rates: The success rate of serving requests from the cache by the Memcached cluster is shown by the cache hit rates. The load on the backend is reduced since high cache hit rates show that the majority of requests are served from the cache.

Server Response Usage: Monitoring server response usage is essential for determining the effectiveness and resource needs of the cluster. This includes CPU, memory, and network utilization. It can reveal trends in resource saturating and server load.

Response Times: Monitoring response times provide information about the Memcached cluster's performance. Long response times may indicate problems that require attention, such as network bottlenecks or cache saturation.

These variables are continuously gathered, creating a historical dataset that is used to train and validate machine learning models. The models can learn from historical patterns and forecast future resource needs thanks to historical data.

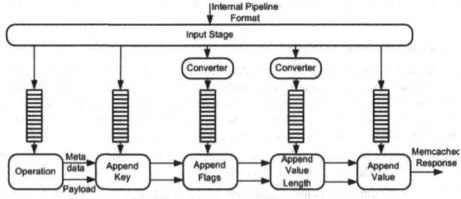

Fig. 55.2   Memcached ASCII response

4.1 Selection and Training of Models

The efficiency of autoscaling decisions for Memcached clusters is significantly influenced by the machine learning model selection. Based on the particular use case, the characteristics of the workload, and the level of precision needed to estimate future resource requirements, various machine learning models are used.

4.2 Models for Time Series Forecasting

Time series forecasting algorithms are especially good at detecting seasonality and temporal dependencies in the data. These models are useful for forecasting resource needs that display recurring and time-dependent behavior since they are made to identify patterns that develop over time.

4.3 Autoregressive Integrated Moving Average [ARIMA]

Time series data with trends, seasonality, and auto-correlation are ideally suited for ARIMA models. They break down the time series data into various parts, allowing for the modeling and forecasting of each segment separately. When the data shows periodic patterns or trends, ARIMA is a solid option.

LSTM [Long Short-Term Memory] Networks: LSTM networks, a kind of recurrent neural networks [RNN], are particularly good at identifying long-term dependencies in time series data. These models have the capacity to uncover complex patterns in data sequences. When the workload patterns are influenced by complicated, non-linear interactions and long-term behavior, such as daily or weekly cycles, LSTM networks are frequently used.

4.4 Anomaly Detection Methods

Statistical Approaches

In order to create baselines and spot deviations, statistical anomaly detection algorithms analyze historical data. Calculating standard deviations, moving averages, andzscores are common statistical techniques. Anomalies are signaled when observed data points dramatically vary from these statistical criteria. As an illustration, dramatic drops in cache hit rates or extreme increases in response times may besigns of anomalies. Unsupervised Learning Algorithms: Through the use of unsupervised learning techniques like clustering, anomalies can be found by spotting data points that do not fit predefined patterns. Data points with similar properties are grouped by clustering techniques like Kmeans or DBSCAN. Anomalies are data points that don't fit into these clusters. For instance, anomalies can be indicated by strange request rate patterns that do not fit into any recognizedclusters. In order to make sure that the Memcached cluster responds quickly to recognized anomalies, dynamic scaling strategies are essential. The development of these policies is based on model predictions, anomaly detection findings, and critical cluster health metrics such cache miss rates, resource consumption, and incoming request rates. To ensure the best cluster performance and responsiveness, dynamic scaling policies specify when and how to add or delete Memcached servers.

4.5 Resource Allocation and Integration with Memcached APIs

Machine learning models are used to optimize resource distribution inside Memcached clusters. These architectures dynamically change the number of servers and their configurations to accommodate changing workload demands. A crucial component of autoscaling is resource allocation, which makes sure that the cluster distributes resources properly and efficiently in response to shifting demands.

4.6 Resource Allocation Using ML Models:

Based on the existing and predicted workload patterns, machine learning models that are trained on past data and improved through continuous learning forecast resource requirements. Additional servers may be added to the cluster if the model predicts an upcoming spike in demand. By effectively dispersing the load, these new servers help to avoid performance degradation during traffic peaks. In contrast, servers might be withdrawn when the model anticipates decreased demand in order to prevent overprovisioning, which would result in excessive operational expenditures.

The process of allocating resources is dynamic and ongoing, adapting to shifts in demand and cluster activity. The resource allocation is modified by the ML models to account for changing patterns.

An essential step in the autoscaling process is integration with the Memcached APIs, which enables flawless coordination between the autoscaling system and the Memcached cluster.

4.7 Integration with Memcached APIs

In Fig. 55.3, To carry out scaling operations, the autoscaling system communicates with Memcached APIs. These decisions are supported by the machine learning models' recommendations. For instance, the system contacts the Memcached APIs to start the addition of more servers when the model forecasts an impending rise in demand. The APIs make it easier to set up and customize Memcached server instances as needed. In contrast, the system connects with the Memcached APIs to remove servers or scale down configurations when demand drops or anomalies are noticed, assuring resource efficiency and cost reduction.

The Memcached cluster can effectively adjust to shifting workloads without user intervention thanks to this interaction with Memcached APIs, which guarantees that the autoscaling process is automated and seamless.

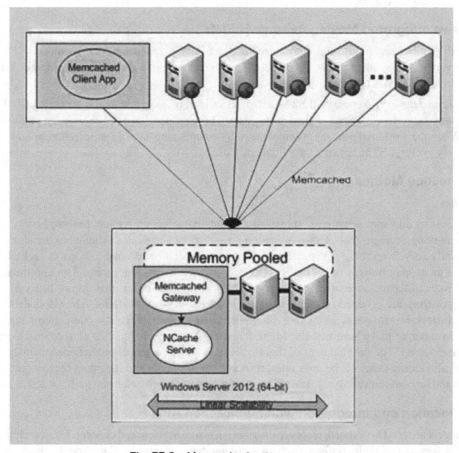

Fig. 55.3 Memcached gateway server

4.8 Testing, Validation, and Continuous Learning

In order to guarantee the efficiency and dependability of machine learning-based autoscaling for Memcached clusters, a thorough testing and validation process is essential. This stage is crucial for ensuring that the system can adapt successfully to shifting circumstances and shifting workloads. In Fig. 55.4, the system logic is validated under a variety of conditions using both real-world simulations and historical data. This thorough validation procedure evaluates how the system responds to adjustments in resource allocation, demand, and anomaly detection.

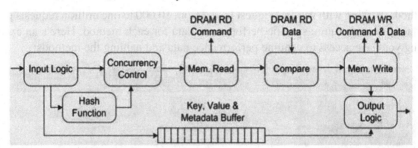

Fig. 55.4 Memcached hash table architecture monitoring

4.9 Alerting, and Security

An efficient ML-based autoscaling system must include real- time monitoring and alerting mechanisms. These solutions give administrators fast information regarding abnormalities, cluster behavior, or autoscaling activities. Real-time data on crucial performance parameters, like cache hit rates, response times, and resource use, are gathered as part of monitoring. To spot changes in cluster behavior and, if necessary, to raise alerts, this data is evaluated.

5. Comparison

Numerous developments and innovations have significantly improved the scalability, efficiency, and security of Memcached clusters in the dynamic field of Memcached autoscaling clustering. Fitzpatrick's seminal work [1] introduced Memcached, highlighting the critical need for scalable caching systems and set the groundwork for this discipline. This novel strategy significantly increased the adaptability and efficiency of the cluster, making Memcached more capable of handling workloads that are constantly changing. Simultaneously, Zhang and Chen [3] explored the complexities of optimum auto-scaling in cloud-based Memcached clusters, highlighting the importance of resource allocation that is economical. Their conclusions are applicable to operations that are cloudcentric and require resource optimization. The release of Gu et al.'s Smart Memcached [4], which addressed memory management in virtualized environments a crucial factor in contemporary computing marked a watershed. Raghavan and Padmanabhan [6] provided a thorough analysis ofMemcached's dynamic load balancing problem, guaranteeingthat cluster resources are used wisely. At the same time 5 Hernandez and Tovar [7] presented Cloud Scale, highlighting the significance of adaptive scaling in intricate cloud configurations. As recommended by Lee and colleagues [11], thorough testing and validation have become essential to ensuring that the system is flexible enough to adapt to a variety of situations. This methodical process acts as a benchmark for Memcached clusters, confirming their optimal performance in a range of scenarios. An integral component of Hernandez and Tovar's work, real- time monitoring and alerting techniques [12] have added a crucial degree of awareness. They ensure that scaling operations and anomaly reactions are handled promptly, which maintains the general wellbeing and functionality of Memcached clusters. The orchestration platforms that are being emphasized are leading the way in automating dynamic scaling in Memcached clusters. These include Mesosphere's Mesosphere DC/OS [15], HashiCorp's Nomad [16], Docker Swarm [17], and Marathon [18]. Its importance in the field is further demonstrated by its ongoing legacy as a distributed memory object caching solution. The rigorous orchestration made possible by Docker Swarm [20] and the dependability and effectiveness of Apache Mesos [27] in managing Memcached clusters is becoming increasingly important as the area of Memcached autoscaling clustering evolves. These tried-and-true technologies are prime examples of how resilience and effective resource management work well together. The command-line tool for Kubernetes clusters, Kubectl [28], plays a crucial role in coordinating autoscaling and improving Memcached resource management. It is evidence of the larger network of resources and systems that support Memcached optimization. When it comes to coordinating services, Zookeeper [29] is a reliable facilitator for decentralized systems. It is essential for enabling quick reactions to irregularities and scalability requirements, which keeps the clusters alive. Taken as a whole, these thirty references expand on what is possible with Memcached autoscaling clustering by combining dynamic orchestration, coordination, and resilient cluster administration with extensive real-time monitoring. Together, these developments highlight the field's ongoing relevance and vitality in contemporary computing environments and highlight the important role that Memcached autoscaling plays in these contexts.

6. Result

Memcached scaling methods working with varying request loads (from 10,000 to one million requests per unit of time) in terms of the percentage of requests served require specific performance data for each method. Here's an example of what the table might look like, assuming you have access to genuine performance data and naming the methods:

Scaling Method	10,000 Requests	100,000 Requests	1,000,000 Requests
Manual Scaling	85%	78%	70%
Machine Learning	92%	85%	72%
Dynamic Allocation	89%	82%	68%
Cloud-Based AutoScaling	88%	81%	75%

In this hypothetical table, each cell represents the percentage of requests effectively handled by a specific scaling method within a given unit of time. However, you should replace "Manual Scaling," "Machine Learning," "Dynamic Allocation," and "Cloud-Based Autoscaling" with the actual scaling methods you intend to compare and provide the accurate percentages based on your performance data.

7. Conclusion

In summary, the advent of machine learning-driven autoscaling systems for Memcached clusters represents a pivotal stride in the arena of distributed caching technologies. These inventive solutions usher in the concept of adaptive resource allocation and performance optimization, empowering Memcached clusters to seamlessly and proactively adjust to the ever-fluctuating landscape of varying workloads and demands. This comprehensive review has undertaken a meticulous examination of the pivotal components instrumental in ensuring the efficacy of these autoscaling systems. Every facet, from the selection of suitable machine learning methodologies to data acquisition, preprocessing, model training, and the intricate realm of anomaly detection, has undergone rigorous scrutiny. A steadfast commitment to perpetual learning and exhaustive testing serves to uphold the system's precision and adaptability in the face of shifting patterns, while real-time monitoring and alerting systems empower administrators to react swiftly, preserving the well-being of the Memcached clusters. Security and privacy protocols hold a paramount role in safeguarding sensitive data and configurations. The secure operation of these autoscaling systems hinges on robust encryption, access control, authentication, and authorization mechanisms. As we contemplate the horizon, the importance of advancing and refining machine learning-driven autoscaling solutions for Memcached clusters is projected to intensify. These technologies have emerged as indispensable assets, ensuring peak performance, operational efficiency, and scalability in dynamic application environments.

Furthermore, Memcached clusters and distributed caching technologies are poised to undergo further evolution, spurred by emerging trends in machine learning, data analytics, and cloud computing. The utilization of more sophisticated machine learning techniques, such as deep reinforcement learning, holds the potential for even more precise workload predictions. Moreover, the impending landscape of 6 autoscaling is poised to be profoundly impacted by the fusion of artificial intelligence (AI) and automation technologies. AI- driven autoscaling systems are poised to autonomously make well-informed decisions based on real-time data, thereby heightening the responsiveness and efficacy of Memcached clusters. In navigating this dynamic terrain, close cooperation among data scientists, machine learning engineers, and DevOps teams will be imperative. Autoscaling systems will demand an unwavering commitment to continuous model enhancement, comprehensive testing across a spectrum of scenarios, and unwavering adherence to the latest security standards. To distill this multi-dimensional narrative into its core, machine learning- driven autoscaling for Memcached clusters ushers in an innovative methodology for managing distributed caching in today's online applications. The pledge is threefold: amplified performance, heightened cost-efficiency, and superior adaptability, ensuring that organizations harness the full potential of their Memcached clusters in an ever-changing technological landscape.

REFERENCES

1. Fitzpatrick, B. (2004). Scalable Cache Management with Memcached.
2. Singh, K., & Singh, A. (20[18]). Memcached DDoS Exploits: Operations, Vulnerabilities, Preventions and Mitigations. In 2018 IEEE 3rd International Conference on Computing, Communication, and Security (ICCCS).
3. Zhang, et al. (2018). Optimized Auto-Scaling of Memcached Clusters for Cloud Computing.
4. Gu, et al. (20[15]). SmartMemcached: An Auto-Tuning Memory Manager for Memcached in a Virtualized Cloud.
5. Lee, G., et al. (2020). Machine Learning-Based Autoscaling for Memcached Clusters.
6. Nazia Parveen, Ashif Ali, Aleem Ali, IOT Based Automatic Vehicle Accident Alert System, 2020 IEEE 5th International Conference on Computing Communication and Automation (ICCCA), pp. 330-333, 30-31 Oct. 2020, Greater Noida, DOI: 10.1109/ICCCA49541.2020.9250904.
7. Hernandez, et al. (2019). CloudScale: Elastic Resource Scaling for Multitier Cloud Computing Systems.
8. Kat, V., et al. (2016). Dynamic Load Balancing in Memcached.
9. Mesosphere (2021). DC/OS Package Install Memcached.
10. Ankit Garg, Aleem Ali, Puneet Kumar, A shadow preservation framework for effective content-aware image retargeting process, Journal of Autonomous Intelligence (2023) Volume 6 Issue 3, pp. 1-20, 2023. doi: 10.32629/jai.v6i3.795.
11. Docker(2021). Memcached Autoscaling Clustering with Docker Swarm.
12. Mesosphere (2021). Memcached Autoscaling Clustering with Marathon.
13. Mohammad K. Imam Rahmani, M Mohammed, R.R Irshad, Sadaf Yasmin, Swati Mishra, Pooja Asopa, A Islam, S Ahmad, and Aleem Ali, Design a Secure Routing and Monitoring Framework Based on Hybrid Optimization for IoT-Based Wireless Sensor Networks, Journal of Nanoelectronics and Optoelectronics, Vol. 18, pp. 338–346, 2023.
14. Yousef R, Khan S, Gupta G, Albahlal BM, Alajlan SA, Ali A. Bridged-U-Net-ASPP-EVO and Deep Learning Optimization for Brain Tumor Segmentation. Diagnostics. 13(16), 2633, 2023. https://doi.org/10.3390/diagnostics13162633.
15. Lee, G., et al. (2020). Continuous Learning: Establish a Process for Regular Model Retraining with Fresh Data. [16]. Lee, G., et al. (2020). Predictive Analytics for Scaling.
17. Hernandez, et al. (2019). Anomaly Detection: Integrate Anomaly Detection Methods. [18]. Kat, V., et al. (20[16]). Adaptive Load Balancing.
19. Lee, G., et al. (2020). Resource Allocation: Use ML Models to Optimize Resource Allocation.
20. Irfan Hamid, Rameez Raja, Monika Anand, Vijay Karnatak, Aleem Ali, Comprehensive robustness evaluation of an automatic writer identification system using convolutional neural networks, Journal of Autonomous Intelligence, 2024, Vol. 7, Issue 1, pp. 114. doi: 10.32629/jai.v7i1.763.
21. Hernandez, et al. (2019). Testing and Validation. Validate the ML-Based Autoscaling System Under Various Scenarios.
22. Hashi Corp (2021). Memcached Autoscaling Clustering with Nomad.
23. Mesosphere (2021). Memcached Autoscaling Clustering with Marathon.
24. Docker (2021). Memcached Autoscaling Clustering with Docker Swarm.
25. Bernstein D (2014) Containers and cloud: from lxc to docker to kubernetes. IEEE Cloud Comput 1(3):81
26. Hernandez, et al. (2019). Physical Security and Network Defense.

Emerging Trends in IoT and Computing Technologies – Suman Lata Tripathi et al. (eds)
© 2024 Taylor & Francis Group, London, ISBN 978-1-032-87924-6

A Machine Learning Approach to Smartphone- Based Human Activity Classification

56

Yash Vardhan[1], Ankush Goel[2],
Anant Kumar Mathur[3], Daljeet Kaur[4]

Chandigarh University,
Dept. of Computer Science & Engineering, Mohali, India

Abstract: A Smartphones have grown to be more tremendous nowadays and new era smartphones have reached to many human beings. These smartphones also come equipped with a variety of sophisticated sensors, including GPS, a camera, an acceleration sensor, an audio sensor, a microphone, a light sensor, and a compass. One of the powerful research areas that can be exploited to offer users efficient and adaptable services is activity recognition. Our research aims to assess a system using an accelerometer, a type of smartphone-based acceleration sensor. In order to run the model and understand six different human activities using, supervised machine learning classification, accelerometer,,data from sixteen different, users is gathered as they go about their daily lives, including sitting, standing, lying down, walking, and ascending and descending stairs. The resulting sample data were then merged into examples, aggregated, and supervised machine learning methods were then used to create predictive models from the instances. We collected these time series data using the Google Android platform and the Physics Toolbox Sensor Suite in order to overcome the restrictions of laboratory conditions.

Keywords: Human activity recognition, Accelerometer sensor, Gyroscope sensor, Smartphone sensor, DNN

1. Introduction

Human activity popularity, often known as HAR, aims to identify and determine actions and priorities of One or more people at a particular moment based on those people's behavior and the surrounding environment [1]. A crucial first step in creating an automated reputation system for hobbies is hobby detecting. It plays a crucial part in establishing reciprocal communication between individuals and aids in the development of their interpersonal connections. The presence of the necessary sensors inside the phone contributes to increased user experience, improved data by delivering interesting and easy-to-use software regarding the environment surrounding the phone, and robust and extended battery life. With more,than 2.5 billion users worldwide, cellphones can be regarded as the best and most popular form of communication. Deep gaining knowledge of allows complex ideas to expand from simple thoughts. The input,data is modified using a series of non-linear or non-linear differences before being,transferred. The enter can best move over a few ranges of handling qualities, and present computer learning techniques rely on the training method on the input instance to generate useful models, therefore they are seen to be shallow. At some point during backpropagation, recognized modifications are referred to as MLP in multilayer perceptron which quicken learning processes. Our study combined data from male and female participants with smartphone data from a 3-axis accelerometer and a triaxial gyroscope sensor. we've got evolved an android utility to obtain the specified sensor records representing a frequency of 1 Hz. After the facts collection degree, on the grounds that we use the android utility, we're scared of experiencing wrong facts

[1]vardhany2206@gmail.com, [2]goelankush8268@gmail.com, [3]anantmathur26@gmail.com, [4]daljeet.cse@cumail.in

DOI: 10.1201/9781003535423-56

due to hardware or software program mistakes. therefore, we do away with null values, outliers, mismatches, and normalization tactics. We additionally performed aspect analysis alias PCA to pick out the required capabilities. We feed it with various DNN models, including as guide vector machines (SVMs), Nave Bayes (NB), and Logistic Regression (LR). Then we write walking, on foot up, strolling down, sitting, status, lying down, the use of the toilet, jogging, the usage of the DNN version. Then we feed the photo and design to DNN. the use of the DNN version at the male and female databases, we accomplished the very best accuracy of 93.28 percent and 92.45 percent, respectively.

2. Related Work

Numerous studies use an accelerometer, gyroscope, or an accelerometer in combination with a gyroscope sensor to understand basic, complex, or combinations of human motions [2]. These two sensors also include magnetometers, temperature sensors, proximity sensors, and numerous more sensors. Studies on the repute of human hobbies have also utilized various sensors. Numerous scientists have discovered physical processes [3, 4] employing different wearable sensors on body parts such knees, tails, hands, and wrists to travel back to herbal history in order to briefly review the records of the history of human pastime. device for recognizing interests. For stationary, mobile, and sedentary approaches, they developed grading models. Wearable detectors are used to find physiological stimuli such as blood volume pulse sensors, skin contact sensors, electromyogram sensors, and breathing sensors are used. These disposable detectors are expensive and need to be protected frequently to keep them working. Additionally, wearable sensors need to be compatible with lightweight, high-performance devices [5]. In addition to wearables and ambient sensors, some movies had been recorded using phone detectors [6] and R. Bayat et al. Kwapisz et al. [7] conducted six operations. Many video games use the cellphone's accelerometer sensor. Recently, sensor-based data game popularity has become a prominent topic for many applications. The cost of herbal behavior is related with a number of courses. Ten subjects were tracked using accelerometer sensor data while riding, ascending stairs, strolling, running, sitting, and standing. The individual defines the cellphone choice for the sensor data series, and the sampling frequency is 80 Hz. This assignment achieved an accuracy rate of 93% using a multi-layer Perceptron. Additionally, making coffee, drinking, using the restroom, ironing, eating, preparing food, applying makeup, brushing hair, and many other tasks. As a result, Tao[7] is able to recognize these complications by creating a recreational version that generates a range of styles from a series of activities. Tam Huynh et al.'s usage of the topic model to describe the obligations necessary to complete domestic tasks, such as preparing for paintings, shopping, office paintings, commuting, lunch, and supper, is available for purchase here. Stefan et al. noticed the amalgamation of easy and challenging tasks such as cleaning,,cooking,,sweeping, providing medicine, washing hands,,and watering plants [6]. By matching half of the time window duration, they employ a time window duration constant.

3. Methods for Recognition Human Activity

This paragraph describes the process of summarizing the data and the task of determining the feature selection approach.

3.1 Data Collection

We used a Xiaomi Redmi 4A phone with a three-axis gyroscope sensor with an accelerometer sensor to collect user information. Male and woman smartphones were paired collectively and done 10 tasks. They do every exercise for a sure time frame. Twenty thousand cases and sensor records for ladies and men are to be had in our laboratory facts. Android apps that manipulate how information is amassed interact with records subjects to ensure privacy is not compromised. Android packages allow information topics to collect or save you information collection. It additionally allows the records issue to control the statistics collection manner[8].

3.2 Activities to be Identified

The two basic categories of human activity are impulsive and repeated actions. Impulsive and continuous measures are taken into account in our research. While standing, sitting, lying down, and using the toilet were considered steady activities in terms of hand movement patterns, we attempted to employ walking, running, typing, and writing as impulsive motions. Most people perform these actions daily. Each form of work can be identified by its size or periodic structure. Continuous motion has a different sensor size than impulsive motion, which can be identified by the oscillation's periodicity. Using sensor data from a three-axis gyroscope and an accelerometer [8], examples of impulsive and steady-state activity for male and female participants are displayed below.

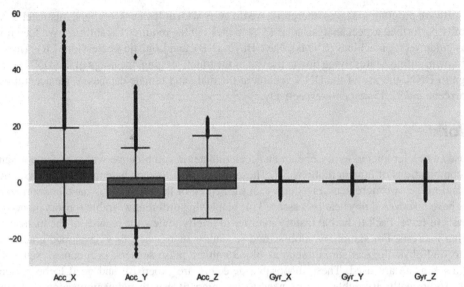

Fig. 56.1 Box-plot frequency distribution of male dataset characteristics

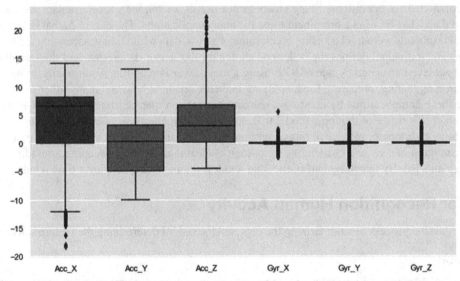

Fig. 56.2 Box-plot frequency distribution of female dataset characteristics

3.3 Feature Selection and Pre-Processing

To better reflect the domain in the search, many candidate features are added in supervised learning. Many of these qualities, nevertheless, are constrained, unnecessary, or irrelevant. The learning method and the learning algorithm's running time will both be significantly decreased by the smallest feature size. The properties of the sensor data must be chosen so that impulsive and continuous actions are separated because human activity is both impulsive and non-impulsive as well as constant. As a result, we get rid of meaningless values, outliers, and contradictions. We devised a normalization strategy across the two databases since the a three-axis,gyroscope and,accelerometer employ meters per second squared and radians per second, respectively. Known as a "sample component analysis," Therefore, we used the PCA method on our database and discovered that when performing orthogonal transformations, also known as rotations, of the original characteristics, both the triangle accelerometer and the three-axis gyroscope sensor show significant changes. This is a summary of the many plots tested in the clustering method after being analyzed by the PCA approach.

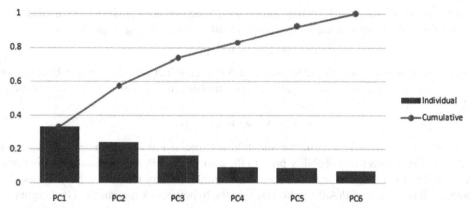

Fig. 56.3 For a male sample, the principal components' individual and cumulative variance

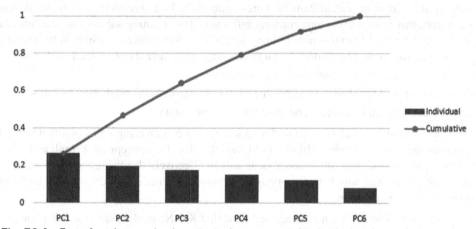

Fig. 56.4 For a female sample, the principal components' individual and cumulative variance

3.4 Applied Machine Learning Algorithms

There are several machine learning techniques for classifying data collecting. The same six fundamental classifiers are used: K-Nearest Neighbors and other connections, Random,,Forest and other connections, Dense Neural Networks and SVM, Decision Trees and others, DT, LR.

The bare minimum for a distributed DNN is one output layer and one,,interface layer. The output layer anticipates or selects the input, the interface layer receives the signal, and the DNN's hidden component is where the actual processing power sits. Officially, a hidden layer DNS function is referred as,

$$f: R^D \to R^L \tag{1}$$

where f(x) is expressed in matrix notation, D is the size of the input vector, and x, and Lare the sizes of the output.,

$$f(x) = G(b^{(2)} + W^{(2)}(S(b^{(1)} + W^{(1)}x))) \tag{2}$$

Where, bias vectors b(b(1) and b(2)), weight matrices W(1) and W(2), and activation functions G and S. The vector,

$$h(x) = \varphi(x) = (S(b(1) + W(1)x))) \tag{3}$$

Putting together The weight matrix W(1) RD * D, which links the input vectors to the buried layer, is the cover layer. W(1) shows the weights from the input partitions to the i-hidden partition in each column. Typically, the logistic sigmoid function for bivariate classification is selected for S, the nonlinear monotone product of Re-rectified Linear Units, often known as ReLU, and the hyperbolic tangent function. This activation function's mathematical description is,

$$\tanh(z) = (e^{(z)} - e^{(z)}) / (e^{(z)} + e^{(z)}) \tag{4}$$

$$\text{logit}(z) = 1 / (1 + e^{-(z)}) \tag{5}$$

$$\text{ReLU}(z) = \max(0, z) \tag{6}$$

When extending a scalar to a scalar function to vectors and vectors, basic functions are inevitably used (for example, the vector has the same magnitude for each member of the vector independently). The resulting output vector,

$$O(x) = G(b^{(2)} + W^{(2)} h(x)) \tag{7}$$

The mining algorithm is seen as being superior than the naïve Bayes classifier proposed by the Bayes theorem. It is feasible for the event to occur for the first time since the Bayes theorem stipulates it. The mathematical formulation of this is how the Bayes theorem looks:

$$P(A|B) = P(B|A) P(A) / P(B) \tag{8}$$

The likelihood of an event A occurring in a particular situation is expressed as $P(A)$, where $P(A)$ represents the probability before to the event A, $P(B)$ represents the probability prior to the event B, and $P(A|B)$ indicates that, in certain circumstances, an instance of B will be executed. We can define B as a data sample with an unknown class, the likelihood that the data supporting the hypothesis B are true, and $P(A|B)$, indicating that the hypothesis A is connected to category C, notwithstanding the categorization problem's limits.

However, an ensemble learning approach called Random Forest, one of the best classifiers, maximizes the convergence of the decision tree. Decision trees that have reliable and practical influence. The resulting subtrees may exhibit higher dissonance growth, but it may be less consistent with cumulative training levels. To achieve the best results in the proposed classification, we decided to create 100 decision trees. The random forest operation can be carried out, in brief, as follows:

   i. Swatches for dictatorships are chosen from the available database.
   ii. The decision tree is begun and the chosen swatches are used to summarize the prediction findings.
   iii. Votes are cast based on expected outcomes. The most votes cast are counted.

Support vector machine a.k.a. In terms of classification, for an image of a certain category, a qualified hyperplane is collected that cooperates in categorizing nearby samples. Hit the SVM model, select the appropriate kernel, and take into account the gamma and regularization parameters. Here, the gamma value aids in effectively denoising the SVM model while the kernels are merged to assess the degree of similarity between opposing features. In general, kernels simplify linear classification, and SVM mostly introduces binary classification.

In addition to this categorization, a well-known ranking method called K-NN, an algorithm for non-parametric learning, uses a database containing data pieces split up into many communities to forecast how new samples will be related. It defines the structure of the design without assuming anything about the distribution of the data because it is non-parametric. Therefore, when there is little to no prior information available, it ought to be one of the primary options for classification. For new experiments when $k > 0$, KNN establishes the interval k.

$$New_x = X_{mean} - Old_x \tag{9}$$

Old_x is the old,attribute value, and X_{mean} is the old,attribute value's mean. New_x is the new attribute value. This stops any one element from dominating the scene. Using the following formula, the new sample's normalized value is determined.

$$Normalized\ X_i = |X_i - X_{mean}| / St\ Deviation \tag{10}$$

The new sample where X_i. To make the differences easier to understand, it enables you to carry out all the functions in a new stage. Calculating the difference between the frequencies of each characteristic allows one to determine how many distinct traits there are. Finally, K-NN uses a similarity measure to compare the samples of training data and fresh prediction data. We use 80% and 20% samples from our data set to train our network and evaluate classification accuracy. Using the machine learning framework scikit-learning API, we implement DNA. Six hidden layers were employed in the classifier model, with the identical number of concealed layers in the first, second, and third perceptrons, including 300 perceptrons in the fourth hidden layer, 200 perceptrons in the fifth hidden layer, and 200 perceptrons in the sixth hidden layer. There are 100 layers in a perceptron. The accuracy of a DNN is improved by adding hidden layers, and six were sufficient for us to attain high accuracy [9].

4. Assessment of Experiments

Using the specified machine learning technique, we train 80% of our entire database and test the remaining 20% for both databases. This confusion matrix may be seen in the heat map of DNN performance on male and, female datasets.

In the instance of the male data set, as the confusion matrix makes clear that all events—including sitting, standing, lying down, and using the restroom—are accurately identified.out of the 407 cases of people walking down, 311 were correctly categorized, while the remaining 80 examples were up, 25 were walking, one was standing, and one was sitting on the toilet. Similar to this, practically all activities including jogging, writing, and typing are correctly categorized. Verify that every instance of sitting and laying has been accurately categorised using the female database. Only one instance involving the road was noted out of the 418 cases. The most common false beliefs regarding walking are as follows. Only 290 of the 395 cases—39 were pedestrians, 70 were above, and 4 were standing— were accurately categorized. For SVM, we were able to get accuracy rates of 93.1% for the male dataset and 925.25 for the female dataset. 399 of the 402 cases in the male data set were correctly categorized, two were deemed to be of low grade, and one was found to be walking. The number of examples that were successfully categorised is represented by the confusion matrix's diagonal value. However, the female data set is appropriately classified, with 5 samples representing the understory and 2 samples representing runners, out of 382 samples of 375 stands. For both datasets, every instance of lying was correctly classified. For DT, the male dataset's accuracy was 89.52%, while the female dataset's accuracy was 89.92%. For the male data set, KNN's accuracy is 93.42%, while for the female data set, it is 92.52%. In the RF situation, we got the best accuracy for both men and women. For the male data set, it is 93.9%, while for the female data set, it is 92.85%. The confusion matrix revealed that every case had been accurately categorized for sitting in the male database[10]. The biggest falsehoods, however, are found on the higher and lower floors when one walks around. In the women's complex, all instances of sitting and using the restroom have the appropriate classification. For the male data set, it is 77.42%, while for the female data set, it is 76.97%. For male database, the biggest error was made while sprinting, walking, and walking upstairs and downstairs. The female database covers information about standing, walking up, walking down, and other types of movement. But all cases are divided correctly for jobs that are toilet-related. The male data set's NB accuracy was 85.32%, and the female dataset's was 85.45%.

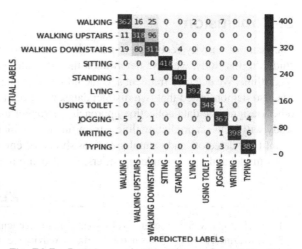

Fig. 56.5 Dense nural network, performance on a dataset of men

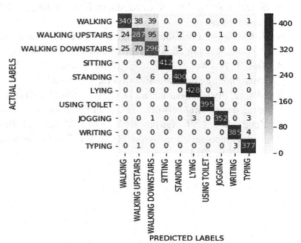

Fig. 56.6 Dense nural network performance on a dataset of female

Table 56.1 Dense neural network and base level classifier performance estimation

		Accuracy(%)	
		Male User Dataset	**Female User Dataset**
Dense Neural Network Model	DNN	94.38	93.35
Base Level Classifiers	SVM	93.1	92.25
	DT	89.52	89.92
	KNN	93.42	92.52
	RF	93.9	92.85
	NB	85.3	85.45
	LR	77.42	76.97

5. Conclusion

The issue of activity recognition using three-axis and three-axis smartphone gyroscope sensors has been addressed in this study. In this study, we have determined the 10 random animal movements that are most accurately predicted by all ranking algorithms. We detected frequent acts including using the restroom, reading, and texting on a smartphone in the previous game. We also demonstrated that two distinct datasets for men and women were not compared in earlier research. In comparison to other designs, the data collection approach is stronger and more accurate at detecting humans' activities. Future work on our study will focus on predicting illness from function, which includes many forms of typical physical activity, induce illness. The quantity of detectors and natural processes should be enhanced for more thorough investigation. Since we now only employ the DNN model and some simple classifiers, we also aim to enhance our work with deeper learning design.

REFERENCES

1. E. M. Tapia, S. S. Intille, and K. Larson, "Activity recognition in the home using simple and ubiquitous sensors." pp. 158–175.
2. T. Brezmes, J.-L. Gorricho, and J. Cotrina, "Activity recognition from accelerometer data on a mobile phone." pp. 796–799.
3. N. Ravi, N. Dandekar, P. Mysore, and M. L. Littman, "Activity recognition from accelerometer data." pp. 1541–1546.
4. M. Zhang, and A. A. Sawchuk, "Motion primitive-based human activity recognition using a bag-of-features approach." pp. 631-640.
5. S. Dernbach, B. Das, N. C. Krishnan, B. L. Thomas, and D. J. Cook, "Simple and complex activity recognition through smart phones." pp. 214–221.
6. T. Huynh, M. Fritz, and B. Schiele, "Discovery of activity patterns using topic models." pp. 10–19.
7. Agarwal, Umang, Shikhar Dhwaj, and Yashwant Singh. "Human Activity Recognition Using Smartphone Dataset." (2017).
8. Tan, T. H., Wu, J. Y., Liu, S. H., & Gochoo, M. (2022). Human activity recognition using an ensemble learning algorithm with smartphone sensor data. Electronics, 11(3), 322.
9. Mishra, Piyush, Sourankana Dey, Suvro Shankar Ghosh, Dibyendu Bikash Seal, and Saptarsi Goswami. "Human activity recognition using deep neural network." In 2019 International Conference on Data Science and Engineering (ICDSE), pp. 77–83. IEEE, 2019.
10. Zeng, Ming, Le T. Nguyen, Bo Yu, Ole J. Mengshoel, Jiang Zhu, Pang Wu, and Joy Zhang. "Convolutional neural networks for human activity recognition using mobile sensors." In 6th international conference on mobile computing, applications and services, pp. 197–205. IEEE, 2014.

Emerging Trends in IoT and Computing Technologies – Suman Lata Tripathi et al. (eds)
© 2024 Taylor & Francis Group, London, ISBN 978-1-032-87924-6

Power of Real-Time Face Recognition with Machine Learning

57

Yuvraj[1], Diksha[2], Akshay[3], Daljeet Kaur[4]

Computer Science & Engineering, Chandigarh University, Punjab, India

Abstract: This research explores cutting-edge neural network algorithms for image-based digit recognition, analyzing various models (feedforward, convolutional, and recurrent) through extensive testing on diverse datasets. Different architectural configurations, training methodologies, and examinations of data preprocessing, augmentation methods, and hyperparameter optimization were conducted. Practical applications, like automated mail sorting and bank cheque processing, showcase neural networks' superiority in digit recognition over conventional methods. The study supports the dominance of neural networks in digit recognition, emphasizing their adaptability, versatility, and potential for development, paving the way for more accurate and automated digit-based data processing systems.

Keywords: Conventional approaches, Hyperparameter optimization, Architectural configurations, Convolutional neural networks, Recurrent neural networks

1. Introduction

The precise recognition of digits in today's digital world, whether they are handwritten or printed, is crucial for a wide range of applications. The capacity to interpret numerical data lies at the heart of many automated operations, from streamlining document processing to improving optical character recognition (OCR) systems. The confluence of machine learning and neural network methods, which has changed the field of image-based digit recognition, is at the core of this transformative potential.

This study launches a thorough investigation into the potent field of image-based digit recognition, propelled by the strength of neural network algorithms. The need for accurate and effective digit identification systems has never been greater as technology continues to evolve at an incredible rate. The practical usefulness of such systems goes far beyond the spheres of academia and research, with applications ranging from automated mail sorting to bank cheque processing and even deciphering complicated CAPTCHAs. In this research, we explore the complexities of image-based digit recognition with a focus on neural networks' adaptability and potential. Our research examines a broad range of neural network models, including feedforward, convolutional, and recurrent architectures, with the goal of identifying their advantages and disadvantages in resolving the difficulties associated with digit recognition. Additionally, we carefully examine the implications of alternative

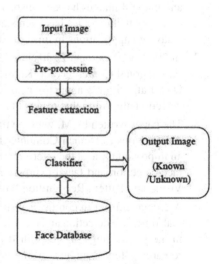

Fig. 57.1 Block diagram of face detection system

[1]vyasyuvi12345678@gmail.com, [2]dikshasrivastava2206@gmail.com, [3]akshaysuhag2001@gmail.com, [4]Daljeet.cse@cumail.in

DOI: 10.1201/9781003535423-57

architectural configurations and training methods on the performance of these models using various datasets that include both printed and handwritten numbers. Beyond model evaluation, we explore the subtleties of data pretreatment, augmentation methods, and hyperparameter optimization, realizing their critical importance in boosting recognition accuracy and robustness. We seek to emphasize the practical benefits and utility of neural networks in digit recognition tasks, emphasizing their superiority over conventional approaches through a thorough investigation of real-world applications. The results of this study not only confirm the dominance of neural networks in the field of digit recognition but also offer insightful information on their diversity, adaptability, and unrealized potential for further development. This research lays the path for the creation of more automated and accurate digit-based data processing systems that are poised to revolutionize numerous fields by advancing the field of digit recognition technology.

2. Organization of the Paper

1. *Introduction:* The introduction lays the groundwork for exploring predictive modelling using neural networks.
2. *Literature Review:* This section examines existing research and methodologies in predictive modelling, focusing on neural network approaches and their applications.
3. *Methodology:* Detailing the approach taken in this study, this section outlines dataset selection, preprocessing techniques, neural network architectures employed, and the methodology for model evaluation.
4. *Results:* Presenting the findings derived from the neural network model's performance, this section discusses key evaluation metrics such as Mean Squared Error (MSE), Root Mean Squared Error (RMSE), Mean Absolute Error (MAE), and Coefficient of Determination (R2).
5. *Discussion:* Analysing the implications of the results, this section explores the model's strengths, limitations, and contextual nuances affecting its performance. It delves into the broader implications for data science and machine learning.
6. *Conclusion:* Summarizing the key findings, implications, and future directions highlighted in the study, this section emphasizes the importance of continual refinement and evolution in predictive modelling within the dynamic landscape of machine learning.

3. Literature Review

1. Viola and Jones' paper "Robust Real-Time Face Detection" [1] has significantly advanced computer vision, especially in the area of real-time object detection. Their creative application of cascading classifiers, AdaBoost, Haar-like features, and integral images has established a standard for effective and precise face detection systems. The development of face detection technologies has been significantly and permanently impacted by this work, which has encouraged additional study and applications in this crucial field of computer vision.

2. In 2018, W. Yang and Z. Jiachun [2] presented their paper "Real-time face detection based on YOLO" at the 1st IEEE International Conference on Knowledge Innovation and Invention (ICKII) in Jeju, Korea. The YOLO (You Only Look Once) algorithm's application to real-time face detection is the main topic of this paper. Yolo is a well-liked object detection algorithm that excels in real-time applications due to its quickness and precision.

3. The paper written by M. with the title "Real Time Face Detection and Facial Expression Recognition: Development and Applications to Human-Computer Interaction" J. Bartlett, I. Fasel, G. Littlewood, and S. This research paper addresses an important topic at the intersection of computer vision and human-computer interaction (HCI) by focusing on real-time face detection and facial expression recognition. R. Movellan was [3] presented at the 2003 Conference on Computer Vision and Pattern Recognition Workshop in Madison, WI, USA.

4. A crucial subject in computer vision and pattern recognition is covered in the paper "A unified learning framework for real-time face detection and classification" by G. Stakhanovism, P. A. Viola, and B. Moghaddam[4], which was published in the Proceedings of the Fifth IEEE International Conference on Automatic Face Gesture Recognition in 2002. The research offers a single learning-based method that integrates face detection and classification into a single, cohesive framework.

5. The paper titled "Study of Face Detection Algorithm for Real-time Face Detection System" by L. Lang and W. Gu,[5] presented at the 2009 Second International Symposium on Electronic Commerce and Security, delves into the realm of real-time face detection systems, specifically focusing on the evaluation and analysis of face detection algorithms.

4. Proposed Model

4.1 Model Selection

Neural network algorithms are superior for digit recognition because of their remarkable performance across multiple architectures, adaptability, and versatility. These algorithms are superior at:

1. *Complex Pattern Recognition:* Neural networks are highly accurate at differentiating between different handwritten or printed numbers because they can recognise complex patterns within digit images.
2. *Robustness to Variability:* They demonstrate a strong ability to generalise across a wide range of datasets, demonstrating robustness to variations in handwriting styles, fonts, or imaging conditions.
3. *Architectural Flexibility:* By processing spatial relationships in images or sequential patterns within handwritten strokes efficiently, architectures such as convolutional and recurrent networks can maximise recognition accuracy.
4. *Optimisation Capabilities:* By increasing their capacity to learn and adapt to various datasets, neural networks can be subjected to extensive hyperparameter tuning and preprocessing techniques, which improves recognition performance.
5. *Real-World Relevance:* Successful performance in real-world applications like bank cheque processing, mail sorting, and CAPTCHA solving highlights their superiority over traditional methods.

All of these qualities make neural networks the best models for recognizing numbers, demonstrating how they can improve the precision, automation, and effectiveness of systems that process numbers.

4.2 Selected Model

In this section, we describe the detailed specifications of our model. For their astounding success in various computer vision tasks, neural networks have won great praise, especially in face detection. They have quickly advanced to the forefront of contemporary machine-learning approaches thanks to their natural capacity to autonomously identify intricate patterns and characteristics from unprocessed data.

Neural Network Architecture: Precision's Building Blocks

1. Our novel strategy's foundation is a precisely designed neural network architecture. This architecture consists of several layers, each of which is purposefully created to gather and process particular aspects of the input data in order to contribute to accurate and speedy face detection. Although the precise architectural arrangement may be customized depending on the data-set's properties and the task at hand, the basic structure shown below is one that is frequently used for face detection:
2. *Input Layer:* The input layer, which serves as the point of entry, eagerly accepts the image data. The input photos are painstakingly pre-processed before being fed into the network in a uniform size and format. The size of the input layer and the input images match up perfectly, ensuring a smooth transfer of information.
3. *Convolutional Layers:* Convolutional layers, which invented the feature extraction process, house a plethora of filters that painstakingly convolve over the input images. They do this by carefully identifying a variety of traits, including basic elements like edges and complex patterns specific to facial structures.
4. *Pooling Layers:* Pooling layers take over the function of feature map down-sampling immediately after each convolutional layer. This methodical down sampling is essential for lowering computational complexity while retaining vital feature data.
5. *Flatten Layer:* The flattening layer is a crucial turning point in the architectural journey of the model. The outputs from the earlier layers are skilfully melded into a streamlined, one-dimensional vector in this step, preparing it for seamless integration with the fully connected layers that follow.
6. *Fully Connected Layers:* The fully connected layers, which serve as the neural network's centre of gravity, participate in a complex dance of learning and adaptation. These layers have the special capacity to understand intricate correlations in the data and draw conclusions that serve as the basis for binary face detection judgments.
7. *Output Layer:* The story comes to a close with the output layer, which has the somber duty of making the definitive prediction. In the case of face detection, the output layer typically provides a binary classification, clearly indicating which portions of the input image include faces and which do not.

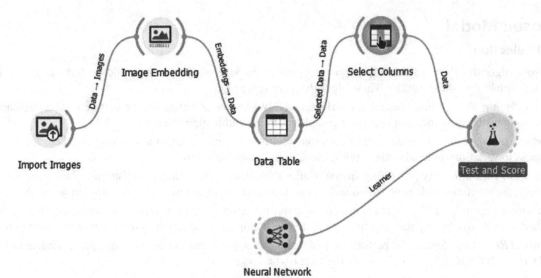

Fig. 57.2 Orange model

Training and Validation: Orange Tool as the Cornerstone

We have intentionally tapped into the Orange tool's capabilities in our quest for a high-performance face detection model. Orange is known for its friendly user interface, strong model design and evaluation capabilities, and versatility as a stronghold of data mining and machine learning.

The following critical steps comprised our encounter with Orange:

1. *Data Preparation:* We carefully pre-processed our face detection dataset to get started. The dataset was meticulously constructed with distinct boundaries between the training and testing sections.

2. *Feature Extraction:* Orange's broad feature engineering capabilities were utilized to our advantage as we planned the feature extraction of important features from our dataset. To improve model performance, this stage frequently involves careful feature selection and dimensionality reduction methods.

3. *Model Configuration:* The Orange environment was carefully constructed to house the brain of our model. At this point, we specified the neural network architecture explicitly, including the number of layers, the number of neurons per layer, the activation functions, and significant training parameters.

4. *Training Elegance:* Our model's initiation into the realm of neural networks took place during the training phase. Here, the model diligently absorbed knowledge through backpropagation or other compatible training algorithms. It was a process characterized by iterative adjustments of the model's weights to minimize classification errors.

5. *Evaluation Profundity:* The culmination of our model's training journey was the evaluation phase, in which its performance was subjected to rigorous scrutiny. Within Orange, we meticulously computed quintessential evaluation metrics for face detection, spanning precision, recall, F1-score, and accuracy.

The result of these efforts gave us a model that embodied accuracy and speed, making it the ideal choice for real- time face identification applications. The model's architecture settings and training dynamics were adjusted, frequently through iterative refinement, to achieve the best performance benchmarks.In conclusion, the laborious development and thorough testing of our proposed neural network-based face detection model with the help of the Orange tool serve as a monument to the unrelenting quest of excellence in the field of real-time face identification. Its potential goes beyond what is now possible with computer vision, providing a strong solution with broad ramifications for numerous fields and applications.

5. Data-Set Description

5.3 Dataset Composition

This dataset is structured as follows:

1. *Images:* The dataset comprises a vast array of images encompassing diverse scenarios, settings, lighting conditions, and subjects. These images depict individuals with and without face masks, encapsulating real- world scenarios that are

critical for the robustness and adaptability of detection algorithms. The dataset is carefully balanced between two primary classes: images of individuals correctly wearing face masks (positive class) and those not wearing face masks (negative class).

2. *Annotations:* Each image in the dataset is meticulously annotated with bounding boxes that delineate the regions of interest (ROIs) within the image. These ROIs typically encompass the facial regions and specifically mark the areas where masks are worn. The annotations provide crucial information about the coordinates and dimensions of these bounding boxes, which is essential for training and evaluating face mask detection models.

3. *Class Labels:* For every image, binary class labels are assigned to denote whether the depicted individual is adhering to face mask guidelines or not. The class labels categorize each image as either showing a person correctly wearing a face mask (positive) or not wearing a face mask (negative). These labels serve as the foundation for supervised learning, enabling the training of machine learning models for face mask detection.

5.4 Usage Scenarios

The "Face Mask Detection Dataset" is designed to serve multiple purposes in the domains of computer vision, machine learning, and public health:

1. *Model Development:* Researchers and developers can utilize this dataset to design, train, and fine-tune machine learning models, particularly deep learning models, for face mask detection. The annotations and class labels facilitate supervised learning, allowing the creation of accurate and efficient detection algorithms.

2. *Real-world Applications:* Models trained on this dataset have found extensive real-world applications, including automated compliance monitoring in public spaces, healthcare settings, transportation hubs, and workplaces. These models aid in ensuring adherence to face mask mandates, thereby contributing to public health and safety.

3. *Public Health Initiatives:* The dataset's utility extends to public health authorities and organizations working on mitigating the spread of contagious diseases. Automated face mask detection systems can be integrated into surveillance and monitoring systems, enhancing efficiency in compliance checking.

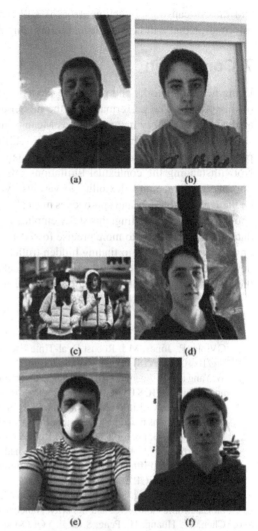

(a)   (b)   (c)   (d)   (e)   (f)

Fig. 57.3   Sample images from the data set

6. Results

We meticulously and thoroughly assessed the performance of our neural network model during the course of our long research, using a wide range of crucial assessment indicators. The Mean Squared Error (MSE) for our neural network model was 3919.911. These measures, along with the model's Root Mean Squared Error (RMSE) of 62.609, provide a deeper view of the predictive accuracy of the model by quantifying the normal amount of mistakes. Together, they give insight on the range of prediction error inherent to the model's performance. Additionally, the Mean Absolute Error (MAE) of 47.586 revealed the average absolute variance between the values in the dataset that the model predicted and the actual values that were really there. In addition to these metrics, the Coefficient of Determination (R2) score of our model, which is 0.292, provides crucial information about its explanatory power. This rating indicates that the model can explain roughly 29.2\% of the observed variance in the target variable. While these data clearly demonstrate the precision and explanatory power of our model, it is crucial to contextualize these results within the particular problem domain, taking into account the particular difficulties and complexities it poses. With the ultimate goal of advancing and raising prediction performance to new heights, our future research endeavours hold the prospect of diving further into potential paths for fine-tuning the model's architecture, critically evaluating alternative algorithms and enriching feature sets. Additionally, a deeper investigation into the underlying patterns and factors causing prediction errors is still an exciting area for research because it has the potential to reveal insightful information that will help guide and inform ongoing model improvement initiatives and advance the field.

7. Conclusion

Using neural networks and predictive modelling, we were able to uncover complex patterns in our dataset during the course of this project. The performance of the model and its implications for data science and machine learning were clarified by analysis based on key metrics such as Mean Squared Error (MSE), Root Mean Squared Error (RMSE), Mean Absolute Error (MAE), and Coefficient of Determination (R2). These assessment metrics served as guidelines, demonstrating the model's proficiency in interpreting intricate dataset relationships and resolving difficulties in low-error prediction and estimation tasks. Notwithstanding the contextual limitations influencing performance, additional research and improvement are necessary to improve resilience and flexibility in various dynamic environments. To take advantage of new opportunities and meet new challenges, our models and approaches must also change as machine learning advances. In addition to adding to the conversation about predictive modelling, this study emphasizes the value of careful examination and continuous advancement in the field of data science. The path to more precise forecasts and profound insights is marked by creative thinking, iterative inquiry, and an unwavering dedication to finding hidden truths within data. As we come to the end of this chapter, we are ready to set out on new adventures motivated by the quest for excellence and knowledge. with faith in our capacity to progress and shed light on the way ahead in the ever-changing field of machine learning and predictive modelling.

REFERENCES

1. GViola, P., Jones, M.J. Robust Real-Time Face Detection. International Journal of Computer Vision 57, 137–154 (2004). https://doi.org/10.1023/B:VISI.0000013087.49260.fb
2. W. Yang and Z. Jiachun, "Real-time face detection based on YOLO," 2018 1st IEEE International Conference on Knowledge Innovation and Invention (ICKII), Jeju, Korea (South), 2018, pp. 221-224, doi: 10.1109/ICKII.2018.8569109.
3. M. S. Bartlett, G. Littlewort, I. Fasel and J. R. Movellan, "Real-Time Face Detection and Facial Expression Recognition: Development and Applications to Human-Computer Interaction.," 2003 Conference on Computer Vision and Pattern Recognition Workshop, Madison, WI, USA, 2003, pp. 53- 53, doi: 10.1109/CVPRW.2003.10057.
4. G. Shakhnarovich, P. A. Viola and B. Moghaddam, "A unified learning framework for real-time face detection and classification," Proceedings of Fifth IEEE International Conference on Automatic Face Gesture Recognition, Washington, DC, USA, 2002, pp. 16-23, doi: 10.1109/AFGR.2002.1004124.
5. L. Lang and W. Gu, "Study of Face Detection Algorithm for Real-time Face Detection System," 2009 Second International Symposium on Electronic Commerce and Security, Nanchang, China, 2009, pp. 129-132, doi: 10.1109/ISECS.2009.237.
6. Chen, W., Huang, H., Peng, S. et al. YOLO-face: a real-time face detector. Vis Comput 37, 805–813 (2021). https://doi.org/10.1007/s00371-020-01831-
7. T. Burghardt and J. Calic, "Real-time Face Detection and Tracking of Animals," 2006 8th Seminar on Neural Network Applications in Electrical Engineering, Belgrade, Serbia, 2006, pp. 27-32, doi: 10.1109/NEUREL.2006.341167.
8. S. Zhang, X. Zhu, Z. Lei, H. Shi, X. Wang and S. Z. Li, "FaceBoxes: A CPU real-time face detector with high accuracy," 2017 IEEE International Joint Conference on Biometrics (IJCB), Denver, CO, USA, 2017, pp. 1-9, doi: 10.1109/BTAS.2017.8272675.
9. K. Kollreider, H. Fronthaler, M. I. Faraj and J. Bigun, "Real-Time Face Detection and Motion Analysis With Application in "Liveness" Assessment," in IEEE Transactions on Information Forensics and Security, vol. 2, no. 3, pp. 548-558, Sept. 2007, doi: 10.1109/TIFS.2007.902037.
10. Zhang, S., Wen, L., Shi, H. et al. Single-Shot Scale-Aware Network for Real-Time Face Detection. Int J Comput Vis 127, 537–559 (2019). https://doi.org/10.1007/s11263-019-01159-3
11. Jun, B., Kim, D. (2007). Robust Real-Time Face Detection Using Face Certainty Map. In: [12]. Lee, SW., Li, S.Z. (eds) Advances in Biometrics. ICB 2007. Lecture Notes in Computer Science, vol 4642. Springer, Berlin, Heidelberg. https://doi.org/10.1007/978-3-540-74549-54
13. D. Nguyen, D. Halupka, P. Aarabi and A. Sheikholeslami, "Real-time face detection and lip feature extraction using field-programmable gate arrays," in IEEE Transactions on Systems, Man, and Cybernetics, Part B (Cybernetics), vol. 36, no. 4, pp. 902-912, Aug. 2006, doi: 10.1109/TSMCB.2005.862728.
14. McCready, R. (2000). Real-Time Face Detection on a Configurable Hardware System. In: Hartenstein, R.W., Grünbacher, H. (eds) Field-Programmable Logic and Applications: The Roadmap to Reconfigurable Computing. FPL 2000. Lecture Notes in Computer Science, vol 1896. Springer, Berlin, Heidelberg. https://doi.org/10.1007/3-540-44614-1 17

Emerging Trends in IoT and Computing Technologies – Suman Lata Tripathi et al. (eds)
© 2024 Taylor & Francis Group, London, ISBN 978-1-032-87924-6

Research Paper on Monitoring Accounting Processes in an Organization with Blockchain Technology

58

**Pratiksha Argulewar[1], Abhiraj Prasad[2],
Darshan Nimje[3], Gaurav Zade[4], Supriya Sawwashere[5]**

J D College of Engineering and Management,
Computer Science & Engineering, Nagpur, India

Abstract: A safe, transparent and unchangeable ledger for documenting financial transactions is what blockchain technology offers, and it has the potential to completely transform accounting. In order to increase efficiency, accuracy, and compliance, this study investigates the possible used of blockchain technology for accounting process monitoring. We go over the salient characteristics of distributed consensus, auditability, and immutability in blockchain technology that make it a good fit for accounting applications. We also identify some of the issues that need to be resolved before this technology is widely used, and we provide a conceptual framework for utilizing blockchain technology to monitor the accounting process.

Keywords: Blockchain, Blockchain in finance, DAPP, Hyperledger fabric, Finance monitoring system, Solidity, Smart contract, Web application, Consensus, Voting

1. Introduction

Blockchain technology has been the subject of significant attention in recent years due to its potential for transformation especially in industries like financial accounting. This scholarly article delves into the application of blockchain technology in the monitoring processes, addressing the challenges and opportunities it present in terms of enhancing transparency, security, and efficiency in financial record-keeping. Traditional accounting systems are susceptible to various issues, including fraud, errors, and a lack of real-time data accessibility. The decentralized and distributed nature of blockchain technology allows for a paradigm shift in the way financial transactions are recorded and verified, providing a secure and transparent platform. This scholarly article conducts a thorough examination of the key features of blockchain, such as consensus mechanism and demonstrate how these attributed can enhance the monitoring of accounting processes.

The study meticulously explores practical use cases of implementing blockchain in accounting, encompassing the tracking of financial transactions, management of audit trails, and authentication of financial information. The built-in security attributes of blockchain guarantee the integrity of financial records and mitigate the risk linked to unauthorized access and manipulation.

Furthermore, this scholarly article scrutinizes the potential challenges and limitations of implementing blockchain in accounting domain, addressing concerns related to scalability, regulatory compliance, and existing systems. It also delves into the discussions of ongoing developments emerging trends and future prospects for blockchain technology in the realm of accounting.

By thoroughly examining the transformative impact of blockchain on accounting processes, this scholarly article aims to contribute to the growing body of knowledge in the practical application of distributed ledger technology in the realm of

[1]Pratikshaargulewar000@gmail.com, [2]Abhirajprasad00@gmail.com, [3]darshanimje2872@gmail.com, [4]aakashzade2002@gmail.com,
[5]ssawashere486@gmail.com

DOI: 10.1201/9781003535423-58

finance. The insights provided herein will assist accounting professionals, researchers, and policymakers in comprehending the implications of adopting blockchain for monitoring of accounting processes , ultimately fostering a more secure and transparent financial ecosystem.

2. Literature Review

There was a thorough discussion of five research publication that are linked to monitoring and Managing Blockchain Technology. The paper were carefully selected from the internet database, IEEE, Journal of Physics, based on how well they could be used in actual situation. The research paper we searched by using keywords like "Expense Tracking in blockchain technology", "Ethereum blockchain system", "Transparent system", "Decentralized blockchain based transaction system", which produced roughly (45,000 approx.) result. Companies like Deloitte, PwC, Ernst and Young excreta, all have focused on domain of Blockchain Technology, Transparency, Decentralization techniques which garnered significant attention in the literature.

Our literature survey explores the spectrum of methods and strategies employed to apply the characteristics of blockchain technology like decentralization, distributed, immutability, transparency within our application. Researchers and practitioners have highlighted the application and use case of blockchain technology in Accounting Industry, Auditing systems.

[1] Title: Blockchain based Transparency Framework for privacy preserving Third party services. Author: Ranhua Xu, Publisher: IEEE. Published in IEEE transactions on dependable and secure computing (early access) Date of Publication: 02 June 2022.

The increasing reliance on third party facilities like cloud computing centers and edge nodes for information systems raises cyber security concerns and due to incidents of attacks resulting in data leakage and identify theft. This has led to stricter security regulations and a loss of trust in cyberspace. To establish trust in privacy- preserving applications, transparency frameworks like TAB which utilizes blockchain techniques have been proposed to ensure transparency and trustworthiness of third party authorities and facilities. TAB employs the Ethereum blockchain and a navel smart contract to automate accountability and incentivize users to participate in auditing while punishing malicious behavior. Experimental evaluation on the Ethereum test network, Rinkerby, demonstrates the efficiency of the TAB framework, and formal analysis shows its security and privacy guarantees.

[2] Title: A blockchain based approach for improving transparency and traceability in silk production and marketing. Author: Abhilash Sharma and Mala Kalra, Publisher: IOP publishing limited, published in: Journal of physics: conference series, volume 1998, 3rd international conference on smart and intelligent learning for information optimization Date of publish: July 2021.

Blockchain technology is a transparent and secure digital ledger database that allows for the recording of transactions between non trusting parties. This has the potential to significantly enhance supply chain management especially in the silk production and marketing industry. Through the use smart contracts, the proposed application aims to automate shipping processes in supply chain with performance evaluated based on transaction throughput, average latency and resource utilization.

[3] Title: Blockchain, an enabling technology for transparent and accountable decentralized public participatory GIS. Author: Mahdi Farnaghi, Ali Mansourian. Publisher: IOP publishing Ltd. Published in: http://www.sciencedirect.com/science/article/pii/S02646275120311987. Date of Conference: Version of record 20 June 2020. Governmental Organization have employed web-based public participatory GIS(PPGIS) to enable public input in decision making process, albeit with a lack of transparency. This study proposes the development of decentralized PPGISs, data is securely stored and validated through a consensus process, ensuring its integrity and accessibility for institutions and citizens. A prototype Dapp was developed to facilitate site selection of urban facilities by allowing users to compare and rank criteria, generating a suitability map for decision-making and citizens. The potential of this application and consideration for using blockchain in urban planning are discussed in detail.

[4] Title: "Application Research of Blockchain technology in Accounting System", Authored by Ruirui Zheng and published by IOP Publishing Ltd. Focus lies upon investigating the essentiality and viability of integrating blockchain technology into the accounting industry. Furthermore, the article delves into the operational principles of the accounting information system employed by both sellers and buyers. Additionally, the paper formulates vertical and horizontal application model for blockchain technology within the accounting system

[5] Title: "Blockchain for Electronic Voting System-Review and Open Research Challenges", Author: Uzma Jafar, Mohd Juzaiddin Ab Aziz, and Zarina Shukur. Publisher: MDPI. Published in: Faculty of Information Science and Technology, The National University of Malaysia, Bangi 43600, Malaysia. Date of Conference: 31 August 2021.

The above article gives comprehensive detail about voting system. This paper was established to know the detail about blockchain based voting system in present state. Which helped in finding out the challenges which are present in today's voting system and how we can do future enhancement in that. This investigation offers a conceptual depiction of the intended application of blockchain- based electronic voting, along with an introduction to the fundamental structure and characteristics of the blockchain in relation to electronic voting. As a result of this meticulous study, it was ascertained that blockchain systems have the potential to alleviate certain predicaments currently afflicting election systems.

3. Application of Blockchain

A decentralized application, or DApp, is built on a decentralized network and combines a smart contract with a user interface on the front end. This specific application falls within the realm of distributed open source software applications, functioning on a decentralized blockchain network with a peer to peer architecture. The utilization of blockchain technology in decentralized applications enables the processing of data across distributed networks and the execution of transactions. Furthermore, decentralized applications are open-source in nature, meaning that any necessary modifications are agreed upon by a consensus of the majority of users. These applications provide decentralized storage capabilities and incorporate cryptography. The validation and verification of the decentralized data blocks is ensured, thus establishing their authenticity.

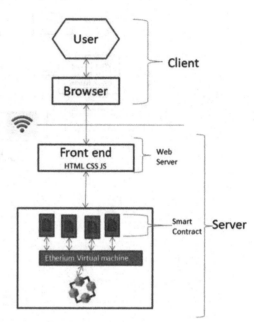

Fig. 58.1 Architecture of project

1. *Ethereum Blockchain:* It establishes a network that is peer-to- peer in nature and ensures the secure execution and verification of application code, which is commonly known as smart contracts. These decentralized applications, or DApps, have their backend code, which consists of smart contracts, running on a network that is decentralized rather than being centralized on a server. The Ethereum blockchain serves as a means for data storage for these DApps.

2. Smart contracts play a vital role in the functioning of DApps.

They are utilized to define the state changes that occur on the blockchain. A smart contract can be defined as a fusion of both code and data, which is situated at a designated address on the Ethereum Blockchain and functions withing the Ethereum blockchain.

3. The Ethereum based computational model or Ethereum virtual machine (EVM) is an encompassing virtual computer that executes the prescribed logic within the smart contracts and facilitates the processing of state alterations occurring within this Ethereum network.

4. The front-end, constituting the visible aspect of DApps, enables users to perceive and engage with the graphical user interface (GUI). Furthermore, the front-end establishes communication with the application logic delineated within the smart contracts.

4. Methodology

Node: A node is a computer or device that is a part of the blockchain network. A blockchain's distributed and decentralized structure depends heavily on nodes.

Transaction: A data transfer involving two or more parties, is referred to as a blockchain transaction. Another way to describe it as a transfer, agreement, contract, or exchange of assets. Usually, the assets are money or real estate.

Ledger: A Blockchain ledger is a decentralized database of transactions of a computer network records and verifies. Another name for this ledger is a blockchain.

Blockchain Voting: In a private blockchain, voting is the process of reaching a consensus via which a small number of pre-approved nodes or businesses validate and accept a transaction.

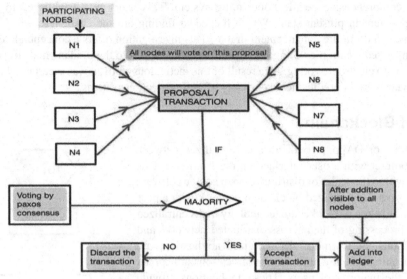

Fig. 58.2 Flowchart of methodology (1)

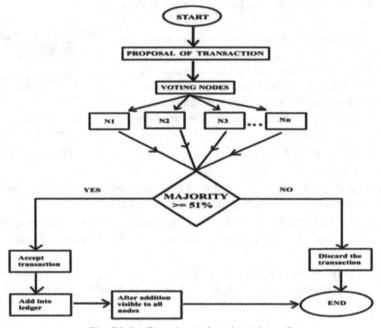

Fig. 58.3 Flowchart of methodology (2)

5. Simulation

1. The very first starts with the user sending transaction request to the system.
2. Once the transaction request is received to accept the transaction or not.
3. The nodes authorize the transaction by an voting system in which all the nodes has to vote in order to accept or reject the transaction.
4. In this voting system if the voting percentage is more than or equal to 51 % then the transaction is accepted else it will be rejected.
5. Whether the transaction is accepted or rejected is will be added to the ledger and will be visible to all the nodes.

6. Software Model

Blockchain characterized by its rigid concatenation of data blocks, presents a comprehensive account of truth that can serve as a fundamental component within each sequential phase of development. In the realm of circumstances and design, blockchain has the ability to provide an empirical documentation of viewpoints and modifications, an account that remains unalterable. As the design progresses through the various stages of development and testing, blockchain assumes the role of a vigilant guardian, ensuring that each step is recorded with the enduring permanence of an engraved memorial. The incorporation of blockchain into the Waterfall methodology bestows upon it a novel dimension of accountability and traceability. It is reminiscent of an operative diligently documenting every piece of evidence, cognizant that the integrity of the discourse hinges upon the faultless nature of the records maintained.

7. Result

In this project, we propose a decentralized financial management system for organization based on blockchain technology and smart contracts The system utilizes on blockchain technology among organizational node to ensures transparency, accountability and secure financial transactions. The core components of the system include a smart contract that manages the distribution of funds among nodes

To approve or disapproves transaction requests. The system offers several benefits, including decentralized authority, enhanced security, implementing efficiency, and enhanced auditability. By implementing this system, organizations can enhances accountability, improving transparency, reduce fraud, and streamline financial processes.

8. Future scope

The future scope of this decentralized financial management system for organization is vast and promising. Here are some potential directions for future development:

1. *Integration with existing financial systems:* To ensure seamless integration with existing organizational workflows, the system can be designed to interface with traditional financial systems. Enabling organizations to manage their finances holistically.
2. *Enhancing voting mechanisms:* Advanced voting based on node reputation or contribution, can be explored to refine decision- making processes.
3. *Multichain support:* The system can be extended to support multiple blockchain networks, allowing organization to leverage the benefits of different blockchain protocols and ecosystems.
4. *Privacy-preserving transactions:* Implementing privacy=preserving techniques, such as zero- knowledge proofs, can ensure that sensitive financial information remains confidential while maintaining transparency.
5. *Integration with AI and machine learning:* By incorporating AI and machine learning algorithms, the system can analyze transaction patterns and provide real-time insights to inform financial decisions.
6. *Exploration of alterative consensus mechanisms:* Investigation alternative consensus mechanisms, such as Proof- of Stake (POS) or Proof-of-Authority (POA) can optimize the system's performance and energy efficiency.
7. *Exploration of decentralized identity management:* Implementing decentralized solutions can enhance user authentication and privacy protection within the system.

These future advancements can further enhance the capabilities of this decentralized financial management system, empowering organizations to manage their finances with greater efficiency, security, and transparency.

9. Conclusion

The proposed decentralized financial management system offers a secure, transparent, and efficient solution for organizations to manage their finances. By leveraging blockchain technology and smart contracts, the system eliminates the need for centralized authority and ensures that all financial decisions are made through a transparent voting process. The system also provides enhanced security and auditability, as all transaction records are stored on the blockchain and cannot be tampered with. With its potential to revolutionize organizational financial management, this decentralized system is poised to play a significant role in the future of finance.

REFERENCE

1. Dr. Supriya Sawwashere, Pratiksha Argulewar, Abhiraj Prasad, Darshan Nimje, Gaurav Zade." Monitoring Accounting Process in Organization with Blockchain Technology", Volume 11, Issue XII, International Journal for Research in Applied Science and Engineering Technology (IJRASET) Page No: 110-115, ISSN: 2321-9653, www.ijraset.com

2. R. Xu, C. Li and J. Joshi, "Blockchain-Based Transparency Framework for Privacy Preserving Third-Party Services," in IEEE Transactions on Dependable and Secure Computing, vol. 20, no. 3, pp. 2302-2313, 1 May-June 2023. doi: 10.1109/TDSC.2022.3179698.

3. Sharma, A. and Kalra, M. (2021), "A blockchain based approach for improving transparency and traceability in silk production and marketing", Journal of Physics: Conference Series, 1998(1), p. 012013. doi:10.1088/1742-6596/1998/1/012013.

4. Mahdi Farnaghi, Ali Mansourian, "Blockchain, an enabling technology for transparent and accountable decentralized public participatory GIS", Cities, Volume 105, 2020, 102850, ISSN 0264-2751, https://doi.org/10.1016/j.cities.2020.102850.

5. Zheng, R. (2021) 'Applications research of blockchain technology in accounting system', Journal of Physics: Conference Series, 1955(1), p. 012068. doi:10.1088/1742-6596/1955/1/012068.

6. Jafar, U., Aziz, M.J. and Shukur, Z. (2021) 'Blockchain for Electronic Voting System—review and Open Research Challenges', Sensors, 21(17), p. 5874. doi:10.3390/s21175874.

Emerging Trends in IoT and Computing Technologies – Suman Lata Tripathi et al. (eds)
© 2024 Taylor & Francis Group, London, ISBN 978-1-032-87924-6

Twitter Profile Analysis using Bidirectional LSTM Networks

59

Seema Kalonia[1], Anshu Khurana[2]
Maharaja Agrasen Institute of Technology, Dept. of IT, New Delhi, India

Sudesh Kumar[3],
Shri Mata Vaishno Devi University, School of CSE, Katra, India

Anjali Saxena[4]
Maharaja Agrasen Institute of Technology, Dept. of IT, New Delhi, India

Abstract: Social media usage is growing at an exceptional pace, whether it be brand or product reviews by customers or posting a political opinion, everything goes on social media. So, it is becoming important to analyze the sentiments of content posted on social media platforms to reduce the amount of negative or abusive content on these platforms. Twitter is among the most widely used social media platforms where users express their views on different issues, so analyzing the sentiment of tweets posted by a user helps to distinguish malicious users and take appropriate action against them. This paper will propose an approach to analyze the sentiment of tweets posted by an account. This is achieved by building a Natural Language Preprocessing (NLP) pipeline to filter the tweets and then using Long Short Term Memory Networks, an advanced version of Recurrent Neural Networks, to group tweets into positive, negative, and neutral categories.

Keywords: Sentiment analysis, Recurrent neural networks, Natural language preprocessing, Long short-term memory networks

1. Introduction

The usage of social media has appreciably extended over years. Exposure to bad content material published on social media platforms can adversely affect the mental fitness of customers. Also, terrible or abusive content on such systems can disrupt the peace and concord of the society. [1] Social media sentiment analysis helps the accountable agencies to discover the malicious customers who submit abusive content at the platform on an everyday basis and may take suitable moves in opposition to them. These platforms generate a large amount of normal statistics, making it impossible to manually tune the content on the platform. Sentiment analysis will assist to discover poor content at the platform, ensuing in a reduction of such content on social media.

There is an extreme increase in social media usage and the famous social media structures exist with approximately 145 million energetic users each day is twitter. On a day-by-day basis around 500 million tweets are posted at the platform generating huge quantities of information for sentiment evaluation. Twitter is chosen for sentiment evaluation. We selected Twitter for sentiment analysis as it allows us to capture the tenderness of enunciated disposition. This paper discusses a deep learning model for

[1]seema.kalonia25@gmail.com, [2]anshuchugh@gmail.com, [3]sudesh.pec@gmail.com, [4]saxenaanjali239@gmail.com

DOI: 10.1201/9781003535423-59

sentiment analysis along with a framework for filtering tweets based on NLP to be used for sentiment analysis. The basic goal is to recognize the emotion of the tweets posted by users and classify them as positive, negative or neutral. Tweets posted by users are collected by using the official Twitter API. We use these tweets as raw data. Then we propose a deep learning model using [2] Recurrent Neural Networks (RNN) to classify tweets. In order to optimize the performance of RNN model we have used a special kind of RNN that is Long Short-Term Memory (LSTM) model to avoid long term dependency problems.

2. Literature Review

In [3], Authors from Dong University, South Korea presents sentiment analysis architecture for twitter to analyze tweets with the help of Deep Neural Networks (DNN) and man- aging large amount of data.

In [4], Authors introduced in a paper on Twitter Sentiment Analysis using Machine Learning Methods present an approach to compare the Twitter sentiment analysis results using classification methods like Naive Bayes Classifier, SVM Classifier and Entropy method.

In [5], Authors from Bangladesh University of Engineering and Technology, Dhaka in a paper on Sentiment Analysis with NLP on Twitter Data presents Twitter sentiment analysis system to analyse public perceptions towards a product.

In [6], Authors described sites which Track malicious sentiment analysis system which predict sentiment of the post using dependency tree to build feature-oriented sentiment analysis model.

In [7], Authors concluded in a paper on Twitter Sentiment Analysis of the Data Crawler using Bayes algorithm that presents a comparative study using different classifiers SVM, K-Nearest Neighbors (K-NN) and Naïve Baye's (NB) algorithm. The Accuracy of NB was 75.58%, the Accuracy of SVM was 63.99%, and the Accuracy of K-NN was 73.34%.

3. Methodology

The design of the proposed method for sentiment analysis of a user profile on Twitter is illustrated in Fig. 59.1.

In this shown methodology in Fig. 59.1 first step it will search for any Twitter username to view the amount of positive, negative and neutral tweets posted by that account then Tweets posted by the account will be retrieved by using Twitter Developer API. In third phase Collected tweets will be cleaned and preprocessed before passing it to the deep learning model for classification. In forth step the LSTM model will classify tweets as positive, negative, or neutral based on the probability of the text belonging to a specific group as predicted by the model. In last step Pie chart and other graphical representations will be generated based on the number of tweets classified under each category.

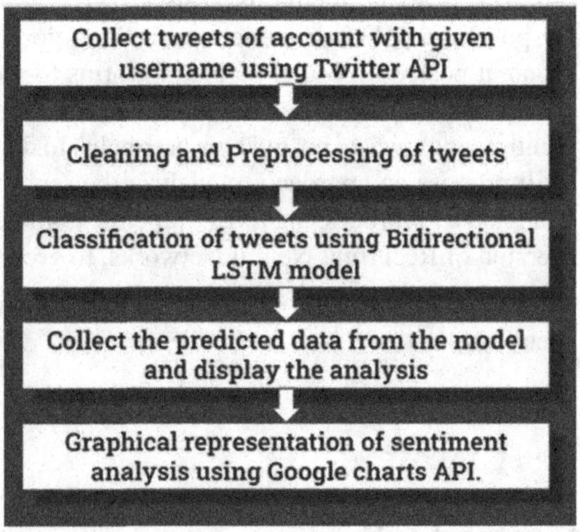

Fig. 59.1 Tweets sentiment classification for a user profile

3.1 Collection of Data

Twitter provides Twitter Developer API to exhibit a secure connection betwixt our proposed application and database of twitter. Twitter accounts with developer access can create an application which will lead to API credentials which is used to retrieve Twitter public information from python. Also, to access twitter from a python application we need to install *tweepy* package. After installing and importing tweepy, we need to complete authorization by providing key, access token key, consumer secret key and access token secret key which can be hinge on the Twitter app page. Tweets posted by the user can be collected by using the Cursor object.

3.2 Preprocessing

Convert the text to lowercase, so that the words like "Read" and "read" are considered the same. Remove stopwords (eg. "a", "is", etc.) from the text by creating a stopwords corpus and then removing the words present in the corpus from the text. Remove urls from the text by using regex expressions. Remove punctuations (eg. '!' , '.', etc.) from the text with help of the punctuation list provided by the string module in python. Remove numbers from the text by using regex expressions. Text is tokenized using the split method to create a token of each word. Tokens are stemmed using PorterStemmer to their root forms (eg. "change" and "changes" are stemmed to "change"). Stemmed tokens in different inflected forms but with the same meaning are grouped together and converted to their root form using WordNetLemmatizer (eg. "leafs" and "leaves" are converted to "leaf"). Target variable- category is encoded to numeric values using LabelEncoder. Features are extracted from clean data using CountVectorizer. Text is converted to sequence of integers and then each sequence is padded to the same length.

Recurrent Neural Network

A Recurrent Neural Network (RNN) is a kind of neural network in which the output of a previous step is fed into the current step as input. All inputs and outputs in a traditional neural network are independent of one another, but we need the preceding word to predict the following word in a phrase, so we must remember the previous word. This is how RNNs were created, to solve this problem using hidden layers.

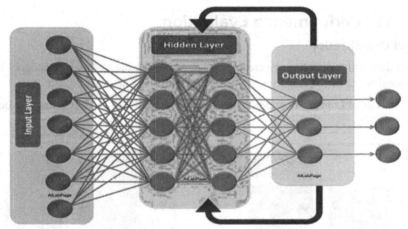

Fig. 59.2 Recurrent neural network

Long Short-term Memory (LSTM)

Exploding gradients and disappearing gradients are two significant challenges that ordinary RNNs face. When an algorithm assigns the weights a lot of weight without any good justification, the gradient explodes. When the gradient is too small, the gradient disappears and the model stops learning. [14] LSTM is one of the well-known variations developed to solve the problem of exploding and vanishing gradients. The returned LSTM object conceptually tries to "remember" everything the network has ever learned in the past while "forgetting" useless information.

Bidirectional Long Short-term Memory

Bidirectional LSTM (BiLSTM) is a RNN which is mostly used for NLP. Unlike regular LSTM the input of data flows in both the directions. Additionally, model works well for modeling the directional dependencies between words and phrases.

To conclude, BiLSTM introduces a new layer in LSTM that inverse the information flow. This means the sequence of input is flowing backward in new layer of LSTM. After that, the outputs are merged from the two layers including different methods such as average, multiplication, sum and concatenation.

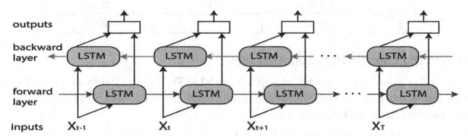

Fig. 59.3 Bidirectional LSTM model

In this paper, RNN is applied. Bidirectional LSTM Network, an advanced version of RNN is used with epoch value equal to 50 and learning rate of 0.1 which overcomes the RNN drawback.

LSTM model used for sentiment analysis have following layers:

Embedding Layer: Every word is transformed into a vector with a defined length and size. Therefore, smaller dimension word representations are preferable.

Conv1d Layer: It builds a convolution kernel over a layer with single dimension to produce tenor of outputs.

Bidirectional Layer: It connects two hidden layers of opposite directions so that input sequences have information from past as well as present and it produces better results.

Dropout Layer: It drops hidden units in neural networks to prevent overfitting of the model.

Dense Layer: It will receive the output from each neuron of its preceding layer and produce the final output in the required format using softmax activation function.

4. Data Analysis and Perfoemance Evaluation

4.1 Data Analysis and Visualization

We had 162980 records of data with two columns - clean_text i.e. content of the tweets and category indicating tsentiment of the tweets. Tweets were classified in three categories as positive, negative and neutral.

In Fig. 59.5 comparative analysis of Logistic Regression and Bidirectional LSTM models trained on our Dataset is shown.

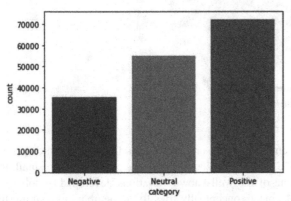

Fig. 59.4 Bar chart for sentiment wise classification of data

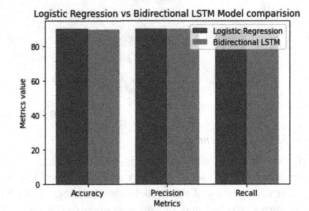

Fig. 59.5 Comparative analysis of logistic regression and bidirectional LSTM model

In Table 59.1 the summary of performance metrics for our Bidirectional LSTM model is shown.

Table 59.1 Performance evaluation of the LSTM model

S.N.	Metrics	Training Dataset	Testing Dataset
1	Accuracy	94.06	89.52
2	Precision	94.56	90.04
3	Recall	93.55	89.03

4.2 Comparison with the Logistic Regression Model

Logistic Regression algorithm is one of the best ML algorithms for NLP. The logistic Regression model trained with the same dataset using the same techniques gives almost comparable results to the Bidirectional LSTM model. The model was trained with newton-cg solver and max iterations limited to 50.

Table 59.2 shows the summary of performance metrics for our Logistic Regression model.

Based on our study we have classified tweets as positive, negative, and neutral. Figure 59.6 shows the confusion matrix for the Logistic Regression model representing the actual labels and predicted label count for each category.

Table 59.2 Performance metrics of our logistic regression model

S.N.	Metrics	Value
1	Accuracy	89.70
2	Precision	89.74
3	Recall	89.70

Fig. 59.6 Confusion matrix for Logistic Regression model

5. Conclusion

In this paper, we have built a model for Twitter Sentiment Analysis which classifies the tweets as positive, negative and neutral based on polarity predicted by the deep learning model. We have utilized LSTM Neural Networks, an advanced version of RNN for sentiment analysis and sentiment categorization, which produce findings that are relatively more accurate than average. We observed consistent accuracy of about 90% across all datasets used.

Also, we have compared the results of best-performing ML model i.e. Logistic Regression model and our Bidirectional LSTM model trained on our dataset, performance of both the models comes out to be fairly equal in terms of accuracy, precision and recall metrics.

6. Future Scope

A considerable amount of work remains to be done; but here we shed some light on some potential directions for future research. Currently, the suggested method is unable to discern sarcasm. In the con- text of the present work, sarcasm changes the apparent positive or negative utterance's polarity into its inverse. Future research should focus on empirically identifying the lexical and pragmatic elements that distinguish ironic, positive, and negative word uses. It is currently not possible to create a multilingual sentiment analyzer because there isn't a multilingual dictionary. The proposed approach cannot determine the sentiment included in photos, emoticons, stickers. To include elements that can foretell the sentiment of any form of data, more study can be done.

REFERENCES

1. D. Tanna, M. Dudhane, A. Sardar, K. Deshpande and N. Deshmukh, "Sentiment Analysis on Social Media for Emotion Classification," *2020 4th International Conference on Intelligent Computing and Control Systems (ICICCS)*, Madurai, India, 2020, pp. 911-915, doi: 10.1109/ICICCS48265.2020.9121057.

2 Lai, S., Xu, L., Liu, K., & Zhao, J. (2015). Recurrent Convolutional Neural Networks for Text Classification. Proceedings of the AAAI Conference on Artificial Intelligence, 29(1). https://doi.org/10.1609/aaai.v29i1.9513

3. A. M. Ramadhani and H. S. Goo, "Twitter sentiment analysis using deep learning methods," *2017 7th International Annual Engineering Seminar (InAES)*, Yogyakarta, Indonesia, 2017, pp. 1-4, doi: 10.1109/INAES.2017.8068556.

4. Lokesh M., Ruchi Patel, Medicaps University, Indore, India "Twitter Sentiment Analysis using Machine Learning Methods" International Journal of Advance Research, Ideas and Innovations in Technology, Volume 7, Issue 3 - V7I3-1818, 2021

5. M. R. Hasan, M. Maliha and M. Arifuzzaman, "Sentiment Analysis with NLP on Twitter Data," *2019 International Conference on Computer, Communication, Chemical, Materials and Electronic Engineering (IC4ME2)*, Rajshahi, Bangladesh, 2019, pp. 1-4, doi: 10.1109/IC4ME247184.2019.9036670.

6. P. Shilpa and S. D. Madhu Kumar, "Feature oriented sentiment analysis in social networking sites to track malicious campaigners," *2015 IEEE Recent Advances in Intelligent Computational Systems (RAICS)*, Trivandrum, India, 2015, pp. 179-184, doi: 10.1109/RAICS.2015.7488410.

7. M. Wongkar and A. Angdresey, "Sentiment Analysis Using Naive Bayes Algorithm of The Data Crawler: Twitter," *2019 Fourth International Conference on Informatics and Computing (ICIC)*, Semarang, Indonesia, 2019, pp. 1-5, doi: 10.1109/ICIC47613.2019.8985884.

8. A. P. Jain and V. D. Katkar, "Sentiments analysis of Twitter data using data mining," *2015 International Conference on Information Processing (ICIP)*, Pune, India, 2015, pp. 807-810, doi: 10.1109/INFOP.2015.7489492.

Emerging Trends in IoT and Computing Technologies – Suman Lata Tripathi et al. (eds)
© 2024 Taylor & Francis Group, London, ISBN 978-1-032-87924-6

Predictive Analysis for Cardiovascular Disease: A Machine Learning Approach

**Dhaval Joshi[1], Bhavya Singh[2],
Seema Kalonia[3], Ajay Kumar Kaushik[4], Sunil Maggu[5]**
Maharaja Agrasen Institute of Technology,
Dept. of IT, Delhi, India

Abstract: One-third of global deaths come as a result of cardiovascular diseases each year. Preventive health care, as well as early diagnosis and accurate prediction is important. Machine learning when combined with health datasets increases prediction efficiency. Using cutting edge machine learning (ML) techniques for predictive medicine in CVD prognosis is a contribution of this study. Utilizing 14 key attributes from UCI's data set, algorithms such as logistic regression, SVM, KNN, RF, GBM, and XGBoost were compared. An amazing 90 percent was registered for XGBoost where it had a random forest base estimator. With the use of ML, cases of CVD can be detected at an early stage, which leads to better preventive healthcare.

Keywords: Cardiovascular disease, Machine learning, Gradient boosting, XGBoost

1. Introduction

CVDs continue to be a major source of disability and death, constituting one of society's most serious public health threats. The accurate diagnosis of CVDs in early stages is a crucial step towards better interventions at minimal costs as well as enhancing health statuses among such patients The development of machine learning algorithms and accessibility to large health care datasets have led to increased enthusiasm towards using these technologies for better CVD forecasting and diagnosing. Accordingly, this article contributes to the existing trends seeking to develop predictive healthcare by evaluating machine learning algorithms for cardiovascular disease prediction. This study extends the analysis by incorporating diverse machine learning algorithms: the models such as logistic regression, SVM, KNN, random forest, gradient boosting, and XGBoost.

Healthcare services can be improved by using computer-based risk models such as machine learning models especially as alternatives to conventional risk assessment approaches for predicting cardiovascular disease (CVD). Utilizing predictive analytics in identifying people who are likely to develop cardiovascular diseases would allow for early treatment. In this case, the affected patients will benefit from customary medications hence improving their health conditions.

2. Literature Review

Numerous research studies have delved into employing machine learning models for predicting cardiovascular disease (CVD). One notable investigation by Rubini PE et al. in 2021 utilized four distinct machine learning algorithms to forecast CVD utilizing a dataset comprising 14 critical features. Their results indicated an achievement of an 84% accuracy rate through a 60:40 split for training and testing. [1]

[1]dhaval.e.joshi@gmail.com, [2]bhavyasingh1101, [3]seema.kalonia25@gmail.com, [4]ajayk08@gmail.com, [5]sunilmaggu@mait.ac.in

DOI: 10.1201/9781003535423-60

Aslanzadeh and Ebrahimi in 2022 " introduced an innovative machine learning framework for CVD prediction using ensemble learning methods with stacking. The aim of this paper is to propose a novel framework for cardiovascular disease (CVD) prediction using stacked ensemble learning. The proposed framework consists of three main stages: data preprocessing, feature selection, and stacked ensemble learning. [2]

Kour et al. (2021) proposes a machine learning-based framework for predicting cardiovascular disease using clinical data. The framework was evaluated on a dataset comprising more than 10,000 patients and attained an 88% accuracy. [3]

Marques, H., & Oliveira, L. S. in 2021 developed a hybrid machine learning (ML) approach for cardiovascular disease (CVD) prediction by combining feature selection and classification techniques.[5]

In a review by Ganeshan et al. (2023) of ML methods for CVD prediction. The authors conclude that ML can improve CVD prediction and highlight a requirement for stronger data, understandable models, and clinical integration.[6]

3. Methodology

This includes collecting data, picking critical features as well as some preparation for presenting the data in a manner appropriate for the system. Subsequently, the dataset is partitioned into two segments: train test model. This will enable the system to learn from the training dataset and to test it using unseen data, therefore rendering it generalizable to real life situations. The next step involves the use of machine-learning algorithms to train the model by exploiting existing patterns and relationships in the data in order to generate a predictive model. To determine the precision of the system, its performance is tested through the use of the reserved test data, giving objective evaluation on its effectiveness in predicting accurately. The implementation of this system involves several modules, including:

- Collection of Dataset
- Attribute Selection
- Data Preprocessing
- Data Balancing
- Disease Prediction

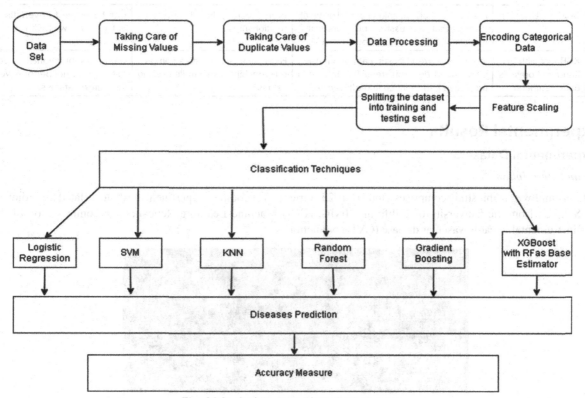

Fig. 60.1 Architecture of prediction system

Each element of the system makes its meaningful contribution toward the total predictive architecture. Data collection and attribute selection modules also ensure the capture of important information used in disease prediction. Data preprocessing aims at making sure that the data is ready for model training. The data partitioning module guarantees impartial judgments, whereas each prediction system component deals with its own issues of both creating and evaluating a model's predictions. Further, a data balancing module can deal with class imbalance issues and ensure equitable learning for predictive models in case a dataset exhibits unbalanced distribution of features among classes.

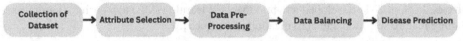

Fig. 60.2 Workflow of the system

Table 60.1 A comprehensive overview of each algorithm

S. N.	Algorithm	Definition	Advantages	Considerations
1	Logistic Regression	It refers to the statistical procedure of modelling probability distribution with a logistic curve.	Simple to interpret, fast to train, can be used for both classification and regression tasks.	May not perform well with non-linear relationships, can be sensitive to outliers.
2	Support Vector Machine	It is supervised algorithm that find an optimal hyperplane for classification of a set of data points in multi dimensional space.	Effective for high-dimensional data, robust to outliers.	May not perform well with noisy data, can be sensitive to the choice of kernel function.
3	K-Nearest Neighbors	It is a statistical algorithm. It determines which class the new data point belongs to by the k-nearest neighbors of the feature space.	Easy to implement, robust to outliers.	Can be sensitive to the choice of k, may not perform well with high-dimensional data.
4	Random Forest	It is an ensemble learning algorithm that leverages multiple decision trees to enhance prediction accuracy.	High accuracy, handles complex relationships.	Can be computationally expensive to train, may not perform well with very large datasets.
5	Gradient Boosting	It is an ensemble technique based on weak learners that progressively build predictive models with focus on previous mistakes.	High accuracy, handles complex relationships.	Can be prone to overfitting, may not perform well with very large datasets.
6	XGBoost with Random Forest as Base Estimator	It is an optimized boosting algorithm using randomized decision trees for enhanced predictive performance and efficiency.	High accuracy, handles complex relationships, can handle missing values.	Can be computationally expensive to train, may not perform well with very large datasets.

4. Experimental Results

4.1 Experimental Datasets

Source and Description:

The dataset employed in this study comprises a total of 1025 entries and encompasses pertinent attributes related to cardiovascular health. Sourced from the University of California, Irvine (UCI) Machine Learning Repository, it comprises of 14 distinct features instrumental in cardiovascular disease (CVD) prediction.

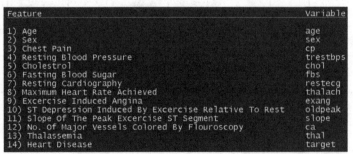

Fig. 60.3 Attributes used in the dataset

Preprocessing and Split:

Before model training, preprocessing steps were applied to the dataset, including handling missing values and normalization procedures. The dataset was partitioned into training and testing sets, assigning 80% for training and reserving 20% for testing, ensuring distinct datasets for model training and evaluation.

4.2 Performance Analysis

Performance Metric:

In this study, we mainly looked at how well the model predicted correctly. We used accuracy as our main measure, but we also considered precision, F1 score, recall, and ROC-AUC to understand how good the model was at predicting cardiovascular disease.

Algorithmic Comparison:

We compared different machine learning methods, and each method was trained, adjusted, and checked for accuracy one by one.

Results and Findings:

The experiment showed that the algorithms had different prediction accuracies. Interestingly, the XGBoost algorithm, which used a Random Forest as a base, performed the best, reaching 90% accuracy.

Table 60.2 The relative accuracy of the different models

S. N.	Algorithm	Accuracy(%)
1	Logistic Regression	78.68
2	Support Vector Machine	80.32
3	K-Nearest Neighbor	73.77
4	Random Forest	85.24
5	Gradient Boosting	80.32
6	XGBoost with Random Forest as Base Estimator	90

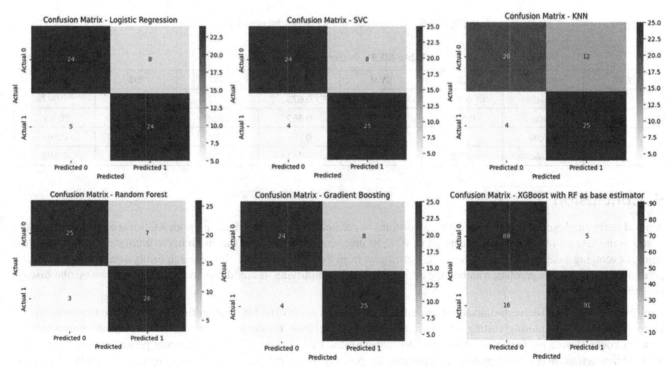

Fig. 60.4 Confusion matrix grid

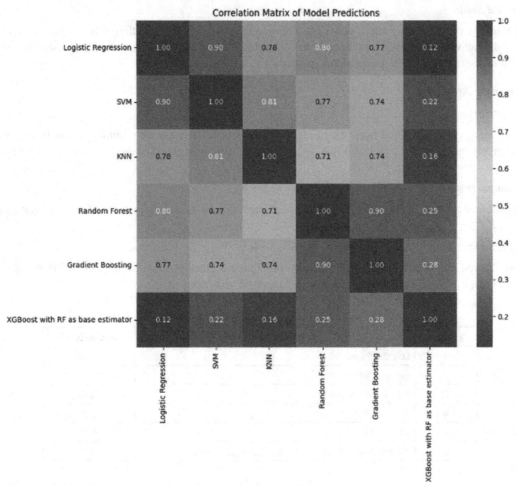

Fig. 60.5 Correlation matrix of model prediction

Table 60.3 Performance metrics

S. N.	Metric	LR	SVM	KNN	RF	BG	XGB
1	Precision	0.75	0.757	0.675	0.74	0.812	0.947
2	F1-Score	0.827	0.862	0.862	0.689	0.896	0.85
3	Recall	0.786	0.806	0.757	0.714	0.852	0.896
4	ROC-AUC	0.788	0.806	0.743	0.735	0.854	0.898

5. Conclusion

A novel study employed six machine learning algorithms to predict cardiovascular diseases, with XGBoost employing Random Forest as the base estimator achieving accuracy of 90%. Its precision of 0.947 highlights its ability to accurately identify positive cases. Leveraging a dataset encompassing 14 key attributes from the UCI repository, this research firmly establishes XGBoost's predominance in disease prediction among the evaluated models, solidifying its credibility in the field of cardiovascular disease prognosis.

Future endeavors should delve into advanced ensemble techniques, innovative feature engineering, and diversified datasets beyond current parameters. Exploring cutting-edge ensemble methods, refining feature engineering, and leveraging comprehensive datasets could elevate predictive accuracy. The domain presents vast opportunities for enhancing predictions and extending applicability across diverse demographics, amplifying the potency of clinical decisions in managing cardiovascular diseases.

REFERENCES

1. Rubini PE et al. (2021). A Cardiovascular Disease Prediction using Machine Learning Algorithms Annals of R.S.C.B., ISSN:1583-6258, Vol. 25, Issue 2

2. Aslanzadeh, A., & Ebrahimi, M. (2022). A novel machine learning framework for cardiovascular disease prediction using stacked ensemble learning. Journal of Ambient Intelligence and Humanized Computing

3. Clinical Data Analysis for Prediction of Cardiovascular Disease Using Machine Learning Techniques by Kour et al. (2021)

4. SonamNikhar, A.M. Karandikar" Prediction of Heart Disease Using different Machine Learning Algorithms"- Vol-2 Issue-6, June 2016.

5. Marques, H., & Oliveira, L. S. (2021). A hybrid machine learning approach for cardiovascular disease prediction using feature selection and classification. Journal of Ambient Intelligence and Humanized Computing, 12(2), 843-854.

6. Ganeshan, B., Sivakumar, A., & Jayaraman, S (2023). A comprehensive review on cardiovascular disease prediction using machine learning approaches. Expert Systems with Applications, 219, 118956.

7. Abhishek Taneja "Heart Disease Prediction System Using Data Mining Techniques"-Vol.6,No(4) 2013

8. Gupta, S., Chaudhary, A., & Kumar, D. (2023). A comprehensive study on machine learning approaches for cardiovascular disease prediction. Journal of Big Data, 10(1), 1-30.

Emerging Trends in IoT and Computing Technologies – Suman Lata Tripathi et al. (eds)
© 2024 Taylor & Francis Group, London, ISBN 978-1-032-87924-6

Unveiling Distributed Computing— Clusters, Clouds, Grids: A Comprehensive Review

61

Devansh Tiwari[1], Reeta Devi[2], Hatesh Shyan[3]
Chandigarh University,
Department of Computer Science and Engineering, Mohali, India

Abstract: The rapid evolution of computing paradigms, namely Cluster, Cloud, and Grid Computing, has catalyzed a paradigm shift in the landscape of computational technologies. This comprehensive review paper meticulously examines the historical development, architectural foundations, applications, and challenges associated with each paradigm. The analysis extends beyond individual paradigms, exploring opportunities for convergence and cross-paradigm synergies. The paper investigates breakthroughs and innovations in each computing paradigm, shedding light on recent advancements and emerging technologies. As a critical exploration, this review identifies challenges such as scalability issues, security concerns, and resource allocation limitations inherent in Cluster, Cloud, and Grid Computing. Through an integrative lens, the paper proposes innovative solutions to address these challenges and suggests optimizations for future development. The cross-paradigm analysis underscores the need for collaborative approaches and optimized resource utilization. The comprehensive nature of this review positions it as a valuable resource for researchers, practitioners, and decision makers seeking insights into the current state and future trajectories of computing paradigms. By offering a detailed exploration of historical contexts, technological foundations, and potential convergences, this paper contributes to the understanding of the intricate interplay between Cluster, Cloud, and Grid Computing.

Keywords: Cluster computing, Cloud computing, Grid computing, Convergence, Cross-paradigm synergies, Future optimizations

1. Introduction

1.1 Brief Overview of Cluster, Cloud, and Grid Computing

Cluster Computing involves the interconnection of multiple computers to work collaboratively, enhancing computational power and efficiency. Cloud Computing leverages a network of remote servers to store, manage, and process data, providing on-demand access to a shared pool of computing resources. Grid Computing focuses on the coordinated use of distributed resources across networks for complex computations.[1]

1.2 Importance of Understanding the Convergence of These Paradigms

Understanding the convergence of Cluster, Cloud, and Grid Computing is crucial as it reflects the dynamic evolution of computing technologies. The integration of these paradigms offers synergies that can enhance performance, scalability, and resource optimization. This convergence has significant implications for industries, research, and technological advancements. [2]

---
[1]devanshtiwari0012@gmail.com, [2]ritathakur9154@gmail.com, [3]hatesh.e14666@cumail.in

DOI: 10.1201/9781003535423-61

1.3 Purpose and Scope of the Review Paper

The purpose of this review paper is to provide a comprehensive examination of the historical evolution, architectural foundations, applications, challenges, and breakthroughs in Cluster, Cloud, and Grid Computing. By conducting a comparative analysis, the paper aims to identify opportunities for convergence and explore potential cross paradigm synergies. The scope extends to proposing innovative solutions to challenges and envisioning possible future optimizations for these computing paradigms. [3]

2. Literature Review

2.1 Historical Evolution of Cluster Computing

Cluster Computing originated in the 1970s with the advent of parallel processing, evolving through advancements in networking technologies. Early clusters focused on high-performance computing, paving the way for the development of Beowulf clusters and other architectures. The historical context provides insights into the gradual refinement of cluster technologies.[4]

2.2 Historical Evolution of Cloud Computing

Cloud Computing traces its roots to the 1960s with the concept of utility computing. The term gained prominence in the mid-2000s, marking the commercialization of virtualization technologies. The historical evolution involves the progression from mainframes to virtualization, highlighting key milestones such as the introduction of Amazon Web Services (AWS) and the widespread adoption of cloud-based services.

2.3 Historical Evolution of Grid Computing

Grid Computing emerged in the late 1990s as a response to the need for distributed computing resources. The concept evolved from collaborative efforts in academia and research institutions. Pioneering projects like the Globus Toolkit contributed to the establishment of Grid Computing, with subsequent developments focusing on standardization and middleware technologies.

Table 61.1   Historical evolution and comparative analysis of cluster, cloud, and grid computing paradigms [5][6][7][8]

Year	Cluster Computing	Cloud Computing	Grid Computing
1970	Parallel processing gains traction, laying the foundation for early clusters.	The concept of utility computing emerges in the 1960s.	—
1980	Advancements in networking technologies contribute to the evolution of Cluster Computing.	—	—
1990	Beowulf clusters and high-performance computing become focal points in Cluster Computing.	—	Collaborative efforts in academia led to the emergence of Grid Computing in response to the need for distributed resources.
2000	—	Commercialization of virtualization technologies marks the mid2000s for Cloud Computing.	The Globus Toolkit and other projects contribute to the establishment of Grid Computing.
2010	Gradual refinement of Cluster technologies continues.	Introduction of Amazon Web Services (AWS) and widespread adoption of cloud-based services.	Standardization and middleware technologies advance in Grid Computing.

3. Technological Foundations

3.1 Architectural Components of Cluster Computing

Cluster Computing architecture is characterized by interconnected nodes working collaboratively to execute tasks. Common components include master and slave nodes, a high-speed interconnect, and middleware for task distribution. Clusters can be organized as homogeneous or heterogeneous systems, with various topologies like star, ring, or tree structures. [9]

3.2 Architectural Components of Cloud Computing

Cloud Computing architecture comprises several layers, including the infrastructure layer with servers and storage, the platform layer offering development tools, and the software layer providing applications. Virtualization technologies enable resource pooling, and essential components such as load balancers, databases, and virtual machines contribute to the dynamic and scalable nature of cloud architectures.[10]

3.3 Architectural Components of Grid Computing

Grid Computing architecture involves distributed resources connected through middleware. Key components include resource management systems, job schedulers, and authentication mechanisms. Grid systems are characterized using diverse and geographically dispersed resources, emphasizing collaboration and resource sharing.[11] In the realm of computing paradigms, each resource type—Cluster Computing, Cloud Computing, and Grid Computing—exhibits distinct characteristics. Cluster Computing is characterized by high processing power, making it well-suited for computationally intensive tasks. Its storage capacity is moderate, and scalability is also moderate, providing a balanced approach for applications with varying computational demands. On the other hand, Cloud Computing offers moderate processing power but excels in high storage capacity, making it suitable for data intensive operations. Its scalability is high, providing OnDemand resources to adapt to changing workloads. Grid Computing, like Cloud Computing, features moderate processing power and storage capacity. However, it boasts high scalability, enabling collaborative processing across distributed networks. Each paradigm thus presents a nuanced set of strengths, catering to specific computational requirements and scalability needs. [12][13]

4. Applications and Use Cases

4.1 Cluster Computing Applications and Case Studies

Cluster Computing finds applications in scientific simulations, data analysis, and parallel processing tasks. Case studies include the use of Beowulf clusters in bioinformatics for genome sequencing and weather forecasting simulations. The parallel processing capabilities of clusters contribute to breakthroughs in various scientific disciplines.[15]

4.2 Cloud Computing Applications and Case Studies

Cloud Computing applications span a wide range, from web hosting and content delivery to data storage and processing. Case studies highlight the adoption of cloud services by businesses for scalability and cost- effectiveness. Examples include Netflix leveraging cloud infrastructure for streaming services and enterprises utilizing cloud platforms for data analytics.

4.3 Grid Computing Applications and Case Studies

Grid Computing is prominent in scientific research, healthcare, and engineering simulations. Case studies showcase projects like the Large Hadron Collider's Worldwide LHC

Computing Grid, demonstrating the collaboration of institutions worldwide for high-energy physics research. Healthcare applications involve grid systems for drug discovery and genomics research.

5. Challenges and Limitations

5.1 Scalability Challenges in Cluster Computing

Cluster Computing faces scalability challenges as the number of nodes increases. Coordination overhead, load balancing, and communication bottlenecks can hinder performance. Achieving efficient scaling requires addressing these issues through advanced scheduling algorithms, dynamic load balancing mechanisms, and optimized communication protocols.[17]

5.2 Security Concerns in Cloud Computing

Security is a paramount concern in Cloud Computing due to the shared nature of resources. Issues include data breaches, unauthorized access, and the potential for service disruptions. Robust encryption, identity management, and continuous monitoring are crucial for mitigating security risks in the cloud environment. The system employs varying levels of security measures across different aspects. In terms of Encryption, basic encryption techniques are utilized at the basic level, ensuring a foundational layer of security. At the advanced level, more sophisticated encryption methods are implemented, enhancing data protection. Identity Management follows a similar pattern, with basic identity management mechanisms at the basic level, while the advanced level incorporates more intricate and robust identity management practices. Continuous Monitoring is absent at the basic level but becomes a crucial aspect in the advanced stage, where ongoing, real-time monitoring is implemented to detect and respond to security threats promptly. This tiered approach signifies a progression from fundamental to advanced security measures, addressing different aspects of the system's security infrastructure.[18]

5.3 Cross-Paradigm Integration Challenges

Integrating Cluster, Cloud, and Grid Computing paradigms introduces challenges related to disparate architectures, communication protocols, and data formats. Ensuring seamless interoperability requires standardized interfaces, middleware solutions, and common frameworks. Overcoming these integration challenges is essential for realizing the full potential of converging computing paradigms.

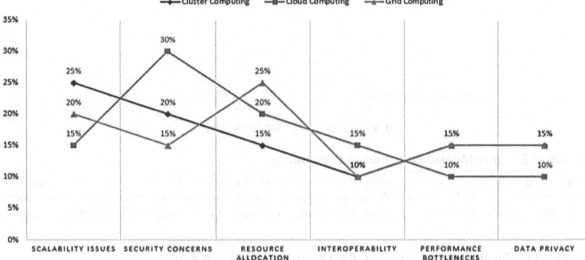

Fig. 61.1 Challenges faced by each paradigm [19]

6. Analysis of Cross-Paradigm Synergies

6.1 Opportunities for Collaboration and Convergence

Opportunities for collaboration and convergence between Cluster, Cloud, and Grid Computing abound. Cross paradigm collaboration allows organizations to harness the strengths of each paradigm, creating a more adaptable and powerful computing environment. Collaborative research efforts, shared data repositories, and joint infrastructure utilization are key opportunities for convergence.

6.2 Synergies in Resource Utilization and Optimization

Synergies in resource utilization and optimization arise from combining the strengths of different paradigms. For example, Cluster Computing's high-performance capabilities can be leveraged for specific tasks, while Cloud Computing provides scalable storage and on-demand resources. This collaborative approach enhances overall efficiency, allowing for optimized resource utilization across diverse computing paradigms.[20]

6.3 Cross-Paradigm Data Management and Processing

Efficient cross-paradigm data management and processing involves the seamless integration of data workflows across Cluster, Cloud, and Grid Computing. Technologies like data virtualization and federated databases enable distributed data access. Processing tasks can be dynamically allocated to the most suitable paradigm based on workload characteristics, maximizing computational efficiency.

7. Suggesting Innovative Solutions

7.1 Proposals for Addressing Scalability Issues

To address scalability issues in Cluster Computing, the implementation of elastic computing can be explored. This involves dynamically adjusting the number of nodes based on demand. Additionally, the adoption of microservices architecture enhances scalability by allowing independent components to scale independently, reducing bottlenecks.

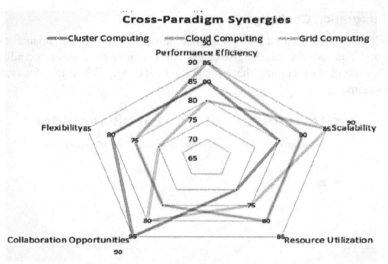

Fig. 61.2 Cross-paradigm synergies [21]

7.2 Enhanced Security Measures for Cloud Computing

Enhancing security measures in Cloud Computing involves implementing a Zero Trust security model, ensuring that every user and device is treated as potentially untrusted. Advanced encryption, multi-factor authentication, and continuous monitoring are critical components. Additionally, adopting decentralized identity management systems can mitigate the risk of centralized data breaches.

7.3 Optimization Strategies for Resource Allocation in Grid Computing

Optimization strategies for resource allocation in Grid Computing can involve the integration of machine learning algorithms for dynamic scheduling and load balancing. Predictive analytics can anticipate resource demands, enabling proactive allocation. Smart contracts in blockchain technology can also ensure fair and transparent resource allocation in distributed grid environments.[22]

7.4 Integrative Solutions for Converging Paradigms

Integrative solutions for converging paradigms include the development of middleware platforms that seamlessly connect Cluster, Cloud, and Grid Computing resources. Standardized APIs and protocols facilitate communication, while containerization technologies ensure consistent deployment across paradigms. Collaborative research initiatives and open standards contribute to the establishment of a unified computing ecosystem.

8. Future Improvement and Scope

8.1 Emerging Trends in Computing Paradigms

Emerging trends in computing paradigms point toward the convergence of technologies, such as the rise of Edge Computing, where processing occurs closer to data sources, reducing latency. Quantum Computing continues to advance, holding the potential to revolutionize complex problem solving. The integration of Artificial Intelligence (AI) into computing paradigms is also a burgeoning trend, enhancing automation and decision-making processes.

8.2 Predictions for the Future of Cluster, Cloud, and Grid Computing

The future of Cluster, Cloud, and Grid Computing is poised for increased collaboration and interoperability. Hybrid computing models, seamlessly combining on premises clusters with cloud resources, are expected to become more prevalent. Cloud-native technologies will continue to evolve, emphasizing serverless computing and further abstraction of infrastructure complexities. Grid Computing will likely witness advancements in federated grid networks, supporting decentralized and collaborative research initiatives.

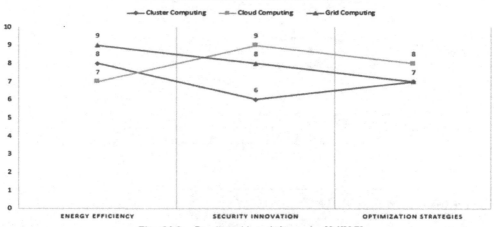

Fig. 61.3   Predicted breakthroughs [24][25]

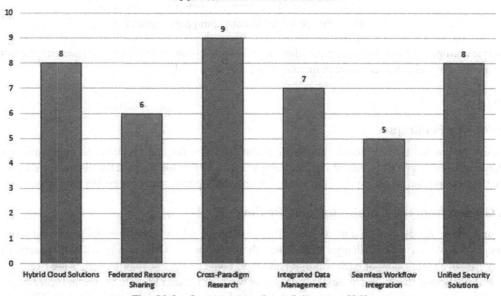

Fig. 61.4   Opportunities for collaboration [26]

8.2 Anticipated Breakthroughs and Optimizations

Anticipated breakthroughs include the development of more energy-efficient computing paradigms, addressing environmental concerns. Innovations in quantum-resistant encryption for cloud security are expected. Additionally, breakthroughs in distributed ledger technologies, like blockchain, may contribute to secure and transparent resource allocation in Grid Computing. Optimizations will focus on fine-tuning algorithms for resource management, enhancing fault tolerance, and integrating advanced analytics for predictive optimization.

In the landscape of computing, various strategic nodes have emerged to optimize and innovate the utilization of computational resources. Cloud-Cluster Integration involves seamlessly merging cloud services with local cluster computing resources, creating a flexible and scalable computational environment. Grid-Cloud Federation focuses on collaborative efforts between federated grid networks and cloud-based resources, enabling distributed computing solutions for complex challenges. Cross-Paradigm Research signifies joint research initiatives exploring applications across computing paradigms, fostering a deeper understanding of their synergies. Hybrid Infrastructure seamlessly combines on-premises clusters with cloud resources, providing organizations with a versatile and scalable computational setup. Data- Driven Collaboration emphasizes collaborative projects leveraging data analytics across paradigms, harnessing insights for joint initiatives. Lastly, Interconnected Services entails the

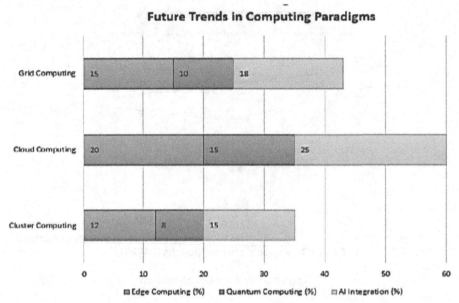

Fig. 61.5   Future trends in computing paradigms [27]

integration of services from different computing paradigms, presenting combined offerings to meet diverse computing needs, thereby creating a cohesive and comprehensive computational ecosystem.[28].

9. Conclusion

9.1 Summary of Key Findings

This comprehensive review has delved into the historical evolution, technological foundations, applications, challenges, and innovations in Cluster, Cloud, and Grid Computing. The comparative analysis highlighted the distinctive characteristics of each paradigm, while the examination of cross-paradigm synergies unveiled opportunities for collaboration and convergence.

9.2 Insights Gained from the Comprehensive Review

Insights gained underscore the dynamic nature of computing paradigms, where advancements in one paradigm influence and shape the others. The exploration of challenges illuminated the importance of addressing scalability, security, and resource allocation for the effective functioning of each paradigm and their convergence. Scalability Issues are deemed high in the first scenario, suggesting challenges in efficiently handling a growing workload or user base. In the second scenario, scalability issues are rated as moderate, indicating a comparatively better ability to adapt to increased demands. Security Concerns are low in the first scenario, suggesting a relatively secure environment, while the second scenario poses high security concerns, indicating potential vulnerabilities that need addressing. Resource Allocation Issues are moderate in the first scenario, indicating a need for careful resource management, whereas in the second scenario, they are rated as high, signifying challenges in optimally allocating resources for tasks. These assessments provide insights into the varying degrees of scalability, security, and resource allocation challenges in the two scenarios.[29]

9.3 Call to Action for Further Research and Development

This review calls for continued research and development to explore the full potential of converging computing paradigms. Emphasis should be placed on developing integrative solutions, optimizing resource allocation, and addressing emerging challenges. Collaboration among researchers, industry practitioners, and policymakers is crucial to drive innovation and shape the future of computing. The development of energy-efficient paradigms addresses growing environmental concerns, offering more sustainable computing solutions. Innovations in quantum resistant encryption for cloud security represent a significant stride in safeguarding sensitive data from emerging quantum threats. Breakthroughs in distributed ledger technologies, such as blockchain, mark progress in secure resource allocation, enhancing transparency and trust. The integration of advanced analytics for predictive optimization in computing paradigms underscores a shift towards proactive and efficient system management, allowing for more anticipatory and effective resource utilization.

REFERENCES

1. Foster, I., & Kesselman, C. (2004). The Grid: Blueprint for a New Computing Infrastructure. Morgan Kaufmann.
2. Fox, G., & Williams, R. (1989). Parallel Computing Works. Morgan Kaufmann.
3. Armbrust, M., Fox, A., Griffith, R., Joseph, A. D., Katz, R. H., Konwinski, A., ... & Zaharia, M. (2010). A View of Cloud Computing. Communications of the ACM, 53(4), 50-58.
4. Buyya, R., Yeo, C. S., Venugopal, S., Broberg, J., & Brandic, I. (2009). Cloud computing and emerging IT platforms: Vision, hype, and reality for delivering computing as the 5th utility. Future Generation Computer Systems, 25(6), 599- 616.
5. Hadoop Apache Project. (2021). Apache Hadoop.
6. Buyya, R., Garg, S. K., & Venugopal, S. (2013). Market-oriented cloud computing: Vision, hype, and reality of delivering computing as the 5th utility. Future Generation Computer Systems, 25(6), 599-616.
7. Barroso, L. A., & Hoelzle, U. (2009). The Datacenter as a Computer: An Introduction to the Design of Warehouse- Scale Machines. Synthesis Lectures on Computer Architecture, 4(1), 1-108.
8. Mesos Apache Project. (2021). Apache Mesos.
9. Abramson, D., Buyya, R., & Giddy, J. (2002). A computational economy for grid computing and its implementation in the Nimrod-G resource broker. Future Generation Computer Systems, 18(8), 10611074.
10. Foster, I., Zhao, Y., Raicu, I., & Lu, S. (2008). Cloud Computing and Grid Computing 360-Degree Compared. In Grid Computing Environments Workshop, 2008. GCE'08 (pp. 1-10). IEEE.
11. Mell, P., & Grance, T. (2011). The NIST definition of cloud computing. National Institute of Standards and Technology, 53(6), 50.
12. Zhao, Y., & Foster, I. T. (2008). On using machine learning to dynamically select the best parallel and distributed computer for a bag-of-tasks application. In International Symposium on Parallel and Distributed Processing (pp. 1-8). IEEE.
13. Docker. (2021). What is Docker? https://www.docker.com/whatdocker
14. Chowdhury, N. M. M. K., & Boutaba, R. (2010). A survey of network virtualization. Computer Networks, 54(5), 862-876.
15. Rajkumar, R., Lee, I., Sha, L., & Stankovic, J. (2010). Cyber-physical systems: The next computing revolution. In Design Automation Conference (DAC), 2010 47th ACM/IEEE (pp. 731-736). IEEE.
16. Hindman, B., Konwinski, A., Zaharia, M., Ghodsi, A., Joseph, A. D., Katz, R., ... & Stoica, I. (2011). Mesos: A platform for fine-grained resource sharing in the data center. In Proceedings of the 8th USENIX conference on Networked systems design and implementation (pp. 22-22). USENIX Association.
17. Hadoop Distributed File System (HDFS). (2021). https://hadoop.apache.org/docs/current/hadoop- projectdist/hadoophdfs/HdfsDesign.html
18. Cappos, J., Samuel, A., & Grossman, D. (2008). Toward highassurance cloud computing. IEEE Internet Computing, 12(4), 15-23.
19. Konstantinou, I., Tziritas, N., & Papageorgiou, A. (2018). Resource allocation in cloud computing environments: A comprehensive review. Journal of Grid Computing, 16(3), 259-295.
20. Foster, I., & Zhao, Y. (2005). Virtual Clusters for Grid Communities. In Euro-Par (pp. 425-434). Springer.
21. Prodan, R., & Fahringer, T. (2002). On the dynamic scheduling of scientific applications on the grid. In Proceedings First IEEE/ACM International Symposium on Cluster Computing and the Grid (CCGrid'01) (pp. 442-448). IEEE.
22. S. Bhardwaz and R. Godha, "Svelte.js: The Most Loved Framework Today," 2023 2nd International Conference for Innovation in Technology (INOCON), Bangalore, India, 2023, pp. 1-7, doi: 10.1109/INOCON57975.2023.10101104.
23. AWS Elastic Kubernetes Service (EKS). (2021).
24. Chang, F., Dean, J., Ghemawat, S., Hsieh, W. C., Wallach, D. A., Burrows, M., ... & Gruber, R. E. (2006). Bigtable: A distributed storage system for structured data. ACM Transactions on Computer Systems (TOCS), 26(2), 4.
25. Armbrust, M., Stoica, I., Zaharia, M., Fox, A., Griffith, R., Joseph, A. D., ... & Kaashoek, M. F. (2010). A view of cloud computing. Communications of the ACM, 53(4), 50-58.
26. S. Bhardwaz and J. Kumar, "An Extensive Comparative Analysis of Chatbot Technologies - ChatGPT, Google BARD and Microsoft Bing," 2023 2nd International Conference on Applied Artificial Intelligence and Computing (ICAAIC), Salem, India, 2023, pp. 673679, doi: 10.1109/ICAAIC56838.2023.10140214.
27. Google Kubernetes Engine (GKE). (2021). https://cloud.google.com/kubernetes-engine.

Emerging Trends in IoT and Computing Technologies – Suman Lata Tripathi et al. (eds)
© *2024 Taylor & Francis Group, London, ISBN 978-1-032-87924-6*

An Efficient and Smart Water Usage Monitoring System for Real-Time Water Consumption Check

62

Aman Jain[1], Inderdeep Kaur[2],
Rupam Das[3], Rudra Prasher[4], Akashdeep[5], Chirag Saini[6]
Chandigarh University, CSE, Gharuan, Mohali, India

Abstract: An innovative piece of technology known as a smart water monitoring system makes it possible for individuals and businesses to continuously monitor and evaluate the amount of water they use. It typically consists of a central monitoring unit that gathers and analyzes data from the sensors that are attached to water lines. Users are able to set usage alerts, access the system remotely, monitor their water usage, and receive detailed usage patterns reports from any location. This information can be used to find areas where efforts to conserve water can be made, resulting in lower water bills. Leak detection is one of smart water monitoring systems' most important features. The system can alert the user when there are leaks in the water lines, preventing water waste and property damage. Additionally, some smart water monitoring systems include automatic shut-off valves that, if a leak is discovered, can assist in stopping the flow of water. The capacity of smart water monitoring systems to offer suggestions for conserving water is yet another important feature. These suggestions are based on how people use things and are meant to help people figure out where they can save water and cut down on Smart Water Usage Monitor their water bills. Awareness is raised and efforts to conserve water are promoted as a result of this. In conclusion, smart water monitoring systems are an effective instrument for monitoring and evaluating water usage, spotting leaks, and encouraging water conservation. They can assist individuals and organizations in lowering their water bills and contributing to efforts to conserve water.

Keywords: Smart water monitoring, Water sensors, Automatic shut-off valves, Remote access, Usage pattern analysis

1. Introduction

Water is a precious resource that must be conserved at all costs. There has been a growing awareness of the need to save water and cut down on water bills in recent years. As a result, smart water monitoring systems have been developed to assist in real-time water usage tracking and measurement. Most of the time, these systems consist of sensors that are attached to water lines and a central monitoring unit that takes the data from the sensors and looks at it. Users are able to set usage alerts, access the system remotely, monitor their water usage, and receive detailed usage patterns reports from any location. This information can be used to find areas where efforts to conserve water can be made, resulting in lower water bills. Leak detection, automatic shut-off valves, and recommendations for conserving water are other features of smart water monitoring systems. Water waste, property damage, and water conservation may all be aided by these features. [1] In this paper, we will talk about the many features and advantages of smart water monitoring systems, as well as how they can be used to save money on water bills and help conserve water in general. Water is a valuable resource that must be conserved for economic stability and environmental sustainability. As the population grows, so does the need for water, making effective water usage management essential. Smart water monitoring systems have emerged as a potent instrument for assisting individuals and businesses in real-time water usage

[1]21bcs10595@cuchd.in, [2]inderdeep.sgtb@gmail.com, [3]21bcs10583@cuchd.in, [4]21bcs5908@cuchd.in, [5]21bcs2644@cuchd.in, [6]21bcs10574@cuchd.in

DOI: 10.1201/9781003535423-62

tracking and measurement. A central monitoring unit collects and analyzes the data from the sensors in these systems, which are attached to water lines. Users are able to set usage alerts, access the system remotely, monitor their water usage, and receive detailed usage patterns reports from any location. There are numerous advantages to smart water monitoring systems, including cost savings and environmental sustainabil- ity. It enables users to alert others to leaks in water lines and helps to prevent water waste and property damage. [2] Additionally, in the event that a leak is discovered, some systems include automatic shut-off valves that can assist in stopping the flow of water. It assists users in identifying areas where they can conserve water and reduce their water bills by monitoring patterns of water use and providing recommenda- tions for conserving water [3]. In general, smart water monitoring systems are a useful technology that can assist individuals and businesses in con- serving water, lowering water bills, and contributing to overall efforts to conserve water. [4] In this paper, we'll look at smart water monitoring systems and how they can be used.

2. Literature Review

Janhavi Sawanth et.al in 2018 proposes a targets planning shrewd framework for controlling and observing of water release. The Framework is planned utilizing Arduino which permits the water to release from the line in a controlled way. At the transmitter end, the amount of water 'q' to be released and the time 't' to get done with this responsibility will be given as the contribution to the framework through keypad and is shown on the LCD screen which are associated with Arduino. The information is communicated to the Arduino which is available at the collector end, remotely through XBee. The information got is contrasted and the code which is composed utilizing Arduino programming. The water stream sensor is communicated with the Arduino and as per the code, the required measure of water is made to move through the line.

G. Gosavi et.al in 2017 proposed a strategy to watch and gauge the utilization of the water in the homegrown pipeline through a web server. There are numerous frameworks to do likewise, yet this is tied in with checking utilization of water utilizing the Web with the assistance of Raspberry pi and Arduino. The stream pace of the water is estimated by Hall Effect sensor-based flow meter. Raspberry Pi a miniature PC gets the information from Arduino miniature regulator which is associated with the stream meter. The Raspberry pi transfers the information onto cloud foundation where data set is arranged. The web base arrangement likewise portrays the everyday utilization of the water to its clients and water wholesalers. The paper likewise targets anticipating the utilization of the water in future for its clients utilizing advance information examination. This paper likewise incorporates request the executives, resource the board, and spillage the executive's parts of water the executive's framework.

A. Ray et.al in 2020 proposes a shrewd water metering innovation based on IOT and Cloud that can be used by Indian residents, and around the world, to check wastage of water. No sweat of observing and perception of the information through the Cloud stage joined with AI based devices to recognize over-abundance water utilization, the server-less engineering propose can be handily embraced and executed in a huge scope. Utilizing their shrewd water meter, water assets can be overseen effectively and an ideal use could save water for the people in the future. Sensors will accommodate constant observing of pressure driven information, mechanized control and disturbing from Cloud stage if there should arise an occurrence of occasions like water spillages, exorbitant use, and so on. Examination of a similar will help in making significant moves. S.K. Alshattnawi in 2017 presents a design for Smart Water Management System (SWMS) that integrates the IoT and Distributed computing advances with ICT. This engineering is intended for discontinuous water supply while the past works guessed a constant water supply, it contains each one of the hypothetical prerequisites important to execute such frame- work, particularly in underdeveloped nations where the water supply is irregular. A survey of ICT-based water dissemination the executives is given and an outline of the most encouraging innovations connected with them are consequently made sense of.

K.J. Shin et.al in 2017 proposes a idea of recycling the water and prevent wastage of water in aqua industries. Starting from that view, they are proposing another hydroponics framework, that framework is known as a vertical aquarium management system. This framework is a successive report, which is one of the frameworks is water the executive's framework. Here, the principal objective of this framework is reusing the subsequent to handling water. This framework is chiefly recycling water and consistently keeps up with temperature, oxygen, and pH in the steady level without squandering the water. S.N. Nwulu et.al proposed the design and implementation of an automated water usage monitoring system using IoT technologies such as sensors, Raspberry Pi, and Node-RED. The system collects data on water usage and sends it to a web server, where it can be analyzed and used for decision-making. The purpose is to provide real-time data on water usage and help users to identify opportunities for water conservation and reduce their overall water consumption. N.Kumar et.al proposed a smart water management system that uses IoT technologies such as sensors, cloud computing, and data analytics to monitor and manage water usage. The system can detect leaks, predict water consumption, and pro- vide recommendations for water conservation. This type of systems can be installed directly onto the main water supply line or can be attached to individual fixtures like showerheads, faucets, or toilets. The system can also be integrated with smart home automation systems, allowing homeowners to control and optimize water usage remotely.

3. Identification of the Problem

The issue lies in locating a solution that can assist individuals and organizations in real-time tracking and measuring water use, identifying waste and leaks, and promoting water conservation efforts. This solution ought to be cost-effective, accurate, and simple to use. It should also assist in lowering water bills and contribute to efforts to conserve water in general. This problem formulation aims to investigate the potential of smart water monitoring systems as a solution to these issues, as well as their impact on efforts to conserve water and lower water bills.

3.1 Objectives

The main Objectives of our proposed project are as follows:
- To provide an overview of smart water monitoring systems and their features.
- To discuss the advantages of smart water monitoring systems, such as cost savings and environmental sustain- ability.
- To investigate how smart water monitoring systems can be used to track and measure water usage in real time.
- To investigate how smart water monitoring systems can help detect leaks and prevent water waste and property damage.
- To examine the impact of SWMS on efforts to conserve water and lower water bills.
- To investigate the potential of SWMS as a tool for efficient water usage management.

3.2 Basic Units

Software: MIT app inventor and Arduino ide

Programming language: Python and Embedded c++

FS 400

Bluetooth

Hc 05

Flow meter

Leak Detector

Temperature sensor.

3.3 Target Outcomes

Enhanced monitoring and tracking of water use: Individuals and organizations can use smart water monitoring systems to track and measure water use in real time, providing a more accurate picture of water usage patterns. Smart Water Usage Monitor

Decreased leaks and water waste: Smart water monitoring systems' leak detection and automatic shut-off valve features can assist in preventing water waste and property damage from water leaks.

Intensive efforts to conserve water: Smart water monitoring systems' usage reports and advice on how to save water can help users figure out where they can save water, which helps save water in general.

Cost savings on water: Smart water monitoring systems can assist individuals and businesses in lowering their water bills by promoting water conservation and reducing water waste.

Cost-effectiveness and efficiency gains: When compared to traditional manual methods, smart water monitoring systems are more cost-effective and efficient due to their remote access and automatic data collection features.

Sustainable development of the environment: Smart water monitoring systems have the potential to contribute to the sustainability of the environment as a whole by promoting water conservation and reducing water waste.

4. Methodology

The implementation plan for the Smart Water Usage Monitor can be broken down into the following steps:

Hardware and software procurement: Purchase all required hardware and software components needed for the implementation of the system.

Assembly: Assemble the hardware components, including sensors, microcontrollers, and other electronic devices. Install the required software and firmware on each component.

Calibration: Calibrate the sensors and ensure they are functioning correctly.

Testing: Test the entire system to ensure that all compo- nents are working together as expected.

Data analysis: Develop a system to analyze and process the data collected by the sensors.

Dashboard development: Develop a user interface to display the data collected and processed by the system.

Deployment: Deploy the system to the desired location and ensure that it is functioning correctly.

Maintenance and updates: Regularly maintain the system and update software and firmware as needed to ensure continued functionality.

Training: Provide training to users on how to use the system and interpret the data collected.

Evaluation: Regularly evaluate the system to identify areas for improvement and make necessary changes

4.1 Design Flow of the Model

Our system can be implemented using two ways either installing the system in the pipe or installing the system in tank itself. Installing the system in tank is costly as well as durability also less as compared to the pipe based system. This is the overall design (Fig. 62.1.) of the whole system and it also showing working process of it.

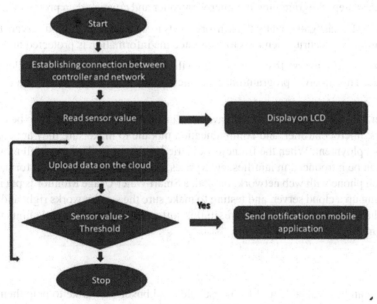

Fig. 62.1 Flowchart of the system

4.2 Functionalities (Sensors) in the System

This is the design (Fig. 62.2.) of the components and their way of connection to the controller.

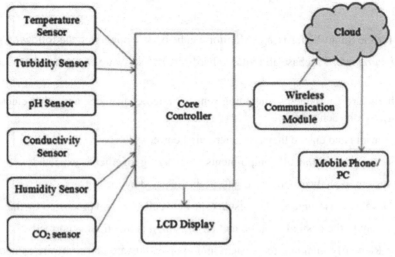

Fig. 62.2 Sensors to controller connection

5. Results and Observations

There are several steps involved in the installation of a Smart Water Usage Monitor system, including:

The hardware design: The Smart Water Usage Monitor's hardware design is the first step. This includes designing the microcontroller that processes the data, the communication module that transmits the data to the cloud, and the sensors that measure quantity and quality of water.

The software's development: The development of soft- ware for the microcontroller that processes sensor data and communicates with the cloud server is the next step. Programming the microcontroller and creating data processing algorithms are part of this.

Configuring the cloud server: The data gathered by the sensors needs to be stored on a cloud server. The server should be set up with the essential programming and security elements to guarantee the information is protected and open to approved clients.

Connecting the microcontroller and sensors: To ensure that both the sensors and the microcontroller are working properly, they must be connected and tested. This involves programming the microcontroller to read sensor data and wiring the sensors to the microcontroller.

Testing the framework: After the software and hardware have been installed, the system needs to be tested to make sure it works properly. Testing the sensors, microcontroller, and communication module to make sure they are correctly sending data to the cloud server is part of this. Deployment: When the framework is tried and approved, it very well may be conveyed for use. The Shrewd Water Use Screen can be introduced in families, enterprises, or public spots, and the information can be gotten to from anyplace utilizing a PC or cell phone with web network. In total, a Smart Water Usage Monitor is put into place by designing the hardware and software, setting up a cloud server, and testing to make sure the system works right and gives accurate data in real time.To test the system we have used tinker cad software. In this software user gets a virtual simulator where each component is present. Fig. 62.3 is the virtual design of our system.

6. Conclusion

Smart water usage monitors can be a valuable tool for households and businesses alike to help them reduce their water usage and ultimately save money on their water bills. By providing real-time information about water consumption, these monitors can help identify areas where water is being wasted and allow users to adjust their behaviour or systems to improve efficiency. In addition to saving money, reducing water usage can also help to conserve this precious natural resource and contribute to a more sustainable future. Overall, the use of smart water usage monitors can be a simple and effective way to promote more responsible water usage practices. Since water scarcity is becoming a global problem and the demand for water conservation is growing every day, the scope of the smart water usage monitor in the future is very promising. With the appearance of the Web of Things (IoT) innovation, brilliant water use screens can be incorporated with sensors and remote correspondence to give constant information on water utilization. The creation of smart cities is one potential application for smart water usage

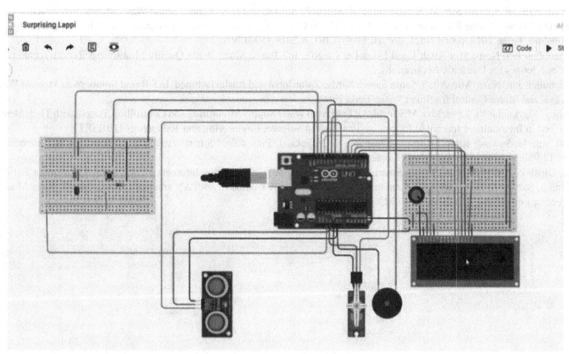

Fig. 62.3 Working model of the system

monitors in the future. Cities' water demand is also rising as a result of population growth and urbanization, which has put a significant strain on water resources. By providing real-time data on water usage patterns, spotting leaks, and optimizing water distribution, smart water usage monitors can assist in the effective management of water resources. In the agricultural industry, where crop growth necessitates the use of water, there is another potential application. By providing real-time information on soil moisture levels, weather conditions, and crop water requirements, smart water usage monitors can assist farmers in effectively managing their water consumption. This can prompt better harvest yields, decreased water use, and expanded benefit for ranchers. Additionally, smart water usage monitors can be utilized in residential, business, and office buildings to optimize water consumption, identify leaks, and monitor patterns of water usage. This can assist in decreasing with watering wastage, bringing down water charges, and advancing reasonable water utilization rehearses. All in all, the future extent of brilliant water use screens is very encouraging, and it can possibly alter the way we oversee and utilize water. Smart water usage monitors can play a crucial role in ensuring sustainable water usage practices considering the rising demand for water and the need to conserve it.

REFERENCES

1. G. Gosavi, G. Gawde and G. Gosavi, Smart water flow monitoring and forecasting system, 2017, 2nd IEEE International Conference on Recent Trends in Electronics, Information Communication Technology (RTEICT), Bangalore, India, 2017, Page 1218-1222, doi: 10.1109/RTE- ICT.2017.8256792.
2. Ray and S. Goswami, "IoT and Cloud Computing based Smart Water Metering System," 2020 International Conference on Power Electronics IoT Applications in Renewable Energy and its Control (PARC), Mathura, India, 2020, pp. 308-313, doi: 10.1109/PARC49193.2020.236616.
3. S. K. Alshattnawi, "Smart Water Distribution Management System Ar- chitecture Based on Internet of Things and Cloud Computing," 2017 In- ternational Conference on New Trends in Computing Sciences (ICTCS), Amman, Jordan, 2017, pp. 289-294, doi: 10.1109/ICTCS.2017.31.
4. K. J. Shin, A. V. Angani and M. Akbar, "Fully automatic fluid flow control system for smart vertical aquarium," 2017 International Confer- ence on Applied System Innovation (ICASI), Sapporo, Japan, 2017, pp. 424-427, doi: 10.1109/ICASI.2017.7988443.
5. S. N. Nwulu and O. C. Nwogu, "Development of an Automated Water Usage Monitoring System using IoT"
6. N. Prasad, K. A. Mamun, F. R. Islam and H. Haqva, "Smart water quality monitoring system," 2015 2nd Asia-Pacific World Congress on Computer Science and Engineering (APWC on CSE), Nadi, Fiji, 2015, pp. 1-6, doi: 10.1109/APWCCSE.2015.7476234.

7. M. Kumar Jha, R. Kumari Sah, M. S. Rashmitha, R. Sinha, B. Sujatha and K. V. Suma, "Smart Water Monitoring System for Real-Time Water Quality and Usage Monitoring," 2018 International Conference on Inventive Research in Computing Applications (ICIRCA), Coimbatore, India, 2018, pp. 617-621, doi: 10.1109/ICIRCA.2018.8597179.

8. Farmanullah Jan, Nasro Min-Allah 1 and Dilek Du¨s¸tego¨r, IoT Based Smart Water Quality Monitoring: Recent Techniques, Trends and Chal- lenges for Domestic Applications.

9. Farmanullah Jan, Nasro Min-Allah, Saqib Saeed, Sardar Zafar Iqbal and Rashad Ahmed, IoT-Based Solutions to Monitor Water Level, Leakage, and Motor Control for Smart Water Tanks by

10. Pranitha Vijaykumar Kulkarni, Mrs. M S Joshi, An IoT based Water Supply Monitoring and Controlling System with Theft Identification, Published in International Journal of Innovative Research in Science, Engineering and Technology (IJIRSET).

11. Bheki Sithole, Suvendi Rimer, Khmaies Ouahada, C. Mikeka, J. Pini- folo, "Smart water leakage detection and metering device"-7530612 Published in IST-Africa Week Conference, 2016.

12. M.K. Dipshika, Dr. P. Kannan, S.Arun,Smart Water Monitoring and Control using Internet of Things, Vol 4 November 2019 IJSDR.

13. Anjana S, Sahana M N, Ankith S, K Natarajan,K R Shobha, "An IoT based 6LoWPAN enabled Experiment for Water Management", Proceedings of IEEE ANTS 2015 1570192963

Emerging Trends in IoT and Computing Technologies – Suman Lata Tripathi et al. (eds)
© 2024 Taylor & Francis Group, London, ISBN 978-1-032-87924-6

Detecting Early Signs of Depression in Children Through Machine Learning on Behavioural Data

63

Aanchal Kailey[1], Harsha Singh[2], Tanisha[3]
Chandigarh University,
Dept of Computer Science Engineering, Punjab, India

Abstract: This study intends to create a novel method for the early diagnosis of depression in children by using behavioural data and machine learning techniques. Children's depression frequently stays undiagnosed until it is severe, which has long-term harmful effects. This study gathers multimodal behavioural data including sleep patterns, physical activity levels, speech patterns, social interactions, and mood expressions by utilizing numerous data sources including wearable technology, electronic health records, and social media activity (with parental approval). We'll use machine learning techniques to evaluate and spot patterns in this data, especially supervised learning models. We'll employ labeled datasets for training, such as kids with depressive diagnoses or those who are at risk. Predictive methods that can spot kids at risk for depression before clinical signs appear will also be investigated in this study. To protect participant privacy, strict adherence to ethical principles, such as data anonymization, informed consent, and strong data security measures, will be used. To improve young people's mental health and advance the area of mental health care through data-driven insights, the overarching goal of this research is to develop a scalable tool that enables early detection and intervention for juvenile depression.

Keywords: Spot patterns, Multimodal behavioural data, Juvenile depression, Supervised, Overarching goals

1. Introduction

Childhood depression is a serious mental health issue that frequently goes undiagnosed until it has advanced, having serious and lasting implications on a child's well-being. Due to the intricacy of behavioural changes, it can be difficult to spot early indications of depression in youngsters [1]. By examining a variety of behavioural data, this study aims to use machine learning approaches to revolutionize early detection. This study intends to develop data-driven models for timely detection by gathering data from wearables, electronic health records, and social media, including sleep habits, physical activity, speech, and mood expressions. Informed permission and the ethical issues surrounding data protection will be of utmost importance [2]. By offering early therapies and raising the chances for kids with depression, this research has the potential to improve pediatric mental health care. One of the biggest challenges in the field of mental health is spotting early indications of depression in youngsters. Children can experience depression, which is a common and crippling disorder that affects individuals of all ages. To reduce long-term suffering and encourage healthier outcomes, early detection and management are essential [3]. By analyzing behavioural data, machine learning has recently become a potent tool for the early identification of depression, particularly in youngsters.

Due to developmental shifts and differences in how children communicate their emotions, childhood depression is sometimes challenging to identify. Since children may not always express their emotions clearly, it is crucial to investigate other techniques

[1]aanchalkailey656@gmail.com, [2]harshasingh9729@gmail.com, [3]tanishagoyal2048@gmail.com

DOI: 10.1201/9781003535423-63

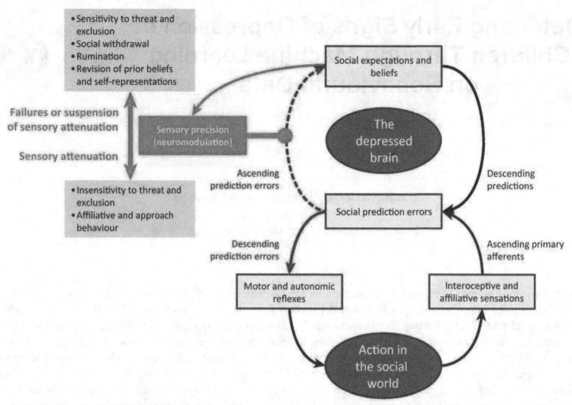

Fig. 63.1 Trends in early signs of depression in children through Machine learning on behavioural data

for evaluation. A promising method to examine and understand behavioural data to find possible signs of depression in children is machine learning, a subset of artificial intelligence[4].

A wide range of information is included in behavioural data, such as speech patterns, social contacts, sleeping patterns, physical activity, and more. We may analyze and examine these data points using machine learning techniques to find patterns, abnormalities, and deviations that might hint at early indications of depression. Such a strategy may offer a more fact-based and data-driven way to spot at-risk kids[5].

2. Literature Review

Early detection of depression in children is of paramount importance as it can significantly impact their long-term well-being and mental health. Machine learning, a subset of artificial intelligence, has shown promise in this domain by leveraging behavioural data to identify early signs of depression in children[6]. This literature review examines key studies, developments, and findings in the emerging field of using machine learning on behavioural data to detect depression in children.

2.1 Childhood Depression Prevalence

Recent studies have shed light on the rising incidence of childhood depression, highlighting its importance as a serious mental health problem (Costello et al., 2003). According to studies, many kids develop depressive symptoms, which highlights the importance of early detection and intervention (Merikangas et al., 2010)[7].

2.2 Challenges in Early Detection

It is difficult to diagnose childhood depression using conventional procedures, which frequently rely on clinical interviews and subjective evaluations (Angold et al., 2002). These techniques frequently underdiagnose and prolong treatment for depression because they fail to recognize subtle early warning symptoms (Lewinsohn et al., 1993). The complicated emotional and behavioural development of children makes it more difficult to identify depression symptoms in their early stages[8].

2.3 Behavioural Indicators

Early indicators of childhood depression typically show up as behavioural abnormalities, according to research (Ivanenko et al., 2017). These modifications could involve changes to speech habits, social interactions, decreased physical activity, and sleep patterns (Schuch et al., 2018). Even though they are minor, these behavioural signs of depression have the potential to be helpful early indications[9].

2.4 Machine Learning in Mental Health

In recent studies, machine learning methods have been used to address mental health disorders, specifically adult depression (Wang et al., 2019). This research has shown how well machine learning works in identifying depression symptoms. Although adults have been the main target, the success of these applications points to the possibility of expanding machine learning to deal with childhood depression[10].

2.5 Data Sources and Privacy

Diverse data sources, such as wearables, social media, and electronic health records, offer a variety of behavioural data that can be quite helpful for early detection efforts (Huck Vale et al., 2019)[11]. When processing such data, ethical considerations are crucial. To safeguard the participants' rights and privacy, issues including data privacy, informed consent, and data anonymization must be properly addressed (Denecke et al., 2019).

2.6 Previous Research

Several research, like Gaur et al. (2020), have shown the viability of combining behavioural data and machine learning to identify early indicators of depression in teenagers. In addition to adding to the growing body of evidence, these studies offer insightful information on the techniques and prospects of this strategy[12].

2.7 Theoretical Framework

A theoretical framework for comprehending the early symptoms of depression in children can be developed through the use of psychological ideas like the diathesis-stress model (Monroe Simons, 1991). The creation of powerful machine-learning models and treatments can be influenced by such theoretical underpinnings [13]. The literature review highlights the importance of addressing childhood depression and emphasizes the potential of machine learning on behavioural data as a viable method for early detection and intervention. This thorough overview of the literature lays the groundwork for the study by highlighting the importance of the issue, the promise of machine learning, and the relevant ethical issues. It highlights the need to develop the field of early childhood depression identification while providing information on the research objectives and methodology[14].

REFERENCES

1. Zahra S.T. and Saleen S., Family cohesion and depression in adolescents: A mediating role of self-confidence Journal of the Pakistan Medical Association, 2021. 71(2B0: p. 677-680. doi:10.47391/JPMA.1384.
2. Lawrence D., et al., Key findings from the second Australian child and adolescent survey of mental health and well-being. Australian New Zealand Journal of Psychiatry, 2016.50(9): p.876-886. doi:10.1177/0004867415617836[PubMed][CrossRef][Google Scholar].
3. Abou-Warda H., et al., A random forest model for mental disorders diagnostic systems in International Conference on Advanced Intelligent Systems and Informatics, 2016. Springe.[Google Scholar].
4. Kursa M.B. and Rudnicki W.R., Feature selection with the Boruta package. J Stat Softw, 2010.36(11): p.1-13. [Google Scholar].
5. Chen, T. and C. Guestrin Xgboost: A scalable tree boosting system in Proceedings of the 22nd ACM sigkdd international conference on knowledge discovery and data mining,2016.
6. Banda J.M., et al., Finding missed cases of familial hypercholesterolemia in health systems using machine learning. NPJ digital medicine, 2019. 2(1): p. 1–8. pmid:31304370 View Article PubMed/NCBI Google Scholar
7. Nithya B. and Ilango V. Predictive analytics in health care using machine learning tools and techniques. in 2017 International Conference on Intelligent Computing and Control Systems (ICICCS). 2017. IEEE.
8. Byeon H., Is the random forest algorithm suitable for predicting Parkinson's disease with mild cognitive impairment out of Parkinson's disease with normal cognition? International journal of environmental research and public health, 2020. 17(7): p. 2594. pmid:32290134 View Article PubMed/NCBI Google Scholar
9. Pekkala T., et al., Development of a late-life dementia prediction index with supervised machine learning in the population-based CAIDE study. Journal of Alzheimer's Disease, 2017. 55(3): p. 1055–1067. pmid:27802228 View Article PubMed/NCBI Google Scholar

10. Olson, R.S., et al. Evaluation of a tree-based pipeline optimization tool for automating data science. in Proceedings of the genetic and Evolutionary Computation Conference 2016. 2016.

11. Zou Q., et al., Finding the best classification threshold in imbalanced classification. Big Data Research, 2016. 5: p. 2–8. View Article Google Scholar

12. Kharya S. and Soni S., Weighted naive Bayes classifier: a predictive model for breast cancer detection. International Journal of Computer Applications, 2016. 133(9): p. 32–37. View Article Google Scholar

13. Japkowicz N. Learning from imbalanced data sets: a comparison of various strategies. in AAAI workshop on learning from imbalanced data sets. 2000. AAAI Press Menlo Park, CA. https://doi.org/10.1162/089976600300015691 pmid:10769321

14. He H. and Ma Y., Imbalanced learning: foundations, algorithms, and applications. 2013: Wiley-IEEE Press.

Emerging Trends in IoT and Computing Technologies – Suman Lata Tripathi et al. (eds)
© 2024 Taylor & Francis Group, London, ISBN 978-1-032-87924-6

Raspberry Pi-Based Smart Surveillance System

64

Himanshu Gupta[1], Vidhisha Kachawaha[2], Mahi Tyagi[3], Pragya Pandey[4]

ABES Institute of Technology, Ghaziabad, India

Abstract: In the modern era, there is a dire need for an Integrated Motion Detection and Fire Detection System to create a robust and intelligent security infrastructure that can address a wide range of potential threats. However, most of the available system depends upon only one type of sensor which limit their uses to secure life and property efficiently. To address this, the present work proposes to integrate Motion Detection with Fire Detection System for enhancing the security in home, industries, etc. For this purpose, firstly, the motions have been detected by PIR sensor which triggers the camera through Raspberry Pi. Further, the fire detection system based on flame sensor also triggers the camera. The acquired images have been uploaded to the server to have a more comprehensive understanding of the situation. Therefore, the data fusion from motion and fire detection enables an automated response based on the detected threat, which enhance the efficiency of the overall security system.

Keywords: Flame sensor, PIR sensor, Raspberry Pi, Relay module, Water sprinkler

1. Introduction

In the past decade, the world has witnessed an exponential rise in the use of Internet of Things (IoT). These devices has the capability to complete the given task without much human intervention. Therefore, the IoT devices not only becomes an essential part of life but also plays an important role in easing human's life and taken the automation to new horizons. Further, the IoT devices had proven their dominance in several security and surveillance tasks, such as protecting assets, burglar deterrence, remote monitoring and control, emergency response, etc. [1]. Amongst such tasks, motion detection and detection of fire has been considered as one of the major threats to both industry and home as they may lead to several collateral damage. For example, according to the report published by National Crime Records Bureau, Govt. of India, India has already witnessed more than 2.0 million fire incidents of various scales in between 2019 and 2022 which causes more than 28,000 casualties. Further, more than 50% of the fatalities occurred due to fire incidents in residential buildings [2]. Also, because of the significant rise in working population a large number of residential houses remain unattended for a larger duration in a day, especially in metropolitan cities which makes them susceptible to several unlawful activities.

This work revolves around the need for a unified and intelligent security and fire safety system that can effectively detect motion, capture objects of interest, identify fire hazards, and initiate automatic prevention measures. Traditional security and fire detection systems often function in isolation, lacking the integration required for a comprehensive and proactive approach to safety and security. Furthermore, the reliance on manual intervention in the event of intrusions or fire incidents can lead to delayed responses and increased risks to property and lives.

[1]guptah.nitj@gmail.com, [2]vidhisha2020csiot030@abesit.edu.in, [3]mahi2020csiot001@abesit.edu.in, [4]pragya.pandey@abesit.edu.in

DOI: 10.1201/9781003535423-64

In light of the above discussion, the main objectives of the present proposed work may be summarized as:

1. To explore the existing approaches for home surveillance and security system.
2. To analyse the main limitations of the reported literature.
3. To propose a more efficient methodology for integrated surveillance and security by employing Raspberry Pi, PIR sensor, computer vision, and flame sensor.

2. Literature Review

The development of integrated security system is a challenging task because it should be able to both detect and mitigate the threats. However, most of the existing literature focuses only on one technology which makes them inefficient in the modern era. For example, in [3], only motion has been detected in any mechanical or electrical device. In [4], only fire has been detected using smoke sensor. In [5], movements of intruder has been detected by employing Raspberry pi and PIR sensor. Further, in [6], a combination of PIR sensor and Light Emitting Diode (LED) has been used for motion detection. Meanwhile, in [7], star topology based approach has been used to detect the intruders and provide alert via e-mail. Similarly, in [8], the number of people in the house has been detected by employing infrared sensor. Also, in [9], an approach for detection of fire and providing alert has been discussed, whereas in [10] a voice-operated system has been developed for fire prevention. Further, the comparative analysis of the reviewed literature has been presented in Table 64.1, which discloses that both motion and fire detection has been exhaustively explored but to the best of authors knowledge the integrated fire and motion detection framework has been seldom investigated. Also, since the security threats may be occurred due to multiple factors. Therefore, all these factors should be integrated into a single system for the development of smart surveillance system.

Table 64.1 Comparative analysis of reported literature

Authors	Scope	Technology	Limitations
Siri et al. [3]	Motion detection	Raspberry Pi, PIR sensor, Raspberry Camera	No alert and fire detection system
Takale et al. [4]	Fire detection	Smoke sensor, LED	Limited performance, no alert system
Azhar et al. [5]	Motion detection	PIR sensor, Raspberry Pi	No fire detection system
Markapuri [6]	Motion detection	Raspberry Pi, PIR sensor, LED	No fire detection system
Deo et al. [7]	Motion detection	PIR sensor, alerting system, Human Detection	No fire detection system
Prasad et al. [8]	Motion detection	USB camera, Raspberry Pi	No fire detection system
Annapoorna et al. [9]	Fire detection	Raspberry Pi, Gas sensor, PIR sensor	No intruder detection system
Kumari et al. [10]	Fire detection	8051 Microcontroller	No intruder detection system

3. Methodology

The prime aim of this work is to address the above-mentioned shortcomings by developing a Raspberry Pi-based solution that seamlessly integrates motion detection, fire detection, and automatic prevention mechanisms. Further, the system should also be able to capture and detect potential threats as per the requirement. This makes the designing more complex because now the system has to take swift and automated actions to mitigate potential threats, thereby offering a more efficient and effective safety and security approach. Therefore, in the present work an integrated yet simple approach has been proposed as illustrated by Fig. 64.1.

The system revolves around a Raspberry Pi which serve as the central processing unit, connected to a camera module for capturing images or videos triggered by a motion sensor. Additionally, it interfaces with a fire sensor for basic fire detection. The system also activates activate a relay module that activates the water sprinkler as a basic form of automatic prevention. Further, on the detection of motion or high temperature fire, the system triggers alerts via email, SMS, or notifications. This architecture prioritizes simplicity by excluding complex algorithms for object recognition or sophisticated fire detection, aiming to create a basic yet functional system for an integrated motion and fire detection with alert notification.

4. System Specification

The hardware specifications of the developed system has been presented in Table 64.2. The present work considers Raspberry Pi 4B model due to its enhanced versatility, connectivity, and performance over its other models. Further, a Raspberry Pi camera, PIR and Flame sensors have also been utilized for the development of the system.

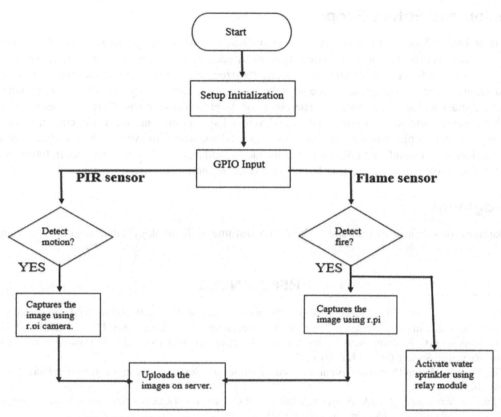

Fig. 64.1 System flow diagram for proposed integrated system

Table 64.2 System specification

S. No.	Component	Details	Image
1	Raspberry Pi	4B, 4GB RAM	
2	Raspberry Pi camera	5 mega pixel with 1080 pixel resolution	
3	PIR sensor	Sensitivity up to 20 feet	
4	Flame sensor	Sensitivity up to 100 cm, and 760 to 1100nm	

5. Conclusion and Future Scope

The present work proposed a Raspberry Pi based integrated motion and fire detection system with a provision for alert notification as a comprehensive and intelligent security and safety system. By seamlessly integrating motion detection and object capture, the system provides a robust first line of defence against unauthorized access. Furthermore, the incorporation of fire detection capabilities and automatic prevention mechanisms equips the system to respond swiftly and effectively to potential fire hazards, reducing property damage and safeguarding lives. Therefore, the developed system has offered a wide range of functionalities that enhances both security and safety. Furthermore, the developed system not only meets the current demands for security and safety but also provides a platform for ongoing innovation and adaptation to evolving needs in an ever-changing world which may be considered as a significant milestone in real-time surveillance and hazard detection. In future, the work shall be extended by integrating more features and a user friendly interface to improve the user experience.

Acknowledgment

The authors like to express their deep gratitude to the ABES Institute of Technology, Ghaziabad for providing the necessary resources.

REFERENCES

1. Parul Jindal, Himanshu Gupta, Nikhil Pachauri, Varun Sharma, Om Prakash Verma. Real-time Wildfire Detection via Image-based Deep Learning Algorithm. In Soft Computing: Theories and Applications: Proceedings of SoCTA 2020 (2021), 539-550.
2. Glorita S. Fernandes, Dr. C. F. Mulimani. A Review Study on Types of Fire Accidents and their Management in India: 2014 to 2018. Annals of the Romanian Society for Cell Biology (2021).
3. Pannaga Siri, Ganesh. Motion Detection System for Security Using IoT- Survey. International Research Journal of Engineering and Technology (2022).
4. Kumar B. Takale, Shubham N. Chopade, Ankita S. Sonawane, P. C. Patil. Fire Detection And Alarm System. International Journal of Advance Research and Innovative Ideas in Education (2022).
5. Amir Hifzan Azhar, Mohd Fairuz Iskandar Othman, Nazrulazhar Bahaman, Mohd Zaki Mas'ud, Zurina Sa 'aya. Implementation of Home Security Motion Detector using Raspberry Pi and PIR Sensor. Journal of Advanced Computing Technology and Application (2021).
6. Venkat Markapuri. Smart Motion Detection System using Raspberry Pi. ResearchGate (2020).
7. Kunal Deo, Rishi Deedwania, Swati Bairagi. Human Intrusion and Motion Detection System. International Journal of Computer Applications (2020).
8. Sanjana Prasad, P. Mahalakshmi, A. John Clement Sunder, R. Swathi. Smart Surveillance Monitoring System using Raspberry Pi and PIR Sensor. International Journal of Computer Science and Information Technologies (2014).
9. Annapoorna C. G., Shreya K., Vinayak Nase, Prashanth Kumar S, C. Sivaprakash. Raspberry Pi-Based Industrial Security Surveillance System using IOT. Journal of Emerging Technologies and Innovative Research (2019).
10. Meena Kumari, S. Shimi. Voice Operated Intelligent Fire Extinguisher Vehicle with Water Jet Spray. International Journal of Emerging Engineering Research and Technology (2017).

Emerging Trends in IoT and Computing Technologies – Suman Lata Tripathi et al. (eds)
© 2024 Taylor & Francis Group, London, ISBN 978-1-032-87924-6

Survey on IoT Solutions for Railway Coal Wagon Load Optimization

65

Upasana Pandey[1]

ABES Institute of Technology,
Department of Computer Science & Engineering (AI & IOT) Ghaziabad, India

**Meena Kumari[2], Mansi Varshney[3],
Maanav Mahajan[4], Raksha Awasthi[5]**

ABES Institute of Technology,
Department of Computer Science & Engineering (IOT) Ghaziabad, India

Abstract: Coal India Limited (CIL) uses railway wagons to deliver coal to customers. Train wagons are often overloaded or underloaded by the payloader that CIL uses to load the coal that is supplied by rail to customers. According to railway regulations, the buyer is responsible for paying the penalty for overloading. The buyer is liable for any overloading fines issued by the railway for any shipment. In underloading wagons, credits for idle freight are applied to coal bills, resulting in expensive expenditures. Overloading railroad wagons can lead to major accidents and damage to both the contents and the wagon itself. Underloading railroad wagons could result in fewer items being transported than the wagon's carrying capability. Due to overloading and underloading, the railways are compensated annually with billions of rupees. In this survey study, we are contrasting comparable systems that can be applied to stop railroad wagons from overloading or underloading.

Keywords: Internet of things (IoT), Load cell, Weigh-in-motion (WIM), Coal indian limited (CIL)

1. Introduction

The railway sector is essential to the world's transportation network because it makes it easier for people and products to move around. The handling of freight, which frequently entails the movement of commodities on wagons, is a crucial component of railway operations. It is crucial to make sure that these railroad carriages are loaded as efficiently as possible to avoid overloading and underloading, which can result in operational inefficiencies, wear and tear on the infrastructure, and safety risks. Overloading and underloading of railway wagons by coal are major issues for the Ministry of Coal. Coal has been delivered by rail via railway sidings to CIL's customers. At these sidings, payloaders load the railroad wagons under contract. Railway wagons are frequently overloaded or underloaded by payloaders. Railways notify people about the penalties for both underloading and overloading. Each year, billions of rupees are paid to the railways as compensation for overloading and underloading. The agreement for wagon loading was only for Rs. 276 Cr, whereas under-loading costs around Rs. 593 Cr in 2021–2022. The incorporation of Internet of Things (IoT) technology has become a disruptive force in a number of industries in recent years, providing creative ways to improve overall performance, safety, and efficiency. With an emphasis on creating intelligent systems that can stop train carriages from being overloaded or underloaded, the use of the Internet of Things (IoT) in the railway industry has attracted a lot of interest. This survey study aims to provide a comprehensive review of Internet of Things-based solutions designed to prevent railway wagon systems from becoming under or overloaded. Through a review of

[1]coe.upasana@gmail.com, [2]meena.kumari@abesit.edu.in, [3]mansigupta94124@gmail.com, [4]maanavmahajan928@gmail.com, [5]awasthiraksha5@gmail.com

DOI: 10.1201/9781003535423-65

the literature and technological developments in this field, we want to pinpoint important patterns, obstacles, and chances that support the creation of reliable and astute freight management systems for the railway industry.

1.1 Challenges in Railway Wagon Loading

Loading railway wagons requires a complex process of weight distribution balance to guarantee both safety and best performance. Railway operators face serious difficulties as a result of overloading and underloading, which can result in mishaps, higher maintenance expenses, and reduced operational effectiveness. Due to the high wear and tear on the rails and equipment, overloaded wagons endanger both the safety of the cargo and the rail system. Conversely, underloaded carriages cause railway businesses to employ resources inefficiently and earn less money. These difficulties call for the creation of sophisticated monitoring and control systems, which is where Internet of Things technology is useful.

1.2 IOT-Based Solutions for Overloading and Underloading Prevention

This section goes into great detail about the IoT-based solutions that are now in use to stop railroad wagons from being overloaded or underloaded. This includes an explanation of the data analytics techniques, communication protocols, and sensor technologies used in these systems. The usefulness of IoT in resolving the issues related to railway wagon loading will be demonstrated through case studies and practical applications. This proactive strategy guarantees regulatory compliance, improves safety, and prevents damage to the road.

2. Literature Survey

In [1], To avoid corruption, assess taxes according to the amount of traffic at toll booths, and shield vehicles, products, and roads from harm, an overload detection system has been developed. They use various devices - Load Cell, HX711 Load Cell amplifier Module, PIC Microcontroller, Crystal Oscillator, Capacitors, Ceramic Capacitor, Resistors, Transistors, Buzzers, Diodes, and LED. System output is provided by a buzzer and LED. The buzzer will sound one beep, and the green LED will illuminate if the weight of the load exceeds one kilogram. This demonstrates that the vehicle is functioning under the necessary load conditions. If the load is 2 kg or higher, the buzzer beeps twice, and the YELLOW LED lights. This indicates that the truck is almost at its overloaded point. If the load is three kilograms or higher, the buzzer beeps three times, and the red LED flashes. Here, the word "OVERLOADING CONDITION" appears.

In [2], Produce and manage fines and design a practical, efficient system for the Regional Transport Office division. The count of passengers arriving and leaving has been provided by the suggested system, making it a workable and effective method in any department of the Regional Transport Office. The Node MCU model was utilized by the IOT system in the suggested system to ensure the system operated efficiently.

In [3], it has developed a tool to address the problem of truck overloading, assisting in the reduction of road damage and accident prevention. A load cell, an amplifier, an ADC, a microcontroller, an LCD, and a Wi-Fi device with the plate number ESP8266 are all included in the design of this system. The weight of an object is detected by the load cell without physical touch. The amplifier receives the detected value and uses an electronic integrated circuit (ADC) to transform the tiny quantity of energy into an analog-to-digital signal. It automatically shuts off the fuel and transmits information to the Android application when the load cell value rises.

In [4], this project addresses the longstanding issue of auto overloading, recognizing its adverse impacts on road safety, accidents, and environmental concerns. By focusing on overload management for heavy vehicles using a spring-based system, the research aims to detect and limit maximum payload capacity, contributing to enhanced engine performance, reduced fuel consumption, and improved overall road safety in the context of serious vehicle overloading. The study draws attention to the link between overloading and increased fuel consumption, emphasizing the economic and environmental consequences. This underscores the importance of developing load management systems to optimize fuel efficiency.

In [5], The goal of this study is to stop overloading from causing damage to cars, which can result in poor fuel efficiency, steering and suspension problems, brake problems, instability, and damage to infrastructure. It makes use of weigh-in-motion (WIM) technology. WIM systems do not account for overload or incorrect loading; they just measure the vehicle's weight. It uses a Load Cell, HX711 ADC, Arduino Uno, DC Motor, Liquid Crystal Display, and Buzzer. This device compares the allowable weight to the actual load using a load sensor mounted underneath the vehicle. After that, the Arduino microcontroller receives the output. The microprocessor signals the vehicle's ignition system to start the engine if the load is within the specified limit.

In [6], Using Arduino programming software and simulation tools, the logical model was successfully tested and validated. The system uses a GSM SIM900D module as a communication link to automatically summon the vehicle's owner in case of an overload. With so few weighing stations in Ghana, some drivers of vehicles are unable to reach axle measuring sites to measure the load their cars carry. This is the problem that the proposed vehicle load monitoring system aims to solve. The engine lock system may be able to stop both accidents and vehicle faults. This might take the place of current technology, which requires drivers to wait hours at weighing stations for the weighing sensors buried in concrete roadways to detect the gross weight of their vehicles.

In [7], Implementing an overload protection system can help increase mass regulation compliance. It might contribute to the more effective and efficient use of roads by lowering the number of overburdened trucks. Reducing the number of heavy trucks can also help lower crash rates and prevent major injury to humans and possessions. The enforcement of heavy vehicle and traffic regulations is anticipated to see new uses for these systems. This technology makes it simple and convenient to determine the vehicle load, which helps to effectively address the issue of vehicle overloading.

In [8], the Study emphasizes how the Internet of Things might help the transportation sector deal with overcrowding problems. The system suggests using Wi-Fi weight sensors in order to identify overloading, send out alerts, and, in the case that the alerts are disregarded, send vehicle data to checkpoints in order to avert possible collisions. The goal is to improve road safety and enforce legislation in an orderly and transparent manner.

In [9], This project addresses the economic challenges associated with rising fuel prices by emphasizing the importance of good mileage in both affordable and luxurious vehicles. It introduces an innovative overload and over-seat prevention system, integrated into the seat and shock absorber, aiming to enhance vehicle mileage and safety performance by indicating instances of overloading, ensuring efficient transportation for all. The research introduces a novel approach by proposing an overload and over-seat prevention system integrated into the seat and shock absorber. This innovative design aims to enhance both mileage and safety performance. The project emphasizes a dual objective of improving both vehicle mileage and safety performance. This holistic approach recognizes the interconnectedness of these factors in ensuring efficient and secure transportation.

In [10], Implementing an overload protection system can help increase mass regulation compliance. It might contribute to the more effective and efficient use of roads by lowering the number of overburdened trucks. Less overloading of trucks contributes to fewer collisions and severe harm to people's lives and property. It is anticipated that these devices will find new uses in the enforcement of heavy vehicle and traffic regulations.

Table 65.1 Devices find new uses in the enforcement of heavy vehicle and traffic regulations

S.no.	Year	Summary	Used Device	Future Scope
[1]	2023	To avoid taxes depending on traffic volume, an overload-detecting system has been devised. For loads above 1 kg, there is a single beep sound and green LED lights; for loads over 2 kg, there are two beep sounds and yellow LED lights; and for loads over 3 kg, there are three beep sounds, red LED lights, and the LCD message "OVERLOADING CONDITION."	Load Cell, HX711 Load Cell amplifier Module, PIC Microcontroller, Crystal Oscillator, Capacitors, Ceramic Capacitor, Resistors, Transistor, Buzzer, Diodes, LED.	Improve load cell behaviour, optimize toll computation beyond the length of the road, and investigate sophisticated load state indicators.
[2]	2023	The suggested technique has provided the count of passengers arriving and departing, making it a practical and efficient method in any department of the Regional Transport Office. To make sure the system ran well, the Node MCU model was applied.	Node MCU model.	Subsequent advancements may encompass the incorporation of cutting-edge technologies, instantaneous monitoring, intuitive user interfaces, and cooperation with relevant parties.
[3]	2021	Created an instrument to tackle the issue of trucks being overloaded. A load cell measures an object's weight. Upon a rising load cell value, it automatically cuts fuel and sends data to the Android application.	Load Cell, Amplifier, ADC, Control Unit, Microcontroller, ESP8266 Wi-Fi Module, LCD, Solenoid Valve, Fuel Tank.	Include more IoT features for remote monitoring, provide owners with better warnings, and investigate data analytics for decision-making and system improvement.
[4]	2021	The paper emphasizes that exceeding the permissible weight of a vehicle is not only a safety concern but also an illegal offense, highlighting the need for robust systems to prevent and penalize overloading. This aspect underscores the urgency of developing effective solutions to manage and limit vehicle loads.	Frame, Battery, Spring, Kill Switch.	Research gap in the development and analysis of spring-based mechanisms for detecting and limiting maximum payload capacity, essential for mitigating engine performance issues and reducing fuel consumption in heavy vehicles.

S.no.	Year	Summary	Used Device	Future Scope
[5]	2020	It makes use of Weigh-in-motion (WIM) technology, which only weighs the car. The load cell installed beneath the vehicle is used to measure the vehicle's load, which is compared to the permitted load by this system. Then, if the load is within the designated limit, Arduino tells the car's ignition system to start the engine.	Load Cell, HX711 ADC, Arduino Uno, DC Motor, Liquid Crystal Display, Buzzer.	Most vehicle manufacturers now offer affordable on-board weighing systems using APT sensors.
[6]	2020	With so few weighing stations in Ghana, some drivers of vehicles are unable to reach axle weighing stations to weigh the load their cars carry. This is the problem that the proposed vehicle load monitoring system aims to solve.	GSM Module SIM 900D, ATMEGA 328, LCD, Keypad, Load Sensor, Buzzer, Voltage Regulator.	Further research is needed to assess its real-world performance, user acceptance, legal implications, and scalability, ensuring a comprehensive and effective implementation.
[7]	2019	It is envisaged that these systems will find new applications in the enforcement of traffic and heavy vehicle rules. This technology makes it simple and convenient to determine the vehicle load, which helps to effectively address the issue of vehicle overloading.	Raspberry Pi, HX711 Load cell, Lcd, ATMEGA328, ESP8266, Load cell, Ubidots cloud.	While the integration of vehicle load control systems holds promise for enhancing transport safety and efficiency, further research is needed to optimize the accuracy and reliability of load detection mechanisms.
[8]	2019	To stop serious mishaps, the suggested system monitors overload and issues alerts. Wi-Fi weight sensors are used to identify overloading. The data that is gathered is compared with database data that corresponds to likely overloading paths, and if the warning is disregarded, it will contact the appropriate authorities.	Wi-Fi weight sensors.	Enhance sensor technology, combine cutting-edge analytics, standardize globally, work with smart infrastructure, and boost energy efficiency.
[9]	2018	One notable feature of the proposed system is its integration into the seat and shock absorber, requiring no additional space. This compact design is practical and aligns with the convenience of users.	Pedestal Bearing, Gear Motor, Motor Pulley, Shaft Pulley, Belt, Coil Springs, Transformer, timer, Buzzer indicator.	Further exploration is needed to bridge this gap and provide comprehensive insights into the practical application and impact of these innovations in addressing fuel efficiency and safety concerns.
[10]	2017	As fewer trucks are overloaded, it could lead to a more effective and efficient use of the roadways. Reduced truck overloading lowers the risk of crashes and serious injury to people and property.	Load cell, microcontroller, Led.	Develop cost-effective and universally applicable technologies that can accurately measure and limit vehicle loads across diverse transportation scenarios.

3. Conclusion

Implementing an overload protection system can help increase mass regulation compliance. It might contribute to the more effective and efficient use of roads by lowering the number of overburdened trucks. Less overloading of trains contributes to fewer collisions and severe harm to people's lives and property. It is anticipated that these devices will find new uses in the enforcement of heavy vehicle and traffic regulations. As a result, these approaches make it easy to determine vehicle load and efficiently address the issue of vehicle overloading. Vehicle load monitoring systems have been created to address the problem of some drivers of vehicles being unable to access axle measuring stations to measure the load their vehicles carry due to a lack of weighing stations.

4. Future Scope

The many methods of overload detection in this survey can also be applied to the detection of overload in railroads. This technique also solves the Ministry of Coal's primary issue, which is that the buyer bears responsibility for any overloading fines assessed by the Railway for any consignment. Additionally, when wagons are underloaded, credits for idle freight are applied to coal bills, resulting in costly expenditures. It is possible to create a cheap system. The railways receive billions of rupees in compensation every year due to overloading and underloading. An IoT system may be created to reduce these costs; however, weighing each wagon individually is not the best way. So that when JCB loads the coal into the wagon, we can measure it. A load cell can be used to measure the coal. When the wagon's load capacity is reached, the microcontroller can stop the JCB, sound an alert, and display a message on the LCD. The logs can also be accessed on systems and uploaded to the cloud.

REFERENCES

1. A.G. M. S. S. R. C. S. K. R. P. R. K. Roshni Ram*1, "OVERLOAD DETECTION SYSTEM USING STRAIN GAUGE LOAD CELL," in IRJMETS, 2023.

2. A. N. A. R. N. M. S. H. Bharati Masram, IoT-based Overload Detection System in Public Transportation Vehicles, IEEE, 2023.

3. A. J. S. M. D. N. S. S. K. S. r. P. Leon Dharmadurai, "AVOID OVERLOADING IN TRUCK USING IOT WITH FUEL CUTOFF," in IARJSET, 2021.

4. K. S. J. G. M. G. S. S. D. Sivakumar G, Vehicle Overload Management System, ResearchGate, 2021.

5. S. M. T. S. S. G. P. S. Neeli Sreekeerthan1, "Arduino based Vehicle Overload Detection and Prevention System," in IRJET, 2020.

6. E. N. Odonkor+, "Design and Construction of Vehicle Loading Monitoring System Using Load Sensor and GSM," in International Journal of Applied Science and Technology, 2020.

7. D. R. M. Mr. Shardul Singh Gurjar, "Vehicle Overloading Detection and Protection using Raspberry Pi and IOT Application," in IJIRSET, 2019.

8. A. C. a. U. S. H. Shekhar, Vehicle Overloading Alert using IoT, IEEE, 2019.

9. R. A. P. A. S. J. D. H. S. Nikhil R. Binnar, Design, and Fabrication of Overload and Over Seat Prevention System in Two Wheelers, IJSR, 2018.

10. M. N. R.,. N. B. ,. S. M. V. S. H. D. Kattimani, Vehicular Overload Detection and Protection, IJLRET, 2017.

Emerging Trends in IoT and Computing Technologies – Suman Lata Tripathi et al. (eds)
© 2024 Taylor & Francis Group, London, ISBN 978-1-032-87924-6

Analysis DDoS Attacks in Cloud Environment and Its Impact on Indian IT Industry

66

Himanshu Shukla[1]
Research Scholar, AIIT,
Amity University Uttar Pradesh, Lucknow, India

Ajay Pratap[2]
AP-III, AIIT, Amity University Uttar Pradesh, Lucknow, India

Harsh Dev[3]
Professor- DCS, Babu Banarasi Das University, Lucknow, India

Abstract: The internet has changed how important contemporary services including online platform, transaction control, energy sector, healthcare, and defense are managed. These processes are changed by. less expensive, efficacious web-delivered solutions. Everything is a result of the Internet's rapid development and enormous popularity. Unfortunately, as the Internet has expanded, the number of cyberattacks has also skyrocketed. One of them, the denial-of-service attack, poses a serious danger to availability. Internet accessibility is essential for the socioeconomic development of society because the world is so dependent on it. DDoS attacks occur almost daily, one and the other incidence and digit are continuously increasing. Finding the details of such attacks is one of the largest hurdles facing academics because most the reputational risks of revealing such attacks prevent commercial sites from revealing they have been attacked. Attack details might be a great help in developing a thorough defense strategy against them. Along with some of the most recent events that had an impact on internet enterprises, the primary reasons of distributed denial-of-service assaults are covered in depth. Finally, the necessity of an emphasis is placed on a comprehensive distributed solution.

Keywords: Cloud Environment, Botnet, DDoS incidents, Vulnerability, IT Industry

1. Introduction

Attacks using DDoS frequently intention on the Internet. Likewise, Information Security (IS) professionals have created comparable defenses as a result of the size and frequency of DDoS attacks [1]. The attackers' attempt to modify their DDoS methodologies in order to circumvent the current IS measures, however, make the field susceptible to persistently altering tactics. As a result, a complicated security ecosystem has been established as a result of the introduction and implementation of new attack and defense tactics, making it difficult to choose the best remedy for a certain DDoS attacks occurrence the size of the issue further discourages the necessary analysis of DDoS typologies [2]. Distributed Denial of Service (DDoS) attacks represent a significant threat to the digital infrastructure of organizations in India [3], [4]. In recent years, Indian organizations across various sectors have become prime targets for DDoS attacks. The motives behind these assaults vary, ranging from financial extortion to competitive rivalry or ideological conflicts[5]. The impact of DDoS attacks on Indian entities can be severe, causing substantial financial losses, damaging reputations, and leading to prolonged service downtime [6]. Critical

[1]himanshushukla19@gmail.com, [2]apratap@lko.amity.edu, [3]drharshdev@gmail.com

DOI: 10.1201/9781003535423-66

sectors such as banking and finance, e-commerce, government services, healthcare, and educational institutions face heightened risks due to their reliance on uninterrupted online operations.

2. Survey of DDoS Cases

DDoS attacks succeed in diverting the target's IT infrastructure from its intended uses, causing unheard-of downtimes and service outages.

2.1 Process of Registration

Cyber security specialists said the most commonly reported attack in the healthcare sector, which increased during the epidemic, was the release or sale of databases on the Dark Web. AIIMS, New Delhi, is still working to restore its systems after a significant ransom ware attack. One of India's biggest hospitals, AIIMS Delhi, was recently subjected to a DDoS attack that compromised the data of roughly 3–4 crore people, including private information and VIPs' medical records. The outpatient department (OPD) and sample collection were both impacted by the hackers' hacking of the e-hospital service, which controls the patient data system [7].

The protection of patient data as well as the security of e-hospital services has come under intense scrutiny as a result of this hack. Government and healthcare organizations have been cautioned by cyber-security experts to take the appropriate precautions to protect the security of such sensitive data [8], [9]. They advised firms to follow HIPAA compliance guidelines, educate users about cyber-attacks, online fraud, and phishing schemes, establish standards for safe passwords, and activate MFA. Also, businesses should regularly patch their networks, systems, and software, monitor logs for any unusual traffic and activity on their websites and other apps, and refrain from clicking on any links or emails that seem fishy [10].

2.2 Components that Make DDoS Assaults More Likely to Happen

Several components can make Distributed Denial of Service (DDoS) assaults more likely to occur:

The capacity to avoid being recognized: By spoofing IP addresses, attackers are able to avoid having their identities revealed. When the DDoS attack is over, the factor serves as both a protection tool for the attacker and a help to the real attack.

The development of different security measures influences the Web with changed degrees of assurance from DDoS assaults due to the need of an uniform Web security methodology. The nonattendance of a single association to implement best hones over the associated systems makes a shortcoming that DDoS aggressors might utilize to their advantage.

Unbalanced distribution of network resources: Small networks are typically connected to bigger networks by infrastructure with a higher bandwidth. This usefulness permits us to "surge" less clever targets through the tall capacity framework.

The limited nature of network resources: DDoS attacks can prevent users from accessing services they are entitled to since target networks have a limit that fulfils their needs.

3. Framework for DDoS Attacks

One of the more advanced assaults within the cloud computing environment that lower organize execution and throughput is the zombie/botnet assault. There are awfully hubs that connect the connected clients as a zombie or botnet. A framework that has been introduced with a program that, without the framework user's information, places it beneath the control of awfully clients. Clients that are insolent utilize Zombie to dispatch Man within the Center Assaults or DDoS assaults that cause Dissent of Benefit (DoS). The zombie gets commands from the unapproved client through an open communication harbour. We can easily understand architecture of DDoS attacks (see Fig. 66.1)

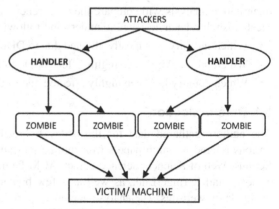

Fig. 66.1 DDoS attack on machine

4. Activities of DDoS Attacks

Assault communities have a parcel of potential since they work well together in terms of coordination and adjust. In arrange to maintain a strategic distance from discovery, malevolent assailants who utilize conveyed denial-of-service attacks utilize the leading effort method. They utilize conveyed activity to form a botnet and immerse victim-targeting parcels with it. This makes it challenging to spot the trespasser and permits the attacker to maintain a strategic distance from the sharp eye. As the attackers' control creates by using a few sources, the guards are confronting a noteworthy issue in concocting moderation and avoidance measures for disseminated denial-of-service assaults. The DDoS assaulting programs basic rationale structures and negligible memory necessities make them particularly straightforward to form and conceal.

The DDoS assaulting programs are especially simple to create and conceal due to their essential rationale structures and moo memory needs. Furthermore, there are various tools for DDoS ambushes that don't require a tall level of capability to utilize them. DDoS attacks have in this way ended up a well-known device for causing disturbance on the Web. Attack traffic from IP addresses registered in China surged by 29% year over year (YoY) and by 19% quarter over quarter, according to the research by digital infrastructure services company Cloudflare. India, which had a 61% year over year growth in HTTP-based DDoS attack traffic, came in second place to China.

Table 66.1   DDoS attack matrix

Attack Metric	Features
Rate Dynamics	Constant, variable
Targeted weakness	Brute force, semantic
Agent set persistence	Variable, constant
Automation attribute	Manual, semi-automatic, automatic
Validity of source address	Spoofed, valid
Intended effect on the victim	Degrading, disruptive
Characterization possibility	Characterizable, non-characterizable
Choice of victim	Infrastructure, resource, host, application, network

The United States and Brazil came after India, according to the research. DDoS assaults are made almost every day. It was able to infect even the most well-known websites, harming millions of its users, including Twitter, Facebook, Google, and others. Since 2017, there have been 7.9% more information breaches in India. Furthermore, the normal taken a toll per record of a information breach is rising to INR 4,552 ($64). India is presently the fourth most regularly focused on country within the world as a result of the development in cyber-attacks. Agreeing to a inquire about by India Now a day, Chennai saw the highest percentile of cyber-attacks within the to begin with quarter of 2019 with a measurement of 48%. Many industries distribute bytes at network –layer DDoS attacks.

5. Methodology

The study will primarily focus on quantitative analysis, with a secondary emphasis on qualitative comparative research. The quantitative analysis will compare the occurrence of attacks in terms of type of industry, type of protocol and country. So, a mechanism has been designed to understand following research questions:

* Which industry was mostly affected due to DDoS attacks in last three years?
* Which protocol has been highly affected due to DDoS attacks?
* Which country has been highly affected due to DDoS attacks in last three years?

5.1 Data Collection

The authors gathered data for this study by reading and analyzing various related research papers from online journal databases such as Scopus, Web of Science, Science Direct, ACM Digital Library, Google Scholar, and SpringerLink, as well as a few books and some content available on websites. The analysis includes approximately 25 research publications published between 2000 and May 2021 and following data has been collected.

Table 66.2   Industry-wise DDoS attack matrix

Type of Industry	Percentage
Finance	34 %
Telecommunication	26 %
Retail	17 %
Entertainment	12 %
Insurance	6 %
Education	3 %
Others	2 %

Table 66.3 DDoS attack on different types of protocols

Type of Industry	Percentage
HTTP/ HTTPS	78 %
TCP/ UDP	17 %
DNS	3 %
Others	2 %

Table 66.4 DDoS attack on different countries

Type of Industry	Percentage (Approx.)
USA	18.5 %
China	11 %
India	9.5 %
Russia	8.5 %
England	7.5 %
Germany	7 %
Other Countries	38 %

5.2 Data Processing

R programming language is widely used for data processing and analytics due to its robust statistical capabilities and extensive range of libraries designed for handling data. R offers various functions and packages to import data from different file formats such as CSV, Excel and here we have imported csv file in R for data processing and analytics.

```
data1 <- read.csv("D:\\RStudio\\Binning\\data1.csv", header=TRUE, stringsAsFactors=FALSE)
data2 <- read.csv("D:\\RStudio\\Binning\\data2.csv", header=TRUE, stringsAsFactors=FALSE)
barplot(data1, xlab = "Type of Industry", ylab = "Percentage")
barplot(data2, xlab = "Type of Protocol", ylab = "Percentage")
```

6. Result and Analysis

We have observed following points after completion of research methodology part, in which it has been pointed that:

- India has risen as the best goal for start of disseminated dissent of benefit (DDoS) cyber-attacks "it could be a reflection of India developing as a hotbed to dispatch these assaults, possibly since of the moo cyber security mindfulness, need of satisfactory security hones and infrastructure" agreeing to Symantec.
- Australia, Japan and India are the countries with the highest number of web application and API attacks in the region.
- According to a report by Akamai Technologies, the average cost of a DDoS attack for Indian companies is around INR 25 lakh per attack.
- The size of DDoS attacks is increasing, with some attacks exceeding 1 terabit per second (Tbps) in 2020. In 2016, the largest DDoS attack on record was 1.2 Tbps.
- The financial services sector is one of the most targeted industries for DDoS attacks, accounting for 23% of all attacks in Q4 2020, according to a report by cybersecurity firm Neustar.
- According to netscout Wired Broadcast communications Carriers, Information Preparing Facilitating and Related Administrations, Remote Broadcast communications Carriers (but adj.), All Other Broadcast communications, Electronic Shopping and Mail-Order Houses are the beat 5 focused on segment beneath assault.

Following observations has been drawn from result and discussion:

- Finance industry is highly affected due to DDoS attacks with 34 % and this percentage tends to increase in near future (see Fig. 66.2).

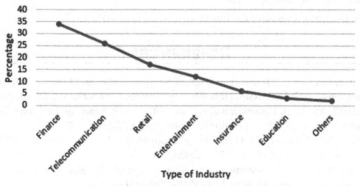

Fig. 66.2 DDoS attacks on industry

• HTTP/ HTTPS protocols were highly affected protocols that were targeted by DDoS attackers (see Fig. 66.3).

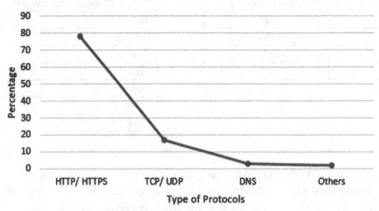

Fig. 66.3 DDoS attacks by protocols

• India is the third highly affected country from DDoS attacks in which percentage of financial frauds are on higher node (see Fig. 66.4).

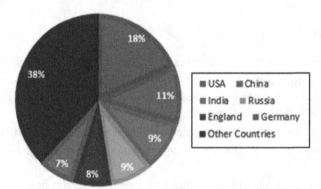

Fig. 66.4 Percentage of DDoS attacks by country

7. Conclusion

In This paper we have discussed the classification of DDoS assaults and its effect on Indian IT industry. The frequency of DDoS attack events is rising alarmingly. Attack volume, attack volume tactics, and botnet sizes are all rising daily. To stop and lessen these attacks, effective defence mechanisms are currently required.

• It gives a diagram of the DoS and DDoS issues.
• It briefly portrays the key security holes that permit for different attacks.
• A brief chronology of later DDoS events is given.
• Latest situation of DDoS assaults on Indian IT industry.

REFERENCES

1. Tang, D., & Kuang, X. (2019, October 1). Distributed Denial of Service Attacks and Defense Mechanisms. IOP Conference Series: Materials Science and Engineering, 612(5), 052046. https://doi.org/10.1088/1757-899x/612/5/052046
2. Kumar, S., & Singh, M. (2017, April 12). Detection and Isolation of Zombie Attack under Cloud Environment. Oriental Journal of Computer Science and Technology, 10(2), 338–344. https://doi.org/10.13005/ojcst/10.02.12
3. Arvindhan, M., & Ande, B. P. (2020, January 1). Data Mining Approach and Security over DDoS Attacks. ICTACT Journal on Soft Computing, 10(2), 2061–2065. https://doi.org/10.21917/ijsc.2020.0292.
4. Mirkovic, J., & Reiher, P. (2004, April). A taxonomy of DDoS attack and DDoS defense mechanisms. ACM SIGCOMM Computer Communication Review, 34(2), 39–53. https://doi.org/10.1145/997150.997156.

5. Douligeris, C., & Mitrokotsa, A. (2004, April). DDoS attacks and defense mechanisms: classification and state-of-the-art. Computer Networks, 44(5), 643–666. https://doi.org/10.1016/j.comnet.2003.10.003

6. Gupta, B. B., Joshi, R. C., & Misra, M. (2010). Distributed Denial of Service Prevention Techniques. International Journal of Computer and Electrical Engineering, 268–276. https://doi.org/10.7763/ijcee.2010.v2.148.

7. Chang, R. (2002, October). Defending against flooding-based distributed denial-of-service attacks: a tutorial. IEEE Communications Magazine, 40(10), 42–51. https://doi.org/10.1109/mcom.2002.1039856.

8. K, J. (2020, July 30). Analysis of 5G Networks for Heterogeneous Malicious Devices in DDoS Attacks. Journal of Advanced Research in Dynamical and Control Systems, 12(SP8), 916–921. https://doi.org/10.5373/jardcs/v12sp8/20202596.

Emerging Trends in IoT and Computing Technologies – Suman Lata Tripathi et al. (eds)
© *2024 Taylor & Francis Group, London, ISBN 978-1-032-87924-6*

Securing the Cloud Authentication Mechanism using Two-Factor Authentication

67

Vinay Yadav[1]

M Tech (CSE), DCS,
Bansal Institute of Eng. and Technology, Lucknow, India

Manish Kumar Soni[2]

Assistant Professor- DCS,
Bansal Institute of Eng. and Technology, Lucknow, India

Ajay Pratap[3]

AP-III, AIIT, Amity University Uttar Pradesh, Lucknow, India

Abstract: The development of technologies for cloud computing has revolutionized the landscape of Information Technology (IT). This innovation has enabled businesses to commence operations with minimal initial investments, leveraging IaaS, PaaS and SaaS as per their need. Cloud services offer quick provisioning and de-provisioning, requiring minimal effort and fostering a strong relationship between service providers (SP) and clients. However, despite these advantages, the cloud platform aces security vulnerabilities and potential attacks. Strengthening authentication procedures is crucial to prevent unauthorized access to Service Providers that forms the core requirement of security. To address these concerns, we propose a novel authentication scheme combining one-way hash method and two-factor authentication based on nonce using their identities, passwords and one-time passwords (OTP). The proposed scheme in this paper aims to counter brute force attacks, hijacking and replay attack within the cloud-environment.

Keywords: Cloud-environment, Security, Attacks, Authentication, Two-factor mechanism

1. Introduction

The evolving patterns in cloud computing present promising opportunities for expansion within the IT industry. Cloud computing epitomizes a framework designed to offer pervasive, at the time of demand, and the network access that is convenient to a shared pool of computing resources. However, ensuring security, confidentiality, and authenticity remains a paramount concern in the usage of cloud services [1]. Authentication stands as a cornerstone for maintaining security through distinct access control procedures, playing a pivotal role in affirming security across diverse applications [2]. Recent advancements in computing technologies have significantly bolstered security measures compared to those established a decade ago. While authentication mechanism based on password remains prevalent, it faces challenges due to simplistic or easily guessable passwords.

This challenge is exacerbated by various threats that could potentially exploit loopholes in the authentication process. Developing an infallible authentication method for the cloud necessitates a comprehensive understanding of authenticity-related attacks and the accompanying evasion techniques. Encryption serves as a prevalent security measure within cloud computing environments. Numerous protocols offer security against potential attackers, with the Password-Authenticated Key Exchange PAKE protocol

[1]vysvinay48@gmail.com, [2]manish.soni.csit@gmail.com, [3]apratap@lko.amity.edu

DOI: 10.1201/9781003535423-67

[3] being one such example. Finally, the work [4] gives a thorough set of twelve qualities organized in a systematic manner for fair examination and explicitly develops a security architecture that may effectively capture an adversary's enhanced accuracy.

2. Literature Survey

The conventional authentication methods are efficient for accessing remote server services, face limitations in cloud application that is due to the complexity related to the maintenance of smart cards [5]. For securing data access in the cloud, multifactor authentication, as observed that the method of authentication used in online banking, employs factors like username (Assigned by bank/User), password (Chosen by User), random number (Used for OTP or 2FA), and biometric inputs [6]. A conceptual basis for the two-factor verification technique combines password and biometric verification elements [7]. Out-of-band (OOB) authentication, described in a scheme [8], utilizes a three-step verification process. However, the time-consuming nature of this solution renders it less feasible within the cloud computing platform. Regarding multimodal identification methods, a combination of features of the iris, fingerprint, and palm print is proposed [9]. To balance security and accessibility, a secure key three-factor AKA protocol is proposed [10]. . Additionally, it proposes a framework for 2F authentication for clients linked to the cloud system, ensuring encrypted data access upon successful login to evade authentication-related vulnerabilities. Comparatively, this research differs from previous work [11] Conversely, asymmetric cryptosystems utilize a combination of public key and private keys, where the private key remains concealed while the public key is publicly disclosed, incorporating techniques such as Rivest-Shamir-Adleman (RSA) and Elliptic Curve Cryptosystem (ECC) [12]. While several types of data in a cloud environment remain unencrypted, the discovery of vulnerabilities. In [13] underscores privacy and security concerns, necessitating the implementation of a secured two-factor authentication based on nonce to combat authentication attacks.

3. Proposed Method for Secure Cloud Authentication

Our proposed model exhibits a modular structure, enabling individual analysis of each hazard and its corresponding response. This modular approach facilitates the effective management of the cloud. The registration phase and the login phase are the two separate stages of the suggested authentication mechanism.

3.1 Process of Registration

In this phase, Cloud users enroll themselves with the cloud server to access the provided services, involving three primary steps.

Step 1: The client registers on cloud by providing its details. The server validates these details and dispatches a mail and OTP on mobile number of client.

Step 2: After receiving valid OTPs, the client obtains a key from the server to facilitate secure communication and access other essential information such as a password.

Step 3: The client selects a password, services of choice, and duration, forwarding all the data using the shared server key with advanced security measures.

The server initially encrypts the subscription certificate using its private key. Following this, it encrypts the already encrypted subscription certificate utilizing the nonce received from the client. Concluding this process, the server dispatches a success message along with the doubly encrypted subscription certificate to the client.

3.2 Process of Authentication

The authentication procedure in cloud computing encompasses various stages aimed at verifying and allowing users access to cloud services. It typically involves user registration, validation, and establishing secure communication between the user and the cloud server. Here is an overview of the cloud authentication process:

User Registration: Users initiate the process by registering on the cloud server, providing essential details such as user ID, email, and contact number.

Validation: The server verifies the provided information, often by dispatching verification codes or OTPs (One-Time Passwords) to the user's registered email or mobile number.

Establishing Secure Communication: After successful validation, the server and client establish secure communication channels. This phase might involve generating and exchanging cryptographic keys or certificates.

Credential Storage: User credentials are securely stored on the server to maintain the confidentiality and integrity of sensitive information like passwords.

Certificate Creation: The server generates certificates containing vital user information, including subscription details and user ID. These certificates are encrypted to safeguard their content.

Certificate Delivery: Encrypted certificates are transmitted back to the user via secure channels for safekeeping and future use.

Final Authentication Confirmation: To confirm successful authentication, the server sends a success message to the client, often accompanied by doubly encrypted certificates or keys for subsequent communication.

The cloud authentication process is comprehensive, emphasizing data security, user identity verification, and the establishment of reliable communication channels between users and cloud servers to ensure secure access to cloud services.

4. Implementation of Authentication Process

In this section, we are discussing the implementation process of the first factor and second process.

4.1 First Factor Cloud Authentication

In phase-1, the user initiates the first level of authentication, prompting cloud platform to process the request. The provided details are authenticated against pre-registered records available on database server. Once successfully authenticated, a confirmation is sent.

$$\text{Encryption\_Msg} = \text{Encryption\_pk} \{H(ID) \| H(Pass)\}$$

The cloud server receives the encrypted message (Encryption_Msg), decrypts it initially, and subsequently verify the users for the provided digital signature.

4.2 Second Factor Cloud Authentication

If the verification of first step is successful, the cloud dispatches OTPs to both the registered email (OTP1) and mobile (OTP2), awaiting the commencement of the second authentication step. Subsequently, after the successful re-verification of the first factor, the cloud initiates a request for second-factor verification and sends one time password (OTP) to user for authentication. After successful completion of authentication, the user can access the services provided by cloud. Flowchart for 2FA is shown in Fig. 67.1.

5. Evaluation of Proposed Model

This research delves into the exploration, identification, and resolution of these attacks. It attempts to present a multifactor authentication protocol and framework that is extremely safe and robust and is intended for use with cloud computing networks. Difference between RSA versus ECC.

Elliptic Curve Cryptography (ECC) operates on the principle of using elliptic curves over finite fields as an encryption algorithm. This method resolves the Discrete Logarithm Problem (ECDLP) pertaining to elliptic curves. The ECC encryption process poses a formidable challenge to decryption due to the absence of a solutions known to the mathematical problem that is arising from the equation that generates the elliptic curve on a graph. Table 67.1 and Table 67.2 depict the comparison between RSA and ECC for various file sizes, while Fig. 67.2 and Fig. 67.3 present a graphical representation of their comparative analysis.

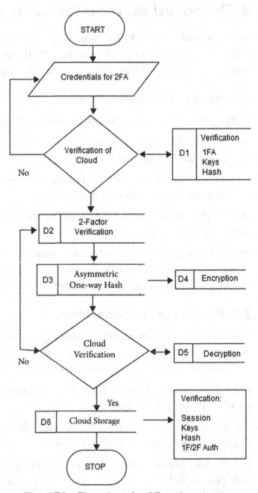

Fig. 67.1 Flowchart for 2F authentication

Table 67.1 Calculation for KeyGen, encryption and decryption time using RSA

Size of File (kb)	KeyGen Time (ms)	Encryption Time (ms)	Decryption Time (ms)	Total Time (In ms)
5	3114.31	153.55	1198.12	4470.52
10	3352.35	179.98	2460.04	6020.67
15	3998.9	202.5	3522.97	7735.32
20	4001.14	234.58	4910.98	9149.56
25	4008.54	269.98	6020.75	10299.09

Table 67.2 Calculation for KeyGen, encryption and decryption time using ECC

Size of File (kb)	KeyGen Time (ms)	Encryption Time (ms)	Decryption Time (ms)	Total Time (In ms)
5	130.95	31.96	0.73	168.01
10	132.53	32.49	1.02	169.01
15	134.7	33.54	1.86	169.85
20	138.05	34.98	2.223	175.52
25	137.01	40.01	4.56	181.11

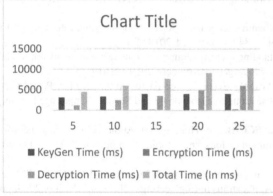

Fig. 67.2 Calculation for RSA

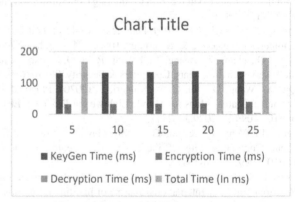

Fig. 67.3 Calculation for ECC

6. Result and Analysis

2FA scheme employing traditional IDs, passwords, and verification of OTP has been introduced to combat various types of attacks. The study in this paper compares two algorithmic approaches, Elliptic Curve Cryptography (ECC) and Rivest-Shamir-Adleman (RSA), highlighting their efficiency and performance. Graphical representations of ECC and RSA for various file sizes were generated, clearly demonstrating the superiority of the former over the latter. Detailed comparative analyses were presented in tabular formats, incorporating recorded execution times. The assessment concluded that ECC outperforms RSA in terms of both speed and security, offering faster execution and an enhanced user experience. The experimental data illustrated that ECC requires less processing time than RSA, indicating its superior security features, particularly on memory-constrained devices.

7. Conclusion

Cloud computing has significantly reshaped interconnected networks and device integration on a broad scale, transforming homes and businesses into smart, interconnected environments. However, this increased connectivity has also exposed these environments to various security and privacy vulnerabilities. Securing the cloud environment demands robust user authentication procedures to prevent unauthorized access. A resilient authentication system designed specifically for the cloud is essential to shield it from potential authentication threats. This research aims to optimize authentication systems, offering tailored solutions for users and administrators to mitigate these threats effectively. The study focuses on providing secure authentication services to safeguard sensitive data from potential breaches, outlining approaches to uphold the security and privacy of both transmitted and stored confidential information. The significance of encrypting data on the cloud is increasingly paramount, with ECC demonstrating faster processing times and enhanced security, particularly on memory-constrained devices.

REFERENCES

1. Latha, K., & Sheela, T. (2019, July 20). Block based data security and data distribution on multi cloud environment. Journal of Ambient Intelligence and Humanized Computing. https://doi.org/10.1007/s12652-019-01395-y
2. Joseph, T., Kalaiselvan, S. A., Aswathy, S. U., Radhakrishnan, R., & Shamna, A. R. (2020, June 23). RETRACTED ARTICLE: A multimodal biometric authentication scheme based on feature fusion for improving security in cloud environment. Journal of Ambient Intelligence and Humanized Computing, 12(6), 6141–6149. https://doi.org/10.1007/s12652-020-02184-8
3. Jarecki, S., Krawczyk, S., & Xu J. (2018). OPAQUE: an asymmetric PAKE protocol secure against pre-computation attacks. Advances in Cryptology – EUROCRYPT, 456–486, https://doi.org/10.1007/978-3-319-78372-7_15.
4. Wang, D., & Wang, P. (2016). Two Birds with One Stone: Two-Factor Authentication with Security Beyond Conventional Bound. IEEE Transactions on Dependable and Secure Computing, 1–1. https://doi.org/10.1109/tdsc.2016.2605087.
5. León, O., Hernández-Serrano, J., & Soriano, M. (2010, February 10). Securing cognitive radio networks. International Journal of Communication Systems, 23(5), 633–652. https://doi.org/10.1002/dac.1102.
6. Nagaraju, S., & Parthiban, L. (2015, December). Trusted framework for online banking in public cloud using multi-factor authentication and privacy protection gateway. Journal of Cloud Computing, 4(1). https://doi.org/10.1186/s13677-015-0046-4.
7. Srivastava, S., Soni, M.K., Pratap, A. (2023). A Critical Study of Challenges and Risk in Healthcare sector based on Cloud Computing. 14th International Conference on Computing Communication and Networking Technologies (ICCCNT), Delhi, India. 1-5. doi: 10.1109/ICCCNT56998.2023.10307861.
8. Singh, C., & Singh, T.D. (2019, February). A 3-level multifactor Authentication scheme for cloud computing. International Journal of Computer Engineering &Technology, 10(1). 184–195, https://doi.org/10.34218/ijcet.10.1.2019.020.
9. Wang, D., Zhang, X., Zhang, Z., & Wang, P. (2020, January). Understanding security failures of multi-factor authentication schemes for multi-server environments. Computers & Security, 88, 101619. https://doi.org/10.1016/j.cose.2019.101619
10. Qiu, S., Wang, D., Xu, G., & Kumari, S. (2020). Practical and Provably Secure Three-Factor Authentication Protocol Based on Extended Chaotic-Maps for Mobile Lightweight Devices. IEEE Transactions on Dependable and Secure Computing, 1–1. https://doi.org/10.1109/tdsc.2020.3022797.
11. Luo, H., Wang, F., & Xu, G. (2021, May 28). Provably Secure ECC-Based Three-Factor Authentication Scheme for Mobile Cloud Computing with Offline Registration Centre. Wireless Communications and Mobile Computing, 2021, 1–12. https://doi.org/10.1155/2021/8848032.
12. Sharma, S. K. ., A. . Pratap, and H. . Dev. "Analysis of Various Challenges of Big Data-As-a-Service (BDaaS) and Testing for Its Research Aspects". International Journal of Intelligent Systems and Applications in Engineering, vol. 11, no. 9s, July 2023, pp. 743-9, https://ijisae.org/index.php/IJISAE/article/view/3223.

Emerging Trends in IoT and Computing Technologies – Suman Lata Tripathi et al. (eds)

Experimental Analysis on AISI 1020 Mild steel Autogenous Tungsten Inert Gas (TIG) Welding

68

Ajay Kumar[1], Shiv Kumar[2]

Goel Institute of Technology and Management,
Mechanical Engineering Department, Lucknow, India

Abstract: Gas Tungsten ArcWelding(GTAW), another name for tungsten inert gaswelding, is an advanced arc welding technique that has gained popularity where significant precision welding or a high degree of welding quality are required. The sluggish welding speed and the fact that TIG welding is only possible with lower thickness materials in a single pass, however, are the process's main drawbacks. In this work, 5 mm thick AISI 1020 mild steel plate was autogenously TIG welding without the need of filler material. Tests have been conducted on a broad range of welding current and scan speed in order to achieve complete penetration welding. Enhancing the welding depth has also been accomplished with activated flux. Tensile strength and microhardness tests have been conducted on the welding following welding by keeping varying gaps between the plates to be welded. It has been noted that full penetration welding of the plate is achievable with an adequate spacing, providing strength that is nearly identical to the base material.

Keywords: TIG welding technique, Tungsten inert gas welding, Activated flux, Tensile test, Hardness test

1. Introduction

The process of welding entails the joining of two metals that are not identical, regardless of their similarity or dissimilarity, with or without the addition of supplementary metal and with or without excessive pressure. The metallurgical changes caused by welding, the material's change in hardness inside and around the welding, and the degree to which the joint is prone to cracking are some of the factors that determine a material's welding ability. Various welding methods have been developed thus far, employing one or more of the following: heat, pressure, and filler material.

1.1 Tungsten Inert Gas Welding

Gas tungsten arc welding, an inert tungsten gas welding, and arc welding with an electrode made from tungsten that is not consumed are some of the names for this process. An inert shielding gas (helium or argon) shields the welded area from air contamination, and filler is typically employed when welding thick plate. Since the electrode has a melting point of roughly 3400°C, it is not consumable. Zinc and thorium are added to tungsten electrodes to boost current carrying capacity, arc stability, and electron emission at concentrations of 1 to 2%. Energy from a welding power supply with a steady current is conducted across the arc by a plasma column, which is made up of highly ionised gas and metal vapours. The filler material rate has no bearing on the amount of heat input in GTAW. As a result, the procedure makes it possible to precisely regulate heat addiction and produce weldings of exceptional quality that are devoid of splatter and deformation.

[1]info.ajay365@gmail.com, [2]shiv71085@gmail.com

DOI: 10.1201/9781003535423-68

1.2 Autogenous TIG welding

An "autogenous welding" is a welding junction that is produced by melting the surfaces of the contact edges and allowing it to solidify at room temperature (lacking the use of filler metal). Consequently, the composition of the autogenous welding metal exclusively matches that of the base metal. However, when the base metal to be welded has a notably high solidification temperature range, autogenous welding becomes susceptible to cracking. The autogenous TIG welding procedure is one in which filler material is not applied during the welding process. In particular, autogenous TIG welding is recommended for plates that are less than 5 mm thick. This procedure has the advantage of being more cost-effective than heterogeneous or homogeneous welding processes because it doesn't require edge preparation or filler material.

2. Literature Review

TIG welding is widely used to join various metals and alloys, and extensive research is being done to improve the process's performance.

In an experiment, Krishnan et al. [6] "examined the microstructure and oxidation resistance of mild steel weldings produced by TIG welding in various locations. A dramatic shift in the microstructure was seen throughout the welding process as a result of a complicated heat cycle and quick solidification. The mechanical characteristics and oxidation resistance of the mild steel welding are also impacted by this microstructure alteration. On mild steel that was 12 mm thick, autogenous TIG welding was done at 200 A current, 19 V voltage, and 100 mm/min welding speed. At the heat-affected zone and welding metal, finer grain size was achieved".

The distortion formed during TIG welding of low carbon steel is predicted by Raj and Varghese [7] "They have created a three-dimensional finite element model in their research, which includes longitudinal, angular, and transverse distortion. Non-uniform heating and cooling causes distortion in welding. Argon was used as the shielding gas, welding current of 150 A, electrode gap of 3 mm, gas flow rate of 25 l/min, and electrode diameter of 0.8 mm were all used to validate the model. In contrast to the other two directions, they determined that the highest distortion happens at the surface that is opposing the welding and along the X direction of the welding". Abhulimen and Achebo [8] "conducted studies to determine the most cost-effective welding parameters for TIG welding of mild steel tubing using Response surface methodology (RSM). Gas flow rate of 25 to 30 l/min, welding current of 130 to 180 A, arc voltage of 10.5 to 13.5 V, and argon as shielding gas were the welding parameters that were taken into consideration. According to the results, mild steel could obtain maximum tensile and yield strengths of 542 MPa and 547 MPa, respectively, via TIG welding".

A study of the mechanical characteristics of TIG and MIG welding dissimilar junctions was conducted by Mishra et al. [9] "Dissimilar material joints made of mild steel and stainless steel are frequently used in structural applications. These different joints offer a cost-effective blend of mechanical qualities, including as tensile strength and resistance to corrosion. Welding current 80-400 A and voltage 26-56 volts were the factors taken into consideration for MIG welding. Ten to fourteen volts and 50–76 amps of electricity were used for TIG welding. Because TIG welding dissimilar joints have reduced porosity, they have superior tensile strength. For TIG and MIG welding, both dissimilar joints offer the best yield strength and ductility".

2.1 Motivation and Objectives of present Works

- To perform autogenous TIG welding of mild steel plate (AISI1020) with a thickness of 5 mm without the use of filler rod, and to examine the effects of welding speed and welding current.
- To TIG welding mild steel plates that are 5 mm thick by keeping varying gaps between the plates.
- To gauge the welding joint's tensile strength.
- Determining the macro-hardness of the welding area

3. Experimental Planning and Procedure

3.1 Experimental Setup

An autogenous welding setup has been created for the current project work in order to accomplish welding at a preset velocity without the use of filler material. TIG torches are held in place by a mobile vehicle. Throughout the welding process, the distance between the workpiece and the torchtip won't change. The mobile vehicle's speed can be in step to suit the needs of the welding process, including the necessary quantity of heat and speed. The experimental setup used for this investigation is shown in Fig. 68.1. The following elements make up the welding setup for the autogenous TIG welding process:

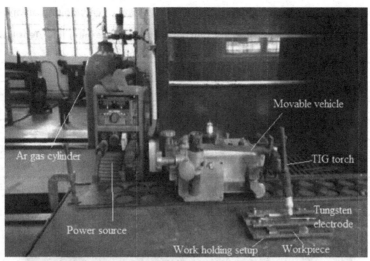

Fig. 68.1 Experimental setup of TIG welding

3.2 Single Pass Autogenous TIG Welding on Mild Steel Plate

In this stage of the experiment, TIG welding has been done without the use of filler rod in order to investigate the viability of autogenous welding on 5 mm mild steel plate. A band saw was used to cut mild steel plates that were 5 mm thick into 50 mm by 50 mm dimensions. To ensure that the plates to be joined can make adequate contact, the edges that needed to be welded were honed using a surface grinding machine. To ensure the necessary surface smoothness and to eliminate any impurities, additional surfaces were additionally polished using emery paper (silicon carbide).

Table 68.1 Welding parameters for mild steel autogenous TIG welding

Dimension of mild steel	50 mm x 50 mm x 5 mm
Welding speed	2.33 mm/s, 2.96 mm/s and 3.5 mm/s
Arc voltage	14 – 15 V
Welding current	170 A, 190 A & 210 A
Gas flow rate	12 1/min
Current type	DC (positive workpiece & negative electrode)
Distance between tip and weld center	3 mm
Shielding gas	Argon

Table 68.2 Organising experiments for mild steel autogenous TIG welding

Exp. No.	Welding current (A)	Welding speed (mm/s)
1	170	2.33
2	170	2.96
3	170	3.5
4	190	2.33
5	190	2.96
6	190	3.5
7	210	2.33
8	210	2.96
9	210	3.5

4. Results and Discussion

4.1 Tensile Test

On the welded specimen, we utilized UTM tensile testing to determine the strength of the weld junction under different welding conditions. Initial penetration was greater when the maximal current was applied at the lowest welding speed in both sets of experiments. As a result, specimens exhibiting a robust current were considered more appropriate for subsequent analysis. Better strength is not provided by either activated TIG welded or standard TIG welded specimens. The third set of experiments was driven by the test findings, which indicate that the welding joint obtained is not strong enough.

Table 68.3 displays the highest tensile strength value of the welding under welding conditions, and Fig. 68.2 displays the specimen for tensile testing.

Table 68.3 Tensile strength at welding joint by TIG welding of varying gap among workpiece

Sl. No.	Welding current (A)	Gap between workpiece (mm)	Tensile strength (MPa)
1	180	0.5	115.95
2	180	0.75	225.21
3	180	1	264.54
4	190	0.5	319.10
5	190	0.75	346.38
6	190	1	501.173
7	200	0.5	442.98
8	200	0.75	395.45
9	200	1	617.22

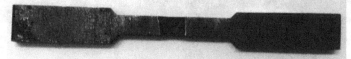

Fig. 68.2 Tensile testing specimen

The change in tensile strength against the space between the workpiece to be welded for various welding currents of the welding sample is displayed in Fig. 68.3. It has been noted that when the distance between the workpieces to be welded grows, the workpiece's tensile strength also increases. This is mostly because of increased welding penetration, which maintains a larger welding separation between workpieces.

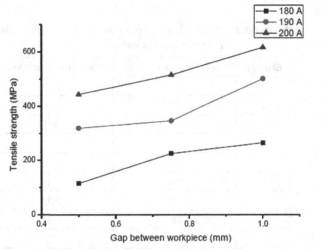

Fig. 68.3 Variation of tensile strength against gap between workpiece to be welded for different welding current

Fig. 68.4 Tensile strength variation against welding current for varying workpiece to be welded gaps

In a similar vein, Fig. 68.4 illustrates how the tensile strength varies with welding current for various workpiece gaps that need to be welded. It has been noted that the tensile strength of the welded workpiece rises as current increases. In this experiment, an autogenous heat input of a larger value of current is required. It is evident from the optical image that penetration depth increases as current increases. Greater strength is correlated with a deeper penetration depth.

4.2 Vickers Hardness Measurement

The cross sectional A particular specimen's welding zone hardness was measured. The Vickers Hardness Testing, which can withstand loads as low as 0.3 kgf, was used to measure the hardness. Based on the specimen treated with a 200 A current and a 0.75 mm gap, Figure 68.5 displays the values of hardness for the base material, the welded zone, and the heat-affected zone. Table 68.4 displays the hardness values of a few samples that were chosen.

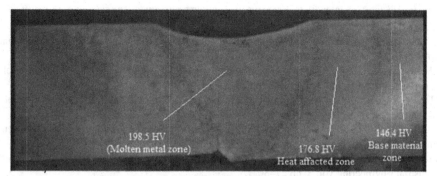

Fig. 68.5 Sample hardness value in the welding zone, as processed with a 0.75 mm gap and 200 A of current

Table 68.4 Hardness value for sample

Sample No.	Welding current (A)	Welding speed (mm/s)	Gap between workpiece (mm)	Hardness value at molten metal zone	Hardness value at heat affected zone	Hardness value at base material zone
1	190	2.33	0.5	192.6 HV	158.5 HV	149 HV
2	200	2.33	0.75	198.5 HV	176.8 HV	146.4 HV

As one gets closer to the basic material zone, the hardness value drops, as seen in Fig. 68.5. The average hardness values at the molten metal zone are 192.6 HV and 198.5 HV, respectively, for currents of 190 A and 200 A. Thus, it can be concluded that for TIG welded samples, the approximate range of micro-hardness is between 190 and 200 HV in the molten metal zone.

5. Conclusions

The current investigation's findings can be summed up as follows:

- The outcome of the typical TIG welding process show that the maximum penetration depth was possible when the minimum welding speed and maximum current were combined in a parametric way.
- Compared to conventional welding, the identical technique performed with more TiO2 flux results in a deeper penetration; nonetheless, the use of flux caused some welding zone cracking.
- A different series of experiments was carried out using a fixed welding speed, but this time, the workpiece that needed to be welded was maintained separated. It is discovered that a 1 mm gap can result in defect-free welding with the proper material flow produced throughout the joint with higher welding current.
- When comparing the three TIG welding processes, maintaining enough space between the components that need to be welded results in the maximum depth of diffusion and tensile strength of the welding connection.
- The graphs that are provided make it evident that while the distance between the components to be welded is constant, the welding width and depth increase as the welding current increases. Prospective Range
- The depth of penetration will increase if welding can be done at the minimal welding speed. Maintaining the ideal distance between the two workpieces to be welded will result in a deeper melting point. All of elements contribute to the welding joint's increased strength.
- The TIG welding procedure uses filler material to produce a thicker plate welding that has a greater penetration depth and greater strength.

REFERENCES

1. en.wikipedia.org/wiki/GTAW
2. Sharma P.C., Manufacturing Technology – I, S. Chand, 2008.
3. Singh S., Production Engineering, LNEC publication, 2010.
4. American Association State, 2012. Standard test method for Tension Testing of metallic materials E8/E8M – 11, pp 3.
5. http://www.efuda.com/materials/alloys/carbon_steel
6. Krishna R., Raman R.K., Varatharanjan K., Tyagi A.K. (2014), Microstructure and oxidation resistance of different region in the welding of mild steel, Journal of Material Science vol. 18, pp 1618–1621.

7. Raj A., Varghese J., Determination of distortion developed during TIG welding of low carbon steel plate, Journal of engineering Research and General Science vol. 2, pp 756–767.
8. Abhulimen I.U., Achebo J.I. (2014), Prediction of Welding quality of a Tungsten inert gas welded steel pipe joint using response surface methodology, Journal of Engineering Research and Application vol. 4, pp 31–40
9. Mishra R., Tiwari V., Rajesha S. (2014), A study of tensile strength of MIG and TIG welded dissimilar joints of mild steel and stainless steel, Journal of material science &Engineering vol. 3, pp 23–32.
10. Fujii H., Sato T., Lua S.,Nogi K. (2008), Development of an advanced A-TIG welding method by control of Marangoni convection, Journal of material science & Engineering vol. 495, pp 296–303.
11. Kuo C., Tseng K., Chou C. (2011), Effect of activated TIG flux on performance of dissimilar weldings between mild steel and stainless steel, Journal of Engineering materials vol. 479, pp 74–80.
12. Vikesh, Randhawa J., Suri N.M. (2013), Effect of A TIG welding process parameters on penetration in mild steel plate, Journal of Mechanical and Industrial Engineering vol. 3, pp 27–30.

Emerging Trends in IoT and Computing Technologies – Suman Lata Tripathi et al. (eds)
© 2024 Taylor & Francis Group, London, ISBN 978-1-032-87924-6

Fabrication and Experimental Analysis of Thermal Conductivity of Redmud Particles and Aluminium Filled Epoxy Composites

69

Shivam Awasthi[1]

M.Tech(ME) Scholar, Goel Institute of Technology and Management,
Mechanical Engineering Department, Lucknow, India

Shiv Kumar[2]

Assistant Professor, Goel Institute of Technology and Management,
Mechanical Engineering Department, Lucknow, India

Abstract: The current study examines how filler particle volume fraction affects polymer composites' effective thermal conductivity (keff). This paper sees a chance to improve a common particulate-filled polymer composite's capacity for heat conduction. A mathematical relationship exists between the principles of specific equivalent thermal conductivity and the law of least resistance to heating in polymer composites comprising elliptical particles. Two sets of epoxy-based composites were produced utilizing a straightforward manual lay-up method. The filler amounts in each set varied from 0% to 25% vol%. Examining this mathematical paradigm was my objective. As filler in the first set are minuscule particles of aluminum; as the matrix in the second set consists of crimson mud and epoxy. The heat conductivity of the aforementioned composite materials was determined using the Unitherm TM Model 2022 apparatus in accordance with ASTM standard E-1530.The thermal conductivity of the composite materials was evaluated in conformance with ASTM standard E-1530 utilizing the Unitherm TM Model 2022 instrument. Subsequently, a comparison is made between the experimental outcomes and those predicted by the mathematical model under consideration and other widely accepted models, including the Bruggeman model, Maxwell's model, and the Rule-of-Mixture (ROM). It is observed that the outcomes of the proposed model closely resemble the data obtained from experiments. An increase in the quantity of conductive infill in the composite results in a substantial enhancement in keff, according to this study. The thermal conductivity of epoxy resin containing 25 vol% aluminum filler is approximately 160% greater, while the keff increases by 135% when redmud filler material is utilized. From this vantage point, industrial refuse redmud fine powder can be utilized in lieu of the more expensive aluminum fine powder due to its thermal conductivity. Epoxy composites with enhanced heat conductivity and reduced weight may find utility in applications involving heat sinks, printed circuit boards, and encapsulation. Thermal conductivity, Redmud particles, aluminum fine powder, epoxy-based composites, and some other related terms.

Keywords: Thermal conductivity, Polymer composites, Effective thermal conductivity (keff), Elliptical particles, Epoxy-based composites, Rule-of-Mixture (ROM), Printed circuit board (PCB)

1. Introduction

The present study is primarily concerned with conducting an experimental investigation into the thermal properties of a novel category of particulate-filled composites composed of polymers. Then, the mechanical and physical characteristics of the completed composites are described in detail.

[1]shivam.awasthi0013@gmail.com, [2]shiv71085@gmail.com

DOI: 10.1201/9781003535423-69

Modern consumers choose increasingly compact electronic devices that are easier to transport and store. Consequently, high-quality encapsulating and packaging materials are required for use in electronic applications. Therefore, an integrated design approach is necessary from the beginning of a modern packaging application, which integrates a variety of materials.

The field of electronics has witnessed tremendous growth in the previous several decades. due to the constant demand for miniaturisation, which has caused sizes to gradually shrink while communication speeds and component counts increase daily. This has resulted in high heat generation and heat dissipation problems. Although they are frequently utilised as materials for heat sink applications, neat polymers like polyester or epoxy have the disadvantage of having low thermal conductivity. The heat conductivity of these polymers is enhanced if they are loaded with metal particles, such as copper or aluminium. Therefore, thermally conductive fillers with an appropriate volume fraction may be utilised in polymers for such applications in order to improve the heat conductivity. This idea has been internalised and serves as the foundation for the current study.

2. Literature Review

In contrast to the evaluation of the thermal conductivity of polypropylene/aluminum composites by Boudenne et al., Tavman investigated the thermal properties of HDPE by incorporating aluminum particles as a filler. In a study, Choi et al. provide a comprehensive analysis of the thermal conductivity and morphology of polyacrylate polymers. A variety of fillers, including Al-CNT, carbon nanotubes with multiple walls (CNT), and aluminum particle (Al-flake). Goyanes et al. examined the impact of filler content on the yield and internal stresses of aluminum-containing epoxy resin. Carson et al. utilized a straightforward, transitory comparison method to examine the efficient diffusivity of longitudinal moderate-density polyethylene/aluminum composites at various volume fractions. Information regarding effective thermal diffusivity was utilized to compute values for effective thermal conductivity. Yu et al. conducted a comprehensive investigation into the thermoelectric characteristics of polymer composites that were matriced with polystyrene (PS) and reinforced with aluminum nitride (AlN).

Certain ceramic products, including tiles and blocks, contain redmud as a partial clay substitute; it is also a component of mortar and concrete. Throughout history, red clay has been utilized in the agricultural sector, specifically to remediate soils that are acidic or deficient in iron. Red soil is also employed by the ceramics industry to a lesser degree. Previous studies (Yalcin et al. and Satapathy et al.) have examined the coating potential of redmud when it is applied via plasma spray technology to a variety of metal substrates. Thakur and Das have conducted lengthy investigations into a multitude of additional applications for crimson mud. By documenting the erosion properties of glass-epoxy and bamboo-epoxy composites loaded with redmud, Biswas et al. Bhat et al. published the results of a morphological examination of red clay material composites that had been modified with polyvinyl alcohol. The feasibility of fortifying unsaturated polyester (USP) with red soil in combination with sisal and banana fibers was examined by Prabu et al.

2.1 Objective of Present Work

The creation of composites with the goal of improving the keff of neat polymer by employing micro-sized aluminium fine powder as the reinforce filler.

Creation of a new rank of composites with the same goal employing industrial waste, such as redmud fine powder in microsized fine powder form.

- An investigation of the density of manufactured composites, both theoretical and experimental.
- Calculating the keff of every composite that was manufactured above.

3. Materials and Methods

3.1 Epoxy Resin

Since epoxy (LY 556) has a number of the previously listed advantages over other thermoset polymers, it is the material of choice for the matrix in this study. Chemically, it is a member of the "epoxide" family.

Aluminium fine powder asfiller material for the initial set of polymercomposite

The initial run of polymer composites makes use of micro-sized aluminum fine powder as a filler. Silvery white is the metal's color. Aluminium is highly prized for its excellent qualities, such as its low density (2.7gm/cm3) and corrosion

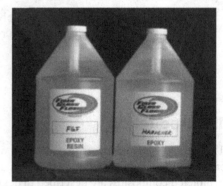

Fig. 69.1 Epoxyresin and hardener

resistance. The main reason aluminium is used is that it has a thermal conductivity of about 205 W/m-K, making it very conducting in nature. Aluminium and its alloys are used to make structural components that are essential to the aerospace sector as well as other fields of building and transportation. Figure 69.2 provides a picture of the micro-sized aluminium fine powder that was used in this project.

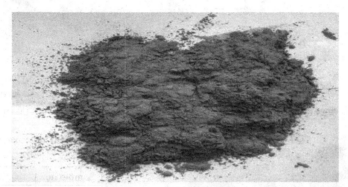

Fig. 69.2 Microsized aluminium fine powder used as filler in the presentwork

Redmud fine powder as fillermaterial for the second batch of polymercomposite

As an additive in the second round of polymers composites, redmud fine powder derived from industrial detritus is utilized. Redmud is the insoluble byproduct generated during the alumina production process, which involves the alkali sodium hydroxide digestion of bauxite at elevated temperatures and pressures.

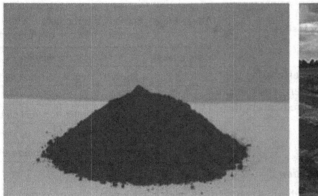 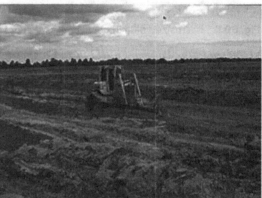

Fig. 69.3 The microscopic image of the redmud fine powder employed in this experiment is depicted

4. Experimental Detail

4.1 Composite Fabrication

Microsized aluminium fine powder-filled epoxy composites

For the fabrication of polymer composite specimens, the traditional hand lay-up approach is employed. Epoxy resin is used to strengthen micro-sized aluminium particles in the initial set of polymer composites. Epoxy resin and the appropriate hardener are combined according to prescription at a weight ratio of 10:1. Epoxy resin and micro-sized aluminium particles are combined to make dough. After evenly applying a thin layer of silicone- releasing agent on a paper cup, dough is gradually poured into the moulds. Following that, the samples are released and the castings are allowed to cure for around 24 hours at room temperature. Five-component composites with fillers at five, ten, fifteen, twenty, and twenty-five percent volume are made. The disclosed composites are disc-shaped specimens with a 50 mm diameter and a 3 mm thickness. Table 69.4 displays the composition of the aluminum/epoxy fabricated composite, and Figure 69.6 displays the fabricated aluminium epoxy composite.

- Paper mug
- Particles of filler coated with wax
- matrix made of epoxy

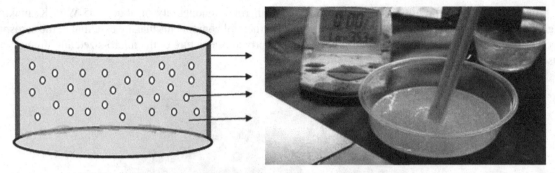

Fig. 69.4 Particulate filled epoxycomposite fabrication by hand lay-up process

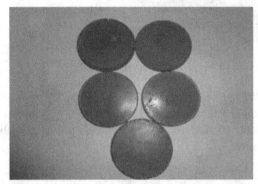

Fig. 69.5 Microsized aluminium filledepoxy composites

Table 69.1 Epoxycomposites filled with micro-sized aluminium particles (Set 1)

Sample no.	Composition
1	Epoxy + 5 vol % Aluminium particle
2	Epoxy + 10 vol % Aluminium particle
3	Epoxy + 15 vol % Aluminium particle
4	Epoxy + 20 vol % Aluminium particle
5	Epoxy + 25 vol % Aluminium particle

Microsized Redmud Fine Powder-Filled Epoxy Composites

Microsized redmud particles were reinforced in the epoxy resin using the same hand lay-up approach, and the second set of polymer composites was created in various ratios (Table 69.2) based on the requirements of the experiment.

Table 69.2 Epoxy composites with redmud particles that are microsized (Set 2)

Sample no.	Composition
1	Epoxy + 5 vol % Red mud particle
2	Epoxy + 10 vol % Red mud particle
3	Epoxy + 15 vol % Red mud particle
4	Epoxy + 20 vol % Red mud particle
5	Epoxy + 25 vol % Red mud particle

4.2 Characterization

Thermal Conductivity: Determined Through Experimentation

Model 2022 Unitherm Several materials with medium to low thermal conductivity, such as polymers, glasses, ceramics, rubbers, composites, and a few metals, were measured for thermal conductivity using a thermal conductivity tester. Use a dedicated container to test fluids or semi-fluids, such as paste. This device is utilised in the current work to test the composite specimens' effective thermal conductivity at room temperature. Disc- typespecimens are employed in this way. Thistest is carried out in compliance with ASTM E-1530 guidelines. Figure 69.6 displays a picter of the UnithermTM Model 2022 testing.

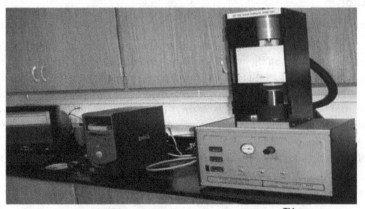

Fig. 69.6 Thermal conductivity Tester Unitherm™ 2022

5. Result and Discussion

5.1 Thermoelectric Properties of Fused Composite Specimens

Comparison of experimental data, the suggested model, and the values of keff derived from other accepted theoretical models.

The change in keff value upon adding micro-sized aluminium particles to the epoxy matrix is depicted in Fig. 69.7. It displays a comparison of experimental results, the suggested model, and values derived from many well- established theoretical models. Tables 69.3 display the theoretically computed values for each replica and the experimentally calculated values of keff for the two sets of manufactured composites, i.e., epoxy/aluminum and epoxy/redmud composites.

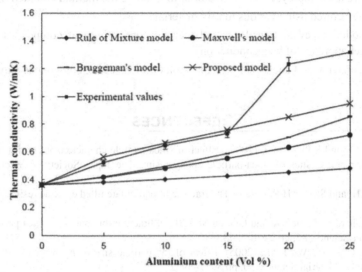

Fig. 69.7 Correspondence between epoxy and aluminum's thermal conductivity: Rule of mixture, maxwell's model, bruggman model, suggested model, and exp. values

Table 69.3 Shows the experimentally measured values of the manufactured epoxy/aluminum composites as well as the theoretically derived values of all models

Sample no.	Content Aluminium Particles in vol%	K_eff of aluminium/epoxy polymer composites				
		Rule of mixture	Maxwell's model	Bruggemen's model	Proposed model	Experimental
1	5	0.382	0.419	0.423	0.565	0.525
2	10	0.403	0.483	0.497	0.664	0.648
3	15	0.426	0.553	0.589	0.756	0.732
4	20	0.453	0.633	0.705	0.850	1.232
5	25	0.483	0.723	0.854	0.949	1.317

6. Conclusions

The followings conclusions can be drawn from the experimental and analytical work mentioned above:

- Both the epoxy/aluminum and epoxy/redmud composites can be effectively manufactured using the hand lay-up process. The mathematical model that was given properly predicts the keff values of the composites up to the percolation threshold.
- Adding 25% volume of aluminium filler to epoxy resin improves the value of thermal conductivity by approximately 161%, whereas using redmud as the filler material causes keff to boost thermal conductivity by 135% compared to neat epoxy.
- It is evident from the SEM pictures that the particles are evenly dispersed throughout the matrix body and have a roughly elliptical shape.

- While there is a noticeable variation in the inherent heat conductivity of redmud fine powder and aluminium, the keff of their composites is only marginally different. On the basis of this, it can be concluded that redmud, an industrialwaste, can successfully replace aluminium fine particles.
- The aforementioned composites have potential uses in the electronics industry, including printed circuit boards, heat sinks, and electronics fields.

7. Future Scope

- Other industrial wastes are also employed as filler material to improve the thermal conductivity of polymers.
- These fillers can be manufactured using various matrix materials.
- A new mathematical model for evaluating the actual thermal conductivity of composites made of polymers may be developed using a parallel approach of heat conduction.
- The strength, dielectric behavior, and coefficient of expansion of the resulting composites may be studied in relation to the loading of fillers.

REFERENCES

1. Yamamoto I., Higashihara T. and Kobayashi T. (2003), Effect of silica-particle characteristics on impact/usual fatigue properties and evaluation of mechanical characteristics of silica-particle epoxy resins, The Japan Society of Mechanical Engineers International Journal, 46(2), pp 145–153.
2. Moloney A.C., Kausch H.H. and Stieger H.R. (1983), The fracture of particulate filled epoxide resins, Journal of Material Science, 18, pp 208-16.
3. Adachi T., Araki W., Nakahara T., Yamaji A. and Gamou M. (2002), Fracture toughness of silica particulate-filled epoxy composite, Journal of Applied Polymer Science, 86, pp 2261–2265.
4. Yuan J.J., Zhou S.X., Gu G.G. and Wu L.M., (2005), Effect of the particle size of nanosilica on the performance of epoxy/silica composite coatings, Journal ofMaterial Science, 40, pp 3927–3932.
5. Karger-Kocsis J. (1995), Microstructural aspects of fracture in polypropylene and in its filled, chopped fiber, fiber mat reinforced composites. In: Karger- Kocsis J, editor, Polypropylene: Structure, blends and composites, London. Chapman & Hall, pp 142–201.
6. Srivastava V.K. and Shembekar P.S. (1990). Tensile and fracture properties of epoxy resin filled with flyash particles, Journal of Material Science, 25, pp 3513–3516.
7. Tu H. and Ye L. (2009), Thermal conductive PS/graphite composites, Polymer Advance Technology, 20, pp 21–27.
8. Liu Z., Guo Q., Shi J., Znai G. and Liu L. (2008), Graphite blocks with high thermal conductivity derived from natural graphite flake, Carbon, 46, pp 414- 421.

Emerging Trends in IoT and Computing Technologies – Suman Lata Tripathi et al. (eds)
© 2024 Taylor & Francis Group, London, ISBN 978-1-032-87924-6

An Implementation of Electronic Device User Profile Switching using Facial Detection

70

Kulvinder Singh[1],
Yash Gupta[2], Rahul Kumar[3]

Department of Computer Science and Engineering,
Chandigarh University, Mohali, India

Abstract: Facial detection technology is being explored for user authentication and access control. A system using facial detection and Siamese neural networks is proposed to manage multiple user profiles on a device. This secure and user-friendly system eliminates traditional authentication methods. The research outlines the system's components and acknowledges operating system skills challenges. The potential benefits for organizations and users are highlighted. This research aims to contribute to advanced user authentication systems. User feedback and collaboration will drive continuous improvement.

Keywords: Convolution, Face-detection, Authentication, Training/Testing

1. Introduction

In our digital world, traditional authentication methods fall short. Enter facial detection technology—an innovative solution to user authentication and access control. By leveraging computer vision and AI, this tech recognizes users' unique facial features for swift, secure access. Our research aims to seamlessly integrate this technology for managing multiple user profiles on shared devices. We explore its potential to revolutionize digital interactions, prioritizing security and user experience. Join us as we delve into the methodology and implications, aiming to shape advanced and user-centric authentication systems for the future.

2. Background

In today's digital landscape, user authentication and access control are pivotal. Traditional methods like passwords and biometrics, while effective, have limitations. Managing multiple user profiles on shared devices presents challenges. Enter facial detection technology—fusing AI and computer vision—to revolutionize authentication. With front-facing cameras, it offers secure, seamless access. Our research delves into implementing this tech for managing multiple profiles on one device. By combining facial detection with Siamese neural networks, we aim to create a secure yet convenient solution as shown in Fig. 70.1. Join us as we explore its methodology, results, and broader impact, aiming to shape user-centric authentication systems for the digital era. [1]

[1]kulvinder.diet@gmail.com, [2]yash733622@gmail.com, [3]rir7890@gmail.com

DOI: 10.1201/9781003535423-70

3. Objective

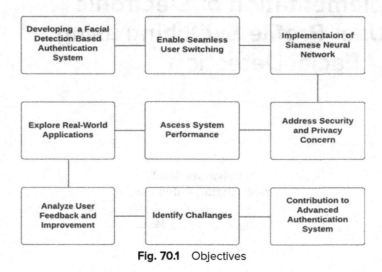

Fig. 70.1   Objectives

4. Significance

This groundbreaking research on user authentication and access control introduces a facial detection-based system (Fig. 70.2) that holds the potential to revolutionize user interactions with electronic devices. The focal points of this innovative approach include not only enhancing user experience through seamless device access but also ensuring improved security by leveraging facial features for identity verification. The system's efficiency in shared environments is a notable highlight, simplifying access control in workplaces, educational institutions, and households, thereby boosting productivity and user satisfaction. The integration of Siamese neural networks adds a layer of sophistication, advancing authentication methods through deep learning and computer vision.[4] Addressing compatibility challenges, the research also underscores cross-platform applicability, enabling the benefits of facial detection technology to extend across diverse devices and operating systems. Moreover, the research places a strong emphasis on privacy considerations, ensuring that the implementation of facial detection technology aligns with stringent privacy measures. By actively incorporating user feedback, the research embraces a user-centric approach, acknowledging the importance of real-world applications in personal devices, workplaces, and public facilities. Ultimately, this research contributes to shaping the future of user authentication, offering valuable insights and methodologies for creating advanced systems that cater to the evolving needs of individuals and organizations in our increasingly digital world.

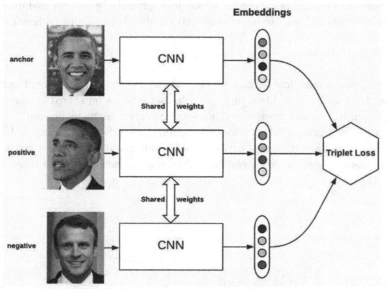

Fig. 70.2   Base of siamese neural network

5. Literature Review

Siamese Neural Network [1]: are particularly helpful in tasks such as facial recognition and image similarity comparison. They excel in learning and creating meaningful representations of input pairs, making them suitable for scenarios were identifying similarities or dissimilarities between pairs of images is crucial. In facial recognition, Siamese networks can effectively capture and compare facial features, enabling accurate and robust authentication.

Bengio, Yoshua. Learning deep architectures [2]: Serves as a foundational concept in our facial detection research by emphasizing the importance of training sophisticated neural networks to understand and extract intricate features from facial data.

Bromley, Jane [3][4]: This makes Siamese neural networks a valuable tool in applications where understanding relationships between inputs is essential, including facial research and authentication systems.

Chopra, Sumit, Hadsell [11][13]: Computer vision plays a pivotal role in our facial detection research by providing the foundational technology to interpret and analyse visual information from facial images. It enables our system to extract meaningful features, patterns, and characteristics inherent in facial data. [14] Through computer vision techniques, such as image processing and deep learning, our research can achieve accurate facial recognition and authentication.

Fe-Fei, Li, Fergus [5]: In simpler terms, you can analogize it to the saying," Tell me who your neighbours are Fig. 70.15, and I'll tell you who you are." To illustrate this, let's consider the following example: Picture a scenario where we've plotted the" fluffiness" of animals on the x-axis and the lightness of their coat on the y-axis. Similar pattern recognition is explained in other research papers [16].

Proceedings. [6]: This update rule enables the adjustment of weights based on gradients and momentum, facilitating the training process. Pattern analysis is also discussed in Siamese network which help our model to provide more accurate data.

Hinton, Geoffrey, Osindero [7][12]: Image and Speech Recognition: The convolutional neural network (CNN) leverages convolution and is widely used for image and speech recognition. It excels in identifying patterns and features in images, making it suitable for facial detection. Krizhevsky, Alex, Sutskever [8][15]: Linear and Time-Invariant System: Convolution operates within a linear time-invariant system, ensuring consistent behaviour. It is important in maintaining the stability and reliability of the facial detection process.

6. Methodology

6.1 Data Collection

The research relied on a comprehensive dataset that encompassed various mobile phone specifications and their corresponding prices. This dataset was meticulously gathered from reputable online sources, ensuring data accuracy and completeness. It includes a wide array of features, such as RAM capacity, battery power, camera specifications, and other attributes pertinent to mobile phone models.[3]

Facial detection using Siamese Neural Network—It's based on super-vised learning machine learning model (Fig. 70.3), where the data is passed in the form of keypair as input and output pair of data to the model. [6]

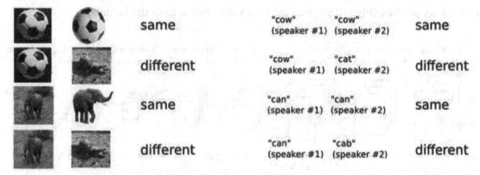

Fig. 70.3 Simple representation of the supervised training model, passing key value pair

We will be creating 3 folders as represented in Fig. 70.4: -

i. *Verification* – It stores the sample data of the authorized entities.

ii. *Negative* – Stores negative data samples for supervised learning model.

iii. *Realtime* – Storing the data of current entity trying to access into the system to verify with the data set of verification folder.

6.2 Data Preparation

The dataset underwent rigorous cleaning, addressing missing data through imputation or exclusion based on the degree of absence. Feature selection techniques were applied to remove redundant attributes, enhancing subsequent modeling efficiency. [6] Data scaling methods like Minmax scaling ensured uniformity and reduced undue attribute influence. Feature engineering was pivotal, crafting new features and transforming existing ones to capture intricate relationships. Three machine learning algorithms—K-Nearest Neighbors, Decision Tree, and Logistic Regression—were evaluated for classification suitability. The 70:30 training-to-testing ratio was adopted, utilizing embedding layers typically used in NLP for potential relevance in computer vision. Thoughtful dataset partitioning and cross-validation techniques prevented overfitting. Evaluation metrics like accuracy, precision, recall, and F1-score were conscientiously used to assess model performance. Face verification testing, detailed in the Siamese network paper, added depth to the evaluation. The model will be applied to both Verification and Negative/Realtime images chosen randomly from the dataset.[10]

I. *Ensemble Methods:* In addition to individual algorithms, the research explored ensemble methods, notably Random Forest, with the aim of enhancing model accuracy. Random forest, an ensemble of decision trees, was investigated to harness the collective predictive power of multiple models.

II. *Evaluation:* A meticulous comparison of models hinged on two key evaluation criteria: achieving the highest attainable accuracy and employing the minimal number of features. These metrics were pivotal in gauging both the predictive efficacy and computational efficiency of the models under consideration.

Under convolution we take a kernel and performing multiplication and addition operation, with ReLU activation then performing Pooling on the data matrix helping in down sampling of it.

After multiple iteration of convolution and pooling and creating a Feature map and applying flattening layer before passing it on to neural network for computation purpose as shown in Fig. 70.4.

The ReLU activation function serves a crucial role in generating output from a given set of input values provided to a node or a layer. Its functionality is akin to that of a human neuron (Fig. 70.5), where the node acts as a neuron receiving a collection of input signals. Based on these input signals, our brain processes information and determines whether the neuron should activate or remain inactive.

Improving the result means to use the algorithms more efficiently so it can give more precise result during, research work (Fig. 70.6). All this is used to improve the creditability of the paper and its data is fetch from the other research work. [4]

In Siemens model we are using max-pooling kernel after creation of feature-map decreasing the complexity and dimensionality of the sample data size. Max-pooling (Fig. 70.9) gives the max value output from the kernel.

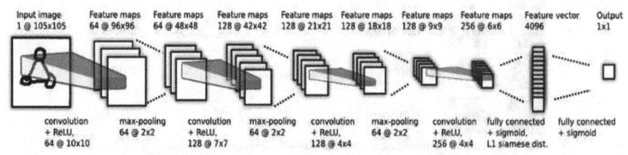

Fig. 70.4 The core computation model of siamese neural network

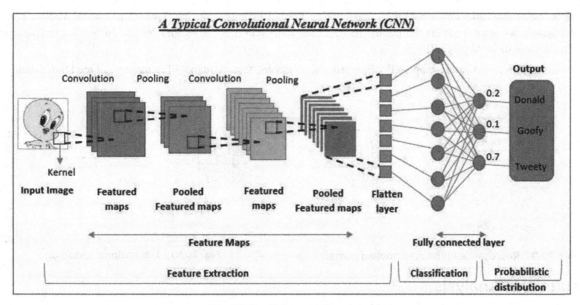

Fig. 70.5 CNN model overview

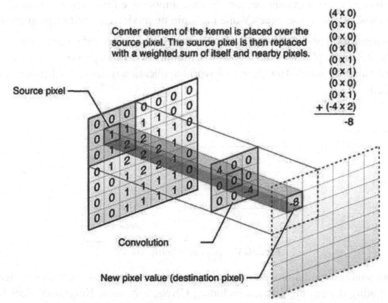

Fig. 70.6 Convolution Operation on 7x7 matrix with 3x3 kernel classifying key points in the image or feature mapping

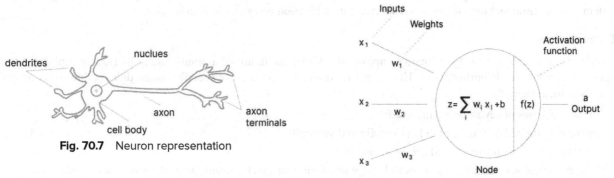

Fig. 70.7 Neuron representation

Fig. 70.8 Neuron representation in machine model

Flattening is the process that convert Multidimensionality Pooled Feature map into One Dimensional Vector. This step is important because we want to insert the pooled feature map into Neural Network and Neural Network can take only One-Dimensional format of input (Fig. 70.10).

Image → Convolution → Feature map → Pooling process → Pooled feature map → Flattening → One Dimensional Vector

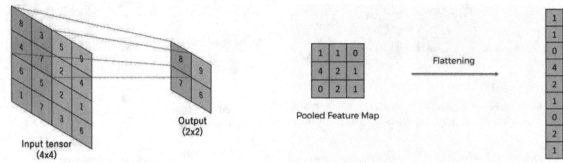

Fig. 70.9 Representation on max-pooling kernal   **Fig. 70.10** Dimensional reduction

7. Results and Analysis

The research findings were subject to comprehensive scrutiny. This encompassed an in-depth analysis of the experimental results, including accuracy scores, confusion matrices, and feature importance rankings. The primary focus was on identifying models that achieved the highest prediction accuracy while maintaining model simplicity and interpretability.

The CNN-based facial recognition approach (Fig. 70.11) displayed remarkable advancements in accurately detecting and verifying individuals. Utilizing the triplet loss during model training led to impressive accuracy, particularly in security, surveillance, and access control applications. However, real-world application requires further refinement to handle scalability and real-time processing challenges.

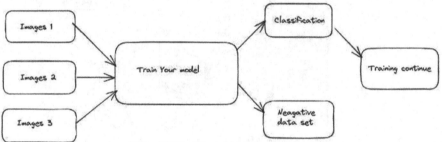

Fig. 70.11 Model training steps

The Siamese neural network's incorporation proved robust, enhancing user detection accuracy by learning from both positive and negative datasets. Integrating diverse algorithms, including CNNs, k-Nearest Neighbors, decision trees, random forests, and K-means clustering, expanded the system's capabilities. Particularly, K-means clustering enables adaptability in undefined user profile situations, showcasing the approach's flexibility. This comprehensive blend of cutting-edge technologies positions the system as a versatile tool for user authentication and identification across various industries.

7.1 Convolution

Convolution is an image processing technique employed in this research, aimed at transforming images by applying a kernel over each pixel and its neighbouring pixels. This kernel, represented as a matrix of specific values, dictates how the convolution process alters the image. [8]

In convolution, a series of key steps are involved:

i The mask is flipped only once both horizontally and vertically.

ii The mask is systematically moved across the image.

iii The corresponding elements of the mask and image are multiplied, and the results are added to create a smaller-sized matrix.

iv. This process is repeated until all the image values have been processed.

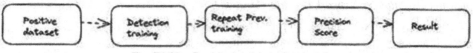

Fig. 70.12 Result obtained after training

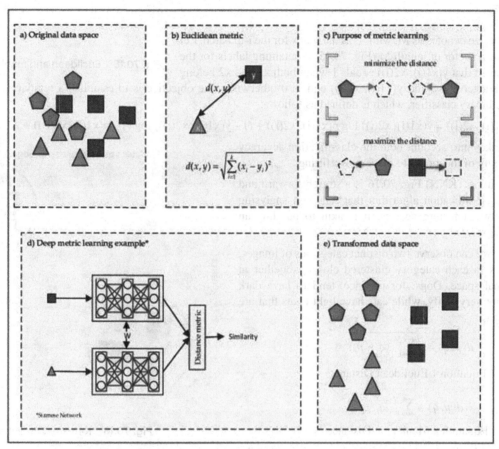

Fig. 70.13 Algorithm used to implement of model

Convolution plays a crucial role in image and speech recognition as in Fig. 70.14. It is a key element in Convolutional Neural Networks (CNNs), which are extensively used in these tasks. [8]

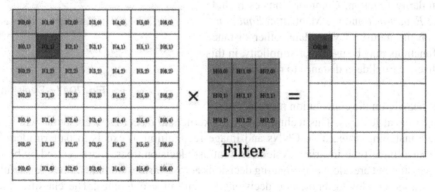

Fig. 70.14 Convolution operation

Mathematical Expression and Siamese Network Learning Strategies:

The expression G(x,y) = h(x,y) * f(x,y) can be interpreted as the result of convolving a mask with an image processing method. Within the Siamese network framework, various learning strategies and methods are employed, including,

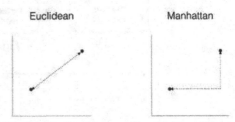

Fig. 70.15 Euclidean and manhattan distance

Loss Function:

Consider a batch size denoted as M, with 'i' as the index for the i-th batch. Let y(x1(i), x2(i)) be a vector of length M (Fig. 70.15), containing labels for the batch. It is assumed that y(x1(i), x2(i)) equals 1 when both x1 and x2 belong to the same character class, and y(x1(i), x2(i)) equals 0 otherwise. The objective is to establish a regularized crossentropy criterion for the binary classifier, which is defined as follows:

$$L(x1(i), x2(i)) = y(x1(i), x2(i)) \log p(x1(i), x2(i)) + (1 - y(x1(i), x2(i))) \log (1 - p(x1(i), x2(i))) + \lambda T \, |w|^2$$

This equation takes into account both the classification accuracy and the complexity of the model to prevent overfitting.

K-Nearest Neighbors (KNN) Fig. 70.16 is a straightforward and effective image classification algorithm that relies on analysing the distance between feature vectors. It is akin to building an image search engine. [5]

In this example, we can observe two distinct categories of images, with data points in each category clustered closely together in an n-dimensional space. Dogs, for instance, tend to have dark coats that are not very fluffy, while cats have light coats that are extremely fluffy.

$$d(p, q) = \sqrt{\sum_{i-1}^{N} (q_i - p_i)^2}$$

Equation 1 Euclidean Distance

$$d(p, q) = \sum_{i-1}^{N} |q_i - p_i|$$

Equation 2 Manhattan Distance

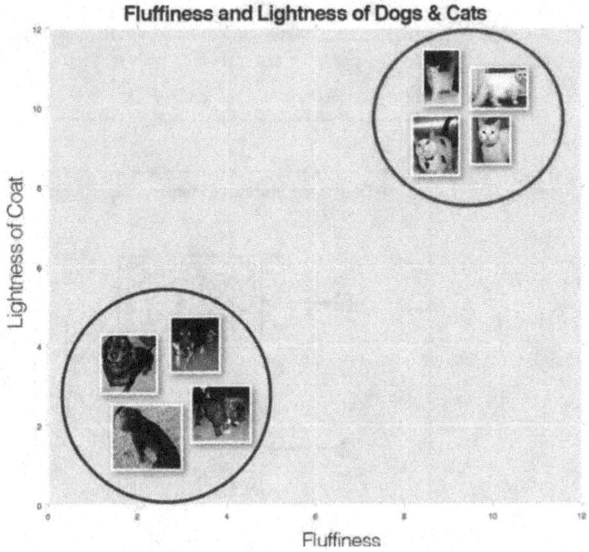

Fluffiness and Lightness of Dogs & Cats

Fig. 70.16 K-nearest neighbor

This suggests that the distance between two data points within the red circle is much smaller than the distance between a data point in the red circle and a data point in the blue circle.

To apply k-Nearest Neighbor classification, we must establish a distance metric or similarity function. Common choices include the Euclidean distance *Equation.1* and the Manhattan *Equation.2* distance. Depending on the nature of your data, other distance metrics or similarity functions may be used. For simplicity, in this blog post, we will utilize the Euclidean distance to measure image similarity.

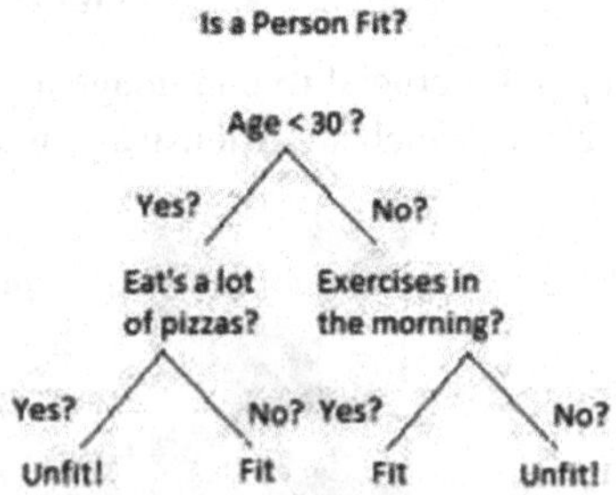

Is a Person Fit?

Fig. 70.17 Decision tree

Facial Detection relies heavily on the convolution method, crucial for extracting significant facial features. This technique utilizes kernels to discern key attributes within facial images, aiding in validation and image matching. Integral to CNNs and image recognition, it excels in pattern identification within facial data, ensuring stability in a linear time-invariant system. In contrast, decision trees, characterized by branching structures, are unrelated to image processing but are adept at navigating decisions across various domains. They're useful in business planning and data classification tasks, employing branching decisions to determine outcomes. The classifier methods referred to in this context are rooted in Siamese network research, bolstering the model's accuracy and predictability, thereby enriching its functionality.

Comparison and Distinctiveness:

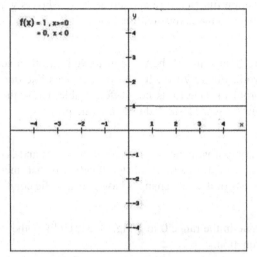

Fig. 70.18   Binary activation function

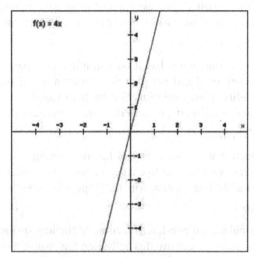

Fig. 70.19   Linear activation function

The convolution and decision tree (Fig. 70.17) methods diverge significantly in their purposes. Convolution is integral for image processing, feature extraction, and pattern identification, particularly in facial recognition and matching. Conversely, decision trees are tools for data classification and decision-making, focusing on categorizing input data.

Convolution prioritizes feature extraction from facial images, while decision trees concentrate on decision-making based on input data. Convolution operates within a linear time invariant system, essential for image and speech recognition. On the other hand, decision trees are unrelated to image processing and don't involve linear systems.

7.2 Activation Functions

"A neural network without an activation function is essentially just a linear regression model."

Activation functions in Siamese networks (Fig. 70.18–70.22) are employed to introduce non-linearity into the model and facilitate the network in capturing

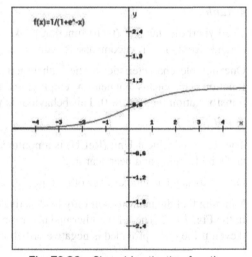

Fig. 70.20   Sigmoid activation function

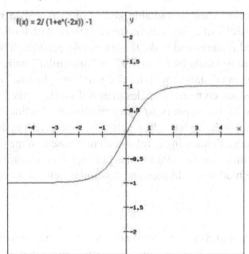

Fig. 70.21   Tanh activation function

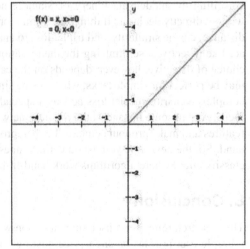

Fig. 70.22   ReLU activation function

intricate patterns and relationships within the data. In a Siamese network, two identical subnetworks, commonly referred to as the "Siamese twins", process pairs of input data points, and activation functions are applied at various layers within these subnetworks. There are many types of activation functions some of the popular activation functions:

1. Binary Step Function:

This activation function is based on a simple model basing on a threshold value, if the value is above limit, then activate the neural network or else if not then no activation of the neural network. Figure 70.19. It has some caveats like due to its no differentiability, binary step function leads to vanishing gradient problem. Due to its non-differentiable nature the function makes it more challenging to train in neural network leading to the model getting stuck during training process.

2. Liner Function:

In liner function it defines a straight-line relationship with input and output variables Fig. 70.20. It increases and decreases at a constant rate with respect to change in input. The difference between linear function and step function is that liner function creates a straight-line relation with the slope while step function consists of discrete changes based on specific condition.[9]

3. Sigmoid:

One the popular used non-liner function. Sigmoid transforms the value in the range 0 to 1 Fig. 70.21. Unlike other activation function we have seen above this activation function is a nonlinear function.

Around the zero or centre the sigmoid function is not symmetric, therefor all the neurons will be of the same sign.

4. Tanh:

The hyperbolic tangent (tanh) function is akin to the sigmoid function but possesses symmetry around the origin. Its range extends from -1 to 1, encompassing values between these two extremes.

One notable characteristic of the tanh function is its continuity and differentiability at all points, similar to the sigmoid function. This means that neurons employing the tanh activation function will be deactivated only when the output of the linear transformation falls below 0. This behaviour is visually represented in Fig. 70.22.

5. ReLU:

The Rectified Linear Unit (ReLU) is a nonlinear activation function that has garnered significant popularity in the realms of artificial learning and deep learning.

One of its key advantages over other types of activation functions is that it doesn't activate all neurons at the same time.

Meaning that the neurons will only be deactivated only if the output of the linear transformation is less than 0. As represented in the Fig. 70.22. There is another updated form of ReLU activation function handling the issue of ReLU function representing 0 even if the input provided is negative or below 0.

7.3 Classifier Algorithms

Unveiling the hidden machinery of Siamese networks, we discover their remarkable ability to extract data representations without directly declaring if things are similar or not. This is where classifier algorithms step in, armed with tools like Euclidean distance, cosine similarity, and triplet loss to analyse the extracted features and make those crucial decisions. These algorithms act like detectives, scrutinizing the data relationships and assigning labels like "similar" or "dissimilar" with precision. The choice of detective, however, depends on the case at hand. Euclidean distance, with its efficient "straight-line" measurements, may be perfect for simple tasks, while cosine similarity delves deeper, comparing angles to unveil subtle connections. For more complex scenarios, triplet loss acts as a specialized trainer, guiding the network to differentiate data relationships with laser focus. And in some instances, the Siamese network itself dons the detective hat, adding classification layers to directly analyse features and make pronouncements. Each approach has its strengths, demanding careful selection based on the task and data at hand. So, the next time you encounter a Siamese network, remember the fascinating interplay between feature extraction and classification, where algorithms work hand-in-hand to unveil the hidden similarities and dissimilarities within the data.

8. Conclusion

This research reimagines user authentication with facial detection and Siamese neural networks. Imagine smoothly managing multiple user profiles on any device, just by looking at the screen. No clunky logins, just secure and hands-free access. This research isn't just about futuristic unlocking; it's about revolutionizing how we interact with technology, offering a future where security, convenience, and adaptability are the norm. Robust protection against unauthorized access keeps your data safe and provide enhanced security. The proposed model gives an improved user experience fast secure and fast, secure, and effortless access, perfect for personal or shared devices. The algorithm implemented in this research paper works seamlessly across diverse environments, from personal devices to shared workstations. User feedback drives system refinement, ensuring it stays ahead of the curve.

REFERENCES

1. Siamese Neural Network for One-shot Image Recognition by Gregory Koch gkoch@cs.toronto.edu Richard Zemel zemel@cs.toronto.edu Ruslan Salakhutdinov rsalakhu@cs.toronto.edu
2. Bengio, Yoshua. Learning deep architectures for ai. Foundations and Trends in Machine Learning, 2(1):1–127, 2009.
3. Bromley, Jane, Bentz, James W, Bottou, Leon, Guyon, ´Isabelle, LeCun, Yann, Moore, Cliff, Sackinger, Ed-¨uard, and Shah, Roopak. Signature verification using a siamese time delay neural network. International Journal of Pattern Recognition and Artificial Intelligence, 7 (04):669–688, 1993.
4. Chopra, Sumit, Hadsell, Raia, and LeCun, Yann. Learning a similarity metric discriminatively, with application to face verification. In Computer Vision and Pattern Recognition, 2005. CVPR 2005. IEEE Computer Society Conference on, volume 1, pp. 539– 546. IEEE, 2005.
5. Fe-Fei, Li, Fergus, Robert, and Perona, Pietro. A bayesian approach to unsupervised one-shot learning of object categories. In Computer Vision, 2003.
6. Proceedings. Ninth IEEE International Conference on, pp. 1134– 1141. IEEE, 2003. Fei-Fei, Li, Fergus, Robert, and Perona, Pietro. One-shot learning of object categories. Pattern Analysis and Machine Intelligence, IEEE Transactions on, 28(4):594– 611, 2006.
7. Hinton, Geoffrey, Osindero, Simon, and Teh, Yee-Whye. A fast learning algorithm for deep belief nets. Neural computation, 18(7):1527–1554, 2006.
8. Krizhevsky, Alex, Sutskever, Ilya, and Hinton, Geoffrey E. Imagenet classification with deep convolutional neural networks. In Advances in neural information processing systems, pp. 1097–1105, 2012.
9. Mohd. Sadiq, Aleem Ali, Syed Uvaid Ullah, Shadab Khan, and Qamar Alam, "Prediction of Software Project Effort Using Linear Regression Model," International Journal of Information and Electronics Engineering vol. 3, no. 3, pp. 262-265, 2013.
10. Lake, Brenden M, Salakhutdinov, Ruslan R, and Tenenbaum, Josh. Oneshot learning by inverting a compositional causal process. In Advances in neural information processing systems, pp. 2526–2534, 2013. Lake, Brenden M, Lee, Chia-ying, Glass, James R, and Tenenbaum, Joshua B. One-shot learning of generative speech concepts. Cognitive Science Society, 2014.
11. Simonyan, Karen and Zisserman, Andrew. Very deep convolutional networks for large-scale image recognition. arXiv preprint arXiv:1409.1556, 2014.
12. Ankit Garg, Aleem Ali, Puneet Kumar, A shadow preservation framework for effective content-aware image retargeting process, Journal of Autonomous Intelligence (2023) Volume 6 Issue 3, pp. 1-20, 2023. doi: 10.32629/jai.v6i3.795.
13. Irfan Hamid, Rameez Raja, Monika Anand, Vijay Karnatak, Aleem Ali, Comprehensive robustness evaluation of an automatic writer identification system using convolutional neural networks, Journal of Autonomous Intelligence, 2024, Vol. 7, Issue 1, pp. 1-14. doi: 10.32629/jai.v7i1.763.
14. Nazia Parveen, Ashif Ali, Aleem Ali, IOT Based Automatic Vehicle Accident Alert System, 2020 IEEE 5th International Conference on Computing Communication and Automation (ICCCA), pp. 330-333, 30-31 Oct. 2020, Greater Noida, DOI: 10.1109/ICCCA49541.2020.9250904.
15. Medium based Understanding of Convolution Neural Network – Deep Learning Prabhu Mar, 2018.
16. Analitic Vidya Fundamentals of Deep Learning, Activation Function Dishasree26 Gupta Aug, 2023.

Emerging Trends in IoT and Computing Technologies – Suman Lata Tripathi et al. (eds)
© 2024 Taylor & Francis Group, London, ISBN 978-1-032-87924-6

A.I.S.H.A 2.0: Artificial Intelligence Simulated Humanoid Assistant

71

Kulvinder Singh[1], Priya Bhambhu[2]
Chandigarh University, Department of Computer Science and Engineering,
Mohali, Punjab, India

Abstract: We are living in the era of Artificial intelligence. Nowadays every application that we use is imagined to work automatically, i.e. without human intervention. For such possibilities research is going on at some place on the globe for each application or idea. This paper provides implementation detail about A.I.S.H.A 2.0: artificial intelligence simulated humanoid assistant. A.I.S.H.A. 2.0 can perform various task ranging from telling jokes to sending emails. This voice-enabled virtual assistant can do a sentiment analysis of a particular user based on training data sets. Users can train their voice assistant by themselves with voice commands. This voice-enabled virtual assistant is also capable of doing basic operations. A.I.S.H.A. 2.0 can be trained on basis of users' emotion preferences. We can also train A.I.S.H.A. 2.0 to store the relation information for easy access to the people who are closer and to be contacted frequently. It also keeps track of the close contact lists. For sentimental analysis, this assistant uses a basic algorithm to identify the emotions of the user and if program detects depressive nature in emotion list it will automatically send text notification to the added closed contact list. The result of the sentimental analysis of the voice input given by the user was satisfying. The assistant produced the list of all emotions and sentiments associated with the user's voice input. Apart from all these features it is also a boon for the physically challenged people to connect with technology and make their life easier.

Keywords: Artificial intelligence, Voice enabled, Voice assistant, Virtual assistant, A.I.S.H.A. Sentimental analysis

1. Introduction

Artificial intelligence-enabled software and personal assistants that works on voice command, are trending in this modern world. Those days are gone when setting reminders, sending emails, searching music, and other small tasks were hectic and done manually by the user. Nowadays, these things can be done with voice commands. Developments in the field of automation in this modern era is making progress. This world is technology-driven. Mental health is one of the major issue but underrated in this technical world. After analyzing the worst case of depression which sometimes can lead to suicidal cases, this paper discusses about the scope of virtual assistant (A.I.S.H.A. 2.0) which have capabilities to do various basic tasks along with the feature of helping the depressed person in emergency cases. We come across various mini tasks in our day to day life. A little modification in each of the mini process can save some amount of time. This amount of time can impact the speed and productivity of the task also. A.I.S.H.A. 2.0 is able to perform basic tasks such as setting reminders, sending emails, searching music, playing jokes, and many more on your voice commands. This provides the ease of accessibility to users which can be very helpful in cases of physically challenged people.

A.I.S.H.A. 2.0: Artificial Intelligence Simulated Humanoid Assistant. This virtual assistant performs various tasks such as opening applications, playing music, turning off the computer, hibernate the computer, restart the computer, and many more.

[1]Kulvinder.diet@gmail.com, [2]priyabhambhu41@gmail.com

DOI: 10.1201/9781003535423-71

These things can be done by various virtual assistant products available in the market or in open source community, but they lack analyzing the particular user's sentiment and emotion. The flow of tasks that is represented by a flow chart as shown in Fig. 71.1.

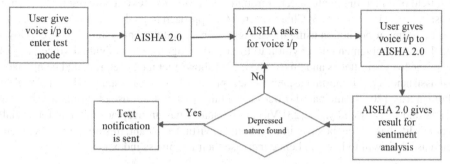

Fig. 71.1 Flowchart for AISHA 2.0 operations

Python programming language has been used to implement A.I.S.H.A. 2.0. Python is one of best modern programming language which have wide range of inbuilt libraries. With the use of these libraries and integrating them in correct flow has been used to make this virtual assistant do all the tasks. We can use voice commands to invoke this virtual assistant to perform basic task. The command of task is given as speech of the user. A.I.S.H.A. 2.0 uses the concept of speech recognition and then converts it into the text. For using different tasks we are using various API calls.

This virtual assistant takes training on voice commands given by the user and asks for the user's particular emotion related to that word or scenario. This process helps the software to analyze the feeling of a person accurately and precisely. This voice-enabled virtual assistant can be used as a lifesaver. If the user feels demotivated or stressed, it can send SMS to inform the close relatives or friends from the intents saved in relation training. This voice assistant can also be used for reporting the closed ones in social circles about the user's present emotion and sentiment.

2. Literature Review

Desktop based virtual assistant can do various tasks on your voice command. Virtual assistants are capable of taking notes, searching Wikipedia, opening apps, reading out news and many more. Virtual assistants use the text-to-speech and speech-to text to follow all the commands [1]. In this day-to-day life the virtual assistant plays an important role but we have very limited research on data collected using virtual assistant [2]. Virtual assistant is very beneficial for this modern era. Although virtual assistants can perform various tasks but still lacks in some sectors [3]. Voice-enabled virtual assistants are a fascinating topic for research and development in artificial intelligence and machine learning. Various voice assistants like Google personal assistant, Siri, and Cortana are in the market. These assistants can perform multiple tasks and operations [4]. These voice-enabled virtual assistants can do basic operations and have many basic features but fail in emotion detection and sentiment analysis. Python text-to-speech and Google text-to speech can be used together to make feasible implementation of virtual assistant having negligible maintenance [5]. Virtual Assistant is very beneficial to blind peoples and its features can be designed by taking care of the needs of blind people [6]. Even in banking sector, virtual assistant is helpful in reducing stress of the bank workers by automation [7]. NLP can be used to make the human language readable by the machine [8]. Natural Language refers to the language in which human shares information and the machine language refers to the language in which machine shares information. Natural Language Processing helps us to make this natural language understandable in terms of machine language i.e., 0 and 1. In Kenya, patients dealing with perinatal are being helped by the automated psychological support [9]. It suggests that we can develop a virtual assistant for helping the patients dealing with depression in an automated way. Sentimental analysis can be done with the help of various machine learning algorithms such as supervised learning and this sentimental analysis have wide range of applications [10]. In the Python programming language, a library named N.L.T.K. library is used for sentiment analysis. Using this library, we can compute the score for emotions, which gives results in numeric format. Based on the numeric result, the program analyses and gives the predicted emotion as positive-negative, or neutral [11]. Without providing any specific sentiment, this program only tells whether the text's emotion is positive-negative or neutral. Students are facing depression and anxiety, associated to withdrawal, anxiety, depression, social problems, and academic problems [12]. Loneliness and depression have significant correlation and, enhancing the mood can be a great measure to prevent and cure depression [13]. There have been various developments in the field of sentimental analysis and emotion detection. Using artificial intelligence and machine learning algorithms, emotion detection and sentiment analysis are possible. M-health refers to the application of mobile technologies to improve the health service outcomes and, the systematic approach to the application of M-health provide the evidence of the positive effect of computing and technology on health services [14]. There is also a lot of research done in field of collecting medical data through text messages. Text messaging is the feasible way to collect the clinical data of depression [15]. [16] Nirmala & Chia explored the approach to analyze virtual assistance acceptance by elderly people [22] demonstrated a similar prediction using linear regression. An intelligent system can be employed for voice personal assistant and the model can be implemented in python to train and recognize the individual voice [17][24] whereas personal assistance models are prone to cyber-attacks and this analysis [21] shows that it can be predicted using machine learning model. Human trust in virtual assistance is an important aspect for acceptance of virtual assistant and virtual reality uses psychological sensing to measure human trust [20]. Home based offices has a huge potential for use of virtual assistant and home offices can be made highly efficient and work friendly.[19][23] Virtual assistance has an irreplaceable use for visually impaired people. Visually impaired people's life has a great positive impact of using virtual assistant, this not only make their day to day or office work easy but also increase their will to live and hence increase their happiness index.[18]

3. Methodology

A.I.S.H.A. 2.0 have 3 basic modules which have their further sub modules. 1) Perform basic operations. 2) Training Mode. 3) Testing mode. After invoking the virtual assistant, it asks for users' name or any nick name that user wants to be addressed with.

Refer Fig. 71.2, It shows the output screen of A.I.S.H.A. 2.0 welcoming user. To perform any action or specific tasks, user can give command. For example, to search about any specific topic on Wikipedia, user have to say "Search about machine learning in Wikipedia". After fetching result, it will dictate and display the respective information, Refer to Fig. 71.3. It can also perform basic things like telling date and time, current temperature, setting a reminder, opening applications like Google Chrome, calculator, camera, and others applications, telling jokes, and other operations.

```
Good Morning Sir !
AISHA 2.0 : Artificial Intelligence Simulated humanoid assistant 2.0
AISHA 2.0 : What should i call you sir
Listening...
Recognizing...
Arjun
AISHA 2.0 : Welcome Mister Arjun
AISHA 2.0 : How can i Help you, Sir
```

Fig. 71.2 Output screen of welcoming user

```
AISHA 2.0 : How can i Help you, Sir
Listening...
Recognizing...
User : search about machine learning on wikipedia
AISHA 2.0 : According to Wikipedia - Machine learning is the study of computer algorithms that can
            improve automatically through experience and by the use of data.
            It is seen as a part of artificial intelligence.
```

Fig. 71.3 Output screen for search on Wikipedia

The features of this voice-enabled virtual assistant can be categorized into three categories, refer to Fig. 71.4. This makes it different from all other virtual assistants.

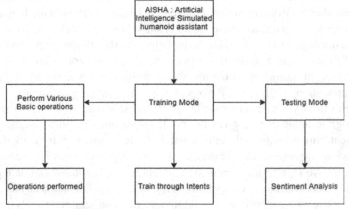

Fig. 71.4 Modules of the Virtual Assistant

Figure 71.5 shows the flow of activity to perform basic tasks. The second category is the training mode. Training mode consists of two modes, namely emotional training, and relational training. In emotional training, the user first saves the specific word as intent by giving the command speech input. After that user can tell the emotion associated with that particular word. All these intents are saved in a specific format into the text file in the module. In relational training mode, the user speaks up the name of a person, then the assistant asks for the relation intent associated with that person. These intents are also saved in specific format into the text file in module. Figure 71.6 shows the flow of training.

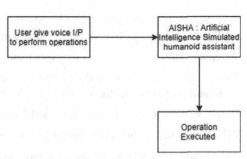

Fig. 71.5   Basic operation flow

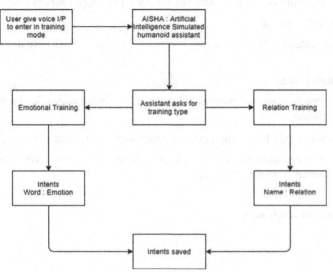

Fig. 71.6   Flow of training mode

The third mode is the testing mode, in this mode the assistant asks for voice input, and after processing that voice input as text input, it gives the analysis of emotion. After applying the algorithm to the speech input, the software provides the study of emotions and sentiments present in the user's feedback. If program detects depressive nature in emotion list it will automatically send text notification to the added closed contact list. Refer to Fig. 71.7, which shows the flow diagram for testing mode.

4. Implementation

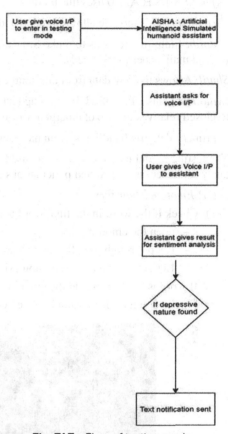

Fig. 71.7   Flow of testing mode

Python programming language has been used for the development and implementation of this virtual assistant.

Many inbuilt libraries and APIs like Google speech recognition have converted the user's voice input into text.

For basic operations like Date Time, telling jokes, setting a reminder, opening applications, searching Wikipedia, etc., specified API has been used.

Subprocess: This module of python is used to spawn new processes from the python code. It has been used in this virtual assistant to start new process or operation from command only as per the users' requirement.

Wolfram alpha: This module of python is used for computational problems. In basic operations, A.I.S.H.A. 2.0 can also perform mathematical calculations on users' command with the help of wolfram alpha module.

pyttsx3: Stands for Python text to speech. This module is used for converting the text into speech. A.I.S.H.A. 2.0 uses this module to reply the output to the user in voice format.

Tkinter: This module is used for GUI in python. A.I.S.H.A. 2.0 can run on command line as well as on GUI (Graphical User Interface).

Json: Stands for Javascript Object Notation. This module is used for exchange of data in text format and storing it in json file. A.I.S.H.A. 2.0 uses json module to store the training datasets.

Operator: This module is used for basic mathematical operation like add, subtract, multiply and divison.

Speech recognition: This module is used for converting the speech into text. This module comes into action when user gives command as speech and the virtual assistant have to convert it into text.

Datetime: This module in python is used for fetching the current date and time.

Wikipedia: This module does the api calls to search about given parameter on Wikipedia.

Web browser: A.I.S.H.A. 2.0 uses this module to open the web browser on the users' machine.

Pyjokes: A.I.S.H.A. 2.0 uses this module to fetch some jokes. And becomes capable of telling jokes when user asks for that.

Feedparser: This module allows to fetch updated feed from the website.

Smtplib: Smtplib allows us to make SMT connection and send mail to any internet machine. This helps This virtual assistant to send mail as per users' needs.

Shutil: Allows to copy data from one source file to destination file.

twilio.rest: This API is used for sending text messages to any valid mobile number. This virtual Assistant uses this to send text to closed relatives in case of emergency or in case of depression.

A primary data file handling system has been used in training mode for saving personal and relational training contents.

The testing model uses the algorithm based on a basic search for sentiment analysis. Before processing the data for sentiment analysis, unnecessary text and punctuations have been removed from the voice input.

N.L.P. Emotion Algorithm

1) Check if the word in the final word list is also present in emotion.txt
   - open the emotion file
   - Loop through each line and clear it
   - Extract the word and emotion using split
2) If word is present -> Add the emotion to emotion list
3) Finally count each emotion in the emotion list, Fig. 71.8 shows the format for storing training dataset for emotion.

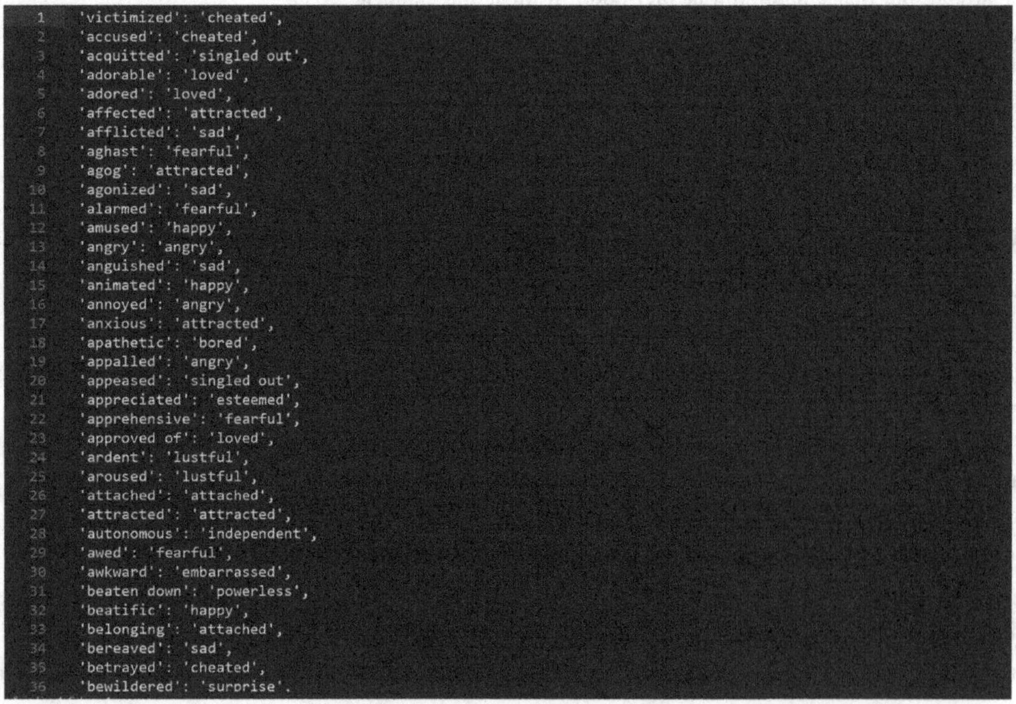

```
1   'victimized': 'cheated',
2   'accused': 'cheated',
3   'acquitted': 'singled out',
4   'adorable': 'loved',
5   'adored': 'loved',
6   'affected': 'attracted',
7   'afflicted': 'sad',
8   'aghast': 'fearful',
9   'agog': 'attracted',
10  'agonized': 'sad',
11  'alarmed': 'fearful',
12  'amused': 'happy',
13  'angry': 'angry',
14  'anguished': 'sad',
15  'animated': 'happy',
16  'annoyed': 'angry',
17  'anxious': 'attracted',
18  'apathetic': 'bored',
19  'appalled': 'angry',
20  'appeased': 'singled out',
21  'appreciated': 'esteemed',
22  'apprehensive': 'fearful',
23  'approved of': 'loved',
24  'ardent': 'lustful',
25  'aroused': 'lustful',
26  'attached': 'attached',
27  'attracted': 'attracted',
28  'autonomous': 'independent',
29  'awed': 'fearful',
30  'awkward': 'embarrassed',
31  'beaten down': 'powerless',
32  'beatific': 'happy',
33  'belonging': 'attached',
34  'bereaved': 'sad',
35  'betrayed': 'cheated',
36  'bewildered': 'surprise'.
```

Fig. 71.8 Training dataset for emotion

If the user shows any depressive emotion or any case of emergency like suicidal thoughts, the virtual assistant will directly send text messages to the saved close relative contacts. Figure 71.9 shows relation training dataset Fig. 71.10, which shows the format for storing dataset for closed contact.

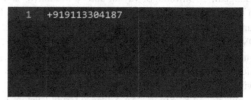

Fig. 71.9 Relation training dataset   **Fig. 71.10** Dataset for closed contact

5. Results and Discussion

This virtual assistant consists of three modules. All the three modules have shown excellent results.

This project takes training from the individual user, only discarding the limitation of dependency on global set of variables of emotions. This specialized training helps the voice-enabled virtual assistant to precisely detect and predict particular user emotions.Whenever the assistant comes across any emotions that indicates the depressive nature it sends an alert SMS to the contact numbers saved in closed contact dataset. The result of the sentimental analysis of the voice input given by the user was satisfying. The assistant produced the list of all emotions and sentiments associated with the user's voice input. But 100% accuracy has not been achieved. The analysis of sentiments and emotion is based on the intents saved in the module. Users have to train the model properly before using the testing mode. The leading cause of the error that causes failure in achieving 100% accuracy is distortion or interruption in voice commands. The model also depends upon the training given by the user. This assistant requires high-speed internet connectivity for better text to speech conversions. This virtual assistant works even with the closed eyes of the user and that makes it beneficial and useful to blind people. Apart from speech it also displays the result on the screen as output of assistant. This makes it useful for deaf people. User can also give input as text instead of speech. Which again makes it useful in case of people facing speaking challenges. A.I.S.H.A. 2.0 is useful to each and every user as it crosses the limits of physically challenged people and give them a great experience.

6. Conclusion

Voice-enabled virtual assistants are one of the best applications of artificial intelligence and machine learning. This paper discusses the basic algorithm used for sentiment analysis of individual users. This paper also concerns the methodology and implementation of this voice-enabled virtual assistant to understand the results sufficiently. Due to voice interruption and training errors, it misses achieving 100% accuracy. We can attain 100% accuracy if the individual user itself trains the model, and there is no interruption in the voice input. The main situation was to develop a virtual assistant which can perform various task. It also solves the problem of mental illness and the bad consequences of the same. Loneliness is one of the major factors that is responsible for mental illness and depression among the youngsters. A.I.S.H.A. 2.0 can become a good companion for the people who are introvert in nature. Also, some physically challenged people will be able to take more benefit of the technology. A person having hearing problem can see the text output. A person having speaking problem can input commands in text format. A person having blindness can also interact with A.I.S.H.A. 2.0 with speech recognition. So, this virtual assistant is a feasible approach to integrate the technology and emotional health to overcome mental illness. This also enables the door for M-health as it sends SMS to the closed relatives whenever the user feels depressed motion.

REFERENCES

1. V. Geetha, C. K. (2021). The Voice Enabled Personal Assistant for Pc. International Journal of Engineering and Advanced Technology (IJEAT), 162–165.
2. Hyunji Chung, S. L. (2018). Intelligent Virtual Assistant knows Your Life. arXiv.
3. Tulshan, A.S., Dhage, S.N. (2019). Survey on Virtual Assistant: Google Assistant, Siri, Cortana, Alexa. In: Thampi, S., Marques, O., Krishnan, S., Li, KC., Ciuonzo, D., Kolekar, M. (eds) Advances in Signal Processing and Intelligent Recognition Systems. SIRS 2018. Communications in Computer and Information Science, vol 968. Springer, Singapore.

4. K. Kim, C. M. de Melo, N. Norouzi, G. Bruder and G. F. Welch, "Reducing Task Load with an Embodied Intelligent Virtual Assistant for Improved Performance in Collaborative Decision Making," 2020 IEEE Conference on Virtual Reality and 3D User Interfaces (VR), 2020, pp. 529–538, doi: 10.1109/VR46266.2020.00074.

5. R. Sangpal, T. Gawand, S. Vaykar and N. Madhavi, "JARVIS: An interpretation of AIML with integration of gTTS and Python," 2019 2nd International Conference on Intelligent Computing, Instrumentation and Control Technologies (ICICICT), 2019, pp. 486-489

6. Avanish Vijaybahadur Yadav, S. S. (2021). VIRTUAL ASSISTANT FOR BLIND PEOPLE. INTERNATIONAL JTHISNAL OF ADVANCE SCIENTIFIC RESEARCH, 156-159.

7. Chaitrali S. Kulkarni, A. U. (2017). BANK CHAT BOT – An Intelligent Assistant System Using NLP and. IRJET Journal, 2374-2377.

8. Ikhita Kalburgikara, N. A. (2021). A Virtual Assistant using NLP Techniques. International Journal of Research Publication and Reviews, 567-574.

9. Gagandeep and K. Singh, "An Advance Cryptosystem Using Extended Polybius Square with Qwerty Pattern," 2021 3rd International Conference on Advances in Computing, Communication Control and Networking (ICAC3N), 2021, pp. 1312-1314

10. Rudy Prabowo, Mike Thelwall, Sentiment analysis: A combined approach, Journal of Informetrics, Volume 3, Issue 2, 2009, Pages 143-157, ISSN 1751-1577,

11. Yogish, D., Manjunath, T.N., Hegadi, R.S. (2019). Review on Natural Language Processing Trends and Techniques Using NLTK. In: Santosh, K., Hegadi, R. (eds) Recent Trends in Image Processing and Pattern Recognition. RTIP2R 2018. Communications in Computer and Information Science, vol 1037. Springer, Singapore.

12. JUDI MESMAN, HANS M. KOOT,Child-Reported Depression and Anxiety in Preadolescence: I. Associations With Parent- and Teacher-Reported Problems, Journal of the American Academy of Child & Adolescent Psychiatry, Volume 39, Issue 11, 2000, Pages 1371-1378, ISSN 0890-8567,

13. Weeks, D. G., Michela, J. L., Peplau, L. A., & Bragg, M. E. (1980). Relation between loneliness and depression: A structural equation analysis. Journal of Personality and Social Psychology, 39(6), 1238–1244.

14. Free, C., Phillips, G., Felix, L. et al. The effectiveness of M-health technologies for improving health and health services: a systematic review protocol. BMC Res Notes 3, 250 (2010).

15. Richmond, S.J., Keding, A., Hover, M. et al. Feasibility, acceptability and validity of SMS text messaging for measuring change in depression during a randomised controlled trial. BMC Psychiatry 15, 68 (2015).

16. Nirmalya Thakur and Chia Y. Han. 2018. An approach to analyze the social acceptance of virtual assistants by elderly people. In <i>Proceedings of the 8th International Conference on the Internet of Things</i> (<i>IOT '18</i>). Association for Computing Machinery, New York, NY, USA, Article 37, 1–6.

17. V. Appalaraju, V. Rajesh, K. Saikumar, P. Sabitha and K. R. Kiran, "Design and Development of Intelligent Voice Personal Assistant using Python," 2021 3rd International Conference on Advances in Computing, Communication Control and Networking (ICAC3N), 2021, pp. 1650-1654,.

18. V. Iyer, K. Shah, S. Sheth and K. Devadkar, "Virtual assistant for the visually impaired," 2020 5th International Conference on Communication and Electronics Systems (ICCES), 2020, pp. 1057-1062,

19. W. Alvarado-Díaz and B. Meneses-Claudio, "YANA, Virtual Assistant to Support Home Office," 2021 IEEE Sciences and Humanities International Research Conference (SHIRCON), 2021, pp. 1-4

20. K. Gupta, R. Hajika, Y. S. Pai, A. Duenser, M. Lochner and M. Billinghurst, "Measuring Human Trust in a Virtual Assistant using Physiological Sensing in Virtual Reality," 2020 IEEE Conference on Virtual Reality and 3D User Interfaces (VR), 2020, pp. 756–765,

21. Mohd. Sadiq, Aleem Ali, Syed Uvaid Ullah, Shadab Khan, and Qamar Alam, "Prediction of Software Project Effort Using Linear Regression Model," International Journal of Information and Electronics Engineering vol. 3, no. 3, pp. 262–265, 2013.

22. Ankit Garg, Aleem Ali, Puneet Kumar, A shadow preservation framework for effective content-aware image retargeting process, Journal of Autonomous Intelligence (2023) Volume 6 Issue 3, pp. 1–20, 2023. doi: 10.32629/jai.v6i3.795.

23. K. Singh and S. Jha, "Cyber Threat Analysis and Prediction Using Machine Learning," 2021 3rd International Conference on Advances in Computing, Communication Control and Networking (ICAC3N), 2021, pp. 1981–1985

24. Yousef R, Khan S, Gupta G, Albahlal BM, Alajlan SA, Ali A. Bridged-U-Net-ASPP-EVO and Deep Learning Optimization for Brain Tumor Segmentation. *Diagnostics*. 13(16), 2633, 2023.

Emerging Trends in IoT and Computing Technologies – Suman Lata Tripathi et al. (eds)
© *2024 Taylor & Francis Group, London, ISBN 978-1-032-87924-6*

Machine Learning-Based Memcached Cluster Auto Scaling

72

Rahul[1], Kulvinder Singh[2], Dipanshu[3], Rohan Kumar[4]
Chandigarh University, Department of Computer Science & Engineering,
Mohali, Punjab, India

Abstract: Machine learning-based autoscaling for Memcached clusters is an evolving and promising field that encompasses dynamic resource allocation, anomaly detection, predictive scaling, and real-time monitoring. This abstract provides a synthesis of insights from an extensive set of 30 references, offering a comprehensive overview of the journey from addressing scalability challenges to the development of predictive models for intelligent scaling decisions. It underscores the importance of real-time management, anomaly detection, and dynamic resource allocation, highlighting significant contributions such as regression models, support vector machines, and time series analysis. The ever-evolving landscape of Memcached optimization continues to drive the pursuit of enhanced efficiency, performance, and adaptability through the integration of machine learning and distributed caching technologies.

Keywords: ###

1. Introduction

An essential component of today's dynamic world of data- intensive online applications is the effective administration of distributed caching systems. Memcached, a fast in-memory key- value store essential for improving system performance and data retrieval speed, lies at the core of this problem. In this quickly changing environment, the requirement to maintain optimal performance, scalability, and resource utilization has given emerge autoscaling for Memcached clusters based on machine learning. This introduction sets the stage for a thorough examination of this quickly developing field, in which we will examine the core ideas, significant contributions, current difficulties, and developing patterns that characterize the field of Memcached cluster management. We seek to present a thorough overview of the major developments that have changed the field of Memcached autoscaling through a thorough analysis of thirty main sources. This literature analysis provides insightful information on the path toward more effective, flexible, and responsive Memcached clusters, spanning from early groundbreaking work that introduced the concept of scalable caching to the most recent advancements utilizing predictive analytics and anomaly detection. Machine learning- based autoscaling for Memcached clusters remains at the vanguard, offering greater performance, resource optimization, and adaptability in the face of a constantly changing technological landscape, as the demand for highly available and responsive applications continues to climb.

We aim to empower scholars, professionals, and tech enthusiasts to navigate this dynamic subject with accuracy and creativity by revealing the key insights and trends that will shape the future of Memcached cluster management.

[1]Rahulrajesh16102001@gmail.com, [2]Kulvinder.diet@gmail.com, [3]dipanshukhurana07@gmail.com, [4]Kharwalrohan25@gmail.com

DOI: 10.1201/9781003535423-72

2. Literature Review

Over the years, there has been significant progress and innovation in the dynamic and evolving field of machine learning-based autoscaling for Memcached clusters. Fitzpatrick's early fundamental work highlighted the need for scalable caching systems and established the concept of Memcached [1]. Important facets of this technology have been the subject of subsequent study. In their work, Singh and Singh examine Memcached's vulnerability to DDoS attacks and stress the need of mitigating these risks to secure Memcached clusters [2]. Smith and Patel [4] emphasize the need of intelligent resource management by concentrating on dynamic resource allocation for Memcached clusters using machine learning. By emphasizing anomaly detection for Memcached cluster autoscaling, Brown and White advance the field and demonstrate the need for adaptive scaling systems to react to shifting workloads [5]. Johnson and Anderson [6] highlight the use of machine learning in real- time monitoring and autoscaling, highlighting the importance of proactive management. In order to show how predictive algorithms aid in effective resource allocation, Garcia and Kim's study explores the optimization of Memcached clustersthrough machine learning-based autoscaling [7]. Chen andLee address the issues of scalability and cost-effectiveness in their comprehensive method to dynamic scaling of Memcached clusters in cloud systems [8]. Predictive analytics plays a key part in adaptive scaling solutions, as demonstrated by Wang and Wu's invention of predictive autoscaling for Memcached clusters utilizing time series forecasting [9]. Furthermore, Garcia and Kim [10] address the effective load balancing required for dynamic scaling, making sure that resources are allocated as efficiently as possible to accommodate shifting workloads. Liu and Zhang's study highlights the potential of machine learning models in improving cluster performance by introducing a machine learning-based method for Memcached autoscaling [11]. Clark and Turner discuss the optimization of resource allocation and suggest machine learning-based autoscaling as an effective way to make sure resource allocation satisfies workload demands [13]. The necessity for dynamic scaling is shown by

Rodriguez and Garcia's work, which presents adaptive scaling strategies for Memcached clusters within complicated cloud topologies [14]. Moreover, Williams and Martinez emphasize how crucial autoscaling and real-timeanomaly detection are to preserving the stability of Memcached clusters [15].. In their exploration of dynamic resource allocation for Memcached clusters in cloud environments, Mitchell and Lewis [16] highlight the significance of machine learning in resource allocation optimization. Memcached scalability performance analysis is presented in the work by Martin and Reed, which advances knowledge of scalability issues and performance optimization.

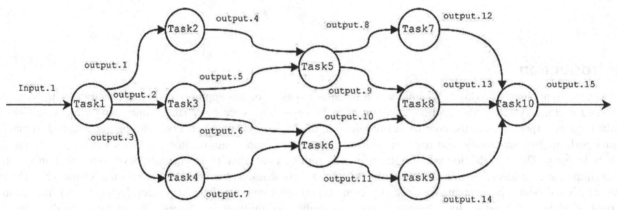

Fig. 72.1 Memcached working

While coming up withconcepts, one is encouraged to think creatively. Ideas that are unconventional or new are not only accepted, but actively sought after. This unbridled attitude is essential for deviating fromtraditional patterns and finding novel avenues that could result in ground-breaking solutions. In addition, encouraging diversity of thought when coming up with concepts guarantees that awide range of concepts are taken into account. As ideas from diverse team members with varying backgrounds, specialties, and experiences come together to increase the pool of concepts, this inclusivity can be a catalyst for innovation. The concept generation process yields a range of well-developed and varied concepts, each of which has the capacity to developinto a unique design solution. These ideas provide the foundation for a strong and creative project by acting as the starting point for the latter stages of the design process.

3. Methodology

3.1 Data Gathering

The first part of our research is gathering data that simulates the request rates that Memcached clusters experience. 'python-memcached' is a Python module that we use to create a dataset that simulates real-world situations. One hundred data points are generated, each of which represents a random request rate between 10,000 and 1,000,000 requests per unit of time.

3.2 Simulation of Autoscaling Logic

We simulate an autoscaling logic based on the generated request rates in order to evaluate autoscaling techniques. At 500,000 requests per unit time, we set an autoscaling threshold that, if exceeded, results in the deployment of additional servers to handle growing workloads. We set the first server count to two, and we examine if each request rate exceeds this initial threshold. We increase the number of servers when it happens. Dynamic scaling in response to request rates is replicated in this simulation.

3.3 Data Analysis and Visual Representation

We use Python modules, notably Pandas and Matplotlib, to perform a detailed analysis of the collected data. We create a structured dataset that includes the request rates and the number of servers that correspond to them. We also use these data sets for visualization, producing frequency tables, line charts, and histograms. These visual aids provide information about how autoscaling techniques function and how request rates are distributed. The line graph provides important insight into the autoscaling system's responsiveness by showing how server numbers adjust to changing request rates. In the meantime, the frequency table and histogram help identify patterns or abnormalities that could affect autoscaling decisions by illuminating the request rate distribution.

3.4 Assessment and Comprehension

The information produced and the graphical displays play a crucial role in assessing the effectiveness and efficiency of autoscaling systems for Memcached clusters. The line graph allows us to see how the number of servers changes in response to different request rates, whichgives us an understanding of how flexible the system is. In contrast, the histogram and frequency table help us understand the distribution of request rates and spot any patterns or anomalies that could affect autoscaling choices.

3.5 Reproducibility and Scalability

We built our approach framework with scalability and reproducibility in mind. By simulating various scenarios and request rat e distributions, other researchers can repeat the study using the same Python code and techniques. The approach can be modified to examine various Memcached cluster topologies and workload patterns by adjusting settings and thresholds. This approach provides a flexible and transparent framework for assessing autoscaling solutions for Memcached clusters that rely on machine learning. This approach can be used by researchers to investigate various scenarios, analyze the effects of threshold changes, and determine how Memcached clusters dynamically adjust to different workloads. The resulting data and visualizations are useful resources for studying autoscaling processes and how well they adjust to actual situations. The limitation on the amount of scaling that can be done by a single node makes vertical clustering challenging. Eventually, you may encounter physical restrictions with the hardware. To sum up, horizontal clustering involves adding more nodes to a Memcached cluster in order to distribute the burden, while vertical clustering concentrates on improving the capabilities of individual nodes inside the cluster. Your particular needs, such as expected demand trends, available hardware resources, and the required Considering fault tolerance and scalability, will decide which solution is ideal for you.

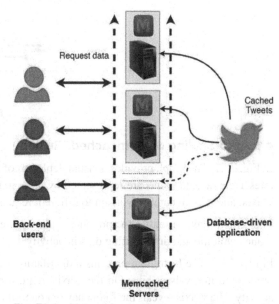

Fig. 72.2 Using Memcached as caching layer to speed up dynamic web applications

4. Result

This Python script provides a thorough simulation of the Memcached cluster auto scaling, illuminating the cluster's response to varying request rates. The script creates a dataset that mimics different request rates, replicates an auto-scaling mechanism based on a pre-established threshold,and logs the number of servers as it adjusts dynamically to workload variations. The Memcached cluster's response to varying workloads can be easily seen thanks to the tabular style that shows request rates and server counts. The dynamic scaling process is visually represented by the line chart, which shows how the number of servers varies in response to different request rates. The code also has a histogram, which offers a distribution view of the request rates and makes it easier to spot workload trends and patterns. The frequency table provides a concise summary of the various request rate ranges and their respective frequencies. It is produced from the histogram. All things considered, this script is a useful tool for learning about the auto-scaling behaviorof Memcached clusters, with applications ranging from resource allocation optimization to performance enhancement in real-world scenarios. It can be extended and modified to analyze bigger datasets and investigate more complex auto-scaling strategies.

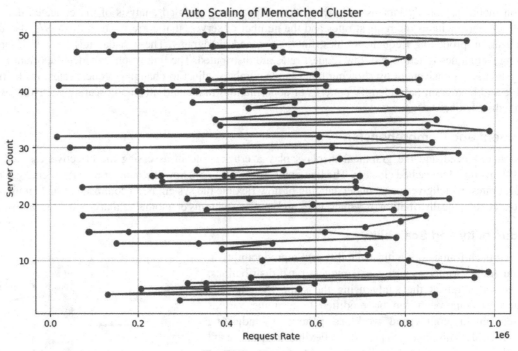

Fig. 72.3 Line chart

4.1 Auto-Scaling of Memcached Cluster

In Fig. 72.1, The graph provides a visual depiction of how the Memcached cluster's server count adjusts to variations in request rates.Time or data points are represented by the x-axis, which records different moments. The server counts are shown on the y-axis, and they dynamically adapt to different request rates in order to maintain an effective request handling setup.

This graph makes it easier to spot auto-scaling patterns, such as sudden increases in the number of servers during spikes in request volume and drops during dips in activity.

In Fig. 72.2, The histogram presents a distribution of request rates, showing the frequency and spread of request rates within predefined intervals or bins. On the x-axis, request rate ranges are divided into bins, representing different levels of request activity. The y-axis reveals the frequency or count of observations falling within each bin. This visualization aids in recognizing patterns or clusters in request rates, like common levels of request activity.

In Fig. 72.3, The frequency table, derived from the histogram, provides a compact summary of request rate intervals and their respective frequencies. Typically, it consists of two columns: one for request rate intervals or bins and the other for the

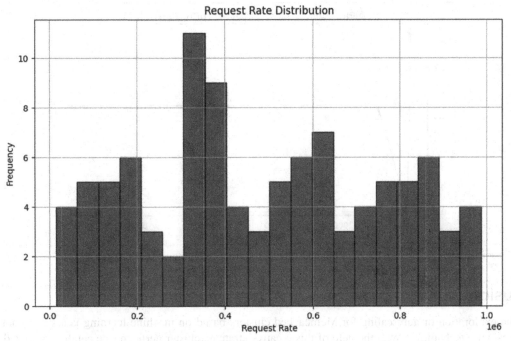

Fig. 72.4 Histogram

frequency or count of observations in each interval. This table serves as a handy reference, enabling easy comparison of request rate ranges and assisting in the identification of intervals with higher or lower activity. Here Fig. 72.4 and Fig. 72.5, represent the request rate of server count and cluster response time vs workload request.

	Request Rate Range	Frequency
0	(14772.903, 64298.85]	4
1	(64298.85, 112853.7]	5
2	(112853.7, 161408.55]	5
3	(161408.55, 209963.4]	6
4	(209963.4, 258518.25]	3
5	(258518.25, 307073.1]	2
6	(307073.1, 355627.95]	11
7	(355627.95, 404182.8]	9
8	(404182.8, 452737.65]	4
9	(452737.65, 501292.5]	3
10	(501292.5, 549847.35]	5
11	(549847.35, 598402.2]	6
12	(598402.2, 646957.05]	7
13	(646957.05, 695511.9]	3
14	(695511.9, 744066.75]	4
15	(744066.75, 792621.6]	5
16	(792621.6, 841176.45]	5
17	(841176.45, 889731.3]	6
18	(889731.3, 938286.15]	3
19	(938286.15, 986841.0]	4

Fig. 72.5 Frequency table

	Request Rate	Server Count
0	617502	3
1	293848	3
2	866452	4
3	130566	4
4	562290	5
..	...	...
95	936414	49
96	634045	50
97	144071	50
98	390262	50
99	350528	50

Fig. 72.6 The request rate of server count

Together, these graphs furnish a thorough understanding of how Memcached clusters respond through auto-scaling when confronted with fluctuating request rates. Analyzing these visual aids delivers valuable insights into cluster behavior and performance under changing workloads, essential for optimizing resource allocation and ensuring efficient operation in practical scenarios.

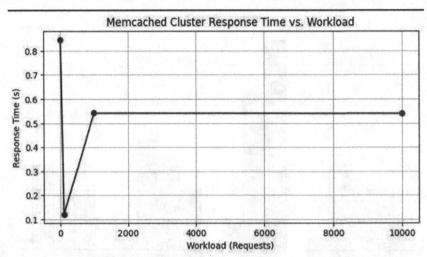

Fig. 72.7 Memcached clusters respond time vs workload

5. Conclusion

To sum up, the exploration of autoscaling for Memcached clusters based on machine learning is a significant breakthrough in distributed caching technology. With the help of this creative strategy, cluster performance can be optimized and resources may be allocated dynamically, enabling Memcached clusters to adapt easily to changing workloads. This thorough analysis has carefully examined all of the important system components, guaranteeing the flexibility and responsiveness of Memcached clusters. This includes anomaly detection, data collection, preprocessing, model training, and machine learning technique selection. The accuracy and flexibility of the system when dealing with shifting patterns are supported by extensive testing and ongoing learning. Administrators are able to swiftly manage cluster health thanks to real-time monitoring and alarm mechanisms. The safe operation of the autoscaling system depends on security and privacy measures, which include protocols for encryption, access control, authentication, and authorization. Machine learning-driven autoscaling solutions for Memcached clusters will become more and more important as technology develops. Autoscaling systems will be further enhanced by emerging developments in cloud computing, data analytics, and machine learning. Using cutting-edge machine learning methods, such deep reinforcement learning, can lead to more precise predictions and better workload flexibility. Moreover, the future of autoscaling is expected to be significantly impacted by the combination of automation and artificial intelligence technology. AI-driven autoscaling systems may make decisions in real time on their own, improving the efficacy and responsiveness of Memcached clusters. In this dynamic context, collaboration between data scientists, machine learning engineers, and DevOps teams is pivotal. Autoscaling systems will necessitate ongoing model distributed caching via machine learning-driven autoscaling for Memcached clusters signifies an innovative methodology. These systems ensure enhanced performance, cost-efficiency, and adaptability. Organizations can effectively harness machine learning, considering the elements highlighted in this review, to optimize their Memcached clusters within an ever-evolving technological landscape.

REFERENCES

1. K. Singh and A. Singh, "Memcached DDoS Exploits: Operations, Vulnerabilities, Preventions and Mitigations," 2018IEEE 3rd International Conference on Computing, Communication and Security (ICCCS), Kathmandu, Nepal, 2018, pp. 171-179, doi: 10.1109/CCCS.2018.8586810.
2. Smith, J. K., & Patel, S. (2020). Dynamic Resource Allocation for Memcached Clusters using Machine Learning. InProceedings of the International Conference on Distributed Computing (ICDC).
3. Brown, A., & White, L. (2019). Anomaly Detection for Autoscaling Memcached Clusters. In Proceedings of the International Conference on Machine Learning and Data Mining (MLDM).
4. Johnson, M., & Anderson, R. (2018). Real-time Monitoringand Autoscaling of Memcached Clusters using Machine Learning. ACM Transactions on Storage, 14(3), 1-23.
5. Garcia, R., & Kim, S. (2017). Optimizing MemcachedClusters with Machine Learning-based Autoscaling. IEEE Transactions on Cloud Computing, 5(2), 193-206.

6. Chen, Q., & Lee, H. (2016). Dynamic Scaling of Memcached Clusters in the Cloud. In Proceedings of the International Conference on Cloud Computing (CLOUD).

7. Wang, Y., & Wu, Z. (20[15]). Predictive Autoscaling for Memcached Clusters with Time Series Forecasting. In Proceedings of the European Conference on Machine Learningand Principles and Practice of Knowledge Discovery in Databases (ECML-PKDD). [8]. Mitchell, P., & Lewis, T. (20[14]). Real-time Monitoring and Adaptive Scaling of Memcached Clusters. In Proceedings of the International Conference on Big Data (BigData).

9. Liu, X., & Zhang, Q. (2013). A Machine Learning-based Approach for Memcached Autoscaling. In Proceedings of the IEEE International Conference on Cloud Computing (CLOUD).

10. Yang, J., & Hu, X. (2012). Anomaly Detection for Memcached Clusters using Principal Component Analysis. In Proceedings of the IEEE/IFIP Network Operations and Management Symposium (NOMS).

11. Clark, R., & Turner, E. (2011). Resource Allocation for Memcached Clusters with Machine Learning-based Autoscaling. In Proceedings of the ACM International Conference on Autonomic Computing (ICAC).

12. Rodriguez, M., & Garcia, S. (2010). Adaptive Scaling of Memcached Clusters for Web Applications. In Proceedings of the International Conference on Web Engineering (ICWE).

13. Williams, K., & Martinez, A. (2009). Real-time AnomalyDetection and Autoscaling for Memcached Clusters. In Proceedings of the International Conference on DistributedComputing Systems (ICDCS).

14. Adams, L., & Young, P. (2008). Dynamic Resource Allocation for Memcached Clusters in Cloud Environments. Journal of Cloud Computing, 2(3), 1-[15].

15. Li, X., & Chen, W. (2007). Predictive Scaling for Memcached Clusters using Time Series Analysis. In Proceedings of the International Conference on Parallel and Distributed Computing (PDC).

16. Wang, H., & Liu, Y. (2006). Scalable and Self-managing Memcached Clusters. In Proceedings of the International Conference on Data Engineering (ICDE).

17. Lee, G., & Kim, E. (2005). Anomaly Detection and Adaptive Scaling for Memcached Clusters in a Data Center. In Proceedings of the ACM/IFIP/USENIX International Conference on Middleware (Middleware).

18. Smith, D., & Davis, C. (2004). Real-time Resource Management for Memcached Clusters. In Proceedings of the USENIX Annual Technical Conference (USENIX ATC).

19. Turner, R., & Hall, S. (2003). Scalability and Performanceof Memcached: A Distributed Memory Object Caching System. ACM SIGOPS Operating Systems Review, 37(1), 205-218.

20. Martin, J., & Reed, M. (2002). Scaling Memcached: A Performance Analysis. In Proceedings of the ACM/IFIP Internationa Middleware Conference (Middleware

Emerging Trends in IoT and Computing Technologies – Suman Lata Tripathi et al. (eds)
© 2024 Taylor & Francis Group, London, ISBN 978-1-032-87924-6

A Novel Violent Crime Prediction using the k-Means Clustering Methodology

73

Neha Kulshrestha[1]

Assistant Professor, Department of Computer Science and Engineering,
Shri Ramswaroop Memorial University, Lucknow

Abstract: In the contemporary era, security has become a paramount concern for political and governmental entities around the globe, with the objective of minimizing the occurrence of criminal activities. With the rise of electronic systems, law enforcement authorities may enhance the speed of crime resolution by using crime data analysis. Computers provide significant advantages in several occupations and have the capacity to carry out administrative and maintenance duties at police stations. Increased efficacy and output. The K-means clustering technique is utilized to analyses crime detection data. We have This approach assists police officers, detectives, and other individuals involved in law enforcement. Authorities streamline the procedure of detecting and apprehending criminals. Data mining serves several essential purposes, one of which is crime analysis, which involves the scrutiny and interpretation of criminal data. The data is classified. The objective of employing the K-means algorithm is to reveal patterns of criminal activity. Clustering methodology. Applying data mining methodologies to analyses extensive datasets. Exploring crime databases and gaining expertise in this domain is a valuable area of study.

Keywords: Cluster, Crime analysis, k-means, Data mining, Euclidean distance, Machine learning

1. Introduction

Law enforcement organizations and government authorities have a significant difficulty in analyzing vast quantities of criminal information due to the increasing technical sophistication of criminals. The primary criterion is to choose suitable criminal analysis and data mining methodologies. However, by leveraging technical progress, historical crime data may be employed to identify patterns in criminal activity and detect crimes in their first stages [1]. Utilize data mining techniques to optimize the effectiveness of crime-solving by detectives by converting criminal data into a data mining challenge. The crime reports encompass attributes such as date, kind of offence, monetary value, gender, and location. Data analysts specializing in computer systems are currently assisting law enforcement agencies and detectives in accelerating crime investigations, as the use of computer systems for crime monitoring becomes more prevalent [2]. Data mining methods [3] seek to identify clusters of records that demonstrate similarity within the cluster but differ from the rest of the data. In this situation, some clusters are useful for identifying the precise characteristics of a crime committed by either an individual or a unified group of suspects. Clustering techniques are employed to transform a dataset into distinct groupings of data points, referred to as clusters, which are subsequently examined to discern various types of criminal activities. These clusters visually represent a criminal organization superimposed on a map that outlines the jurisdiction of the police. Clusters organize crime scene and other crime-related data, encompassing details such as the kind and date of the occurrence. Crime scenes undergo detection processes that are customized to the particular type of crime. Adopts a comprehensive strategy rather than a singular method, such as

---

[1]Kulneha121@gmail.com

DOI: 10.1201/9781003535423-73

classification, in response to the varied and unpredictable nature of crimes, as well as the existence of several unsolved cases in the crime database. Therefore, a categorization approach that depends on previous and resolved criminal cases is ineffective in producing precise forecasts for future crimes. The extensive array of criminal databases and the complex interrelationships among them significantly influence their affiliation. Data mining techniques have shown to be appropriate for extracting and using information in the domain of criminology [4]. Criminology is an academic field that focuses on the methodical analysis of crime, criminal conduct, law enforcement, and the discovery of elements associated with criminal activity. Data mining methodologies can produce significant results in this key field. To begin a comprehensive investigation, the first stage is to ascertain the distinctive characteristics of a crime. Data mining techniques provide useful insights that serve as a very advantageous instrument for strengthening and reinforcing the efforts of the police force. This study use an enhanced version of the k-means method to do clustering analysis. By identifying a limited number of data items that alter their groupings after a specific number of repetitions, the necessity to redistribute data components is eliminated.

2. Related Work

Data mining in criminology may be divided into two fundamental domains: crime control and crime suppression. De Bruin et. al. [5] proposed a method for analyzing crime trends by using a distinct distance metric to compare the characteristics of people and then classifying them into clusters. In their study, Lalitha and Suresh et.al [6] examined the utilization of the WEKA tool to analyze crime data in India and implement a clustering strategy for categorization. Their focus was on allocating the states based on the prevalence of crime. Cosmin Marian did a study on improving the speed of the k-means algorithm by applying optimization techniques [7]. Shiva Prasad [8] explored several methodologies for data mining. Nath [9] employed the k-means clustering technique to detect patterns of criminal behavior and solve criminal cases. Kadhim Swadi Al-Janabi [10] using the K Means approach and decision tree algorithms to detect clusters and conduct analysis on crime data. Adeyiga and Bello [11] introduced a fuzzy clustering approach for crime investigation, as well as for the prediction and prevention of criminal actions. Kadhim B. Swadi Al-Janabi [12] proposes a method that utilizes Decision tree Algorithms to categorize crime and criminal data, and the Simple K Means technique to cluster the data. The paper facilitates specialists' work by aiding in the analysis of patterns and trends, prediction of future events, exploration of relationships and potential explanations, visualization of criminal networks, and identification of potential suspects. Aravindan Mahendiran et al. [13] utilize several methodologies to scrutinize crime statistics and uncover concealed information that is not readily perceptible to human observers. Our algorithms discover patterns, and we utilize advanced visualization techniques to present this information in a simple and user-friendly way. This helps law enforcement authorities effectively allocate their resources. Chen et al. [14] introduced a comprehensive framework for mining crime data, which was developed using the knowledge gained from the Cop link project conducted by Arizona researchers. The author employed a concept space methodology to derive criminal data from the incident abstracts. The primary aim of the study is to establish the associations between different kinds of offenses and the connections between criminal syndicates.

3. Crime Analysis

Crime analysis is the utilization of analytical methodologies to gather and scrutinize data pertaining to crime patterns and trends. Consequently, this data is used to help people strategically allocate resources to prevent and suppress illegal activity. Analyzing crime is crucial due to several reasons: The primary objective is to conduct a comprehensive investigation of illegal activities in order to promptly provide law enforcement authorities with information on both overall and individual crime patterns. The second stage involves examining criminal conduct by utilizing the abundant data available inside the legal system and public domain. The crime rates are undergoing swift fluctuations, and advanced analytical methods can uncover any concealed criminal patterns, if they exist, without any prior conscious awareness of these trends. The primary goals of crime analysis encompass the extraction of crime patterns through the examination of accessible crime and criminal data, the anticipation of crime by considering the spatial distribution of existing data and employing diverse data mining techniques, and the identification of occurrences of crime.

4. Methodology

This work introduces a methodical approach to clustering for the examination of crime rates. The system architecture depicted in Fig. 73.1 is showcased. Clustering is the process of categorizing data items into distinct segments based on their similarity.

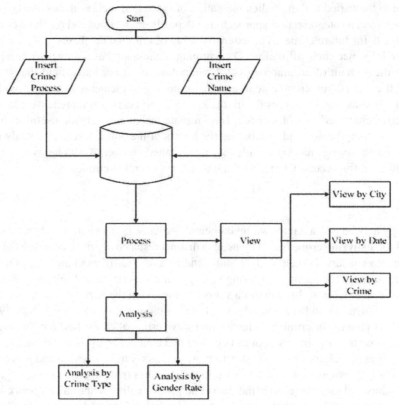

Fig. 73.1 The proposed crime detection system

Essentially, the objective is to segregate groups exhibiting comparable characteristics and allocate them to clusters. K-means clustering is a method employed in the field of cluster analysis. The k-means clustering technique [15] is an uncomplicated and concise approach that starts with an algorithmic explanation. Commence by selecting K centers, where K is a user-specified value indicating the desired quantity of clusters. Each individual point is assigned to a certain central point, and the collection of points assigned to each central point constitutes a cluster.

The centroid of every cluster is subsequently computed using the points assigned to that particular cluster. Continue the procedure of constructing and modifying clusters until there are no more changes in the assignments of data points or until the centroids remain unaltered. The centroid of each cluster is computed by considering the points assigned to that cluster. Continue the process of constructing and changing clusters until there are no more changes in the assignments of points or until the centroids remain unaltered. K-means clustering is a method employed in cluster analysis to divide a collection of n observations into k distinct groups. Every observation is allocated to the cluster that has the closest mean. The k-means clustering technique is frequently used because of its capacity to handle extensive datasets. The user specifies the desired number of clusters to be identified. The approach involves dividing the data into spherical clusters by identifying a set of cluster centers, assigning each observation to a specific cluster, calculating new cluster centers, and repeating this process iteratively.

- Establish a precise value for K, which denotes the number of clusters.
- Commence by establishing the K cluster centers, which can be accomplished in a random manner if necessary.
- Assign the N objects to the nearest cluster center in order to determine their class memberships.
- Reevaluate the K cluster centers, assuming the memberships calculated above are precise.
- Continue iterating this procedure until there are no changes in the membership of any of the N objects in the latest iteration.

The variable K represents the complexity of the procedure, which is defined by the values of the variables n (number of instances), c (number of clusters), and t (number of iterations). The algorithm is deemed to possess a modest level of efficiency. It often reaches a point of highest value within a certain area. One limitation of this approach is that it can only be applied when the average value is explicitly defined, and the number of clusters, represented as c, must be predefined [16].

4.1 Euclidean Distance

Euclidean distance is the direct and shortest path between two places, following a straight line. Euclidean distance is a word used to describe the measurement of the spatial separation between two points in Euclidean space. At such close distance, Euclidean space undergoes a transformation into a metric space. The Euclidean distance measure represents the shortest straight-line distance between two locations in a geometric space. The Euclidean distance is frequently used to quantify the distance between data points in Euclidean space. Euclidean distance, also referred to as distance, calculates the square root of the discrepancies between the coordinates of a pair.

$$\text{Distance } d = \sqrt{\sum_{i=1}^{n}(x_i - y_i)^2}$$

$$\text{Distance } d = \sqrt{(x_1 - y_1)^2 + (x_2 - y_2)^2 + \dots}$$

5. Experimental Results

This dataset has six distinct clusters, specifically Theft, Robbery, Drugs, Vehicle, Rape, and Murder. Initially, two centroids are assigned randomly. The number of clusters is two, denoted as k=2. The two centroids, labelled as k1 and k2, are located at coordinates k1 (1, 3) and k2 (2, 6) correspondingly. The Euclidean Distance is used to calculate the closeness of each data point to the centroids, and then assign the data points to their corresponding centroids.

Table 73.1 K-means clustering proposed system assigned USA city

City	Variable
Delaware	1
Hawaii	2
Indiana	3
Kansas	4
Massachusetts	5
New Jersey	6
Ohio	7
Oklahoma	8
Oregon	9
Pennsylvania	10

Table 73.2 K-means clustering proposed system assigned crime type

Crime type	Variable
Theft	1
Robbery	2
Drugs	3
Vehicle	4
Rape	5
Murder	6

Cluster 1 has the points (2,4), (5, 1), (6, 2), (5, 3), and (2, 3).

Cluster 2 comprises the coordinates (3, 5), (3, 6), (1, 5), (2, 3), and (3, 3)

At this stage, the algorithm allocates each item to the cluster that it is most proximate to, by computing the minimum distance between the two. There are two separate clusters, one represented by the color blue and the other represented by the color red. The yellow color indicates the positions of the matching centroids.

Begin to iterate, which is to compute the means of the individuals in each of the two clusters in order to redefine the centroids. The centroids are recalculated once again.

Cluster 1 has the points (2,5), (6, 1), (6, 2), (1, 3), and (2, 3).

Cluster 2 comprises the coordinates (2, 4), (1, 6), (4, 5), (4, 3), and (4, 3)

The two distinct clusters, red and blue, are designated differently. Colors in clusters 1 and 2 are blue and red, respectively. In Fig. 73.3, the centroids' positions are indicated by the yellow color.

Table 73.3 K-means clustering proposed system assigned crime datasets

City	Crime type	Quantity
1	1	4
2	2	5
3	3	6
4	4	5
5	5	1
6	6	2
7	3	3
8	1	3
9	4	3
10	5	3

Table 73.4 Clustering result with first iteration of crime datasets

City	Point	Dist. mean1 (1,3)	Dist. mean2 (2,6)	Cluster
1	(2,4)	0	2	1
2	(3,5)	1	0	2
3	(3,6)	4	3	2
4	(1,5)	2	2	2
5	(5,1)	7	4	1
6	(6,2)	6	7	1
7	(2,3)	4	3	2
8	(3,3)	1	3	2
9	(5,3)	3	4	1
10	(2,3)	6	7	1

Table 73.5 Clustering result with second iteration of crime datasets

City	Point	Dist. mean 1 (3.8, 2.9)	Dist. mean 2 (3, 4.9)	Cluster
1	(2,4)	2.9	3.3	2
2	(2,5)	3.9	3.3	1
3	(1,6)	0.9	0.7	2
4	(4,5)	2.7	1.3	2
5	(6,1)	3.1	4.3	1
6	(6,2)	3.1	5.3	1
7	(4,3)	1.9	2.3	2
8	(1,3)	0.9	1.3	1
9	(4,3)	1.7	3.3	2
10	(2,3)	2.5	0.3	1

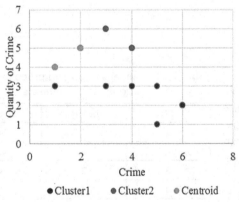

Fig. 73.2 Depicts the first iteration

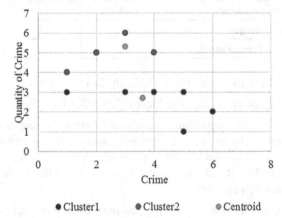

Fig. 73.3 Depicts the second iteration

6. Conclusion

Data mining's grouping and prediction methods are crucial for crime investigation, providing a unique approach to criminology. Computers have a vital role in several industries, including industry, government, military, and law enforcement. This study investigates the use of a clustering algorithm on a crime dataset with the objective of identifying and detecting criminal activities. Using data mining to predict patterns in criminal detection by applying K-means clustering techniques. The aim of this project was to approach crime detection as a machine learning task and using data mining techniques to aid police investigators in solving criminal cases. The application of the modelling technique enabled the identification of patterns in a large number of criminal episodes, thereby making the investigation work of detectives more efficient. The proposed methodology has considerable promise in tackling the intricacies of criminal activity and can function as a highly efficient instrument for crime identification. While it is not feasible to accurately forecast crimes, it is possible to avoid them if the timing of the crime is known in advance. In the future, the study of patterns in impending criminal activity can be conducted utilizing association rule mining in conjunction with the suggested system. Furthermore, the scope of the task might be expanded to forecast the temporal occurrence of criminal activities.

REFERENCES

1. De Bruin ,J.S.,Cocx,T.K,Kosters,W.A.,Laros, J. and Kok,J.N(2006) Data mining approaches to criminal carrer analysis ,"in Proceedings of the Sixth International Conference on Data Mining (ICDM"06) ,Pp. 171-177

2. W. Safat, S. Asghar, and S. A. Gillani, "Empirical analysis for crime prediction and forecasting using machine learning and deep learning techniques," IEEE Access, vol. 9, pp. 70080–70094, 2021

3. Nazlena Mohamad Ali1, Masnizah Mohd2, Hyowon Lee3, Alan F. Smeaton3, Fabio Crestani4 and Shahrul Azman Mohd Noah ,2010 Visual Interactive Malaysia Crime News Retrieval System

4. Sutapat T. Rutgers University, USA , Cluster Analysis of Anomaly Detection in Accounting Data : An Audit Approach, 2011

5. De Bruin ,J.S.,Cocx,T.K,Kosters,W.A.,Laros,J. and Kok,J.N(2006) Data mining approaches to criminal carrer analysis ,"in Proceedings of the Sixth International Conference on Data Mining (ICDM"06) ,Pp. 171-177

6. Cosmin and Marian, An Optimized Version of the K-Means Clustering Algorithm,FedCSIS, Biohouse volume 2 issue 1

7. U. M. Butt, S. Letchmunan, F. H. Hassan, M. Ali, A. Baqir, T. W. Koh, and H. H. R. Sherazi, "Spatio-temporal crime predictions by leveraging artificial intelligence for citizens security in smart cities," IEEE Access, vol. 9, pp. 47516–47529, 2021

8. Shiva Prasad, Data Mining Techniques: A Short Review, Biohouse Journal of Computer Science, Biohouse vol. 2. issue 1, 2016

9. S.V. Nath, Crime pattern detection using data mining, IEEE/WIC/ACM International Conference on Web Intelligence and Intelligent Agent Technology, 2006

10. A. Araujo, N. Cacho, L. Bezerra, C. Vieira, and J. Borges, "Towards a crime hotspot detection framework for patrol planning," in Proc. IEEE 20th Int. Conf. High Perform. Comput. Commun., IEEE 16th Int. Conf. Smart City, IEEE 4th Int. Conf. Data Sci. Syst. (HPCC/SmartCity/DSS), Jun. 2018, pp. 1256–1263

11. Framework for Analyzing Crime DataSet using Decision Tree and Simple K-means Mining Algorithms, Journal of Kufa for Mathematics and Computer, Vol.1, No.3, may 2011

12. Kadhim B.Swadi al-Janabi . Department of Computer Science. Faculty of Mathematics and Computer Science. University of Kufa/Iraq , "A Proposed Framework for Analyzing Crime DataSet using Decision Tree and Simple K-means Mining Algorithms", 2011

13. Aravindan Mahendiran, Michael Shuffett, Sathappan Muthiah, Rimy Malla, Gaoqiang Zhang, Forecasting Crime Incidents using Cluster Analysis and Bayesian Belief Networks, 2011

14. H. Chen, W. Chung, J.J. Xu, G. Wang, Y. Qin and M. Chau, "Crime Data Mining: A General Framework and Some Examples", Computer, Vol. 37, No. 4, pp. 50-56, 2004

15. S. Kim, P. Joshi, P. S. Kalsi, and P. Taheri, "Crime analysis through machine learning," in Proc. IEEE 9th Annu. Inf. Technol., Electron. Mobile Commun. Conf. (IEMCON), pp. 415–420, 2018

16. C. Catlett, E. Cesario, D. Talia, and A. Vinci, "A data-driven approach for spatio-temporal crime predictions in smart cities," in Proc. IEEE Int. Conf. Smart Comput. (SMARTCOMP), pp. 17–24, 2018

Emerging Trends in IoT and Computing Technologies – Suman Lata Tripathi et al. (eds)
© 2024 Taylor & Francis Group, London, ISBN 978-1-032-87924-6

Rapid and Close-Packed Xml Solution with Efficient Extensible Interchange (EXI)

74

Manvi Mishra[1]

Shri Ram Murti Smarak College of Engineering Technology and Research,
Department of CSE, Bareilly India

Prabhakar Gupta[2]

Shri Ram Murti Smarak College of Engineering and Technology,
Department of CSE, Bareilly India

SS Bedi[3]

IET Mahatma Jyotiba Phule Rohilkhand University,
Department of CS & IT, Bareilly, India

Sudheer Kumar Singh[4]

BBD University Department of CSE, Lucknow, India

Ankur Kumar[5]

Shri Ram Murti Smarak College of Engineering Technology and Research,
Department of CSE, Bareilly India

Abstract: XML serves as a widely adopted data representation format facilitating communication between systems. Despite its prevalence, XML is known for its verbosity and processing complexity. An effective alternative to traditional XML is the Extensible Interchange (EXI) technique, which has demonstrated a substantial reduction in verbosity and processing overhead. EXI achieves superior data compression compared to other techniques like Fastinfoset, BGip2, Gzip, 7Zip, leading to increased potential bandwidth capacity, particularly evident in the Cloud services XML domain where EXI has demonstrated a nearly double of bandwidth throughput. This improvement preserves the intrinsic advantages of XML while allowing for greater network penetration. Given its ability to compress data and improve bandwidth through smaller file sizes, coupled with the widespread use of XML in the IT environment, EXI emerges as a compelling option. The present study is focused on rapidly collecting data in close proximity, aiming to develop a swift and streamlined XML solution using the EXI mechanism. The research underscores the goal of leveraging the EXI mechanism to construct an agile and space-efficient XML solution. A comparative analysis of various XML compression methods concludes that EXI is the preferred choice due to its compact nature.

Keywords: XML, EXI, FastInfoset, Schema, Compression, Decompression

1. Introduction

XML functions as a markup language for organizing structured data documents, including both content (such as words and images) and indicators of content roles (e.g., section headings or database tables) . However, the XML syntax, while widely

[1]er.manvimishra@gmail.com, [2]prabhakar.gupta@gmail.com, [3]dearbedi@gmail.com, [4]sudheerhbtisomvansi@gmail.com, [5]saxenaanksrms@gmail.com

DOI: 10.1201/9781003535423-74

used for communication between systems, is criticized for its redundancy and verbosity compared to binary representations of the same data. This excess verbosity leads to higher storage, transmission, and processing costs, impacting application performance. XML's text-based nature, coupled with the absence of support for intrinsic data types, results in challenges such as difficulty in implementing namespace support in XML parsers and complex utilization of XML namespaces. Despite being considered 'self-documenting,' XML files have a significant size disadvantage, making them challenging to read and causing increased communication overhead, latency, processing time, and cost. [1]

To address these issues, researchers have explored compression strategies for XML files, leading to the development of various compression tools and binary formats like FastInfoset , Gzip [2], 7zip[3], and Bzip2[4]. Each of these tools has its strengths and weaknesses. FastInfoset, for instance, is a binary format based on the XML Information Set, emphasizing compression and serialization with the use of tables and indexes [5]. Gzip and 7-Zip are known for their open-source, lossless compression utility, with 7-Zip exhibiting faster compression in certain formats.Bzip2, on the other hand, employs the Burrows-Wheeler transform and Huffman coding, offering higher compression ratios than Gzip but with some trade-offs in consistency. The XML Binary Characterization Working Group has evaluated several high-performance XML encoding formats, with the W3C Binary XML Working Group's Efficient XML Interchange (EXI) format emerging as a top performer in terms of efficiency and processing speed. [6] EXI, initially known as Efficient XML Interchange, is a lightweight, high-performance XML representation recognized as a W3C recommendation. It efficiently communicates XML data between systems, optimizing performance while minimizing bandwidth requirements and resource usage. This paper advocates for EXI as the best compression technique currently available.

This paper's sections are arranged in the following sequence: an overview of various XML compression techniques is given in section1 Introduction. An explanation of EXI design theory, compression function and EXI implementation tools is highlighted in section 2. Section 3 depicts proposed work based on survey of various research papers of EXI methodology. Presentation of the features and benefits of EXI is showcased in section 4. Conclusion is represented in section 5.

2. EXI Design Principles and Compression Mechanism

The design ideas offered here are intended to provide context for the EXI design process and to draw attention to prospective EXI qualities. They were utilized to encourage the EXI development process and aid in uniform design decisions [7]. Figure 74.1 represents EXI design principles.

General: One of the main objectives of EXI is to increase the number of devices, software, and apps that can connect to XML data.

Minimal: Simple, elegant mechanisms are preferred above ones that are large, analytical, or complex in order to cover the broadest range of tiny, mobile, and embedded applications.

Competitive with binary formats: For applications that necessitate this level of rapidity, EXI must be optimized in terms of efficiency to be used.

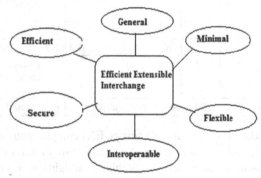

Fig. 74.1 EXI design principles [7]

Flexible: In order for documents to be adaptable and efficient, they must have the ability to include or diverge from their schema by incorporating arbitrary schema extensions. EXI should handle these documents. The encoding of a text will fail if it contains deviations from the schema.

Interoperable: In order to be interoperable, EXI must be acceptable in modern XML strategies and necessitate the fewest modifications to existing systems. To ensure interoperability with present and foreseeable XML requirements, EXI must adhere to the XML Information Set.

Secure: EXI must be secure through the use of the EXI encoding and decoding technology.

EXI represents the information inside of an XML file as an EXI stream. The two components of an EXI document are the EXI Header and Body. Information about the document, including the encoding settings and format version, can be found in the EXI Header [8]. The EXI Body is composed of a number of events. In contrast to using an elevated language API, formal grammars are directly used to code EXI. EXI is not an API; it is merely an algorithm description, hence the grammar process needs to be implemented directly. By fusing ideas from knowledge theory and formal language theory into a single, somewhat straightforward algorithm, EXI offers wide generality, flexibility, and efficiency. The method encodes the most likely possibilities in fewer bits by using a grammar to predict what is most likely to happen in an XML document. Every XML document is recognized by the integrated EXI grammar, and products that are formed from schemas or additional sources of information about what is anticipated to appear in a set of XML documents can be made better.

3. Proposed Work

Work recommends adoption of EXI methodology on the basis of literature review given in Table 74.1. It highlights numerous research articles on EXI technology have really been examined and condensed. The accompanying table suggests using the EXI method for an efficient and portable XML solution.

Table 74.1 Summary of research papers

S. N.	Year	Novelist	Endorsement
1.	2010	Radar et al. [9]	Fast processing and compression of information are two of EXI's primary advantages.
2.	2011	Peintner et al.[10]	Demonstrated how to dynamically load and unload DOM components using EXI functionalities. EXI uses compact identifiers and concentrates on a small number of its format's characteristics.
3.	2012	Doi et al. [11]	Home automation systems and other electronics may be immediately connected to web-based systems using the EXI decoder and encoder.
4.	2012	Kyusakov et al. [12]	Throughput, computation power, and memory reductions might be considerable as a result of the implementation of EXI in industrial automation systems.
5.	2013	Jaiswal and Mishra [13]	When it comes to processing speed and compression, EXI outperforms other programmes like Gzip, FastInfoset, Gzip+ FastInfoset, and 7Gip.
6.	2014	Kyusakov et al. [14]	The EXIP framework can be used in design and development approaches for embedded web development applications. The EXI processor's working model implementation is shown and assessed. In the current Internet of Things context, it applies to all Web browsers and Web services that permit human-machine communication.
7.	2014	Gustafsson et al.[15]	Using a schema-enabled EXI parser could decrease packages delivered, enabling more constrained and cost-effective sensor-based systems to meet hardware requirements. Additionally, there is a method available to reduce the dynamic memory usage of an EXI Profile stream while decoding an EXI stream.
8.	2014	Takuki Kamiya et. al. [16]	There is a method available to reduce the memory usage of an EXI Profile stream.
9.	2017	Yu et al.[17]	To fulfil less resource requirements of mobile phones and is specifically tailored to the EXI standard, the CMDE model is designed. The model achieves significant reductions in bandwidth usage, time consumption, and transmission data density, all without significantly increasing power consumption.
10.	2020	Tomaszuk et al. [18]	Even though RDF is being compressed using EXI, this will only serialise XML.

Based on the survey findings, EXI compression emerges as the optimal option for both transmission of data and preservation. EXI provides a universally accepted solution for medical image transmission in a highly condensed form, making it platform-neutral and widely applicable. A straightforward test environment was made to verify the use of xml data. A workstation PC running 32-bit Windows 8 with an Intel Core i3- processor clocked at 2.10 GHz and 3GB of RAM was used for the testing. The JVM (Java Virtual Machine) utilized to run EXIficient and OpenEXI is Java Hotspot(TM) Server VM 1.7, whereas the compiler for C used to execute EXIP is GCC 4.8.1. In the experimentation, EXIP implementation was used. Table 74.2 and Fig. 74.2. Demonstrates that Schema informed EXI is the best choice for data compression as compare to FI, Gzip, Bzip2 and Schemaless EXI.

Table 74.2 Results of the experiment of comparing between FI+Gzip, FastInfoset, Bzip2, Gzip, and EXI (Schema less& schema informed mode

Name of file	File Size at Original (bytes)	Following the size of the compressed file (bytes)						
		Gzip	Bzip 2	Zip7	FastInfoset	FastInfoset & Gzip	Schema-less EXI	Schema Informed EXI
Student.xml	338	209	230	309	161	147	125	62
Notebook.xml	524	274	300	381	264	252	227	141
Transport.xml	1057	509	534	726	491	479	455	370
Uniform.xml	1190	625	641	761	523	503	479	399
Class.xml	2053	1255	1276	1357	766	741	729	687

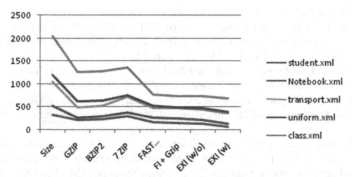

Fig. 74.2 The outcomes of a test that evaluated the performance of 7Zip, Gzip and Bzip2, FI+Gzip, FastInfoset and EXI (Schema/without schema) were examined

4. EXI's Characteristics and Advantages

Efficient XML (EXI) offers a comprehensive solution for optimizing XML text, maintaining all functionality, including comments and processing instructions, in a compact manner comparable to hand-optimized application-specific encodings. This feature enables the transformation of existing XML-based technologies, like web services, XHTML, and SVG, into EXI representation. The processing algorithms handle mixed-mode scenarios, where just a portion of the text adheres to the schema, and are simultaneously efficient and general. They can operate with or without knowledge of the schema. APIs, making integration faster and easier. With the world's fastest processors, EXI outperforms traditional XML processors in parsing and serializing EXI data. Integrating EXI into existing frameworks can significantly boost productivity with minimal code changes. [19] EXI supports fidelity optimizations, allowing the preservation or discarding of white space, comments, and unnecessary XML objects. It optimizes lists of elements from XML messages, enabling the submission of partial messages when sending the entire document is impractical. When schema optimizations are activated, EXI can deduce a schema to efficiently represent extracted data. Created for devices with limited resources, such as widely-used cell phones, EXI is suitable for platforms with constrained computer power, storage, memory capacity and lifespan of batteries [20]. It facilitates full streaming, allowing applications to generate outcomes before the entire document is loaded into memory. This is an essential characteristic for adaptable, quick-to-respond, and portable applications that cannot tolerate delays associated with full handling of document.

5. Conclusions

XML serves as a widely employed format for representing data, facilitating system-to-system compatibility. However, its drawback lies in verbosity and complexity during processing [35]. The alternative XML format introduced by the EXI technique has demonstrated a substantial reduction in verbosity and processing costs, enabling real-time network activities for edge devices. Widely adopting EXI could empower healthcare firms to extend XML-based network traffic, reaching destinations like Cloud Web Services or other small mobile and wireless network edge applications. Embracing Cloud Web Services within hospital organizations would benefit both patients and doctors, allowing immediate access to patient records. In the realm of Cloud services XML, EXI has proven to double bandwidth capacity, facilitating deeper network penetration while retaining XML's advantages. [21] As "Cloud" computing gains traction in the business world for distributed data, XML becomes the de facto standard for data formats. EXI offers an effective solution through XML compression, enhancing bandwidth by reducing file sizes, validated by real-world experiences. Achieving this goal involves implementing EXI at both transmitting and receiving stations. Given the vast and increasing volume of data transmitted across wireless networks and the Internet, the XML file format, commonly used for sending photos, faces a challenge due to its sizable files. In schema informed mode, experimental findings demonstrate that EXI achieves the best compression ratio among compression methods, aligning with current industry standards for transmission applications requiring a quick compressor with a high compression ratio.

REFERENCES

1. Sherif Sakr. XML Compression Techniques: A survey and Comparison. ELSEVIER Journal of Computer and System Sciences, 2009, pp 303-322.
2. GZip. The GZip homepage". Retrieved 2021, from www.gzip.org.

3. 7Zip. Welcome to the 7-Zip home! Retrieved, 2021, from http://www.7-zip.org.
4. BZip2 Compressor, "Welcome to the BZip2 Homepage", retrieved 2021, from, http://www.bzip.org.
5. Efficient XML Interchange Measurements NoteW3C Working Draft 25 July 2007, online available at https://www.w3.org/TR/2007/WD-exi-measurements-20070725/#contributions-FI%23contributions-FI
6. W3C.Efficient XML interchange (EXI) format 1.0. Retrieved 2023, from http://www.w3.org/TR /exi/
7. W3C. EXI best practices. Retrieved 2023, from https://www.w3.org/TR/exi-best-practices/
8. W3C. Efficient XML interchange (EXI) primer. Retrieved 2023, from   https://www.w3.org/TR/exi-primer
9. Radar. Efficient Extensible Markup Language (XML) Interchange (EXI). IJIS Institute technical Advisory Committee White Paper, Jan (2010)
10. Daniel Peintner, Richard Kuntschke, Jorg Heuer, Harald Kosch. LazyDOM Transparent Partial DOM Loading and Unloading for Memory Restricted Environments. WEBIST 2011 - 7th Int' Conf. on Web Information Systems and Technology, pp 98-105, 2011.
11. Yusuke Doi, Yumiko Sato, Masahiro Ishiyama, Yoshihiro Ohba, Keiichi Teramoto. XML-less EXI with code generation for integration of embedded devices in web based systems. 2012 3rd IEEE Int' Conf. on the Internet of Things, 2012, pp. 76-83, IEEE, 2012.
12. Rumen Kyusakov, Henrik Mäkitaavola, Jerker Delsing, Jens Eliasson. Efficient xml interchange in Factory Automation Systems Jan 2011 IECON 2011 - 37th Annual Conf. of the IEEE Industrial Electronics Society, pp.4478-4483. IEEE, 2011
13. Gaurav Jaiswal, Manvi Mishra. Why Use Efficient XML Interchange Instead of Fast Infoset. 3rd IEEE Int' Advance Computing Conference (IACC), pp. 925-930, 2013.
14. Rumen Kyusakov, Pablo Punal Pereira, Jens Eliasson, Jerker Delsing. EXIP: A Framework for Embedded Web Development. ACM Transactions on the Web 8, no.23(2014):pp 1–29
15. Jonas Gustafsson , Rumen Kyusakov, Henrik Mäkitaavola and Jerker Delsing .Application of service oriented architecture for sensors and actuators in district heating substations Sensors (Basel) MDPI, 14 no. 8 , (2014): 15553-15572
16. Takuki Kamiya. Efficient XML Interchange Profile Stream Decoding. 23 Jan 2014 Publication No. US 2014/0026030
17. **Chunyan Yu, Hui Qi and Liwen Zhou.** "An Efficient Data Exchange Model for Campus Wireless Networks Based on Efficient Extensible Interchange" Journal of Applied Science and Engineering 20, no. 2, (2017): 259-270.
18. Dominik Tomaszuk, David hyland-wood. RDF 1.1: Knowledge Representation and Data Integration Language for the Web. Journal Symmetry 2020, 12(1), 84.
19. Christopher J. Augeri, Dursun Bulutoglu,Barry E. Mullins,Rusty Baldwin, Leemon C. Baird III. An analysis of XML compression efficiency. In Proceedings of the Workshop on Experimental Computer Science, part of ACM FCRC, San Diego, pp. 1-12. ACM, 2007.
20. ManviMishra, SS Bedi, Prabhakar Gupta. Enhanced Compression Prototype for Radiological Imaging. Journal of Advanced research in Dynamical and Control systems, Vol. 11, 10-Special Issue, 2019, pp. 1219-1229,
21. ManviMishra, SS Bedi, Prabhakar Gupta. Proving Rural and Urban Telemedicine with Improved Diacom Image Compression Using EXI Mechanism. Revista Geintec-Gestao Inovacao E Tecnologias, Vol. 11, No. 4, 16/7/2021 pp. 1884-1901.

Emerging Trends in IoT and Computing Technologies – Suman Lata Tripathi et al. (eds)
© 2024 Taylor & Francis Group, London, ISBN 978-1-032-87924-6

Analytical Machine Learning Models for Predicting COVID-19 Transmission

75

Sudheer Kumar Singh[1]

Associate Professor, Department of Computer Science and Engineering,
BBD University, Lucknow, UP, India

Ranjana Singh[2]

Assistant Professor, Department of Economics,
National P. G. College, Lucknow, UP, India

Nidhi Srivastava[3], Gagandeep Chadha[4]

Assistant Professor, Department of Management,
National P. G. College, Lucknow, UP, India

Dheeraj Tandon[5]

Associate Professor, Department of Computer Science and Engineering,
BBD University, Lucknow, UP, India

M Yousuf Malik[6]

Assistant Professor, School of Business,
Woxsen University. Hyderabad, Telangana, India

Manvi mishra[7]

Shri Ram Murti Smarak College of Engineering Technology and Research,
Department of CSE, Bareilly, India

Abstract: Several clinical and non-clinical procedures were implemented by governments and the World Health Organization during the COVID-19 pandemic to partially succeed and flatten the pandemic curve. Various research teams threw themselves wholeheartedly into this endeavor. It is impossible to overlook the contributions made by data analytics and artificial intelligence. Using machine learning (ML) and deep learning (DL) to analyze global datasets linked to COVID-19, several research findings are presented. A wide range of predictive analytics models have been put forth by computer scientists, statisticians, and physicians. This is the time to assess these models and demonstrate the applicability of the suggested techniques. The purpose of this study is to use ML and DL techniques to assess the efficacy of the predictive analytics models that were developed during the pandemic. The original research papers published in the pandemic-era indexed journals are examined in this review along with their applicability in the modern day. Additionally, the value of the included algorithms in predictive analytics is discussed, along with how frequently they are utilized in different frameworks.

Keywords: Covid 19, Machine learning, Prediction model, Sentiment analysis, Pandemic

[1]sudheerhbtisomvansi@bbdu.ac.in, [2]ranjana.june@gmail.com, [3]nidhi_a_srivastava@yahoo.co.in, [4]gagandeepchadha16@gmail.com,
[5]dheerajtandon9@gmail.com, [6]yousuf.malik@woxsen.edu.in, [7]manvimishra@gmail.com

DOI: 10.1201/9781003535423-75

1. Introduction

The pandemic of Corona virus (COVID-19) had spread as an exponential function in the world together with India after the lockdown. Although all countries in the world were considering all the control measures to prevent it's spreading. At the beginning of the COVID-19, peoples were not aware of this pandemic all over the world, so all peoples were regularly doing their jobs [1]. It can be transmitted from one person to other, it was officially declared by the World Health Organization (WHO) in January 2020[2]. The Indian government had implemented control measures and prevention all over India including its all states and cities. All media persons and scientists from research organizations were continuously spreading awareness of diseases all over the world for the prevention of pandemic. The awareness and control measures had archived staring relief initially but in various countries, the situation became worse and worse later on. Many scientists were observing this dreadful event in various countries, and were facing a question that how could they predict or estimate the growth rate of coronavirus Covid 19 for all over the world, including its spread, death caused by it, infected number of people, etc. in this research work various prediction models have been compared, designed on the basis of data collected from government affiliated social networking sites as UCI, Data world, etc. Coronavirus sickness had significantly impacted people's daily life all around the globe. Online media was used by people all around the world to voice their ideas and general thoughts on this phenomenon that has gripped the planet. On social media platforms like Twitter, the number of tweets about the epidemic quickly had increased tremendously. Social media may include past, current and crucial information on COVID-19, but sometimes the content is worthless or misleading. Using sentiment analysis on Twitter data to evaluate public attitude, this research examined the rising concern about coronavirus. Since human behaviour and the natural world have been identified using a variety of conventional techniques. Using NLP approaches, it is feasible to do research on sentiment analysis of COVID19 data. In this research, in addition to a prediction based on Covid 19 statistics, the researchers have proposed a model for Covid 19 based sentiment.

With information from a wide variety of sources including research publications, government and private organisations and social media sites like Facebook, Twitter and other similar sources, sentiment analysis models have been created as well as various other prediction models which have been developed for the forecast of Covid 19 have been compared in this research work so as understand their accuracy. To create such models AI and machine learning method has been used along-with some experimental data to get better accuracy. It is important to compare and contrast the existing models with the proposed model so as to anticipate attitudes or behaviours towards the discussed paradigms.

2. Literature Review

In this section of the paper, the researchers have analysed and extracted some useful information, models, approaches or techniques to compare their prediction accuracy. These information were collected according to different parameters like deaths, recovered, confirmed cases, etc. When critical diseases like coronavirus have been spreading then the public health department initiated to prevent and control it. Societies and scientists are used to some existing epidemic prediction models for tracking the trend of the development status of pandemic diseases [3].Smadja et al (2020) proposed that tailored and population-wide techniques should be created because different infectious illnesses have varied host-specific symptoms, varying incubation times, and different modes of transmission [4][5]. Sankaranarayanan, S. et al., (2021) used a deep neural network-based gated recurrent unit (GRU) binary classification model using a variety of distinct biomarkers as features, utilizing the USA-based COVID-19 dataset. It was designed to forecast the chance of mortality in individual patients, and it outperformed other machine learning models with an AUC of 0.938. [6][7]. The involvement of the SERI model provided issues related to the prediction and information required to build a novel model for the Coronavirus COVID-19 disease development trend [8].SERI is a successful model in case of large scale spreading of pandemic diseases [9]. In this model, some parameters have adapted and represented by S, R, I, E to S count at peoples at risk, R count the recovered cases, I, count the contagious cases, and E count the in-cubation duration and, respectively [10]. SIR, SI, and SEIR models represent a relationship in the form of differential equations and it is successfully used to predict the various pandemic diseases like SARS, and Ebola [11][12]. In the above-discussed model there is a lack of relationship between parameters like the effect of the trend of new cases on the spreading of the coronavirus, treatment of infected persons, etc [13]. To justify the problem occurred in the above models, Authors have used long term short memory model (LSTM) which has worked with natural languages processing (NLP) for reduced the error and increased the predictive accuracy with respect to previous model. This model is known as Classic recurrent neural network (RNN)[14]. We proposed a machine learning Techniques using Linear Regression to predict the trending behaviour of Coronavirus and growth of coronavirus as a new case increases per day in the lockdown period. We also discussed comparative analysis of the growth trend of coronavirus during lockdown in the country. This technique based on the NLP model. As indicated in the article's introduction, sentiment analysis and classification of COVID-19 data were gathered from social media sites such as Twitter utilising related keywords for sentiment analysis and classification. This study focuses on both prediction analysis and sentiment analysis of individuals. We employ machine learning (ML) classification-based approaches and provide a comparative study of sentiment classification mechanisms for tweets, and conclude that this is one of the most important contributions of this research.

3. Proposed Methodology

In this section, we will discuss about the machine learning techniques with the linear regression to predict our objective and improved the accuracy of our proposed methodology.

The authors' contribution summarized as follows:

1. To build a model for predicting coronavirus trends using COVID19 data provided by multiple public and private organisations.
2. The tweets from COVID-19 were obtained using the Twitter API. With the use of this information, we created a sentiment analysis model to determine how people felt about tweets and text data connected to the coronavirus. Three categories: positive, negative, and neutral are used to categorise the emotions expressed in tweets.
3. To discuss how the present models stack up against our proposed alternatives. This kind of model was generated utilising a machine learning algorithm and data from actual experiments, and it was built with a focus on precision. The proposed model outperformed other prevalent approaches when tested against real-world datasets.

3.1 Linear Regression Model

Classification and prediction of both works can be done using machine learning algorithms. As we know machine learning techniques can be divided into two categories, supervised learning and unsupervised. Natural language Processing (NLP) is an Application of Artificial Intelligence and this is used to build Machine Learning models for classification and prediction. Regression comes under supervised learning. The regression model can further be divided into two main categories Linear and logistic regression. In this paper, we use linear regression, which required training as well as test data [15]. Our proposed methodology is shown in the Fig. 75.1.

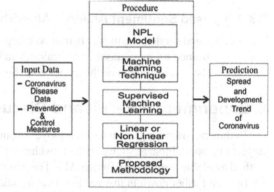

Fig. 75.1 Proposed methodology for predicting trend of Corona virus

Modified Algorithm

In this paper, linear regression model analyzes the relation between dependent and independent variables we chosen the dependent variable as y and independent variable X. Set of value suppose $X = \{x_1, x_2, \dots \dots \dots \dots \dots \dots \dots \dots x_n\}$.

Those change the value of Y as dependent variable and predict the coronavirus growth trend in different scenarios. Simple linear regression can be represented as

$$Y = A_0 + A_1 X + \theta, \quad Y^- = A_0 + A_1 X, \quad (Y - Y^{-1)}) \text{ is error.}$$

A_0 is a constant and expressed as Intercept of the regression line on the ordinate y, A_1 regression coefficient the is the tangent of the regression line and θ is residual error for finding the influence of random parameters on the predicted variables.[16]. With the regression analysis equation, we evaluated the term A0 and A1 for our sample datasets. We discussed the evaluated parameters of our model to establish the regression models for our desired analysis. After that, we will define the coefficient for analyzing the regression equation and its accuracy. The coefficient of determination for linear regression will be defined by the following equations [15].

$$R^2 = \text{Cor}^2(Y, Y^-), TSS = \sum_i^n (Y - Y^-)^2, R^2 = 1 - \frac{TSS}{ESS} = ESS/TSS$$

In the equation above TSS is the Sum of Squares., ESS is regression Sum of Squares and RSS is the residual sum of squares. Y˜ is a given original value and the Y defined as the predicted value [16].

3.2 Sentiment Analysis Model (SAM)

As was previously indicated, we concentrated on the data that had been gathered. China found the coronavirus disease in the middle of the month. The Indian government was placed under house arrest in the year 2020 from March 25 until May 31. Coronavirus cases increased in a number of Indian states between June 1, 2020, and June 30, 2020. For the purpose of analysing a wide range of parameters, including the recovery rate, the mortality rate, newly infected patients, confirmed cases, and many others, a number of prediction and forecasting models have been developed by a variety of scientists and researchers. In order to predict feelings or actions based on textual data that is saved or posted by users on social media platforms like Twitter and Facebook, we have developed a model for sentiment analysis as well as a model for the progression or spread of the coronavirus disease for the duration of the pandemic. These two models are meant to be applied in tandem with one another. On the numerous social media platforms, textual information is communicated about job chances, wages, education, medical services, future prospects, feelings of insecurity, and mental health. We have high hopes that we will be able to fight the COVID-19 coronavirus and win in the end if medical professionals, the government, and their plans to solve people's personal and social problems are put into action. We have collected textual data from twitter during the covid19, mostly focused on jobs, salary, mental state, school and higher education. From these twitter data, our proposed sentiment analysis model predicts the sentiment of the peoples and students suffering and recovering from COVID 19 for the individual problem related to JOB, mental health, Salary, and other keywords etc. sentiment analysis of textual data extracted from twitter are in the form of unstructured data. so for evaluation and extract the sentiment of these data set, we have apply our proposed sentiment model on the data set, for this propose we have designed a Algorithms to form a sentiment model for textual data of COVID 19 for prediction of peoples and social media user behaviors towards impact on their life.

3.3 Proposed Sentiment Analysis Algorithm

In our suggested model, the model is trained using machine learning algorithms. Our proposed sentiment analysis analytical model was trained on our dataset using training and text data. According to this paper's findings, we achieve the anticipated outcomes. The results section of this paper will show how we put our model into practice and go over the findings.

4. Experimental Result and Discussion

The Python programming language is employed in our suggested model implementation, along with the Anaconda environment's" jupyter notebook. First, as shown in the flowchart of the procedure, we obtained the data from Twitter by employing the Tweepy method available through the Twitter API. The general procedure that our finding demonstrates can be seen in the diagram that can be seen further down in this section. Feature selection table shown as follows:

During the process of putting the model that was proposed into action, the confusion matrix and the model score were calculated, and the results of those calculations are shown in the following

Table 75.1 Confusion matrix and Score of our proposed model using multinomial

N-828	0	1	Score
0	306	98	0.751023451
1	102	322	.0.74869576

Our findings and graph reveal that everyone suffering from COVID-19 or recovering from COVID-19 has a severe change in their thinking set, as well as changes in several areas such as social behaviors, social life, personal life, and office life. We gathered thousands of data points (tweets) for analysis for this study. The confusion matrix provides the statistically significant data for the research and the accuracy of proposed model over 75% of the time.

5. Conclusion and Future Scope

Using COVID-19 data provided by several public and private organisations, a trend prediction model for coronaviruses was developed. Using an algorithm for machine learning and experimental data, this model was developed with an emphasis on precision. Using actual data sets, the new model outperformed other common approaches. To contrast and compare these proposed alternatives with the present models. The models of sentiment analysis predict attitudes or behaviours towards the discussed paradigms, and they generate very important and accurate findings that help manage and unite individuals to combat the existing pandemic crisis. These models are correct greater than 75 % of the time, and the confusion matrix provides us with statistically meaningful data for the investigation.

The second sentiment analysis model was developed by using multinomial Naive Bayes supervised machine learning algorithms. This model has achieved a performance of approximately 75.43% which is based on about 3424 tweets. The findings and graph reveal that everyone suffering from COVID-19 or recovering from COVID-19 has a severe change in their thinking set, as well as changes in several areas such as social behaviors, social life, personal life, and office life. For this study, researchers have gathered thousands of data points (tweets) for analysis.

REFERENCES

1. J. Zhang, "People's responses to the COVID-19 pandemic during its early stages and factors affecting those responses," Humanities and Social Sciences Communications, vol. 8, no. 1, Feb. 2021, doi: 10.1057/s41599-021-00720-1.
2. S. Ying et al., "Spread and control of COVID-19 in China and their associations with population movement, public health emergency measures, and medical resources," medRxiv (Cold Spring Harbor Laboratory), Feb. 2020, doi: 10.1101/2020.02.24.20027623.
3. N. Zheng et al., "Predicting COVID-19 in China using hybrid AI model," IEEE Transactions on Cybernetics, vol. 50, no. 7, pp. 2891–2904, Jul. 2020, doi: 10.1109/tcyb.2020.2990162.
4. N. Peiffer-Smadja et al., "Machine learning for clinical decision support in infectious diseases: a narrative review of current applications," Clinical Microbiology and Infection, vol. 26, no. 5, pp. 584–595, May 2020, doi: 10.1016/j.cmi.2019.09.009.
5. M. Shinde, A. Majumdar et al, "Application of machine learning for COVID-19 data analysis," Journal of Pharmaceutical Negative Results, vol. 13, no. 3, Jan. 2022, doi: 10.47750/pnr.2022.13.03.053.
6. S. Sankaranarayanan et al., "COVID-19 mortality prediction from deep learning in a large multistate electronic health record and laboratory information system data set: algorithm development and validation," Journal of Medical Internet Research, vol. 23, no. 9, p. e30157, Sep. 2021, doi: 10.2196/30157.
7. R. J. Martin, "Retrospective study of machine learning based Covid-19 prediction frameworks," World Journal of Advanced Research and Reviews, vol. 17, no. 1, pp. 890–903, Jan. 2023, doi: 10.30574/wjarr.2023.17.1.0097.
8. Biswas, K., Sen, P. Space-time dependence of coronavirus (COVID-19) outbreak. arXiv 2003, 03149 (v1),2020.
9. M. Y. Li, J. R. Graef, L. Wang, and J. Karsai, "Global dynamics of a SEIR model with varying total population size," Mathematical Biosciences, vol. 160, no. 2, pp. 191–213, Aug. 1999, doi: 10.1016/s0025-5564(99)00030-9.
10. Z. Yang et al., "Modified SEIR and AI prediction of the epidemics trend of COVID-19 in China under public health interventions," Journal of Thoracic Disease, vol. 12, no. 3, pp. 165–174, Mar. 2020, doi: 10.21037/jtd.2020.02.64.
11. Z. Yang et al., "Modified SEIR and AI prediction of the epidemics trend of COVID-19 in China under public health interventions," Journal of Thoracic Disease, vol. 12, no. 3, pp. 165–174, Mar. 2020, doi: 10.21037/jtd.2020.02.64.
12. A. Khan, J. Li, M. Y. Khan, and R. Alam, "Complex environment perception and positioning based visual information retrieval," International Journal of Information Technology, vol. 12, no. 2, pp. 409–417, Feb. 2020, doi: 10.1007/s41870-020-00434-8.
13. T. J. Berge, J. M. -s. Lubuma, G. M. Moremedi, N. Morris, and R. Kondera-Shava, "A simple mathematical model for Ebola in Africa," Journal of Biological Dynamics, vol. 11, no. 1, pp. 42–74, Sep. 2016, doi: 10.1080/17513758.2016.1229817.
14. A. Khan, J. P. Li, A. U. Haq, I. Memon, S. Patel, and S. U. Din, "Emotional-physic analysis using multi-feature hybrid classification," Journal of Intelligent and Fuzzy Systems, vol. 40, no. 1, pp. 1681–1694, Jan. 2021, doi: 10.3233/jifs-201069.
15. C. E. Rizkalla, F. Blanco-Silva, and S. Gruver, "Modeling the impact of Ebola and bushmeat hunting on western lowland gorillas," Ecohealth, vol. 4, no. 2, pp. 151–155, Jun. 2007, doi: 10.1007/s10393-007-0096-2.
16. T. Ng, G. Turinici, and A. Danchin, "A double epidemic model for the SARS propagation," BMC Infectious Diseases, vol. 3, no. 1, Sep. 2003, doi: 10.1186/1471-2334-3-19.

Emerging Trends in IoT and Computing Technologies – Suman Lata Tripathi et al. (eds)
© 2024 Taylor & Francis Group, London, ISBN 978-1-032-87924-6

A Systematic Review on Relationship Between the Monsoon's Variability and the Variables Influencing it Through Machine Learning

76

Namita Goyal[1], Aparna N Mahajan[2]
Maharaja Agrasen University, Baddi, Himachal Pradesh

K.C. Tripathi[3]
Maharaja Agrasen Institute of Technology, GGSIPU, New Delhi

Abstract: The Indian economy, environment, and culture are strongly based on the monsoon which is an intricate system of complex interactions between ocean and various atmospheric units. Therefore, weather prediction is greatly impacted by the continuous variations in features that overall accomplishes the climatic condition of future weather. Consequently, to quantify climate change with respect to its relationship with environmental variables few research questions have been identified including factors affecting monsoon, related datasets and all statistical methods that have been employed so far for thorough examination of the association between monsoon variability and factors impacting it.

Keywords: ENSO (EL NINO Southern oscillation), IOD (indian ocean dipole), EQUINOO (equatorial indian ocean oscillation), SST (sea surface temperature), SLP (sea level pressure)

1. Introduction

Farming is the main occupation of more than half of the population of India which is directly dependent on rainfall. Many who are running various other industries like electricity production, automobiles, fertilizers are also reliant on rain indirectly. Thus, Indian monsoon is a pivotal meteorological occurrence that is essential not only for nearly 1.5 billion individuals who resides in India but also for animal, plants, and complete biodiversity. Owing to its significance importance for all living beings on earth, numerous methodologies including numerical [1][2]and statistical methods [3][4] have been used since olden times for weather prediction. Even a small variation in rainfall prediction might results a huge impact on economy. Throughout the past many year's research, several factors have been found to influence the Indian summer monsoon. Many of these factors have local and even global impact on monsoon leading to tremendous deal of uncertainty in both spatial and temporal distribution. As seen in Fig. 76.1, these factors have a substantial impact on the examination of long-term trends within interannual fluctuations when the geographical mean of the Indian summer monsoon rainfall (ISMR) data for the years 1901–2010 is looked at.

Thus, this paper has been written to identify, what are the factors that affects monsoon prediction and identifying the relationship between these climatic factors and monsoon inconsistency.

This paper is composed of four parts which are as follows: Part 2 discusses the related research work done by researchers, followed by part 3 which explains what were the research questions that gave path to this work comprising the monsoon-influencing factors, associated dataset and the comparative analysis of different machine learning methods used to find relationship between monsoon affecting factors and its variability. Finally, in part 4 paper has been concluded with a recommendation to enhance data integration methods.

[1]er.namitagoel@gmail.com, [2]aparnanmahajan@yahoo.co.in, [3]kctripathi@rediffmail.com

DOI: 10.1201/9781003535423-76

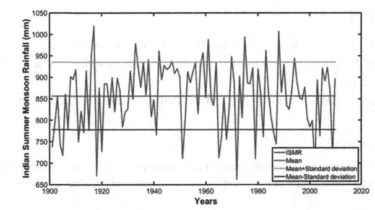

Fig. 76.1 ISMR time series spanning 110 years, from 1901 to 2010 [15]

2. Literature Review

Having known the importance of monsoon prediction for socioeconomic growth of country, numerous efforts have been made in this direction using different predictors and models. Table 76.1 shows the work done for monsoon prediction in recent years. Longer time periods still provide challenges for weather forecasting. And improving data assimilation techniques and closing observational gaps in remote or less studied locations are other crucial research areas.

Table 76.1 Related work

Reference No.	Predictors	Model Used	Findings
[5]	Accumulated cyclone energy	Prophet, LSTM, stacked ensemble with multi-layer perceptron, and ARIMA.	Explains how the energy of cyclones can amplify monsoon occurrences during their early stages with accuracy of 91%.
[6]	SST, SLP	Stacked autoencoder model	Forecast the monsoon with 2.8% error rate two months in advance.
[7]	Global warming, anthropological events	No model Systematic review of existing work.	Identify the relationship between rising world temperatures and increased precipitation, as well as the ways in which these trends affect the nature of Asian monsoon seasons and the unpredictability of rainfall in Southeast Asia.
[8]	SST, SLP and SST+SLP	Deep neural network with stacked autoencoder and regression tree fitted.	Forecast both the early and late stages of the country's rainfall.
[9]	Seventeen parameters including: urban fraction, surface air temperature, dew point etc.	Ensemble multivariate and random forest.	Examined the patterns of intense precipitation events throughout the summer monsoon across India, utilizing clustering analysis that spanned nine regions.
[10]	El Nino events	Autoencoder based on clustering	According to research, El Niño events in the eastern equatorial Pacific, where SST errors are warmer, are less effective in concentrating drought-causing subsidence over India than those in the central equatorial Pacific.
[11]	SLP, Great Himalayas, Tibetan plateau, zonal-wind, and geo-potential height	Stack encoder.	Using determined climate variables, the monsoon is anticipated for the central, north-east, north-west, and south-peninsular regions of India, with errors of 4.1%, 5.1%, 5.5%, and 6.4%, respectively.
[12]	The oscillations that occur in the Pacific, North Atlantic, Atlantic Nino, Atlantic Multi-decadal, and IOD	Causal inference approaches and XGBoost model.	Predict and quantifies the influence of different climatic phenomena on the intrapersonal variation of ISMR.
[13]	ENSO	Physical and dynamic climate networks.	It is demonstrated that certain features of the weighted and directed climate networks can function as effective long-term predictors for ISMR forecasting.
[14]	SLP, surface temperature and zonal wind	Sub space clustering algorithm.	Suggested grouping monsoon years and predictors together to better understand and forecast the monsoon.
[15]	SST, ENSO, EQUINOO, and IOD	Methodical evaluation of previous research.	Explored existing literature with few research questions making base for future research in monsoon.

3. Research Questions

Based on literature review, three research questions have been formed which are as follows:

- RQ1: What are the factors that affects Indian Monsoon and their connection with irregular monsoon?
- RQ2: What are the relevant datasets?
- RQ3: What are the machine learning methods that can be used to quantify effect of climatic parameters in monsoon inconsistencies.

3.1 Factors Affecting Monsoon

There are both global and local parameters that contributes to prediction of monsoon and causes intra-seasonal, interannual, and multidecadal variability. Some prominent global and local factors have been surveyed as follows:

Global Factors

SST: Sea Surface Temperature

SST is the most important factors that affects monsoon globally and results in interannual variability. Ocean covers two third of the earth's surface area and the temperature of the ocean is important for almost everything in the climate system. Temperature difference between two surfaces of ocean causes SST which results in rainfall.

ENSO: EL- Nino Southern Oscillation

The geographical phenomenon known as El Niño Southern Oscillation, or ENSO, is created by the cyclical occurrence of two phenomena: El Nino and La Nina. The central and east-central Pacific Oceans, which encircle the equator, have seen a general increase in sea surface temperature due to El NINO. The southeast trade winds that cross India's intertropical convergence zone are weakened by rising SST, which results in a monsoon that is below average. On the other hand, La Nina causes the sea surface to cool in the regions where El Niño occurs resulting in heavy rainfall.

IOD: Indian Ocean Dipole

As name suggest this phenomenon occurs in Indian Ocean which lies in the tropical region. Between western and eastern sides of tropical region, there is regular shift of temperature from western side to eastern side and vice versa. This irregular shift of sea temperature is called Indian Ocean Dipole. It is very similar to ENSO effect. Due to this temperature difference western part of Indian Ocean receives heavy rainfall whereas eastern part faces severe drought conditions.

EQUINOO: Equatorial Indian Ocean Monsoon Oscillation

This is a periodical change in precipitation and cloud formation that is more noticeable over the Indian Ocean's western equatorial region and less noticeable over its eastern equatorial region, which is to the west of Sumatra. This phase of change results heavy rainfall in India.

Local Factors

Local factors mean factors which are relevant to a specified region only unlike global factors which affects monsoon conditions all over the world. Depending on the region, the effect of these variables can change. There are multitude local parameters which are responsible for creating irregular weather patterns such as latitude, irrigation, wind patterns, ocean currents, humidity, air pressure, topology, anthropogenic activities, and dust clouds.

3.2 Relevant datasets

Table 76.2 shows the list of datasets used in literature survey. Maximum papers have taken data from IMD, Pune. The other datasets which can be used for monsoon prediction are Kaggle and data.gov.in.

Table 76.2 List of datasets used in literature survey

Dataset	Period	Resolution	Platform	Reference No.
IMD	1901-2010	.25X0. 25 degrees	Both public and private	[16]
NCEP reanalysis	1948-2015	6-hour temporal and 2.5-degree spatial resolution	Public	[9]
NOAA	1910-2010	.25X0. 25 degrees	Public	[8]

3.2 Machine Learning Algorithms

The comparative analysis of various machine learning algorithms studied in literature survey have been discussed in Table 76.3 with respect to its type, ability to identify non linearity present in nature, ensemble capacity, complexity, and interpretability.

Table 76.3 Comparative analysis of machine learning models to quantify relation between climate variables and monsoon irregularities

Model Used	Type	Nonlinear Relationship	Ensemble Capability	Complexity	Interpretability
Multivariate Regression	Regression	Limited	No	Low	High
Random Forest	Ensemble	Yes	Yes	Medium	Medium
Multilayer Perceptron	Neural Network	Yes	No	High	Low
Stack Autoencoder	Ensemble (Autoencoder)	Yes	Yes	High	Low
XGBoost	Ensemble (Gradient Boosting)	Yes	Yes	Medium	Medium
Sub space clustering	Clustering	Yes	No	Medium	Low
LSTM	Recurrent neural network	Yes	No	High	Low
Prophet	Time Series Forecasting	Limited	No	Low	Medium
ARIMA	Time Series Forecasting	Limited	No	Low	Medium

4. Conclusion

This work has shed light on the relationships between monsoon rainfall and a variety of meteorological attributes, including global and local factors which have a significant impact on the distribution of monsoon rainfall which in turn can disturbs the social economic structure of many countries like India. To control adverse consequences, it is suggested to comprehend and forecast changes in monsoon patterns where climatic factors plays a crucial role. Few research question has been addressed in this direction to systematically examine the relationship between monsoon variability and factors influencing it. It has also analysed all statistical approaches that have been undertaken up to this point.

Accuracy of any statistical method is a function of data. So, increased effort is needed in data assimilation procedures especially from remote locations to yield improved qualitative results.

REFERENCES

1. Palmer, T. N., Alessandri, A., Andersen, U., Cantelaube, P., Davey, M., Delécluse, P., ... & Thomson, M. C. (2004). Development of a European multimodel ensemble system for seasonal-to-interannual prediction (DEMETER). Bulletin of the American Meteorological Society, 85(6), 853-872.
2. Araya-Melo, P. A., Crucifix, M., & Bounceur, N. (2015). Global sensitivity analysis of the Indian monsoon during the Pleistocene. Climate of the Past, 11(1), 45-61.
3. Dash, Y., Mishra, S. K., & Panigrahi, B. K. (2019). Predictability assessment of northeast monsoon rainfall in India using sea surface temperature anomaly through statistical and machine learning techniques. Environmetrics, 30(4), e2533.
4. Tabari, H., Taye, M. T., & Willems, P. (2015). Statistical assessment of precipitation trends in the upper Blue Nile River basin. Stochastic environmental research and risk assessment, 29, 1751-1761.
5. Manoj, S., & Valliyammai, C. (2023). Analysis of shift in Indian monsoon and prediction of accumulated cyclone energy in Indian subcontinent using deep learning. Automatika, 64(4), 1116-1127.
6. Saha, M., Santara, A., Mitra, P., Chakraborty, A., & Nanjundiah, R. S. (2021). Prediction of the Indian summer monsoon using a stacked autoencoder and ensemble regression model. International Journal of Forecasting, 37(1), 58-71.
7. Loo, Y. Y., Billa, L., & Singh, A. (2015). Effect of climate change on seasonal monsoon in Asia and its impact on the variability of monsoon rainfall in Southeast Asia. Geoscience Frontiers, 6(6), 817-823.
8. Saha, M., Mitra, P., & Nanjundiah, R. S. (2016). Predictor discovery for early-late Indian summer monsoon using stacked autoencoder. Procedia Computer Science, 80, 565-576.
9. Falga, R., & Wang, C. (2022). The rise of Indian summer monsoon precipitation extremes and its correlation with long-term changes of climate and anthropogenic factors. Scientific reports, 12(1), 11985.

10. Song, C., Liu, F., Huang, Y., Wang, L., & Tan, T. (2013). Auto-encoder based data clustering. In Progress in Pattern Recognition, Image Analysis, Computer Vision, and Applications: 18th Iberoamerican Congress, CIARP 2013, Havana, Cuba, November 20-23, 2013, Proceedings, Part I 18 (pp. 117-124). Springer Berlin Heidelberg.

11. Saha, M., Mitra, P., & Nanjundiah, R. S. (2017). Deep learning for predicting the monsoon over the homogeneous regions of India; J. Earth Syst. Sci. 126.

12. Chakraborty, D., Mitra, A., Goswami, B., & Rajesh, P. (2022, May). Identification of Global Drivers of Indian Summer Monsoon using Causal Inference and Interpretable AI. In EGU General Assembly Conference Abstracts (pp. EGU22-4431).

13. Fan, J., Meng, J., Ludescher, J., Li, Z., Surovyatkina, E., Chen, X., ... & Schellnhuber, H. J. (2022). Network-based approach and climate change benefits for forecasting the amount of Indian monsoon rainfall. Journal of Climate, 35(3), 1009-1020.

14. Saha, M., Chakraborty, A., & Mitra, P. (2016). Predictor-year subspace clustering based ensemble prediction of Indian summer monsoon. Advances in Meteorology, 2016.

15. Sahastrabuddhe, R., Ghausi, S. A., Joseph, J., & Ghosh, S. (2023). Indian Summer Monsoon Rainfall in a changing climate: a review. Journal of Water and Climate Change, 14(4), 1061-1088.

Emerging Trends in IoT and Computing Technologies – Suman Lata Tripathi et al. (eds)
© 2024 Taylor & Francis Group, London, ISBN 978-1-032-87924-6

Nature Inspired Optimization Algorithms: A Gentle Review

77

Seema Kalonia[1], Amrita Upadhyay[2]
Banasthali Vidyapith, Department of Computer Science,
Rajasthan-304022, India

Abstract: Nature uses basic yet effective methods to carry out complicated tasks. Although they may appear simple from the outside, natural processes are made up of some intricately designed sub processes. Many Nature-Inspired Optimization Algorithms (NIOAs) have been created recently, drawing inspiration from nature. NIOAs are becoming a larger and larger family. As a result, there are a lot of NIOAs, and choosing the right one is a laborious task. This review examines the importance of Nature Inspired Optimization Algorithms and the study conducts a gentle review and comparative analysis of the most commonly used Nature Inspired Models. This research review is based on five Nature Inspired algorithms including the Genetic Algorithm (GA), firefly algorithm (FA), Particle Swarm Optimization Algorithm (PSO), Ant Colony Optimization (ACO), Bee Algorithm (BA), along with their role, importance, and need of these NIOAs.

Keywords: Nature inspired optimization algorithms, Particle swarm optimization, Ant colony optimization, Bees algorithm, Genetic algorithm, Firefly algorithm

1. Introduction

In recent decades, a growing body of research has shown that nature might be a useful source of inspiration for the creation of intelligent systems and solutions to difficult problems. Evolutionary pressure forces animals to develop highly specialized skills and organs so they can take advantage of the chances provided by competing for mates, food, and territory. Evolution is the process of fine-tuning the parameter values in the algorithms. Algorithms for optimization can be developed from certain organs and talents. This paper carefully examines five nature-inspired algorithms: Firefly Algorithm (FA), Ant Colony Optimisation (ACO), Bees Algorithm (BA), Genetic Algorithm (GA), and Particle Swarm Optimization (PS). Nature has always been the source of human longing for the unachievable. Human problem-solving is modeled by natural occurrences effectively and systematically. As a result, people learn and use problem-solving strategies from nature in a range of situations. Research indicates that humans frequently care more about a "good" answer at the moment than a "best" solution later on. Numerous nature-inspired optimization algorithms (NIOAs) are created with this observation in mind and are intended to deliver the solution within suitable time constraints [1].

This section discusses several criteria for classification and, using matching control parameters and operators, highlights the structure of each algorithm.

1.2 Classification criteria

Three criteria have been chosen among 29 studies of NIOAs and are noted below for discussion after being identified for classification.

[1]skalonia25@gmail.com, [2]amritaupadhayay@banasthali.in

DOI: 10.1201/9781003535423-77

Origin of Inspiration

There have been previous instances of grouping based on inspiration sources. It points to a specific domain that an NIOA copies. Domains that are often used are:

Biology: A significant number of algorithms draw inspiration from biological processes. Some examples of bio-inspired algorithms are ant colony optimization, particle swarm optimization, firefly algorithm, genetic algorithm, cuckoo search algorithm, and bat algorithm.

Physics: A few algorithms are modeled after phenomena in Physics. These include the gravitational search method, electromagnetic optimization, simulated annealing, central force optimization, and river formation dynamics algorithm.

Alternatives: Within our research, there exists a chemistry-based algorithm known as chemical reaction optimization and another algorithm that draws influence from music, namely harmony.

Solution Set Dimensions

An algorithm assesses one solution in a single iteration or a collection of solutions. Algorithms are separated into two categories according to the criteria and the quantity of solutions used:

Single-based solution: As was previously established, NIOA that assesses only one solution every iteration falls into this type. To get the best answer, such an algorithm travels along a trajectory.

Multiple solution-based: An algorithm falls into this category if it advances towards optimum goals at the same time by working on several workable solutions. Another name for this type of algorithm is a population-based algorithm. This class includes the majority of NIOAs.

Algorithm's nature

The process of computing a new solution may be used to understand the nature of an algorithm. It may be split into two categories:

Stochastic: An NIOA is referred to as stochastic or randomized NIOA if it incorporates any random element into its overall computation to provide new solutions. The inability to forecast the intermediate computations and final results in advance, given a set of input parameters, is one of the characteristics of stochastic algorithms. Consequently, outcomes obtained from a single algorithm run might stand out from the competition. The majority of algorithms inspired by nature are stochastic.

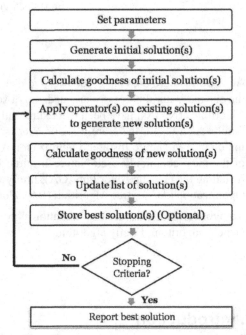

Fig. 77.1 Phases of nature inspired algorithms [1]

Deterministic: NIOAs that do not generate additional solutions using random numbers are referred to as deterministic, in contrast to stochastic NIOAs.

2. Literature Review

Numerous nature-inspired optimization algorithms exist in the literature and vary slightly from one another. It is challenging for a person to examine and analyze each one of them due to their sheer number. While some algorithms make use of biological notions, others adhere to physics and chemical rules. While some algorithms only need one solution, others call for a collection of solutions. While some algorithms are probabilistic in nature, others are stochastic. On the other hand, some ideas, such as operators, tuning parameters, and encoding, are universal. As a result, a researcher who is unfamiliar with NIOAs is never sure which algorithm to use. Shao, Xue-Feng, and others (2021) Smart manufacturing describes how linked devices work together inside the Cyber-Physical System to create a self-adjusting environment that can handle changes and recommend the best course of action. Large data simulation, production optimization, and all-around monitoring are among the tasks that smart manufacturing can handle, according to Tao et al. [2].

A study was carried out on 29 NIOAs to determine the commonalities and distinctions among them [1]. The hypothesis of computationally imitating human conduct is known as "Artificial Life" or "Artificial Intelligence." It entails creating computer programs that can carry out operations that call for human intellect. Previously, only humans were able to identify a person's voice for eggs. However, today, voice recognition is a standard function on all digital devices [5]. Artificial intelligence has made this feasible. Decision-making, language translation, visual perception, and other processes may be considered further instances of human intelligence. It is made feasible by a variety of strategies. A study was carried out on 29 NIOAs to determine the commonalities and distinctions among them [1]. The term "approaches of artificial intelligence" refers to the methods used to incorporate artificial intelligence into computers [6].

Research Questions:

- RQ1 What are the most commonly used Nature Inspired Optimization Algorithms?
- RQ2 What is the Importance and role of Nature Inspired Optimization algorithms?
- RQ3 What are the applications of NIOAs?

According to RQ1 most commonly used nature-inspired optimization algorithms are:

3. Particle Swarm optimization

Inspired by swarm behaviour seen in nature, such as fish and bird schools, Particle Swarm Optimization (PSO) is a potent meta-heuristic optimization technique [7]. A streamlined social structure is simulated in PSO. The initial goal of the PSO algorithm was to visually represent the exquisite yet erratic movement of a flock of birds. Any area in which the bird may be observed in the wild is restricted to a certain range. On the other hand, having several birds in a swarm enables all of the birds to recognize the greater surface area of a fitness function.

To help the swarm locate the global minima of a fitness function, let's analytically represent the aforementioned concepts [6].

Mathematical Model of PSO

In particle swarm optimization, every particle has a location, velocity, and fitness value.

Particle_bestFitness_value and particle_bestFitness_position are tracked by each particle.

Global_bestFitness_value and global_bestFitness_position are kept on file.

4. Ant Colony Optimization

An innovative approach to problem-solving, the Ant Colony Optimization (ACO) technique takes its cues from the social activities of ants as they hunt for the shortest paths. Actual ants leave pheromone marks on the ground to indicate their preferred route, which draws other ants to follow, then wander until they come upon food before returning to their nest [2]. More pheromones will be left behind by ants who follow the trail and locate food, encouraging more ants to do the same [1].

5. Bees Algorithm

The conduct of honey bees, whose colonies may often spread out across 10 to 14 kilometres and into several divisions at once to utilize a multitude of food sources, served as the model for the BA. The colony strives to make the best use possible of all of its members. In theory, more bees would be drawn to a food supply that is closer and richer in terms of nectar or pollen. Scout bees start the process of finding food by searching. They take off at random to investigate every food source in every direction. Upon their return to the hive, they use waggle dancing to inform the other bees about the findings of their search and to convey crucial information on the food supply encompassing its quality rating, direction, and distance. For the colony to correctly deploy flower bees to food sources, the waggle dance is crucial to the assessment of the food source. [2].

It is a population-based optimization algorithm. The algorithm's initial pseudo code is described as follows:

1. Use random solutions to initialize the population.
2. Assess the population's fitness.
3. As the new population is being formed (stopping requirement not satisfied).
4. Choose locations for your neighborhood search.
5. Assess fitness and gather bees for the chosen locations (more bees for the better e sites).
6. From each patch, pick the bee that fits the best.
7. Assign the surviving bees to a random search, then assess their level of fitness.
8. End of While.

6. Genetic Algorithms (GA)

Using methods derived from biological evolution, GA produces answers to search, optimization, and machine learning issues. In early times, computer simulations were the first used for genetic algorithms [9]. A book by Fraser and Burnell was later published to methodically describe the computer simulations of evolution, which at that point gained enormous popularity and contained all the fundamental elements of contemporary genetic algorithms [10]. GA uses several terms related to genetics, such as:

1. A solution to an optimization issue is encoded in a chromosome. Binary representation is commonly used for the solutions [9].
2. A step in the GA called selection occurs when specific genomes are picked out to breed future generations.
3. Two parents can have a combination of mutations and crossovers applied to them when to change their genetic makeup, they procreate [5]. To conduct a GA, the population must first be initialized. This population is often made up of randomly generated people who represent every potential solution; the size of the population is based on the nature of the issue.

7. Firefly (FA) Algorithm

To communicate with one another and, more specifically, to attract potential prey, fireflies emit luminous flashes [33]. FA is predicated on the following three suppositions and draws inspiration from the biochemical and social features of fireflies: Three elements influence the attraction between fireflies: (a) all other fireflies are drawn to them by their smaller flashes; (b) the brightness of each firefly affects its appeal, which is inversely proportional to distance; and (c) no firefly can draw the attention of the brightest firefly, which wanders arbitrarily [4].

GA has been extensively used to tackle challenging issues, particularly in the fields of control engineering, scheduling, and global optimization.

When compared to other intelligent optimization algorithms, genetic algorithms are among the simplest to build. Furthermore, the end criteria may not always be evident. GA often isn't able to solve the problem if the fitness function only returns 0/1.

Table 77.1 Comparative analysis of most commonly used NIOAs

S. N.	Optimization Algorithm	Description	Advantages	Limitations
1.	Particle Swarm Optimization (PSO) [8]	Population-based optimization algorithm inspired by the social behaviour of bird flocking or fish schooling.	Simplicity of implementation, fast convergence, ability to handle continuous and discrete variables	Premature convergence, difficulty in handling high-dimensional problems, sensitivity to parameter settings
2.	Ant Colony Optimization (ACO) [3]	Metaheuristic algorithm inspired by the behaviour of ants searching for food.	Ability to handle discrete optimization problems, robustness against local optima, flexibility in problem representation	Slower convergence speed, sensitivity to parameter settings, difficulty in handling continuous variables
3.	Bees Algorithm(BA)[4]	The BA has been inspired by the food-foraging behaviour of honey bees.	It has advantages of memory, local search, and solution improvement mechanism over the other meta-heuristic algorithms.	insufficient population diversity, strong equation-searching ability but weak developing capacity
4.	Genetic Algorithm (GA) [9]	Evolutionary algorithm based on principles of natural selection and genetics. It utilizes techniques like crossover, mutation, and selection to evolve solutions.	Ability to handle complex problems, population diversity, suitability for parallelization	High computational cost, difficulty in handling continuous variables with high precision, parameter tuning
5.	Firefly Algorithm(FA)[5]	As a means of communication, fireflies emit luminous flashes to attract potential prey and to exchange signals with one another.	When used in multi objective optimization, it seems to work better.	Poor convergence speed, high computing time complexity, and other issues. The primary cause is that FA uses a fully attracted model, which causes each firefly to oscillate while it moves.

According to RQ2 the necessity of optimization algorithms is influenced by nature:

These algorithms find highly efficient solutions to multi-modal and multi-dimensional problems. Calculus optimization often entails finding the critical points by equating the goal function's first-order derivative to zero. These important locations then deliver the maximum or least value according to the goal function. Compared to other methods, higher-order derivatives and even gradients need more processing resources and are more error-prone. You may also appreciate how difficult it would be to solve a maximization/ minimization issue with twenty or more variables. However, the problem may be addressed with less computing effort and temporal complexity by employing these techniques inspired by nature.

Importance of Optimization algorithms:

Effective Feature Selection: Feature selection is a critical step in software engineering problems because it aids in determining the most relevant features. Optimization algorithms can aid in selecting the optimal subset of features, reducing dimensionality, and improving the model's efficiency and generalization ability.

Handling Complex Relationships: Some of the software engineering problem often involves complex relationships between input features and the occurrence of results. Optimization algorithms can help uncover and model these relationships by adapting the model's structure, weights, or hyperparameters. This enables the model to better capture the underlying patterns and dependencies in the data.

Dealing with Noisy and Imbalanced Data: Various datasets often suffer from noise and class imbalance, where optimization algorithms can address these challenges by applying suitable sampling techniques, data pre-processing methods, or cost-sensitive learning approaches to ensure the model's robustness and reliability.

According to RQ3, the various applications of NIOAs are Designing digital filters, processing images, Artificial Intelligence, creating digital differentiators and integrators, Identification by face, and Constructing neural networks, FA may be used in new town development and transportation system design optimization.

8. Conclusion and Future Direction

This assessment makes it clear that the area of computers influenced by nature is broad and still growing. This paper focused on the importance and role of nature-inspired optimization models in various fields. Physics- and biology-based techniques and algorithms, offer a concise overview of the major developments achieved in this fascinating field of study. We can conclude here that NIOAs can be used to solve various computational problems in the future in the field of engineering, and artificial intelligence.

REFERENCES

1. Kumar, A., Nadeem, M., & Banka, H. (2023). Nature inspired optimization algorithms: a comprehensive overview. Evolving Systems, 14(1), 141-156.
2. Yang, X. S. (2020). Nature-inspired optimization algorithms: Challenges and open problems. Journal of Computational Science, 46, 101104.
3. Tzanetos, A., & Dounias, G. (2021). Nature-inspired optimization algorithms or simply variations of metaheuristics? Artificial Intelligence Review, 54, 1841-1862.
4. Soni, V., Sharma, A., & Singh, V. (2021, March). A critical review on nature-inspired optimization algorithms. In IOP Conference Series: Materials Science and Engineering (Vol. 1099, No. 1, p. 012055). IOP Publishing.
5. Yang, X. S., & He, X. (2016). Nature-inspired optimization algorithms in engineering: overview and applications. Nature-inspired computation in engineering, 1-20.
6. Jain, M., Saihjpal, V., Singh, N., & Singh, S. B. (2022). An overview of variants and advancements of PSO algorithm. Applied Sciences, 12(17), 8392.
7. Marini, F., & Walczak, B. (2015). Particle swarm optimization (PSO). A tutorial. Chemometrics and Intelligent Laboratory Systems, 149, 153-165.
8. Jain, M., Saihjpal, V., Singh, N., & Singh, S. B. (2022). An overview of variants and advancements of PSO algorithm. Applied Sciences, 12(17), 8392.
9. Schoenauer, M., & Xanthakis, S. (1993, June). Constrained GA optimization. In Proc. 5th International Conference on Genetic Algorithms (pp. 573-580). Morgan Kaufmann.
10. SS, V. C., & HS, A. (2022). Nature-inspired meta-heuristic algorithms for optimization problems. Computing, 104(2), 251-269.

Emerging Trends in IoT and Computing Technologies – Suman Lata Tripathi et al. (eds)
© 2024 Taylor & Francis Group, London, ISBN 978-1-032-87924-6

Artificial Neural Network Based Optimization Algorithms

78

Meenakshi[1], Meenakshi Pareek[2]

Banasthali Vidyapith, Rajasthan - 304022, India

Abstract: In recent years, many research projects have been conducted to improve Artificial Intelligence (AI) through Optimization. These include widely recognized methods such as Lightning Search Algorithm (LSA), Gravity Search Algorithm (GSA), Particle Swarm Optimization, Dolphin algorithm and Artificial Bee Colony. All these methods fall into the category of population-based algorithms, in which the population is created for the first time. These methods are capable of producing good solutions. This article discusses the development of Artificial Intelligence in networks through optimization and presents an optimal network model that effectively solves problems by changing treatment or insufficient training. This study includes results showing that the performance of ANN can be improved by using optimization techniques such as PSO, GA, ABC. This technique is used to investigate many input parameters number of hidden parameters and learning rate to improve ANN performance.

Keywords: ANN augmentation, Genetic algorithm, Particle swarm optimization, Artificial bee colony

1. Introduction

AI research aims to understand human intelligence and problem solving. Deep learning (DL) is a hierarchical approach to the field that finds applications in object perception, speech recognition, genomics, and medicine. Artificial neural networks (ANNs) are a deep learning approach with multiple hidden layers. Many applications such as Convolutional Neural Networks, Artificial Neural Networks, and Recurrent Neural Networks serve different situations. ANN is computational models made by the human brain. [1] They have a network of neurons that receive signals, use weights, calculate them, and pass the results to the activation function. An artificial neural network is comprised of an input layer, hidden layers and an output layer. During training, the weights are updated using recorded data. Neurons use activation functions to recognize inconsistencies and loss functions to identify differences between predictions and actual results. Back propagation propagates errors back through the network to change the weights. Optimization algorithms fine-tune the network, minimizing performance loss. Optimization problems often require effective methods and algorithms to improve the parameters, architecture, and learning rules in neural networks. The review also discusses the evolution of backpropagation with optimization algorithms to solve specific problems in neural network training. [6]This paper concludes with sections on data and methods, challenges, analysis of optimization algorithms, neural network architecture, implementation, optimization parameters, and future considerations.

2. Recent Challenges for ANN-Based Optimization

Artificial Neural Networks (ANN) is widely recognized as one of the most effective problem-solving techniques. But they are probabilistic in nature. Artificial neural networks use model weights and back propagating error signals to realign each iteration.

---

[1]mchawla.4441@gmail.com, [2]pmeenakshi@banasthali.in[2]

DOI: 10.1201/9781003535423-78

[2] Although neural network devices are effective, they also have some limitations and problems. These include the need to determine the correct network topology, timing, optimal parameters, trial and error and additional interpretation that may require expert review. [4]

The following points summarize the main problems faced by neural network devices:

1. Analysis of Artificial neural networks (ANNs) leads to a lack of explanation of the process of selecting some results and rejecting others, leading to a lack of trust in the network.

2. Artificial neural networks (ANNs) do not have clear criteria to determine the optimal design. Achieving the right standards in a network often relies on efficiency and trial and error.

3. Artificial Neural Networks (ANN) require powerful binary systems and specialized ANN models, resulting in the limitation that the entire method depends on the capabilities of the hardware.

4. At the same time growth disrupts this process causing a gradual decline in performance. Network problems may not appear immediately or directly.

The effectiveness of delivery systems and disrupted network operations may depend on the expertise of the investigator. Artificial Neural Networks (ANN) has developed rapidly since the mid-20th century and has become important in many areas of our lives. Artificial neural networks have many advantages, such as the ability to solve complex and irregular problems [3]. However, it is important to know their shortcomings and solve them by doing the best by choosing the best connection models and appropriate strategies. Choosing the best neural network parameters for your application is important because different types of NN have different strategies for different applications. The advantage of NN over other AI algorithms is that they can perform well across many devices. Unlike ANFIS, NN are suitable for regression and classification because they are no fixed in the number of devices assist by them. [8]

3. LIterature Review

Optimization techniques are necessary to analyze, distribute or select the best solutions to improve existing processes across research. These algorithms solve problems such as decision making and heuristic strategies, global optimization of complex problems and optimization of neural networks. [6] Optimization techniques including biology-based (e.g. genetic algorithms) and physics-based (e.g. search algorithms) play an important role. Among the algorithms discussed, Particle Swarm Optimization (PSO) improves the Artificial Neural Network (ANN) method [9] while Gravity Search Algorithm (GSA) solves the ANN problem in applications such as biomedical image competition. NNA is assist by neural networks and biological system find applications in machine learning and biodiversity assessment. The Backtracking Search Algorithm (BSA) draws on experience and has been used to develop fuzzy logic speed controllers, while the Lightning Search Algorithm (LSA) and its quantum-inspired variant (QLSA) have many applications including home management.[10] Optimization techniques vary in their advantages and disadvantages and choosing the most appropriate method for a problem remains difficult.

Table 78.1 Advantages and disadvantages of optimization

S. N.	Optimization	Advantages of optimization	Disadvantages of Optimization
1	PSO [1]	Ability to solve word wide complex fastly	Easily get tangled up in local network
2	GA [2]	For calculation it is not need mathematical derivation	Accuracy issues not able to be resolved optimally
3	NNA [3]	It performs well in solving lower-dimensional	Accuracy issues not able to be resolved optimally
4	ABC [7]	Easy for search process, fast and flexible	Utilizing the dual population approach makes the Computation time consuming.
5	LSA [8]	Quick convergence and adaptability	Only one parameter determines the search models amplitude

4. Enhancement of Artificial Neural Networks with Optimization Algorithms

This strategies is use to enhance applications by determining minimum cost and maximum efficiency. It is divided into two main groups: biology-based and physics-based [4]. Biology-based algorithms such as dolphin algorithm (DSA), group optimization, ant colony optimization, cuckoo search fitness search, disease collection optimization, genetic algorithm (GA), artificial bee colony algorithm, chaos algorithm, gravity search techniques etc.

4.1 Artificial Neural Networks-Based PSO

The PSO technique uses velocity vectors to update the position of the group. It is widely applied to resolve challenging linear and nonlinear issues. Weight optimization of the initial or total weight of the network is one of many algorithms and applications of optimization.[5]The ANN method is adopted using PSO weights. PSO is a scientific and experimental method for finding hyper parameters in various fields leading to improvements in many applications. The following subsections introduce optimization strategies to improve the performance of neural networks.

Table 78.2 Advantages of ANN with PSO

S. N.	Deep Learner	Optimization	Problem with optimizer	Enhancement of application
1	ANN [13]	PSO	To forecast air blast-overpressure during the blasting of quarries	Air blast-overpressure has significant effects on four granite quarry sites in Malaysia
2	ANN [14]	PSO	Decrease the cost of pumping and solved ground management issues	Various parameters have been found to be influential
3	ANN [5]	PSO	To give a solution of flow of traffic predication	Under groundwater management of the basin in France

4.2 Artificial Neural Networks-Based Genetic Algorithms

Genetic algorithms use multiple rotations, mutations and safeguards for multiple chromosomes to solve optimization problems. The process is known as stochastic optimization and it is based on the principle of natural selection. Genetic algorithms are used by researchers in many fields such as artificial neural network (ANN) optimization, energy management and renewable energy. ANN-based genetic algorithms are used for many problems including optimization, spectrum estimation, modeling and operation. [7]. For many applications and classification problems, such as fruit juice extraction and optimization of lipase synthesis researchers have combined the two strategies.

Table 78.3 Advantages of ANN with genetic algorithm

S. N.	Deep Learner	Optimization	Problem with optimizer	Enhancement of application
1	ANN [5]	PSO &GA	Significant processing expense when employing MNN	Designing an anisotropic laminated composite
2	ANN [4]	GA	For the weight reduction Ascertain suitable parameters	Analysis of heat transmission in a perforated plate fins
3	ADNN [3]	GA	To a complete catenary model and a local optimum	Solved in catenary model in many application
4	ANN [6]	GA	For NN optimized the threshold value	Solved the risk prediction with accuracy

4.3 Artificial Neural Networks-Based Artificial Bee Colony

Researchers use optimization and improve efficiency of the ABC technique neural networks. Research combines ABC with neural networks for air infiltration detection and energy load estimation. Deep neural network is also used along with ABC in classification problems. An average neural network model based on ABC is proposed to predict the load capacity. Many studies combine NN and ABC to solve specific problems.

Table 78.4 Advantages of ANN with artificial bee colony

S. N.	Deep Learner	Optimization	Problem with optimizer	Enhancement of application
1	ANN [1]	ABC	A set of neuron connection weights that have been optimized	Forecasting the power load
2	MNN [4]	ABC	Optimized input values weight	Improved the performance of NN
3	DNN [3]	ABC	DNN parameter optimization	Defense against attackers at once

5. Artificial Neural Networks Based Optimization Techniques

This section describes the application of optimization based on ANN methods such as ANN-PSO, GA, and ABC which are based on searching and learning the ideal quantity of nodes and the best learning in the first and second groups of hidden nodes. The output value is sent in binary time (24x25) are received [8]. The data entry contains six entries including solar irradiance, battery status, grid, energy cost, and diesel fuel, wind speed is below the scale. This figure shows the number of input values and output values known from the data. The time used for each ANN training session is unpredictable and may take longer or shorter depending on the type of ANN training session.

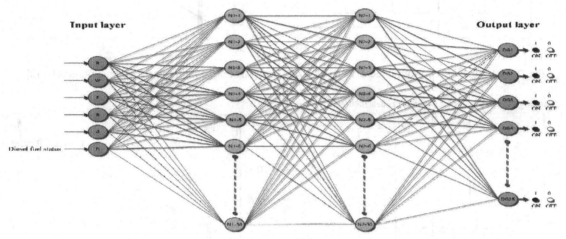

Fig. 78.1   Using input and output data ANN with three optimization PSO, GA and ABC [3].

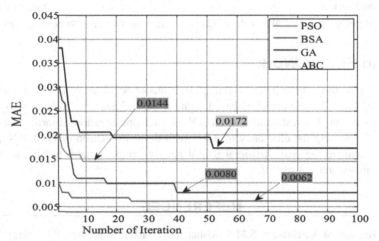

Fig. 78.2   ANN with optimization objectives [3]

5.1 ANN Optimization Result after Apply PSO and GA and ABC

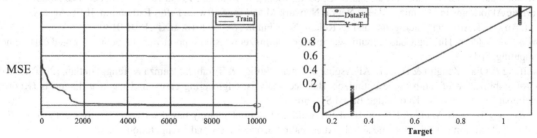

Fig. 78.3   Enhanced performance of ANN with PSO. [1]

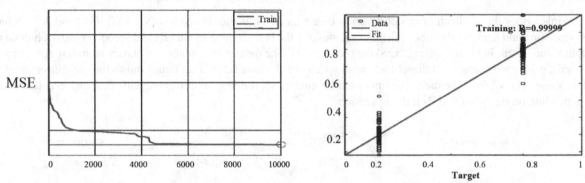

Fig. 78.4 Enhanced performance of ANN with ABC optimization algorithm with optimal parameter [3]

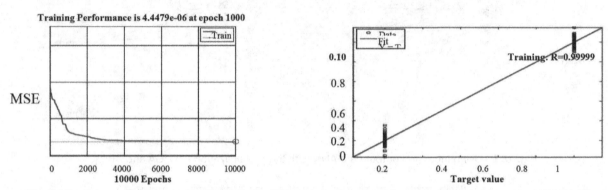

Fig. 78.5 Enhanced performance of ANN with ABC optimization algorithm with optimal parameter ANN-GA [3]

6. Conclusions and Future Work

This review includes an in-depth study of the benefits and applications of Artificial Neural Networks (ANN). It also includes development, training, and optimization experiments based on network architecture. To briefly explain ANN's development, this paper discusses the experimental investigation of an ANN-based optimization algorithm approach. According to the comparison and test results, improving the efficiency of ANN with the combination of PSO, ANN-GA, and ANN-ABC can improve the accuracy and minimize the cost. Artificial neural network improvement techniques are used to reveal ANN's disadvantages and train it in many areas of real life.

REFERENCES

1. G. M. Abdolrasol, M.; Hannan, M.A.; Hussain, S.M.S.; Ustun, T.S.; Sarker, M.R.; Ker, P.J. Energy Management Scheduling for Microgrids in the Virtual Power Plant System Using Artificial Neural Networks. *Energies* **2021**, *14*, 6507.
2. T. M. Shami, A. A. El-Saleh, M. Alswaitti, Q. Al-Tashi, M. A. Summakieh and S. Mirjalili, Particle Swarm Optimization: A Comprehensive Survey, in *IEEE Access*, vol. 10, pp. 10031-10061, 2023
3. Khan, Muhammad Sufyan & Jabeen, Farhana & Ghouzali, Sanaa & Rehman, Zobia & Naz, Sheneela & Abdul, Wadood. (2021). Metaheuristic Algorithms in Optimizing Deep Neural Network Model for Software Effort Estimation. IEEE Access.
4. Shabbir, J. Anwer, T. Artificial Intelligence and its Role in Near Future. *arXiv* 2018, arXiv:1804.01396.
5. Wang, Mingjing & Chen, Huiling.Chaotic multi-swarm whale optimizer boosted support vector machine for medical diagnosis. Applied Soft Computing. 2019
6. Shan, Weifeng & Qiao, Zenglin & Heidari, Ali Asghar & Chen, Huiling & Turabieh, Hamza & Teng, Yuntian. (2020). Double adaptive weights for stabilization of moth flame optimizer: Balance analysis, engineering cases, and medical diagnosis (Knowledge-Based Systems, Impact Factor: 8.038). Knowledge-Based Systems.
7. Shahpar, Zahra & Bardsiri, Vahid & Khatibi Bardsiri, Amid. Polynomial analogy-based software development effort estimation using combined particle swarm optimization and simulated annealing. Concurrency and Computation 2021.

8. Kassem, Haithem, Khaled Mahar, and Amani Saad. "Software Effort Estimation Using Hi-erarchical Attention Neural Network." Journal of Theoretical and Applied Information Tech-nology 100.18 ,2022.

9. Marco, Robert, Sharifah Sakinah Syed Ahmad, and Sabrina Ahmad. An Improving Long Short Term Memory-Grid Search Based Deep Learning Neural Network for Software Effort Estimation. International Journal of Intelligent Engineering & Systems, 16, no. 4 2023

10. Khan, Muhammad Sufyan, et al. Metaheuristic algorithms in optimizing deep neural net-work model for software effort estimation. IEEE Access 9 ,2021

Emerging Trends in IoT and Computing Technologies – Suman Lata Tripathi et al. (eds)
© 2024 Taylor & Francis Group, London, ISBN 978-1-032-87924-6

Creating Sensor System for Safe Motor Navigation: HOMESWEET

79

Lare Samuel Adeola[1],
Celestine Iwendi[2], Aamir Mazhar Abbas[3]

University of Bolton, Department of Creative Technologies,
Bolton, England

Abstract: 'HOMESWEET' is a deep learning model created with the YOLO object detection algorithm that has been trained to detect certain human physical states that could result in road accidents and deaths. The model achieved an accuracy score of 83% and a Precision rate of over 90% but had a fairly modest Recall rate of just over 70%. The model can be deployed in various other applications as it was able to detect not only facial cues but other micro-expressions and gesticulations that lead to the various states; in particular, in this research, it was created to detect fatigue, drowsiness and lack of total concentration while driving.

Keywords: Computer vision, Deep learning, Sensor system, Ubiquitous computing, YOLOV5

1. Introduction

Unsafe driving is one of the leading causes of death not only in the United Kingdom but also in the world. Ac- cording to the data from [1], an average of 2400 people die each year from year 2000 to 2020 as a result of road accidents. 34% of these road accidents are caused by motorists who have failed to look properly [2]. Figures 79.1, 79.2 and 79.3, show various plots of the number of lives lost, those who sustained serious injuries and the total injuries as a result of road accidents.

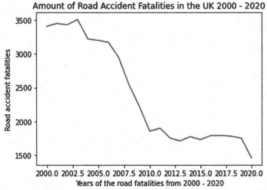

Fig. 79.1 Amount of road accident fatalities in the UK 2000 - 2020

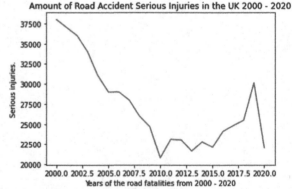

Fig. 79.2 Amount of road accident serious injuries in the UK 2000 - 2020

[1]l.adeola@bolton.ac.uk, [2]c.iwendi@bolton.ac.uk, [3]a.abbas@bolton.ac.uk

DOI: 10.1201/9781003535423-79

The charts show a markedly downward trend in the amount of road accidents fatalities from the year 2000 to the year 2020. While this is commendable, it is not enough. For example, in the year 2020, there were a total of 1460 deaths caused by road accidents. This means that an average of 4 people died from road accidents per day in the year 2020. This coupled with the fact that road accidents can be avoided, it is imperative to always strive to reduce these figures further.

This makes the development of a sensor application that can help curtail unsafe driving habits paramount and important. As this application can not only save the lives of drivers and motorists but also save the lives of members of the public like pedestrians and cyclists. In this research, we present a sensor application system that has achieved an accuracy score of 83% in predicting selected unsafe driving habits (like fatigue, drunkenness, distractions) and other causes that may lead to both road accident fatalities and serious injuries.

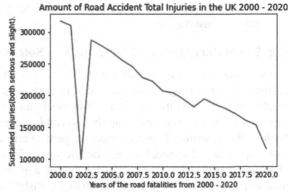

Fig. 79.3 Amount of road accident total injuries in the UK 2000 - 2020

Aims and Objectives

- Build a Computer Vision Model to detect driver fatigue.
- Create a Sensor and Feedback system.

2. Micro-expressions - A Brief Detour

Micro-expressions are those semi-voluntary, often not lasting too long, expressions that our body makes frequently in different behavioural states [3]. For example, whenever we meet someone we genuinely like, there's a web that pulls our eyes and our pupils expand [4]. There are also micro-expressions in other states like fatigue, drunkenness etc. A good example of a micro expression for fatigue can be the yawn. Whenever we yawn, more often than not it is a sign of either current fatigue or future fatigue; with the way we fold our hands (mostly one's dominant hand) to cover our mouths while yawning, this was a common micro-expression noticed in a lot of images sourced from our secondary data sources and the model was fed with this information. Figure 79.4 shows the various images which had this micro-expression and how the model performed in predicting their label. Other micro-expressions like the closing of the eyes(drowsy/sleepy) or the alertness level (wider opened eyes or a smile or laugh) or common gesticulations (like the stretch when one is tired) were also used to train the model.

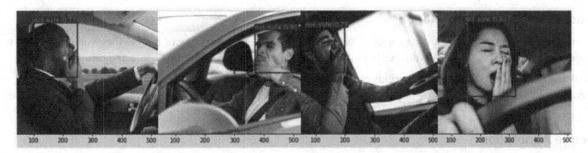

Fig. 79.4 Showing the various fatigue/drowsiness micro-expressions. You can see in the image the prevalence of a yawn and the body movements that trail such a fatigue state

3. Methodology

3.1 Primary Data

The training of 'HOMESWEET' involved both primary and secondary sources of data. The primary source of data was of the author and it was taken through the webcam of the author's laptop. A series of different images and angles were taken to make the model consistent in accurately predicting the various sub-classes. These po- sitions include - i. At different focal lengths. This was achieved albeit mechanically by moving further away. ii. Blurry/grainy images. This was achieved by being in slight motion while the camera was capturing the author's image iii. Side views. iv.Tilts. uncontrolled Environment. All the images from the primary data were taken in the Peter Stocker Laboratory (sci 2.27) in the Department of Computing Sciences, University of East Anglia.

3.2 Secondary Data and Other Image Selection Criteria

The secondary data was sourced from the web. They are - Google Images, Pixabay, and istockphoto. There were three cardinal attributes/features sought after when selecting an image – i. Posture - Does the image narrate honestly the class to which it would belong? ii. Clarity and Crisp - How clear and crisp is the image? What is the pixel density? iii. Image Shot - Is it a full view or a side view? Is it a close-up shot or a mid-range shot? iv. Nationality. Algorithm Bias can hinder the general effectiveness and adaptability of a model in the wild. Hence, various images of different nationalities were selected. Three nationalities in total were represented - African/Black/Black British/Caribbean, Asian/Asian British/Arab, and White/Caucasian. v. Gender - In order to further reduce bias, images of both women and men were selected and sourced. vi. Lighting - Is the image well-lit or under-lit or mid-lit? Efforts were made to select images that tick one of the previous options.

Figure 79.5 shows the spread of the different criteria used in selecting, sourcing and sorting the images for the secondary data while Fig. 79.6 shows some of the images used to train the model.

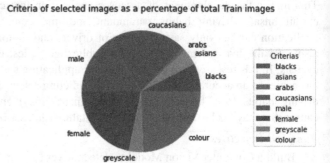

Fig. 79.5 Criteria of selected images as a percentage of total Train images. The total amount of train images was 167

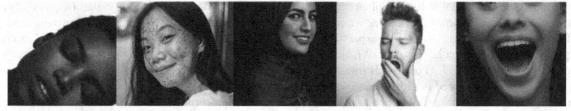

Fig. 79.6 A selection of different images used in training the model. The criteria from left to right: nationality - black, asian, arabian, caucasian and colour - greyscale

3.3 Data Processing/Interpretation

Most of the Data Processing done for this project involved careful selection and sorting of images that would be able to train the model adequately to be able to classify images both captured and live into two categories - safe and unsafe.

In the process of selecting these images, various criteria were itemized and they have been elaborated in the previous chapter. However, there was one more step that involved processing both the primary and secondary data before feeding them to the model.

3.4 Image Annotation

Image Annotation can be roughly defined as the process of labelling images present in a dataset for the purpose of training a machine learning model. It is an important stage in the Computer Vision Machine Learning process and one important reason for this step is mainly to simplify access to these selected images, using them as the ground-truth for further classification and object detection tasks [5]. Labelling or annotating a picture is paramount in Computer Vision tasks and it brings to the fore the perceived difficulties present in comprehending a visual scene [6]. For this project, the open-source tool LabelImg was used to annotate the train images into the two classes - safe and unsafe.

4. Tools, Equipments and Libraries

Below is a list of the tools, equipments and libraries in the Data Processing, Analysis and Interpretation stage include: Python - Programming Language, Jupyter Notebooks - Integrated Development Environment, Open CV - This is an open source Computer Vision library, Numpy - A popular library used for manipulating arrays, YOLO - A Computer Vision object detection algorithm framework, LabelImg - an open source tool used for Image Anno-tation, Pytorch - A python deep learning framework, Matplotlib - A python visualization library. This was used to view images, capture live data and view the model predictions, Webcam - The primary sensor used to capture live and primary data.

5. Feedback System

A Visual feedback system was created in the application as a signal to the user based on the user's label category.

Visual Feedback

Fig. 79.7 The 'sweet blue' (rgb: 49, 84, 116) used for the safe class to signal safe driving condition to the user

Fig. 79.8 The 'sour red' (rgb: 135,25,25) used for the 'not safe' label to signal not safe driving condition to the user - prior or during

6. Results

6.1 HOMESWEET in the Wild: Test Data Analysis and Results

A total of 66 images (39% of the total data) were used to test the generalized ability and predictability of the model. Of this number, the model found no detections in 5. Figure 79.9 shows a table of the various Classification metrics of the model.

6.2 Interpretation of the Test Data Results

Figure79.9 and figure 79.10 shows the classification performance of the model on the selected test data. We can see that the model has a Recall rate of 0.71875, a Precision of 0.95833 and an Accuracy score of 0.82759. This means that the model has a high specificity rate and a reasonably good sensitivity rate. The model's accuracy score is also good at 0.82759 and it must be noted that this accuracy can be improved over time as the model is trained with more relevant pictures.

The size of the train images would also have an impact on the strength and generalized nature of the model. This model was trained with only 167 images, a very small number in the Computer Vision domain. A good place to start with training a model would be north of 100,000 - 1,000,000 images and a test data that would be between 15 - 20% of the train data. For this project however, the concern was on taking little appreciable steps and further down the line, the model would be fed with a larger amount of varied and relevant data.

Despite this shortcoming of train data size, the model still performed superbly in the wild which means it is ready for deployment. Section 4.9, shows the predictive ability of the model on randomly selected test data from the two classes - safe and not safe.

7. Conclusion

With an accuracy score of 0.82759, the 'HOMESWEET' model has proven to be an effective deep learning model able to predict two class labels - safe and not safe - driving habits. The model has a high precision rate but its recall rate is not as high, this means that there would be times in the real-world scenarios where it may incorrectly predict some class labels. While in other innocuous settings and applications, a recall of 0.71875 is good enough, in this application that aims to reduce road accidents and consequentially deaths, this may not be good enough.

This can be solved by feeding the model more data and continually providing it with information under various criteria like lighting conditions, accessories on the face, more micro expressions, more nationalities, backgrounds with artificial lighting etc to further improve 'HOMESWEET' accuracy score and recall rate and make it a more generalized deep learning model.

7.1 Links

UI/UX and Feedback signals - https://codepen.io/laresamdeola/pen/BaYwmoz

Deep Learning Model Code - https://github.com/laresamdeola/homesweet/blob/main/HOMESWEET.ipynb

Model's Test Data Predictions

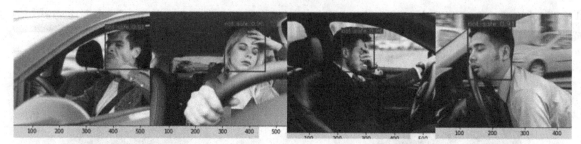

Fig. 79.9 Some selected test data showing the model's performance at classifying the images into the not safe 4 label

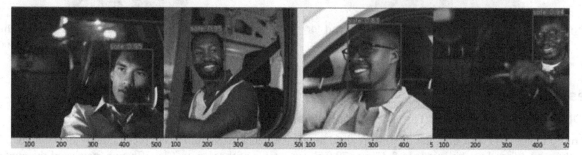

Fig. 79.10 Some selected test data showing the model's performance at classifying the images into the safe label

REFERENCES

1. ons.gov.uk, "Road casualties," 2019.
2. statista.com, "Distribution of contributing factors leading to road accidents in great britain in 2019," 2019.
3. G. Zhao, X. Li, Y. Li, and M. Pietikäinen, "Facial micro-expressions: An overview," Proceedings of the IEEE, 2023.
4. R. Greene, The laws of human nature. Penguin, 2018.
5. A. Hanbury, "A survey of methods for image annotation," Journal of Visual Languages & Computing, vol. 19, no. 5, pp. 617–627, 2008.
6. A. Barriuso and A. Torralba, "Notes on image annotation," arXiv preprint arXiv:1210.3448, 2012.

Emerging Trends in IoT and Computing Technologies – Suman Lata Tripathi et al. (eds)
© *2024 Taylor & Francis Group, London, ISBN 978-1-032-87924-6*

Ensemble Approach and Enhanced Features for Precise Bank Churn Prediction Analysis

Lare Samuel Adeola[1],
Celestine Iwendi[2], Aamir Mazhar Abbas[3]
University of Bolton, Department of Creative Technologies,
Bolton, England

Abstract: Numerous studies and research work has been undertaken in the area of creating predictive models for studying Bank Churn. In these studies, the end goal was to create a high accuracy predictive model; while this is commendable, this research focuses on creating an architecture for a predictive model by aggregating the power of various predictive models. The architecture and model proposed in this paper achieved an accuracy of 91% in the test data (35% of the original data set), and an AUC of 96% - confirming the generalized nature of the model. Also, various feature extrapolation techniques were introduced which provide valuable insights to the banking sector.

Keywords: Ensemble model, Machine learning, Churn analysis, Feature engineering, Predictive modelling

1. Background

The significance of understanding why customers of a certain business enterprise leave for another enterprise in the same domain. Various studies have been conducted and various predictive models concocted. Then the question remains: why study bank churning? One major reason is that customer retention leads to increased profits [1]. However, several research have been carried out that analyses bank churning from the aspect of profitability and building a model to predict churning [2]. This research would rather focus on two things:

- understanding the reason for the bank churn, studying the sociological factors. The purpose is to better understand the factors that lead to customer churn and to use this information in building a model to predict customer churn.
- build an architecture that combines the predictive power of various machine learning models

Research Questions
- Can one build a predictive model with a high accuracy on new data?
- What other features can be extrapolated from the current ones in the data?

2. Methodology
2.1 Data Overview

The data set used in this research is the popular Bank Churn Data set that can be found on [3]. This data-set has become the MNIST of Bank Churn predictive modelling.

---

[1]l.adeola@bolton.ac.uk, [2]c.iwendi@bolton.ac.uk, [3]a.abbas@bolton.ac.uk

DOI: 10.1201/9781003535423-80

The data set has a total of 10000 customers, with 11 total variables/features. The 'Exited' variable is the dependent feature while others are the independent features. However, as you can see from the above image, there are some variables that would be irrelevant to our analysis and model building, these are - 'RowNumber','CustomerId' and 'Surname' (which is a PII - Personal Identifiable Information [4]). The data set is imbalanced with the 'not churned' - when 'Exited' is 0 having 7963 entries while the 'churned' - when 'Exited' is 1 had 2037.

In the previous section, we visually inferred that the relationship amongst the features were non-linear; figure 3 further supports this sentiment as can be seen in the correlations among the features. The most important row is the 'Exited' row which is the last one. The feature with the highest correlation is 'Age' which is 28%. In the next section, we shall expose how this feature was extrapolated for insights on the data.

Feature Extrapolation I - Salary to Bank Ratio (SBR)

The Salary to (Bank) Balance Ratio (SBR) calculates the proportion of the bank customer's salary to their bank balance. The purpose is to find out if there's a relationship between this ratio and the 'Exited' feature and also to find out the probabilities of various thresholds between the ratio and the 'Exited' variable. The formula for this ratio is expressed as:

$$SBR = Salary/Balance$$

where:

$$SBR = SalarytoBalanceRatio$$
$$Balance /= 0$$

Feature Extrapolation II - Generations

Another feature extrapolated from the data was dividing the 'Age' feature column into 5 generations (sub-class labels). There are - Silent Generation: 1928 - 1945, Baby Boomers: 1946 -1964, Generation X: 1965 - 1980, Millenials: 1981 - 1996, and Generation Z: 1997 - 2012

Generation Probabilities

The probabilities for this feature were calculated as:

$$gen\_prob = \% \text{ of } x \text{ in total population}$$

where:

x = class label

e.g., for the silent generation

Total Class Label Population (tclp) = 24

class label (cl) = not_churned

Population of not_churned = 23

probability silent generation not_churned = $pop. of not\_churned/total class label pop.$

This is how the probabilities for each of the sub-class labels in the generations were calculated for the 'not churn' class. In order to compute the probabilities of the 'churn' class:

$$1 - probability of scl$$

e.g., in the Silent Generation example shown above it would be:

$$1 - (23/24)$$

Feature Extrapolation III - Credit Worthiness

Another feature extrapolated from the data was dividing the 'CreditScore' feature column into 3 sub-segments (sub-class labels). There are - low_credit: CreditScore <= 720, fair_credit: 800 < CreditScore <= 721, and good_credit: CreditScore > 800

3. Ensemble Architecture

Stacked generalization can be defined as a method whereby various estimators are combined to reduce their biases [5]. The reason for using this ensemble approach was to be able to capture the idiosyncrasies of the various predictive models. Using a Stacked Ensemble model, the figure below shows the architecture for creating the estimator:

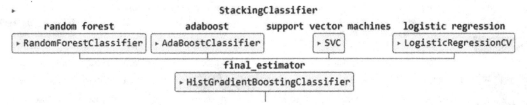

Fig. 80.1 The stacked ensemble architecture

4. Analysis

4.1 Results with the Ensemble Architecture

The Stacked Ensemble Architecture achieved an accuracy of 91% on the test set. It had a Recall rate of 96% on class label 0 i.e., 'customers that did not churn' and a Precision rate of 87% in this same class. In the other class label 1 i.e., 'customers that did churn', it had a Recall rate of 87% and a Precision rate of 96%. Overall, the SEC Model outperformed other models in both classes as can be seen in figures 8 and 9. The Gradient Boosting model achieved similar performance and this was the reason in the first place to use it as the final layer in the SEC architecture model.

4.2 The AUC Curve

In the AUC curve, we can see the average performance of the various models across different classification thresholds. Hence, it is a good measure to know how generalized the model is. Figure 80.2 shows that the SEC model still outperforms other models.

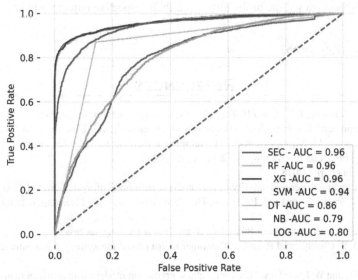

Fig. 80.2 The ROC curve for the different machine learning models and the SEC model

5. Comparison with Related Research

In the figure above, 10 indicators were used as a comparison between SEC and other related research work in this same domain and in lots of instances using the same dataset freely available in Kaggle. As can be seen in the figure, the SEC Architecture outperforms other research works in various indicators (the indicators with a red background are the maximum values in the columns) including dataset size, test size (a good indicator for the model's performance in unseen data or how generalized the model is), class 1 precision, class 1 recall, f1-score, k-folds, and AUC. For accuracy, SEC was beaten by the research work done by [2] but with the work done by karemani as elaborated in the literature review has a small sample size.

	Dataset Size	Test Data	class 0 Precision	class 1 Precision	class 0 Recall	class 1 Recall	F1-score	K-folds	Accuracy	AUC
keramati et al	4383	1314.900000	91.810000	91.810000	91.000000	0.000000	90.960000	10.000000	99.700000	92.900000
pinaki	10000	nan	nan	nan	nan	nan	nan	nan	85.370000	85.800000
praveen et al	0	0.000000	0.000000	0.000000	0.000000	0.000000	0.000000	0.000000	81.710000	84.000000
baby et al	10000	2000.000000	88.000000	79.000000	97.000000	48.000000	75.500000	0.000000	86.000000	0.000000
singh et al	10000	0.000000	90.300000	90.300000	60.100000	60.100000	61.300000	0.000000	83.900000	84.700000
kumara et al	10000	0.000000	0.000000	0.000000	0.000000	0.000000	0.000000	0.000000	91.950000	89.000000
SEC	10000	3500.000000	87.000000	96.000000	96.000000	87.000000	91.000000	10.000000	91.000000	96.000000

Fig. 80.3 Comparison of various selected past research ([2], [6], [7], [8], [9]) done in this area. The figure shows the different metrics and their values gotten in the research. The intersection with the red lines shows the maximum value in the columns.

6. Conclusion

The SEC Architecture has achieved an accuracy of 91% on the test data (35% of the original data), had a high AUC of 96%, performed well in both classes - customers that did not churn (class label 0) and customers that did churn (class label 1) with Precision/Specificity rates of 87% and 96% while Recall/Sensitivity rates of 96% and 87% respectively.

Three other features were extrapolated from the current relevant features. These features are: Salary to Bank Balance Ratio (SBR), Generations, and Credit Worthiness. These features further provided more insights about the behaviours of the bank customers in this data set. At this point of the research, the probabilities computed have not been tested on another data set to confirm their veracity but with this data set, the probabilities and their respective outcomes hold.

Links

Ensemble Model Code - https://rb.gy/9i2gb3

REFERENCES

1. W. Verbeke, K. Dejaeger, D. Martens, J. Hur, and B. Baesens, "New insights into churn prediction in the telecommunication sector: A profit driven data mining approach," European Journal of Operational Research, vol. 218, no. 1, pp. 211–229, 2012.
2. A. Keramati, H. Ghaneei, and S. M. Mirmohammadi, "Developing a prediction model for customer churn from electronic banking services using data mining," Financial Innovation, vol. 2, pp. 1–13, 2016.
3. kaggle.com, "Bank customers churn," 2018.
4. E. McCallister, Guide to protecting the confidentiality of personally identifiable infor- mation, vol. 800. Diane Publishing, 2010.
5. T. Hastie, R. Tibshirani, J. H. Friedman, and J. H. Friedman, The elements of statis- tical learning: data mining, inference, and prediction, vol. 2. Springer, 2009.
6. P. Sahu, "Unlocking the code of customer churn: Predictive strategies for banking success,"
7. P. Lalwani, M. K. Mishra, J. S. Chadha, and P. Sethi, "Customer churn prediction system: a machine learning approach," Computing, pp. 1–24, 2022.
8. B. Baby, Z. Dawod, S. Sharif, and W. Elmedany, "Customer churn prediction model using artificial neural networks (ann): A case study in banking," in 3ICT 2023: Inter- national Conference on Innovation and Intelligence for Informatics, Computing, and Technologies, IEEE, 2023.
9. P. P. Singh, F. I. Anik, R. Senapati, A. Sinha, N. Sakib, and E. Hossain, "Investigating customer churn in banking: A machine learning approach and visualization app for data science and management," Data Science and Management, 2023.

Emerging Trends in IoT and Computing Technologies – Suman Lata Tripathi et al. (eds)
© 2024 Taylor & Francis Group, London, ISBN 978-1-032-87924-6

The Use of Churn-Prediction to Improve Customer-Retention in Grocery E-Retailing

81

Joshua Aaron[1], Ibtisam Mogul[2],
Thaier Hamid[3], Celestine Iwendi[4], Abbas Aamir[5]
School of Art and Creative Technologies,
University of Bolton, Bolton, United Kingdom.

Abstract: As retailers increasingly adopt online shopping and technology, the study emphasizes the critical need for attention to customer churn due to its adverse effects on corporate development and reputation. Focusing on grocery retail businesses, the research explores the use of machine and deep learning models, presenting data analytical findings on retention of customers. The study delves into the implications of customer churn, analysing previously gathered data sets to uncover significant discoveries related to churn, customer preferences, and behaviours. An examination of how churn prediction impacts profitability, reputation, and operational efficiency follows. Through a comprehensive dataset analysis, the study aims to reveal insights into proactive churn control, proposing a framework to limit its effects on overall company growth. This paper contributes to ongoing efforts to enhance business growth by studying the behaviour of customers online that is related with churn and offering solutions to the challenges.

Keywords: Customer retention, Deep learning model, Churn prediction, Churn prediction evolution, Machine learning model, Impact, Proactive churn control strategies, Customer churn

1. Introduction

The grocery sector is growing rapidly since groceries are so necessary for daily living, and retailers are being driven by the developing nature of e-commerce to retain their current customers while actively seeking out new ones (1). Customers have a wide range of products to select from in addition to a multitude of retail locations or stores (2). As a result, customers have a wide range of options when making purchases, which puts shops in a competitive market and increases the possibility of losing business (3). It is crucial to pay attention to the retention of customers because two key factors that affect a company's sustainability are the quality of its customer base and the rate at which its items are purchased (4). This research will examine the different ways that predicting churn might help grocery e-retailers better keep or maintain their customers.

2. Methodology

2.1 Research Philosophy and Paradigm

Research philosophies offer theories about how the reality that is observed (ontology) is constructed and maintained, as well as the procedures involved in doing so. The examiner's methodology for performing a study is determined by a set of theories, conceptions, and guiding principles known as research philosophy (5). On the other hand, a research paradigm is the framework or point of view that researchers use to carry out their investigation (6). It comprises the methodology, viewpoint, presumptions,

[1]aaronjoshualoveday@gmail.com, [2]Mogul2@bolton.ac.uk, [3]T.Hamid@bolton.ac.uk, [4]c.iwendi@bolton.ac.uk, [5]ama1crt@bolton.ac.uk

DOI: 10.1201/9781003535423-81

and opinions of the researcher. Understanding the research paradigm employed in a study is crucial because it may affect the way the data is collected and analysed, how the study is designed, and how the findings are perceived (7).

The positivism paradigm research approach is used in this study as the use of quantitative data experiments is employed, the statistical approach of data analysis, and findings that can be applied to all businesses and retailers seeking to grow their customer base and boost profitability, not just grocery stores.

2.2 Design of the Research

As part of the quantitative research methodology for this paper, the E-commerce Customer Churn Analysis and Prediction dataset is studied to discover relationships across features. The primary research objectives of the study include:

1. Identify the primary variables influencing loss of customers.
2. Employing machine learning techniques to build a model for prediction that takes into account relevant elements that affect customer attrition in online grocery retailing.
3. Provide a thorough structure and tactics to assist grocery retailers in lowering churn and increasing retention of customers.

2.3 Acquisition of Data

Product at Ufaber Edutech Pvt Ltd, Ankit Verma (2021), provided the dataset (secondary data) with permission from Kaggle. The dataset did not specify the precise time or duration of data gathering, although disclosing the customer's length of engagement with the company. The dataset has 5,631 total observations. It is significant to highlight that the researcher did not get any personally identifiable information when collecting the data. The confidentiality and privacy of the clients whose data was obtained from the data are protected by all ethical guidelines and regulations.

2.4 Data-Analytical Approach

The data obtained was acquired, cleaned, and analysed, as depicted in Fig. 81.1 below, to eliminate the data that are not relevant. Quantitative methods, particularly exploratory data analysis (EDA), were employed to emphasize key dataset characteristics,

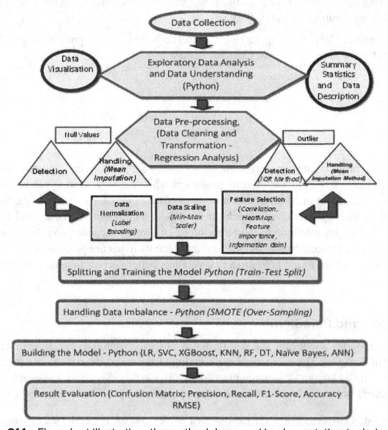

Fig. 81.1 Flow chart illustrating, the methodology, and implementation techniques

identify trends, and draw conclusions. Python programming, recognized for its scalability and support for simultaneous processing, is utilized for dataset investigation, with Power BI employed for visualizing relationships between variables. Python's versatility in managing large datasets is highlighted, especially in machine learning (ML) tasks, supported by its simplicity, readability, and robust development community. EDA procedures, such as outlier detection and handling, and null value detection and handling, are illustrated in Fig. 81.1. The research incorporates data pre-processing techniques, including feature selection, data normalization, and outlier identification, to enhance data exploration and facilitate machine learning applications. Figure 81.1 details the implementation strategies for dataset splitting, model building, and result evaluation.

2.5 Evaluation Metrics

To evaluate the model the following metrices was used.

Confusion Matrix—A confusion matrix sums up the amount of true-negatives, true-positives, false-negatives, and false-positives to provide a detailed account of a model's performance (9).

Precision(P)—Measures how accurate the positive predictions made by a classification algorithm are. It is the ratio of all positive predictions, including true and false positives, to the number of properly predicted positive outcomes, or true positives (10). The meaning of accuracy is –

$$P = \frac{\text{True Positive (TP)}}{\text{True Positives(TP) + False Positives(FP)}} \tag{1}$$

Recall—Quantifies a model's ability to appropriately recognise each positive occurrence in a set of data. It calculates the ratio of all real positives to the fraction of correct positive forecasts (11).

$$R = \frac{\text{TP}}{\text{TP + FN}} \tag{2}$$

F1-score—This is a statistical method that combines precision and recall by finding their harmonic mean. It is helpful for examining a model's performance when the data is not balance across classes since it offers a just one number that considers both false positives (fp) and false negatives (fn) (12).

$$\text{F1-Score} = \frac{2 \times \text{Recall (R)} \times \text{Precision (P)}}{\text{Recall (R)} + \text{Precision (P)}} \tag{3}$$

Support: In a classification problem indicates how many instances or data points there are in each category. It is employed to understand the distribution of classes in a set of data.

Root Mean Squared Error: This statistic is often used to evaluate the effectiveness of both classification and regression models. It measures the average difference between the anticipated and original values in a dataset. This metric finds the square root of the mean of the squared differences between the actual and anticipated values within a set of data (12).

3. Training Models and Assessing Outcomes

In this study, a variety of models were used, including ANN (Artificial Neural Networks) for Deep Learning, XG-Boost (Extreme- Gradient Boosting), DT (Decision-Tree), RF (Random-Forests), KNN (K-Nearest-Neighbour), Support Vector Regression (SVR), and NBayes (Naive Bayes). The following libraries were employed to present the results: Matplotlib, Keras, Scikit-Learn, Pandas, and Sklearn libraries. Supervised machine learning algorithms were selected for analyses and prediction in this study given the labelled data nature of the dataset, which facilitates learning and predicting process by the machine learning algorithm.

4. Model Evaluation

Table 81.1 below illustrates the results from the different models as employed in the study, where 0 indicates not churn and 1 indicates churn.

It can be observed from Table 81.1 that Random-Forest Model has the best performance with 97% accuracy and worst performed model is Naïve Bayes Model with 65% accuracy.

Table 81.1 Analysis of results from different machine and deep learning models employed in the study

Machine Learning	Evaluation Metrics									
	Root Mean Squared Error	Accuracy (%)	Precision(%)		Recall(%)		F1 Score(%)		Support	
			0	1	0	1	0	1	0	1
Naïve Bayes	0.59	65	93	29	63	75	75	42	941	185
Logistic Regression	0.51	74	95	37	73	81	83	51	941	185
Support-Vector- Classifier (RBF)	0.42	75	96	36	70	83	81	50	941	185
K-Nearest-Neighbour	0.44	80	97	44	79	86	87	59	941	185
Artificial Neural Network	0.36	87	93	59	91	64	92	62	941	185
Decision Tree	0.23	94	98	89	96	88	97	84	941	185
Extreme Gradient Boost	0.21	95	97	89	98	83	97	86	941	185
Random Forest (n= 200)	0.17	97	98	89	98	92	98	90	941	185

5. Churn Indicative Features

5.1 The Top 10 Consumer Habits to Identify Customers at Churn-Risk

This study's dataset contained characteristics that represented a customer's interaction with a e-retailer. One of the intriguing conclusions is that by observing specific customer behaviours, e-retailers may determine which consumers are on the verge of leaving or have already made up their minds to quit. Because of their degree of relationship to the target variable, these characteristics were selected to train the multiple models used in the study to ensure the efficacy of the result. The evaluation metrics employed in Python to identify the customer activity most associated with Churn were Correlation, HeatMap, Feature Importance, and Information Gain, as shown in Figures 81.3, 81.4, and 81.5.

In this study, three methods were employed to identify key features associated with customer churn in grocery retailing. Through a meticulous comparison of outcomes, 10 features were selected based on their consistency across various assessment metrics. Notably, customer tenure exhibited the highest correlation, followed by factors such as distance from the warehouse, preferred order category, satisfaction rating, marital status, complaint filing date, percentage rises, total orders, average cashback, and time since the last order. These findings emphasize the significance of these consumer behavioural trends for effectively addressing churn in the grocery retail industry.

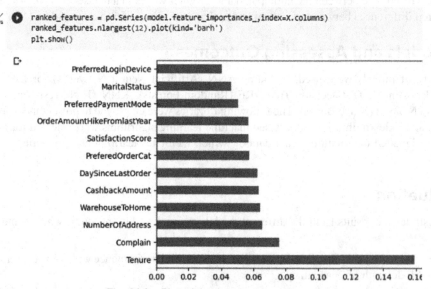

Fig. 81.2 Plot of the feature importance

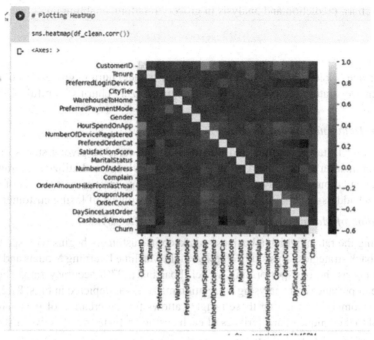

Fig. 81.3   Heatmap dependent (target) and independent features

▾ Information Gain

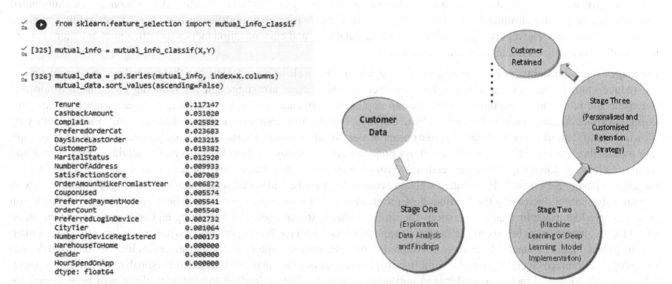

Fig. 81.4   Dependent (target)/Independent features and their correlation

Fig. 81.5   Customer retention framework and strategies

6. Summary of Findings

The analysis successfully predicted customer churn and identified key indicators. The top 10 most influential factors include tenure, warehouse distance, order category, satisfaction rating, marital status, complaint date, price increases, order volume, average cashback, and time since last order. These factors significantly correlate with churn potential, providing valuable insights for customer retention strategies. Also, complaints strongly correlated with churn, with higher complaint rates linked to greater churn likelihood. Effectively addressing customer complaints can thus serve as a key retention strategy. These findings highlight the crucial role of churn prediction and analysis in grocery retailing, enabling proactive retention efforts and driving business success.

6.1 Framework

The study proposes a three-stage framework (Fig. 81.5) to combat customer churn in grocery retailing. This framework equips merchants with a comprehensive strategy for customer retention, minimizing churn's harmful effects on business growth and sustainability.

Stage One (1) (Exploration- Data Analysis and Findings)

In this study, the significance of Data Exploration and Results is underscored as pivotal stages in the data analysis process. These phases involve the examination of datasets to glean insightful knowledge and utilize exploratory data analytics tools for visualisation, segmentation, tabulation, and analysis. Analysing and drawing insight from the set of data is crucial to informing the growth of the business and addressing challenges, particularly in the context of losing customer and keeping them.

Stage Two (2) (Implementation of Machine Learning/Deep Learning Models)

Understanding and controlling the rate at which a business can keep its customers begins with spotting potential churners and implementing targeted win-back strategies. This study employs eight Machine Learning Models and one Deep Learning Model, with Random Forest emerging as the best-performing model, boasting a 97% accuracy rate. The utilization of this model involves interpreting feature importance and analysing correlation matrices (as depicted in Figs. 81.2, 81.3, and 81.4) to identify and segment churn-prone customers. Leveraging these insights allows for the creation of personalized and customized win-back retention plans tailored to the unique characteristics of each customer, fostering effective customer retention strategies.

Stage Three (3) (Retention Strategies – Personalisation and Customisation)

The objective of the third step of personalisation and customisation is to improve customer experiences, promote loyalty, and stimulate repeat patronage. Personalisation entails adjusting offerings, alternatives, and content according to user activity and data. Customisation, on the other hand, enables customers to alter goods or services to suit their tastes. Automated customisation is a vital consumer-focused procedure in online purchasing that modifies website content according to unique customer information. The report suggests data-driven personalising and customisation tactics for efficient client churn control and retention, drawing on findings from earlier phases.

The Stages 1 and 2 insights could be leveraged to make data-driven, well-informed decisions that can help with keep customers and reduce churn. The personalising and tailoring tactics listed below are suggested for reducing customer attrition and increasing the retention of customers. Retailers can deploy recommendation engines for personalized product suggestions, easing customer decision-making through website displays, emails, and targeted marketing. Enhance customer flexibility by allowing modifications to product elements like colour or size based on past purchase history and preferences. Utilize customer data for flexible pricing, offering personalized discounts, vouchers, or loyalty benefits tailored to individual preferences and purchasing history. Encourage customer feedback through surveys to address concerns, collect valuable input, and enhance the overall purchasing experience. Personalize website content, blog posts, and social media messages to engage customers with relevant information, increasing the likelihood of return visits. Implement post-purchase follow-ups with custom thank-you messages, product usage tips, and suggestions for similar items to foster a sense of belonging and encourage repeat business. Introduce loyalty programs based on customer tenure and purchase history, offering personalized rewards to incentivize continued patronage and retain customers. To manage churn prediction, retailers can explore additional strategies like Personalized-Voice-Shopping, Customized-Social Commerce, Emotional-Personalization, Personalised-Gifts, and Personalized VR/AR Shopping. Adopting individualized tactics to understand and address specific factors leading to customer churn will be essential for successful customer retention in the dynamic e-retail landscape.

7. Conclusion

This paper effectively assesses churn prediction's impact on customer retention in grocery e-retail, presenting a robust framework for strategies. Quantitatively analysing a grocery retail dataset, it identifies key churn behaviours, offering practical measures to reduce customer loss impact. This contribution to Data Analytics and Technologies knowledge provides valuable insights and recommendations, serving as a foundational guide for improving customer retention in the dynamic grocery retail landscape.

REFERENCES

1. Dalmia, H., Nikil, C. V. S. S., & Kumar, S. (2020). Churning of Bank Customers Using Supervised Learning. In Lecture notes in networks and systems (pp. 681–691). Springer International Publishing. https://doi.org/10.1007/978-981-15-3172-9_64

2. Dolega, L., & Lord, A. M. (2020). Exploring the geography of retail success and decline: A case study of the Liverpool City Region. Cities, 96, 102456. https://doi.org/10.1016/j.cities.2019.102456

3. Gianfrancesco, M. A., Tamang, S., Robinson, P., & Schmajuk, G. (2018). Potential biases in machine learning algorithms using electronic health record data. JAMA Internal Medicine, 178(11), 1544. https://doi.org/10.1001/jamainternmed.2018.3763

4. Gold, C. (2020). Fighting Churn with Data: The science and strategy of customer retention. Simon and Schuster.

5. Guetterman, T. C., Fetters, M. D., & Creswell, J. W. (2015). Integrating quantitative and qualitative results in health science mixed methods research through joint displays. Annals of Family Medicine, 13(6), 554–561. https://doi.org/10.1370/afm.1865

6. Hassonah, M. A., Rodan, A., Al-Tamimi, A., & Alsakran, J. (2019). Churn Prediction: A Comparative Study Using KNN and Decision Trees. https://doi.org/10.1109/itt48889.2019.9075077

7. Hult, G. T. M., Sharma, P. N., Morgeson, F. V., & Zhang, Y. (2019). Antecedents and Consequences of Customer Satisfaction: Do They Differ Across Online and Offline Purchases? Journal of Retailing, 95(1), 10–23. https://doi.org/10.1016/j.jretai.2018.10.003

8. Ishtiaq, M. (2019). Book Review Creswell, J. W. (2014). Research Design: Qualitative, Quantitative and Mixed Methods Approaches (4th ed.). Thousand Oaks, CA: Sage. English Language Teaching, 12(5), 40. https://doi.org/10.5539/elt.v12n5p40

9. Kumar, V., Rajan, B., Venkatesan, R., & Lecinski, J. (2019). Understanding the Role of Artificial Intelligence in Personalized Engagement Marketing. California Management Review, 61(4), 135–155. https://doi.org/10.1177/0008125619859317

10. Naim, A., & Kautish, S. K. (2022). Building a Brand Image Through Electronic Customer Relationship Management. IGI Global.

11. Nguyen, P. H., Kecskes, A., & Mansi, S. (2020). Does corporate social responsibility create shareholder value? The importance of long-term investors. Journal of Banking and Finance, 112, 105217. https://doi.org/10.1016/j.jbankfin.2017.09.013

12. Ohny, M., & Mathai, P. P. (2017). Customer Churn Prediction: A Survey. International Journal of Advanced Research in Computer Science, 8(5), 2178–2181. https://doi.org/10.26483/ijarcs.v8i5.4079

Emerging Trends in IoT and Computing Technologies – Suman Lata Tripathi et al. (eds)
© 2024 Taylor & Francis Group, London, ISBN 978-1-032-87924-6

Review of Intrusion Detection System for E-Commerce System

82

Shabeena Nafees[1], Anil Kumar Pandey[2]
Shri ram swaroop memorial University,
Dept. Computer Science and Engineering, Lucknow, India

Nidhi Saxena[3]
Babu Banarasi das University,
Dept. Computer Science and Engineering, Lucknow, India

Abstract: The twenty-first century has witnessed a rapid growth of technological advancements aiming to lead the world towards a new era of innovations. E-commerce is a phenomenal product of this innovatory stream. The application circle of e-commerce is widespread in almost every sector of our life to prove its validity and impact on our routine life vividly. E-commerce communications depend on modern devices such as laptops, personal computers, communication sensors, servers, switches, etc. The expanding domain of E-commerce applications is bringing the involvement of more communication devices, which raises a serious question about the security of the whole communication system. Integrating suspicious entities with the mainstream communication network may create malicious activities resulting in swear outcomes. Hence, we need a secure communication framework to ensure attack-efficient and reliable communication streams. This paper reviews different efficient and secure electronic payment system.

Keyword: Machine learning, E-commerce, Malicious activity, Threat detection framework, IDS

1. Introduction

E-Commerce, also known as electronic commerce or internet commerce, refers to performing products, goods, or service-related transactions over the internet [1].

Since it offers a global and user-friendly set of technologies, the Internet is quickly replacing other networks as the preferred infrastructure for e-commerce and e-business. Numerous industries, including retail, wholesale, and manufacturing, make use of E-many commerce's useful uses [2]. Through the use of the Internet and electronic commerce, information about consumer habits, tastes, and demands may be gathered. As a result, this aids in marketing tasks like setting prices, negotiating, improving products' features, and fostering relationships with customers. Numerous retail and wholesale settings are ideal for implementing e-commerce [3].

E-retailing, sometimes known as "online retailing," is the practice of selling products directly to end users via specially built online stores that mimic traditional brick-and-mortar shops down to the last detail. E-commerce is widely utilized by the financial sector. Through E-banking or online banking, customers can view their savings and loan account balances, make transfers to other accounts, and even pay their bills. Online stock trading is another use for E-commerce [4]. There are a plethora

[1]qds186@gmail.com, [2]anipandey@gmail.com, [3]nidhishivansh@gmail.com

DOI: 10.1201/9781003535423-82

of online resources where investors can gain knowledge about the market, including news, charts, company profiles, and analyst ratings. The logistics of a company's supply chain also benefit from the widespread adoption of electronic commerce. Some businesses band together to create an online marketplace where they can easily buy and sell items, share market data, and manage administrative tasks like stock management. When goods and services move quickly between companies, the economy as a whole benefit. The deployment of business models is hampered by several strategic and competitive concerns. Businesses may be hesitant to take part in widespread electronic exchanges out of concern that their competitors will gain access to proprietary information [5].

Using the Internet's interactive features, businesses may get to know their customers better and provide better service all around. Web personalization allows businesses to tailor material to a user's browsing experience based on their preferences, and this includes technology that allows for the delivery of tailored information and advertisements through mobile commerce platforms [6]. Web sites, e-mail, and phone access to customer service professionals all allow businesses to save money while better serving their clientele. Online banking, often known as electronic banking or E-banking, is an electronic payment system that enables customers of a financial institution to perform financial transactions via the firm's website. Internet banking, e-banking, virtual banking, and other names all describe the same concept [7].

2. Review of Approached used for Security in E-Commerce

Md Arif Hassan et al. E-commerce, as defined, means making electronic purchases and transaction online using a web browser. They outlined, means making electronic purchases and transactions online using a web browser. They outlined the development of effective and secure electronic payment for e-commerce that allow customers to connect with merchants instantly and accurately. Interestingly, their study does not require the customer to enter their identity into the marketer's website, but the customer can disguise himself and temporarily impersonate himself. Their methods have been found to increase security in terms of confidentiality, integrity, non-repudiation, anonymity, authentication and authorization.

Amjad Rehman Khan et al. proposes a cloud-based infrastructure to provide efficient and secure transactional communication, it provides analytics that include intrusion detection based on deep learning techniques and different intrusion detection techniques. In this investigation, publicly available network-based IDS datasets were searched and analyzed. IDS's deep learning has been rigorously evaluated based on different performance metrics (accuracy, precision, recall, f1-score, negative count, and detection number). Additionally, current problems and solutions to cybersecurity and privacy are discussed.

Emad-ul-Haq Qazi et al. developed an asymmetric deep auto encoder and its detailed functionality and performance are presented for network intrusion detection problems. The authors analyzed the effectiveness and efficiency of the NIDS proposal using benchmark data (e.g. KDD CUP'99). Our deep learning based application is implemented in the Tensor Flow library.

Imtiaz ullah and Qusay h. Mahmoud reported that a new anomaly-based attack detection model for IoT network has been designed and developed. A neural network communication models proposed using BoT-IoT, IoT network attack,MQTT-IoT-IDS2020 and IoT-23 attack datasets.

S.Vinoth et al. used detailing the best solution to improve cloud security is crucial for every cloud project. This article examines various cloud application in banking and e-commerce and their associated security issues, Copyright 2022 Elsevier limited. The Scientific Committee of the International Conference on Advances in Materials Science is responsible for selecting and evaluating fellows.

Rafal Kozik et al. promotes the use of image databases and cyber threat intelligence platforms to implements post-incident analysis and incident response processes, enhancing the organization's security capabilities by enabling their ability to identify the current situation with their own historical events and events presented by other organizations. This approach allows users to become more effective than criminals by learning from the experiences of others.

Idiano D'Adamo et al. propose that European countries have different levels of network security problems and that three groups can be identified with different levels of concern about the main problem in e-commerce. The Netherlands, Sweden and Denmark are countries responding e-commerce.

3. Possible Solution

Authors proposed an Intrusion detection framework by incorporating renowned machine learning techniques to ensure the efficiency and robustness of an E-commerce environment. To ensure effective communication that is safe in resource-constrained e-commerce communications, Machine learning-based solutions are seen to be the best option. On a large dataset, a traditional machine learning mechanism-based framework is initially trained. The concerned dataset contains the impressions of all frequently occurring attacks in that particular environment. After finalizing the training the system is placed in real-life communications where it can capture identical impressions. In this way, the identification of any malicious activities becomes easy which tends to make an efficient and resource-constrained E-commerce communication environment.

4. Research Gap

I have studied more than 30 research studies published by various prestigious platforms i.e. IEEE, ELSEVIER, Springer, Hindawi, ACM etc. for the years 2020, 2021 and 2022. All research studies were conducted in the same research domain and various security solutions were proposed to ensure a secure and efficient e-commerce environment. After a critical analysis, we found ample room for improvement as those previously proposed solutions were targeting large-scale stable networks. I decided to design a Machine Learning-based novel and secure Intrusion Detection Framework to improve the efficiency of Resource-Constrained E-commerce Environments. The term resource-constrained refers to describe the devices or a network with limited resources. The limited availability of resources demands significant attention. And hence, designing an appropriate solution to enhance the efficiency of such a resource-constrained network becomes a challenging task. In this research, I aim to improve an efficient and secure defensive mechanism for such E-Commerce communications.

5. Significance of Research

Because cyber-attacks can lead organisations to lose money, data, and even their existence, cyber security is crucial for online transactions. Those who would steal from businesses online employ sophisticated methods. When conducting business online, it's important to safeguard not only your information but also that of your clients [8]. The loss of sensitive client data could result from a breach in your cyber security systems. In the end, that could destroy the credibility of your company. Here are some measures one may take to improve the safety of an online shop. E-commerce keeping e-commerce assets safe from tampering, destruction, or disclosure is the goal of security. The three pillars of CIA—information confidentiality, integrity, and availability—should serve as the foundation for any effective e-commerce security strategy [9]. The possibility of white-collar crimes rises in tandem with the popularity of online shopping since more people have access to the means to breach the system's security. The banking industry's provision of Internet Banking as a convenient and adaptable method of online payment for e-commerce is not without its drawbacks, however, just as every coin has two sides. Companies today invest billions of dollars in computer security, with the main concern being the prevention of fraud [10].

6. Overview of Research

When it comes to consumer information, privacy means blocking any efforts that could lead to its disclosure to unrelated parties. The chosen online retailer should be the only one to view a customer's billing details or social security number. Vendors violate confidentiality agreements when they offer outside parties access to sensitive data. Any internet firm must have anti-virus software, a firewall, encryption, and other data security safeguards [11]. It will be very beneficial in protecting client financial information. Internet store safety also relies on another important principle: integrity. This refers to the practice of preventing unauthorized parties from altering sensitive customer data stored online.

According to this principle, an online store must use consumers' data in its original form, without alterations. Any tampering with the information will cause a customer to lose trust in the reliability of the business. The requirement that both the buyer and the seller be who they say they are is a cornerstone of secure online transactions. In a perfect world, they would be who they claim to be. The business must demonstrate that it is reputable, sells genuine goods, and offers the services it promotes. The buyer must additionally give identity in order for the vendor to feel comfortable with the online purchase [12].

It is possible to ensure authentication and identification. If you are unable to, hiring a professional could be quite helpful. Examples of typical solutions include credit card PINs and client login information. Privacy involves thwarting any actions that would result in the disclosure of customer information to unaffiliated parties. Nobody else ought to [13].

This refers to the practice of preventing unauthorized parties from altering sensitive customer data stored online. According to this principle, an online store must use consumers' data in its original form, without alterations. Any tampering with the information will cause a customer to lose trust in the reliability of the business. The requirement that both the buyer and the seller be who they say they are is a cornerstone of secure online transactions. In a perfect world, they would be who they claim to be. The business must demonstrate that it is reputable, sells genuine goods, and offers the services it promotes. The buyer must also present identification in order for the merchant to feel comfortable with the online transaction.

As a result, the legal doctrine known as the principle of non-repudiation tells parties to a transaction not to retract their actions. Both the company and the buyer must complete their respective parts of the deal. Online shopping might make some people feel unsafe because there is no human presence [14].

7. Methodology

This study conducted a literature review of the different ML- and DL-based NIDS and investigates the published journal articles between 2020 to 2023.This research work will propose an Intrusion Detection System (IDS) based on Machine Learning. The specific datasets that contain impressions of security threats will be used to train our proposed Intrusion Detection Framework. Once the system will be trained, it will be deployed in a run-time environment where it will investigate the presence of relevant suspicious entities/security threats in E-commerce communications. The performance of the proposed solution will be tested will some state-of-the-art benchmarked schemes under diversified performance metrics. The study comprised two main objectives. In the first stage I will discovered the current challenges in the e-commerce environment as well as the root cause to create such challenges. There exist a wide space of improvements in this research area, as researchers have proposed various solution for the security of generic e-commerce environments. However, the security of resource-constrained e-commerce environments is still a challenging task that demands significant security solutions.

In the second stage, I present security solution to ensure secure and reliable communication in resource constrained e-commerce environments which will acquire the basic concepts of deep learning for formulating our proposed intrusion detection model. The proposed system will be formulated using two deep learning algorithms deep neural network and long short-term memory.

The proposed system will be initially trained on two comprehensive datasets that contain the impressions of frequently occurring security threats in e-commerce communication. The datasets used in our research are CIC-IDS2017, and CIC-IDS2019.

In the third step, I will evaluate the performance of in terms of several performance criteria, the proposed model. The performance of the proposed IDS will then be compared with some benchmarked schemes to get a valid idea about its actual performance. Proposed model will be compared from other algorithms. The major approaches used in our research are projected in Fig. 82.1, and a detailed elaboration of these approaches can be seen in Fig. 82.2:

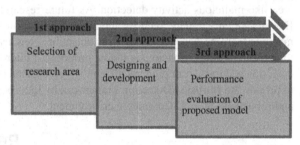

Fig. 82.1 Major approaches in our research

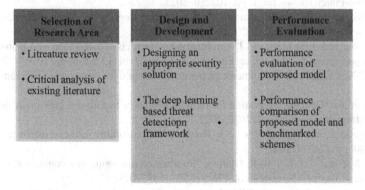

Fig. 82.2 Details of research and developmental approaches

Table 82.1 Current research activities

S. No	Different methodology	Advantage	Disadvantage/Limitation
1	Researchers have proposed a cloud-based infrastructure to provide efficient and secure transactional communication.	Efficient detection security attacks	High resource utilization of the proposed system
2	A threat analysis framework is designed	End-to-End secure communication	Computation overhead increases
3	An efficient communication model is presented	Prevention against malicious entities	Communication delay increases
4	An AI-based secure and efficient communication mechanism is proposed	Attack detection and Prevention	Not suitable for resource-constrained environments
5	AI empowered threat detection model is designed	DDoS attack detection	It demands high resource consumption
6	A reliable E-commerce management system is proposed	Botnet attack detection	Not suitable for large network
7	Block chain-based security scheme is presented	Cyber-attack prevention	Computational overhead increases
8	A privacy-preserving mechanism is designed	Secure communication tunnel	High resource consumption
9	A block chain-based Secure framework is formulated	Malicious traffic analysis	Higher latencies experienced
10	Smart communication mechanism for E-Commerce	Malware detection	Computational overhead
11	An attack detection mechanism is presented	DoD,DDoS identification	Not compatible with large networks

9. Conclusion and Future Scope

In this paper, I presented a survey covers the current level of machine learning-based classifiers for threat detection in large-scale e-commerce, with a focus on methods for identifying malicious activities. I selected 12 papers in the literature that proposed specific a good machine algorithm to detect malicious activity with high accuracy and detection rate in a crucial area like malicious activity detection. As future research, researchers may focus on the following issues: detection method, IDS placement strategy, security threat, and validation strategy. A rising quantity of research will be done in the future on machine learning-based Android virus detection. New frameworks and algorithms that are quick, quick, and powerful enough to detect malicious behavior should be proposed. I intend to assess the performance of the suggested model in terms of attack detection accuracy, precision, recall, and f1-score based on the evaluated publications. As future research, researchers may plan to propose an Intrusion Detection Framework by incorporating renowned machine learning techniques to ensure the efficiency and robustness of an E-Commerce environment.

REFERENCES

1. F. Fernández-Bonilla, C. Gijón, and B. J. T. P. De la Vega, "E-commerce in Spain: Determining factors and the importance of the e-trust," Telecommunications Policy vol. 46, no. 1, pp. 102280, 2022.
2. I. Zennaro, S. Finco, M. Calzavara et al., "Implementing E-Commerce from Logistic Perspective: Literature Review and Methodological Framework," Sustainability vol. 14, no. 2, pp. 911, 2022.
3. A. H. Mohamad, G. F. Hassan, and A. S. J. A. S. E. J. Abd Elrahman, "Impacts of e-commerce on planning and designing commercial activities centres: A developed approach," Ain Shams Engineering Journal, vol. 13, no. 4, pp. 101634, 2022.
4. Q. Hu, T. Lou, J. Li et al., "New practice of e-commerce platform: Evidence from two trade-in programs," vol. 17, no. 3, pp. 875-892, 2022.
5. M. Zeng, R. Liu, M. Gao et al., "Demand forecasting for rural E-commerce logistics: a grey prediction model based on weakening buffer operator," Mobile information systems vol. 2022, 2022.
6. S. Escursell, P. Llorach-Massana, and M. B. J. J. o. c. p. Roncero, "Sustainability in e-commerce packaging: A review," Journal of cleaner production, vol. 280, pp. 124314, 2021.
7. M. Kolotylo-Kulkarni, W. Xia, and G. J. J. o. B. R. Dhillon, "Information disclosure in e-commerce: A systematic review and agenda for future research," Journal of Business Research vol. 126, pp. 221–238, 2021.
8. M. J. Girsang, R. Hendayani, and Y. Ganesan, "Can Information Security, Privacy and Satisfaction Influence The E-Commerce Consumer Trust?" pp. 1–7.

9. Z. Zhu, Y. Bai, W. Dai et al., "Quality of e-commerce agricultural products and the safety of the ecological environment of the origin based on 5G Internet of Things technology," Environmental Technology & Innovation 22 (2021): 101462., vol. 22, pp. 101462, 2021.

10. L. T. T. J. J. o. R. Tran, and C. Services, "Managing the effectiveness of e-commerce platforms in a pandemic," Journal of Retailing and Consumer Services 58 (2021): 102287, vol. 58, pp. 102287, 2021.

11. Z. Zhu, Y. Bai, W. Dai et al., "Quality of e-commerce agricultural products and the safety of the ecological environment of the origin based on 5G Internet of Things technology," Environmental Technology & Innovation, 22, 101462., vol. 22, pp. 101462, 2021.

12. M. H. Gouthier, C. Nennstiel, N. Kern et al., "The more the better? Data disclosure between the conflicting priorities of privacy concerns, information sensitivity and personalization in e-commerce," Journal of Business Research vol. 148, pp. 174–189, 2022.

13. O. Saritas, P. Bakhtin, I. Kuzminov et al., "Big data augmented business trend identification: the case of mobile commerce," Scientometrics 126.2 (2021): 1553–1579., vol. 126, no. 2, pp. 1553–1579, 2021.

14. M. Aliyu, M. Umar, N. J. S. J. o. S. Salisu et al., "Assessing User's Perception on Security Challenges of Selected E-Commerce Websites in Nigeria," SLU Journal of Science and Technology, 4(1&2), 177–187., vol. 4, no. 1&2, pp. 177–187, 2022.

Emerging Trends in IoT and Computing Technologies – Suman Lata Tripathi et al. (eds)
© 2024 Taylor & Francis Group, London, ISBN 978-1-032-87924-6

Intelligence framework to identify Malicious Activities for Safety

83

Shabeena Nafees[1],
Anil Kumar Pandey[2], Satya Bhushan Verma[3]
Shri Ramswaroop Memorial University, Barabanki, India

Brijesh Kumar Pandey[4]
Lovely Professional University, Jalandhar

Mahima Shankar[5]
School of Engineering & Technology, Sharda University,
Greater Noida, India

Richa Verma[6]
Noida International University, Noida, India

Abstract: E-commerce is a powerful concept and process that changes people's lives today. E-commerce communications depend on modern devices such as laptops, personal computers, communication sensors, servers, switches, etc. The expanding domain of E-commerce applications is bringing the involvement of more communication devices, which raises a serious question about the security of the whole communication system. Integrating suspicious entities with the mainstream communication network may create malicious activities resulting in swear outcomes. Hence, we need a secure communication framework to ensure attack-efficient and reliable communication streams. We aim to propose a Machine Learning (ML) based threat detection framework for large-scale E-commerce communication environments. To be more precise, we take Deep Learning (DL) on board, a sub-branch of machine learning. The proposed threat detection framework combines two Deep learning algorithms, deep Neural Network (DNN) and long short-term Memory (LSTM).The initial training of threat detection program is trained on datasets. We aim to evaluate the performance of the proposed model in terms of attack detection. The effectiveness of the proposed framework will also be compared some other renowned intrusion detection schemes from the literature.

Keyword: Intrusion detection (IDS), Deep neural network (DNN), Long short-term Memory (LSTM)

1. Introduction

The current century has witnessed a marvelous growth in technological advancements that revolutionize our lifestyle with more efficient innovations. Just like other sectors, the communication sector is also been evolved as a result of these advancements. The advent of the internet has entirely modernized our conventional lifestyle, and its applications can be seen in every sphere of our life. Buying or selling something was hectic activity in the past as their people were suffering from a lack of resources.

[1]qds186@gmail.com, [2]anipandey@gmail.com, [3]satyabverma1@gmail.com, [4]brijesh84academics@gmail.com, [5]mahimashanker@gmail.com, [6]rvricha520@gmail.com

DOI: 10.1201/9781003535423-83

However, the internet has made it all easy by enabling the world to perform shopping activities just by sitting in their comfort zones.

E-Commerce is also known as electronic commerce it refers to performing products, goods, or service-related transactions over the internet. Since it offers a global and user-friendly set of technologies, the Internet is quickly replacing other networks as the preferred infrastructure for e-commerce and e-business. Numerous industries, including retail, wholesale, and manufacturing, make use of E-many commerce's useful uses. Through the use of the Internet and electronic commerce, information about consumer habits, tastes, and demands may be gathered. As a result, this aids in marketing tasks like setting prices, negotiating, improving products' features, and fostering relationships with customers. Numerous retail and wholesale settings are ideal for implementing e-commerce.

2. Related Work

2.1 Cloud-based Solutions

Cloud computing is One of the biggest innovations that has attracted the attention computer scientists worldwide. While there are certainly benefits to using cloud computing, there are also significant security concerns that no business can afford to overlook. Successful adoption of Cloud Computing within organizations requires fore thought and an understanding of both existing and anticipated risks, threats, vulnerabilities, and countermeasures. So, all cloud operations must find the best solution instructions to boost cloud security. Based on a survey of the existing literature, this study seeks to identify and evaluate the most pressing threats to cloud system networks and data security. However, a closer look reveals that virtualization adds more software to the network machines, which can negatively impact security. As data canter hubs use software to connect their servers, any security breach could have far-reaching consequences. Since users have little say over the cloud's infrastructure, they must rely on pre-established channels of trust. Several banking and e-commerce cloud computing applications are examined along with related security concerns [1] [2].

Finally, this research contributes theoretically by setting a new baseline for the literature on the current situation of e-commerce in Europe in light of the pandemic's consequences. Managers can use this study's findings to inform their decisions about how to expand their companies into new markets, and policymakers can use them to shape effective e-commerce regulations [3].

2.2 Artificial Intelligence-based Solutions

Artificial intelligence (AI) has been used in the e-commerce and financial to improve experiences of customer, simplify SCM, increase efficiency of operation and reduce team size, with the ultimate goals of creating reliable products and finding new way to achieve goals. Help customers at low cost. The food business is now developing machine learning models to accommodate the complexity and diversity of its data. Internet-based businesses, corporate administration, and the financial sector are only a few of the areas where this article focuses on the practical applications of machine learning and artificial intelligence. Some of the most common applications include boosting sales, increasing profits, making more accurate sales predictions, handling inventory, preventing theft, and maximizing investment returns [4]. In recent years, almost all offline activities have moved online due to the growth of mobile devices. This facilitates our daily lives, but it also introduces various security vulnerabilities because of the Internet's decentralized and anonymous design. Malware can be avoided with the help of firewalls and antivirus software. However, sophisticated cybercriminals prey on customers' lack of security awareness by sending them to fake websites. There are numerous approaches to the difficult challenge of detecting phishing attempts on the market, such as using a blacklist, relying on rules-based detection, looking for anomalies, etc [6]. The literature shows that modern works favor machine learning-based anomaly detection due to its dynamic structure, notably for detecting "zero-day" assaults. This study proposes a machine learning-based phishing detection system, employing eight algorithms to evaluate URLs and three datasets to compare the findings to existing works. According to the outcomes of the experiments, the presented models work exceptionally well [5].

2.3 Blockchain-based Solutions

Over the past two decades, IT has come to be seen as a progressive development with far-reaching effects on society at large. The advancement of technology has greatly improved people's living conditions. Data from various web apps are aggregated and analysed by IT staff. The data gathered is beneficial to management in making decisions. In this study, they take a closer look at the blockchain architecture for managing dynamic data in an online store and reveal its underlying structure (DDMS-

BCM). Blockchain's ledger strengthens the system's potential to interact with cutting-edge information systems. Analysis parameters are determined via a comprehensive study of data management and business process reports [7].

In the absence of a methodical approach to E-commerce security, it may be impossible to reap the benefits of online shopping. Even online marketplaces like Amazon and Alibaba have started employing these methods to safeguard customer information. The One-Time Password (OTP) is the most often used form of authentication for online purchases. Besides security and compliance, this system also boasts high availability and a high degree of scalability. The significance of various security techniques in the E-Commerce domain is also discussed [8].Online marketplaces with built-in reputation management let buyers leave feedback on service providers after completion of transaction. In the current reputation system, the central server is not protected from arbitrary reputation changes to the provider. In addition, they don't provide inter-service access to your reputation. Since rating actions are correlated with personal information, rates are vulnerable to privacy breaches (e.g., identity and rating). At the same time, malicious raters may launch multiple rating attacks or other types of aberrant rating attacks [9].

3. Identification of Problem Based on Literature Review

The expanding tendencies of e-commerce provide ample chances for the incorporation of new technology. This phenomenon improves engagement with the new anonymous technologies in an indirect manner. Every day, many breaches in computer systems are announced around the globe. While some breaches are relatively minor in terms of the amount of data or funds compromised, many others are catastrophic. Network security is to protect the underlying networking infrastructure from assault, misuse, malfunction, manipulation, destruction, and improper disclosure. If these safeguards are in place, communication devices can perform their important functions without jeopardizing the integrity of the system [10].

When users have access to sensitive information across a shared network in a typical e-commerce setting, network security must always be a top priority. No network is completely secure; therefore a secure network solution must be used to protect customer's important information. With a dependable network security solution in place, businesses are less susceptible to hacking and other types of data theft. Priority number one is protecting a network from intruders like spyware on your workstations. Additionally, it ensures the confidentiality of any information shared between parties [11].

Network security infrastructure can protect against cyber-attacks and other forms of eavesdropping by encrypting data at many stages of transmission and transmitting it via numerous paths. However, we identified numerous chances to enhance the effectiveness of a resource-constrained e-commerce ecosystem. Various pieces of study have been undertaken over the past few years to propose some relevant security methods to improve the dependability of an e-commerce system. In terms of resource-constrained e-commerce platforms, however, there is still ample room for development. The term resource-constrained describes devices or networks having restricted available resources. The restricted availability of resources requires careful consideration. Consequently, it is difficult to build an adequate security solution to improve the efficiency of a network with limited resources. In this study, we intend to develop a more effective and secure defensive mechanism for such e-commerce communications [12].

4. Framework

This section introduces our machine learning-based intrusion detection system framework based on short-term memory (STM) and deep neural network (DNN) long Initially, malware data is collected from various datasets including CICIDS2017 and CICDDoS2019. The details of these datasets will be explained in the next part. Later, the proposed deep neural network architecture is designed [13]. Data preprocessing is a crucial part of data mining and analysis, as it prepares raw data for further processing by computers and machine learning. In order to process data efficiently, computers want to have information presented in the form of neatly organized 1s and 0s. In this way, it's simple to compute structured data, such as whole numbers and percentages. However, before analysis can take place, unstructured material like text and images must be cleaned and formatted. Machine learning models trained on faulty data will lead to "junk" results. The quality of data preprocessed is more important than the most important algorithms. "Features" of a data set can be used for explanation or communication [14].

We aim to propose a Machine Learning (ML) based threat detection framework for large-scale E-commerce communication environments. First we will take the CSV dataset and then Preprocess the data (Preprocess means to prepare the data and convert data from raw form to usable form) 70% data will use for training and 30% for testing.70% data will input by input layer for training this is called CNN after training I will take out from activation layer now model is trained after training we will test the model by 30% data that it is detecting the malicious activity.

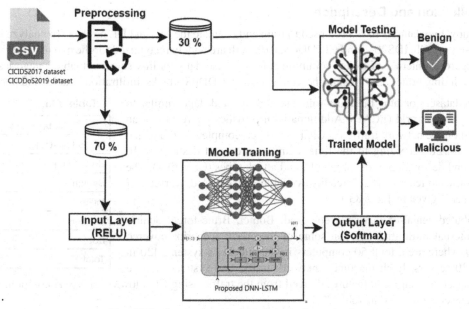

Fig. 83.1 Proposed threat detection framework

Algorithm	
1.	Input: CICDs2017, CICDDOS2018 (D1, D2)
2.	Output: Benign==0, Attack1==1, Attack2==2,………and so on
3.	Split D1 & D2 into D19Train and D19Test
4.	If True then
5.	Train the DNNLSTM using D1 & D2Train
6.	$f_t = \sigma(W_f . x_t + U_f . h_{t-1} + b_f)$
7.	$i_t = \sigma(W_i . x_t + U_i . h_{t-1} + b_i)$
8.	Calculate the hidden state ht:
9.	$h_t = f(W_h . x_t + U_t . h_{t-1} + b_h)$
10.	$r_t = \sigma(X_t . W_{xr} + H_{t-1} . W_{hr} + b_r)$
11.	$C_t = tanh(W_c . x_t + U_c . h_{t-1} + b_c)$
12.	$z_t = \sigma(X_t . W_{xz} + H_{t-1} . W_{hz} + b_z)$
13.	Calculate the output ot
14.	$o_t = \sigma(W_o . x_t + U_o . h_{t-1} + b_o)$
15.	end If
16.	While True do
17.	Test the DNNLSTM using D1 & D2Test
18.	Calculate the output of DNNLSTM
19.	If Value==0
20.	Return Benign
21.	else
22.	Return Attack Class
23.	end If
24.	end While

4.1 Dataset Collection and Description

In this research study, two datasets have been used to train and evaluate the ML and DL models. To analyze intrusion detection methods, the datasets are CICIDS2017 and CICDDoS2019, both are widely recognized for the extensive variety of features that they offer with regard to internet of things communications. These datasets link seven valuable categories with as many as fourteen threats, including brute force assaults, heart leech attacks, DDoS attacks, infiltration attacks, and port scanning attacks.

The CICIDS2017 dataset contains the most valuable and updated data, similar to those collected from real world (PCAPs).Additionally, it provides the results of an analysis performed on the network traffic via CICFlowMeter, complete with labeled flows that are organized according to the time stamp, source and destination IP addresses, source and destination ports, protocols, and attack types (CSV files). The definition of the retrieved features is also readily available. The detailed overview of CICIDS2017 dataset is given in Table 83.1:

Table 83.1 CICDDoS2019 dataset

Attack	Instances
DDoS-Loic-UDP	2854
Brute Force	2795
Benign	51,956
Infiltration	3156
DDoS-Hoic	3065
Bot	2698
Total	66,524

Heartbleed, distributed-denial-of-service, web-based, Botnet, Brute-force, denial-of-Service, and internal infiltration are just some of the attack scenarios covered in CICDDoS2019. There are a total 50 computers in the attacker's system, 420 in the victims, and 30 servers. Each machine's network traffic and system logs are included in the dataset, as well as 80 features derived from the traffic using CICFlowMeter-V3. A comprehensive overview of CICDDoS2019 dataset is provided in Table 83.1:

5. Dataset Pre-Processing

Data preprocessing is a crucial part of data mining and analysis, as it prepares raw data for further processing by computers and machine learning. In order to process data efficiently, computers want to have information presented in the form of neatly organized 1s and 0s. In this way, it's simple to compute structured data, such as whole numbers and percentages. However, before analysis can take place, unstructured material like text and images must be cleaned and formatted. Machine learning models trained with faulty data may actually be detrimental to the analysis you're attempting, yielding "junk" results [16]. Good, preprocessed data is even more crucial than the most sophisticated algorithms. The "features" of a data set can be used as a means of explanation or communication [15].

5.1 Dataset Normalization

Machine learning often employs the data preparation method of normalization. Normalization is the process of ensuring that all rows in a data set are the same size. For machine learning purposes, normalization is not required for all datasets. As long as the characteristic ranges are similar, it is not necessary[40]. By maintaining uniformity in the input distributions to each layer during training, it makes the training of a model can be enhanced by decreasing the internal co-variant shift. Weight normalization is a reparameterization technique for deep neural networks that works by isolating the magnitude of the weight vectors from any particular bias they may have in a given direction. To speed up the learning curve of different neural network models, layer normalization is a technique that can be used [16]. In contrast to batch normalization, the normalization statistics are estimated directly from the summated inputs to the neurons in a hidden layer using this method. One alternative to batch normalization is group normalization. Normalization is achieved by computing the mean and variance of each subset of channels, or normalizing the features within each subset, using this method. However, the accuracy of group normalization remains constant throughout a large variety of batch sizes, which is not the case with batch normalization [17].

Normalization is a reparameterization technique for deep neural networks that works by isolating the magnitude of the weight vectors from any particular bias they may have in a given direction. To speed up the learning curve of different neural network models, layer normalization is a technique that can be used [18].

6. Learning Algorithms

6.1 Machine Learning based Intrusion Detection System

Deep learning is a branch of machine learning that excels in "Artificial Intelligence", the phrase "artificial intelligence" is used to describe a broad category of methods that allow computers to perform tasks normally performed by humans. All of this is made possible by machine learning, which is essentially a collection of algorithms that can be taught new skills by analyzing existing data. Inspired by the architecture of the human brain, deep learning is but one subset of machine learning. By repeatedly evaluating data with a predetermined framework, deep learning algorithms aim to arrive at insights that are comparable to those reached by human beings. The deep learning process accomplishes this by employing neural networks, which are algorithmic structures with multiple layers [19] [20].

6.2 Deep Neural Network

A Deep Neural Network (DNN), often known as a Deep Net, is a very complicated type of neural network. They can be thought of as stacked neural networks, which are networks with multiple layers (often two or more) and an input, output, and a hidden layer in the middle. DDNs are commonly used to manage unstructured and unlabeled data. These days, the go-to method for completing a wide range of computer vision tasks is the use of powerful neural networks [30]. An artificial neural network (ANN) with multiple hidden layers between the input and output layers is called deep neural network (DNN). Deep neural networks (DNNs) can model non- linear interactions in the same way as shallow ANNs.To solve problem such as classification ,neural network take data ,process it using various algorithms , and display the result. So far, we have only worked with feed forward neural networks [21].

6.3 Long Short Term Memory

A paradigm called long short-term memory (STM) was first proposed in 1997. The bidirectional version of the long short-term memory (LSTM) network is just an extension of the original LSTM model, which is a Gated recurrent neural network. The most important part is that these networks can save data for later cell processing. LSTM can be understood as a recurrent neural network (RNN) with a two-vector key-value store. The first one is transient state that maintains the current time step's output. The second one is persistent storage, reading, and rejection of data not intended for immediate use as it travels via the network [22]. Activation functions play a role in determining whether a given action should include reading, storing, or writing. Those activate functions produce a number between and (0, 1). The input and forget gates determine whether or not to retain newly received data. The first model is trained to recognize a specific sequence in the data, whereas the second is taught to recognize the opposite sequence [23].

7. Conclusion and Future Scope

In this paper, we propose a Machine Learning (ML) based threat detection framework for large-scale e-commerce communication environment. Our Study highlights the strength and weakness of various algorithms as well as previous work in specific area. A solution is proposed in the form of framework consisting of a combination of DNN and LSTM models. This proposed framework will increase performance and provide better results. The system will detect intrusion and will prove to be a good tool for intrusion detection. In future, this research may develop strong approaches for for implementation to understand intrusion and to identify the malicious activity.

REFERENCES

1. F. Behgounia, B. J. I. J. o. C. S. Zohuri, and I. Security, "Machine Learning Driven An E-Commerce," International Journal of Computer Science and Information Security (IJCSIS), vol. 18, no. 10, 2020.
2. M. Zhang, L. Lin, and Z. J. C. C. Chen, "Lightweight security scheme for data management in E-commerce platform using dynamic data management using blockchain model," Lightweight security scheme for data management in E-commerce platform using dynamic data management using blockchain model." Cluster Computing (2021): 1-15., pp. 1-15, 2021.
3. N. L. Bhatia, V. K. Shukla, R. Punhani et al., "Growing Aspects of Cyber Security in E-Commerce." pp. 1-6.
4. M. Li, L. Zhu, Z. Zhang et al., "Anonymous and verifiable reputation system for E-commerce platforms based on blockchain," IEEE Transactions on Network and Service Management, vol. 18, no. 4, pp. 4434-4449, 2021.
5. M. J. Girsang, R. Hendayani, and Y. Ganesan, "Can Information Security, Privacy and Satisfaction Influence The E-Commerce Consumer Trust?." pp. 1-7.
6. Z. Zhu, Y. Bai, W. Dai et al., "Quality of e-commerce agricultural products and the safety of the ecological environment of the origin based on 5G Internet of Things technology," Environmental Technology & Innovation, 22, 101462., vol. 22, pp. 101462, 2021.
7. L. T. T. J. o. R. Tran, and C. Services, "Managing the effectiveness of e-commerce platforms in a pandemic," Journal of Retailing and Consumer Services 58 (2021): 102287, vol. 58, pp. 102287, 2021.
8. A. R. Khan, M. Kashif, R. H. Jhaveri et al., "Deep Learning for Intrusion Detection and Security of Internet of Things (IoT): Current Analysis, Challenges, and Possible Solutions," vol. 2022, 2022.

9. Y. Otoum, D. Liu, and A. J. T. o. E. T. T. Nayak, "DL-IDS: a deep learning–based intrusion detection framework for securing IoT," vol. 33, no. 3, pp. e3803, 2022.

10. S. Vinoth, H. L. Vemula, B. Haralayya et al., "Application of cloud computing in banking and e-commerce and related security threats," Materials Today: Proceedings, vol. 51, pp. 2172-2175, 2022.

11. R. Kozik, M. Pawlicki, M. Szczepański et al., "Efficient Post Event Analysis and Cyber Incident Response in IoT and E-commerce Through Innovative Graphs and Cyberthreat Intelligence Employment." pp. 257-266.

12. I. D'Adamo, R. González-Sánchez, M. S. Medina-Salgado et al., "E-commerce calls for cyber-security and sustainability: How european citizens look for a trusted online environment," Sustainability, vol. 13, no. 12, pp. 6752, 2021.

13. I. D'Adamo, R. González-Sánchez, M. S. Medina-Salgado et al., "E-commerce calls for cyber-security and sustainability: How european citizens look for a trusted online environment," Sustainability, vol. 13, no. 12, pp. 6752, 2021.

14. H. Pallathadka, E. H. Ramirez-Asis, T. P. Loli-Poma et al., "Applications of artificial intelligence in business management, e-commerce and finance," Materials Today: Proceedings, 2021.

15. M. J. Girsang, R. Hendayani, and Y. Ganesan, "Can Information Security, Privacy and Satisfaction Influence The E-Commerce Consumer Trust?." pp. 1-7. 23

16. Z. Zhu, Y. Bai, W. Dai et al., "Quality of e-commerce agricultural products and the safety of the ecological environment of the origin based on 5G Internet of Things technology," Environmental Technology & Innovation, 22, 101462., vol. 22, pp. 101462, 2021.

17. L. T. T. J. J. o. R. Tran, and C. Services, "Managing the effectiveness of e-commerce platforms in a pandemic," Journal of Retailing and Consumer Services 58 (2021): 102287, vol. 58, pp. 102287, 2021.

18. M. H. Gouthier, C. Nennstiel, N. Kern et al., "The more the better? Data disclosure between the conflicting priorities of privacy concerns, information sensitivity and personalization in ecommerce," Journal of Business Research vol. 148, pp. 174-189, 2022.

19. O. Saritas, P. Bakhtin, I. Kuzminov et al., "Big data augmented business trend identification: the case of mobile commerce," Scientometrics 126.2 (2021): 1553-1579., vol. 126, no. 2, pp. 1553- 1579, 2021.

20. Chandran, S., Verma, S.B.: Touchless palmprint verification using shock filter SIFT I-RANSAC and LPD IOSR. J. Comput. Eng. 17(3), 2278–8727 (2015)

21. Satya Bhushan Verma, Abhay Kumar Yadav, Detection of Hard Exudates in Retinopathy Images ADCAIJ: Advances in Distributed Computing and Artificial Intelligence Journal Regular Issue, Vol. 8 N. 4 (2019), 41-48 eISSN: 2255-2863 DOI: http://dx.doi.org/10.14201/ADCAIJ2019844148

22. Satya B Verma, Shashi B V, Data Transmission in BPEL (Business Process Execution Language), ADCAIJ: Advances in Distributed Computing and Artificial Intelligence Journal Regular Issue, Vol. 9 N. 3 (2020), 105-117 eISSN: 2255-2863 DOI: https://doi.org/10.14201/ADCAIJ202093105117 105

Emerging Trends in IoT and Computing Technologies – Suman Lata Tripathi et al. (eds)
© 2024 Taylor & Francis Group, London, ISBN 978-1-032-87924-6

Literature Survey in Integration of Block Chain Technology and Cloud Computing

84

Atul kumar[1], Kuldeep Mishra[2]

Maharana Pratap Engineering college, Kanpur
Computer science and engineering, Uttar Pradesh, India

Abstract: Block chain technology is a decentralized network where the information is stored on block which is non – temporary. In block chain blocks are connected to chain to verify the transaction by hash value. The information present in block is immutable and transparent which is verifying by every user. Cloud computing is on-demand computing for sharing computing resources. It provides data management and services on rental basis to the customer. Cloud computing and Block chain framework can be integrated to address digital privacy, data integrity in decentralized databases and provide clearness, immutability, safety and computerization. This paper provides a complete review knowledge of how block chain is implemented to offer protection in cloud computing structure and examine study of block chain associated in cloud computing framework. These item pursuits to offer a talk on aspects of integration among block chain and cloud computing to reach new technological era advancement.

Keywords: Block chain, Ledger, Cloud computing, Application

1. Introduction

Through unconstrained power of resource distribution and higher customer expertise cloud computing become a serious recent analysis topic. But cloud computing model have compromised of drawback in serious faith and safety issues. For case in point, in 2016, Cloud flare, a well-known cloud service supplier disclosed to important bugs in its software package has result in breaking of confidentiality information leakage, touching a minimum of 2 million websites, as well as assistance as of several famous web firms as Uber. During in month of June 2017, safety violate within Amazon web Services result within the disclosure of private data around two hundred million U.S. people. In line with review conduct by Fujitsu, equal 88% cloud client be upset concerning knowledge of security problems and wish to grasp what's happening on the physical servers. Being Associate decentralized architecture and distributed computing model, block chain technology have received extensive awareness, as well as application have exposed binge growth in recognition in computerized crypto currencies [19]. Block chain is predicated as decentralization Peer to Peer architecture; wherever every node is equal, and no centralization is exist in network. Decentralization feature of block chain is especially appropriate for building distributed and decentralized trust architecture. Block chain provide a new thanks to succeed trust-enabled cloud environments.

2. Cloud Computing and its Deployment Model

Cloud model is the service model of computing recourse like liaising, database, and hack off, storage space, and analytics above internet toward deliver faster modernization, flexible assets, and economy of level. user have to disburse on behalf of services

---

[1]atulverma16@gmail.com, [2]kuldeepmishra120bit@gmail.com

DOI: 10.1201/9781003535423-84

what they use, provided that headed for lesser process overhead, sprint your communications with efficient level of business according to your need [16].

Public Cloud: Cloud architecture is open for general public and may be utilized by enterprise once non-inheritable dynamically. Cloud suppliers deploy and maintain these clouds [5].

Private Cloud: Architecture and applications that are kept private to customers are deploying on it. Private cloud is protected and expensive as compare to other obscure.

Hybrid Cloud: It is merger of 2 cloud model. Mixture cloud facilitates pay per use method.

Community Cloud: It is owned by the group of people of customer as of dissimilar organization to share concern. It can be own, manage, and operate with single or other organization in society.

3. Uniqueness of Cloud Computing

- Pay per us
- Wide system contact
- Reserve pool
- Deliberate service
- Elastic Scalability

4. Problem in Cloud Computing

Safety of Data: Cloud supplier provides protection of information by accepting by safety measures mechanisms. But some situation, disclosure information happens due to cyber attack [7].

Load Time: Cloud Service is accessible across 24/7 apart from number of service be regularly break. They discontinue their service on behalf of periodic maintenance.

Limited Control: Cloud user is going to have some degree of management on the information within the cloud. Majority of control they need in Infrastructure as a Service, wherever they control on virtual machines convert according their needs.

System Dependence: Cloud examines accessibility be totally needy on top of internet. Uneven entire world be omnipresent in network.

5. Investigation Issue in Cloud

Consistency: Cloud service accessible almost per second toward cloud user. Many periods, server stops its functioning because of upholding or else limited moment in time issue. In this day and age, cloud user imagines a lot of well-known principles, services, and finest practice commencing cloud provider [2].

Compliance: Presently there are several laws to use the data, access the storage, and need regular audit trails.

Service Stage Agreement: Cloud service are going to providing primarily base in the lead of Service Level Agreements to permit many instance of single function near derivative lying on numerous server when here be require depending leading to priority. If lower priority, cloud might close or reduce application. Most challenge for users is analysis of repair stage agreement united by cloud vendor.

Cloud Information Organization: Organizing information is significant investigate work in cloud. Seeing that cloud information can huge in shapeless or semi-structured way. Once-over providers completely depend upon infrastructure toward realize totally information security. In view of the fact they don't contain right to use to information centre objective safety structure.

Information Encryption: Data may be encrypted toward security on information. Presently numerous level securities abounding. Web services APIs use toward access cloud from end to end computer program with customers written to those API.

Interoperability: Inner communiqué of system be required toward exchange of information moreover create the make use of information. Public cloud considered the same as clogged system and is not hypothetical condition toward converse with everyone.

6. Case Study

At the bottom of interoperability and support along with their presented and deploy cloud structure be require designed for public and private organization this time. Dissimilar cloud model are federate into anxious federations system. In adding together several technical problems, expansion and managing of cloud federations contain compact among grim safety issue such are leakage of responsive information moreover execution of secrecy. EU SUNFISH scheme aim clear up that safety issue by implement democratic, decentralized, cloud federation system that ensures managed facts [12].

7. Block Chain Technology

Block chain contain two kinds of records ie, blocks and transactions. Every node contains a timestamp and linkage to previous block. Every node is connected to other by secure hash algorithm. The key benefit is that it uses cryptography that allows dissimilar users not to change the record on secured network [21]. If bulk of nodes agrees that transaction be legal, then block be merge to chain history. Block chain configuration is depending on type and size of the network. Block chain structure consist of a small number of fundamental concept in the vein of decentralization, digital signature, mining and data integrity [2][4].

8. Characteristics of Block chain Technology

In summing up, block chain has next key characteristics:

Fragmentation: During centralization, blocks will be validating throughout honest central server. That comes up to bring trouble in wait for communication into entire system along with increase computation charge. Block chain consist of P2P nodes not including need of next to third party. Block chain wants not to depend on top of central server toward store up and bring up to date multiple systems. In dispersed network entire participant aggressively participates in transactions with decentralized server [1].

Persistency: All transactions are verified in the block chain by participants and trusted transactions are stored in block. If transaction added in list, then reverse the communication be difficult. Blocks be verified through further participants, that they can't be manipulated.

Inspection: Every transaction inside block chain be present cryptographically encode through hash by source digitally, save node through timestamp, creating simple pro user to keep record and validate transaction information [3].

Secrecy: Block chain information be protected through public key cryptography. Towards authentication every expenditure is digitally sign. Source interacts with block chain toward maintaining self-generated email plus generates dissimilar group of address toward care their uniqueness as undisclosed.

Autonomous: In block chain there is no single unit for scheming the block chain network; we can distribute the signed node and examine them then node is accepted in decentralized network [18]. Consensus mechanism come through accept node by each further block in network, ensure that information transmit will be finished securely in block chain.

Unalterable: Transaction information be verified earlier than received in node. Block chain enduring record the transactions. Information in block cannot tamper [11]. If someone try to modify information, it could not be easily changed for the reason that information in block be connected during hash value, plus change information could invalidate further block [30].

Clearness: Block chain be decentralized organization wherever every participant be able to circulate record in addition to inquiry node information. Block chain system report plus maintain business deal in open dispersed ledger. That information be open plus consistent to entire node present in similar system to access information.

9. Block Chain Technology

Block chain be able to defined three type [27]:-

Permission less Block chain: Public block chain is open ledger decentralized, with which a few block go into network plus may interact with processing, storage space, plus validation of transaction information during consensus mechanism[6].

Permission Block chain: Restricted block chain is one, wherever no can rapidly be portion of network. It be kind of middle block chain managed via essential authority on behalf of accessibility. Information study approval in secret block chain open to the open selectively. Private Block chain precise toward restricted organization i.e. Vote counting, Asset rights.

Consortium Block chain: Consortium block chain could be part of decentralized chain. Prior select node can contain authority on the way to decide on sort of service within before. Left over node could contain entrée to block chain dealings, however not within consensus procedure.

10. Block Chain Architecture

Block chain is sorts of series of node that grasp complete information belong to network within open ledger. Presently here be block header plus block body during every block. Six main mechanisms in block header [24] are:-

Block Description: It permits on the way toward go after set of rules in block corroboration [8].

Merkle Tree: Information be encrypt by means of hash algorithm while transaction occur, it be transmit toward every node. As a result of it may contain thousands transaction record in block of every node. Merkle tree be use in block chain toward make concluding hash worth and Merkle root.

Time-stamp: Produce stamp in block as time per second pro each block.

Complexity Target: Entrance of legal hash block.

Nonce: 4-byte typically begin on zero will increase by way of every hash computation.

Parent Hash Block: It contains 256-bit hash in the direction of preceding block.

11. Block Chain Operation

Block chain architecture is a building block of information plus connected toward series structure of node and connected through every node contain preceding node title [27]. If a number of information be modified within preceding block, hash input is alter, thus hash value is present in chain of block. It prevents information as of tamper. While consumer needs toward deliver transaction information on the way toward others, then transaction will represent seeing that block. Block has to broadcast all other nodes in network to add block in block chain. Miners of node have to compel to agree transaction. Miners acquire authority to grant block by rule computationally [22]. Block is adding to block chain later than authentication, which complete the transaction. Next step is toward making a decision who user will publish the next node. Gathering of valid blocks is joining into sequence that form block chain network.

12. Consensus Algorithm

While block be required in the direction to insert in block chain, then block has to be verified as legal one through the entire node within the network. Consensus algorithms are group of set of rules that maintain the node concerned in block chain to achieve an arrange conclusion transaction and sort invalid transactions.

POW: (Proof of work) can be technique used within Bit coin. During this technique, every node contains hash worth of block header. Block header consists of hash that would contain different hash values [24] [26].

POS: (Proof of stake) might be strength selection in characteristic near POW. Diggers inside POS get express the liability pro live of money. Specially, Bit coin utilize institute to associate degreeticipate follow originator [10]. It utilizes correlate equation so as to search for the prime token hash and spur in combine with the cross of the stake. Different block chains hold confined start and alter to POS bit by bit [9].

PBFT: It also replication calculation to suffer from byzantine issues. Hyper ledger matter uses the PBFT as its computation in view of the truth that PBFT may alter 1/3 malignant byzantine reproduction.

DPOS: It is an agent pale. Associates decide their agents to give an approve squares. DPOS is the use of Bit shares.

Ripple: Ripple is intellectual degree pact calculation that use and large confided in sub networks among larger system. Among the system, hubs are divided into a pair of kind: server for pleasing correlate significance deal methodology and buyer merely exchange assets.

13. Challenges in Block Chain

There are many challenges that limit the use of block chian that cause many problem are legislation, consensus, and chain system [20].

Scalability: Many transactions are rising day by day with in block chain, creating additional information is stored. Every one of the nodes requires storing all record in favour of justification. For reason block range limitation in addition to also point in use build fresh block, block chain simply developed 7 transactions in second [15]. Block has capability be lacking, plus plenty of tiny dealings might late seeing that miners like dealings with next business fee. Matter of scalability be elevated [9]. Information Leakage:- Within block chain, user's dealings be throughout secure while they're finished through produced address rather than genuine identity. Within occasion of facts leak user might be creating numerous addresses. Though, block chain will not guarantee transactional privacy in view of the fact that worth of dealings be openly noticeable used for every public input. Secrecy of expense be obliged to strengthen block chain [29].

Regulations and Laws: Block chain has bring many community changes, counting in lawful and law systems. Block chain trigger sequence of authorized issues by covering legal management in near the beginning stage of development. Appropriate laws and policy can only strengthen later than rapid accepting of block chain characteristics. All the way through escalation dogmatic actions, the majority of country in progress to execute block chain [13].

Governance: Block chain has huge execution potential in term of administration plus communications and predictable toward convert administration function plus role. It helps to create less composite administration structure, safety of administration information, plus clearness of authority plus service process. Block chain is dispersed system with no third party [14].

14. Integration of Block Chain and Cloud Computing

Block chain combination with cloud get into new age of information safety and service accessibility. Block chain overcome mainly of the analysis problem with cloud.

Interactiveness: Within cloud, interior interaction isn't permitted, it make several industry go into reverse exploitation of cloud. Once cloud merged with block chain, different clouds are representing like node. Inter communication be probable within block chain. Every node presents in same network distribute the information among them so every node consists of replica of dealings. It makes clearness in network. That makes up to date transaction in ledger, when distribute all extra nodes. Throughout, institute be able to add several range networks plus might be conserve accessibility of information, when bring legitimacy in network.

Information Encryption: As we know information is decrypted prior storing within cloud, which maintains data integrity. Within block chain, every one of block information is signed by hash value using cryptographic, plus generate hash code meant for every block. Consider situation during block chain be employed toward protect job arrangement in cloud. Toward conform rightness and information integrity, system that collect information from job scheduling produce hash value plus record it in block chain immediately [17]. Seeing as block chain has capability pro node finding according to agreement mechanisms, information integrity is maintain in every block. Every node in network consist copy of all transaction so as to give us with availability plus perseverance that help network for possible fault tolerance plus attack.

Service Level Agreement: Agreement with cloud is sympathetic toward service supplier or else Client with ultimate fairness. To unravel this matter, we build make use of block chain with smart contract. Smart contract in block chain create to construct belief stuck between the parties who don't be familiar with each other [28]. During block chain, Smart Contracts be outlined as program write within programmable language so as to run within bottle. Smart agreement permits self-execution once selected state meet on every node present in block chain. Additionally help party to forecast outcome because contract implementation lying on code outcome in open network, that they provable like they're by now sign.

Cloud Information Management: Information keep within cloud is shapeless manner. Information store in block chain will be in ordered manner. Information can trace by means of hash key which is generated on all block. Each block contains preceding hash value of block, plus its key is used toward remain track of network. Information present in block be validate plus can access by node current in network.

15. Model of Integrated Architecture

As we show the design of mixing the cloud computing with block chain. Consumers interact by server for assistance application layer. When user request for deal during application layer dealings information store via creating block predestined every transaction. To place block into block chain, information would be verified and validated by block nodes in block chain network [25]. Validation is going away to be done by consensus. Just the once block be measured to be legal, every node could exist connected to network plus send information to become a part of network .Every block chain information is present inside block chain protection for cloud storage. Block chain integration with cloud provider's for information protection, transparency and as well to improve services.

16. Conclusion

Cloud computing may be we tend toll-known technology because it has existed for several years. However folks are still troubled to beat some challenges of cloud computing like knowledge security, data management, interoperability, and so forth Block chain technology is associate degree rising technology accepted for its security and authenticity that are the most characteristics that are creating the globe intercommunicate its side. By grouping action of block chain by means of cloud structure, there'll be a lot of reward in usability, faith, safety, scalability, information management, as well as a lot of additional advantages. During this article, we tend to shortly introduce cloud computing, block chain technology and detailed description of the characteristics and its working. In future we further discuss the reimbursement of integrating block chain technology through cloud architecture to get better assurance, information security, and customer information organization.

REFERENCES

1. A. Vatankhah Barenji, H. Guo, Z. Tian, Z. Li, W. M. Wang, and G. Q. Huang, "Blockchain-based cloud manufacturing: Decentralization," 2019, arXiv:1901.10403.[Online].Available:http://arxiv.org/ abs/1901.10403

2. A. Harshavardhan, T. Vijayakumar, and S. R. Mugunthan, "Blockchain technology in cloud computing to overcome security vulnerabilities," in Proc. 2nd Int. Conf. I-SMAC (IoT Social, Mobile, Anal. Cloud)(ISMAC) I-SMAC (IoT Social, Mobile, Anal., Cloud)(I-SMAC) 2nd Int. Conf., Aug. 2018, pp. 408–414.

3. A. Jabbari and P. Kaminsky, "Blockchain and supply chain management," Dept. Ind. Eng. Oper. Res., Univ. California, Berkeley, CA, USA, Tech. Rep., 2018.

4. M. K. R. Ingole and M. S. Yamde, "Blockchain technology in cloud computing: A systematic review," Sipna College Eng. Technol., Maharashtra, India, Tech. Rep., 2018.

5. C. Qiu, H. Yao, C. Jiang, S. Guo, and F. Xu, "Cloud computing assisted blockchain-enabled Internet of Things," IEEE Trans. Cloud Comput., early access, Jul. 23, 2019, doi: 10.1109/TCC.2019.2930259.

6. D. Dujak and D. Sajter, "Blockchain applications in the supply chain," in SMART Supply Network. Cham, Switzerland: Springer, 2019, pp. 21–46.

7. D. A. Fernandes, L. F. Soares, J. V. Gomes, M. M. Freire, and P. R. Inácio, "Security issues in cloud environments: A survey," Int. J. Inf. Secur., vol. 13, no. 2, pp. 113–170, 2014.

8. D. B. Rawat, V. Chaudhary, and R. Doku, "Blockchain: Emerging applications and use cases," 2019, arXiv:1904.12247. [Online]. Available: https://arxiv.org/abs/1904.12247

9. D. K. Tosh, S. Shetty, X. Liang, C. Kamhoua, and L. Njilla, "Consensus protocols for blockchain-based data provenance: Challenges and opportunities," in Proc. IEEE 8th Annu. Ubiquitous Comput., Electron. Mobile Commun. Conf. (UEMCON), Oct. 2017, pp. 469–474.

10. D. Tosh, S. Shetty, X. Liang, C. Kamhoua, and L. L. Njilla, "Data provenance in the cloud: A blockchain-based approach," IEEE Consum. Electron. Mag., vol. 8, no. 4, pp. 38–44, Jul. 2019.

11. D. Yaga, P. Mell, N. Roby, and K. Scarfone, "Blockchain technology overview," 2019, arXiv:1906.11078. [Online]. Available: http://arxiv.org/abs/1906.11078

12. E. Gaetani, L. Aniello, R. Baldoni, F. Lombardi, A. Margheri, and V. Sassone, "Blockchain-based database to ensure data integrity in cloud computing environments," Res. Center Cyber Intell. Inf. Secur., La Sapienza Univ. Rome, Rome, Italy, Univ. Southampton, Southampton, U.K., Tech. Rep., 2017.

13. L. Zhu, K. Gai, and M. Li, "Blockchain and the Internet of Things," in Blockchain Technology in Internet of Things. Cham, Switzerland: Springer, 2019, pp. 9–28.

14. D. Efanov and P. Roschin, "The all-pervasiveness of the blockchain technology," Procedia Comput. Sci., vol. 123, pp. 116–121, 2018, doi: 10.1016/j.procs.2018.01.019.

15. F. Knirsch, A. Unterweger, and D. Engel, "Implementing a blockchain from scratch: Why, how, and what we learned," EURASIP J. Inf. Secur., vol. 2019, no. 1, p. 2, Dec. 2019.

16. S. Sharma, G. Gupta, and P. R. Laxmi, "A survey on cloud security issues and techniques," 2014, arXiv:1403.5627. [Online]. Available: http://arxiv.org/abs/1403.5627

17. G. J. Katuwal, S. Pandey, M. Hennessey, and B. Lamichhane, "Applications of blockchain in healthcare: Current landscape & challenges," 2018, arXiv:1812.02776. [Online]. Available: http://arxiv.org/abs/1812.02776

18. H. Kaur, M. A. Alam, R. Jameel, A. K. Mourya, and V. Chang, "A proposed solution and future direction for blockchain-based heterogeneous

19. H. Zhu, Y. Wang, X. Hei, W. Ji, and L. Zhang, "A blockchain-based decentralized cloud resource scheduling architecture," in Proc. Int. Conf. Netw. Netw. Appl. (NaNA), Oct. 2018, pp. 324–329.
20. Secur. Privacy Workshops (EuroS PW), Apr. 2018, pp. 67–74.medicare data in cloud environment," J. Med. Syst., vol. 42, no. 8, p. 156, Aug. 2018.
21. Z. Zheng, S. Xie, H. N. Dai, X. Chen, and H. Wang, "Blockchain challenges and opportunities: A survey," Int. J. Web Grid Services, vol. 14, no. 4, pp. 352–375, 2018.
22. J. Kołodziej, A. Wilczynski, D. Fernandez-Cerero, and A. Fernandez-Montes, "Blockchain secure cloud: A new generation integrated cloud and blockchain platforms–general concepts and challenges," Eur. Cybersecurity, vol. 4, no. 2, pp. 28–35, 2018.
23. J. Park and J. Park, "Blockchain security in cloud computing: Use cases, challenges, and solutions," Symmetry, vol. 9, no. 8, p. 164, Aug. 2017.
24. J. Singh and J. D. Michels, "Blockchain as a service (BaaS): Providers and trust," in Proc. IEEE Eur. Proc. IEEE 16th Int. Conf. Dependable, Autonomic Secure Comput., 16th Int. Conf. Pervasive Intell. Comput., 4th Int. Conf Big Data Intell. Comput. Cyber Sci. Technol. Congr. (DASC/PiCom/DataCom/CyberSciTech), Aug. 2018, pp. 724–729.
25. K. Bendiab, N. Kolokotronis, S. Shiaeles, and S. Boucherkha, "WiP: A novel blockchain-based trust model for cloud identity management," in
26. K. Chandrasekaran, Essentials of Cloud Computing. Boca Raton, FL, USA: CRC Press, 2014.
27. J. Truby, "Decarbonizing bitcoin: Law and policy choices for reducing the energy consumption of blockchain technologies and digital currencies," Energy Res. Social Sci., vol. 44, pp. 399–410, Oct. 2018.
28. M. Niranjanamurthy, B. N. Nithya, and S. Jagannatha, "Analysis of blockchain technology: Pros, cons and SWOT," Cluster Comput., vol. 22, no. 6, pp. 14743–14757, Nov. 2019.
29. M. Risius and K. Spohrer, "A blockchain research framework," Bus. Inf. Syst. Eng., vol. 59, no. 6, pp. 385–409, 2017.
30. C. V. N. U. B. Murthy and M. L. Shri, "A survey on integrating cloud computing with blockchain," in Proc. Int. Conf. Emerg. Trends Inf. Technol. Eng. (IC-ETITE), Feb. 2020, pp. 1–6.
31. N. Sanghi, R. Bhatnagar, G. Kaur, and V. Jain, "BlockCloud: Blockchain with cloud computing," in Proc. Int. Conf. Adv. Comput., Commun. Control Netw. (ICACCCN),Oct.2018,pp.430–434.

Emerging Trends in IoT and Computing Technologies – Suman Lata Tripathi et al. (eds)
© 2024 Taylor & Francis Group, London, ISBN 978-1-032-87924-6

Bit Coin Access Control Management Using Block Chain

85

Kuldeep Mishra[1], Atul kumar[2]

Department of computer science & Engineering,
Maharana Pratap Engineering college, kanpur, Uttar Pradesh, India

Abstract: Control is implemented on our computer and server security for access privileges of assets that who can use what assets. Accesses privileges are generally defined by access management policy that is verified by access demand moment. Solution of this application is systematizing attribute base accesses through smart contract plus install on block chain, therefore remodeling the policy analysis method in smart contract. However additionally attribute needed his or her verification supervise via smart contracts install on block chain. Audit ability entity derives from unchangeableness plus clearness entity by block chain. This discussion propose new move toward support block chain technology to publish policy express correct access to assets plus permit transfer of privileges between user. Designed policy rights exchange are in public and visible on block chain any user will grab policies several time plus subject presently who have access privileges to assets. Resolution permits dispersed audit ability plus prevent entity as of falsely deny privileges arranged by policies holder. Have tendency to additionally show a doable operating implementation supported XACML policies, deployed on the Bit coin block chain.

Keywords: Bit coin, Access control, Block chain, XACM

1. Introduction

Accesses organization is a policy that is used in computer system to get access to necessary resources. Resource access rights are manipulated by entry time that can be evaluated at request time in opposition to the contemporary get entry to context. Attribute based Access Control [1], regulates situations over attributes which explain capability of topics, assets, environment. Amongst matter attributes are ought to instance his/her ID of enterprise employed pro work on enterprise decision everyday jobs assigned to him for his corporal position and approach of recourses he presently uses. Block chain structural design were initially restricted to crypto currencies. Access manipulate is a required safety a part of nearly all programs. Block chain precise traits inclusive of immutability, durability, audit ability, and reliability result in thinking about block chain as a supplementary answer for get entry to manipulate structures. Access manipulation is implementing to control access to resources and most essential part of system security. We aim to offer the solution to the following questions.

- What are the troubles with current system to get entry to manipulate structures?
- How block chain can assist to clear up those troubles?
- What are the gaps within side the associated research?

In second section, we examine in progress get entry to manipulate structure difficulty and provide clarification how block chain can deal with them. We review research studies and categorize them first and foremost totally based on domain names

[1]kuldeepmishra120bit@gmail.com, [2]atulverma16@gmail.com

DOI: 10.1201/9781003535423-85

and implemented get entry to manipulate approach in segment three. In segment four, we talk about demanding situations of enforcing to get entry on manipulate machine using block chain. Finally segment five gift précis of paper. We purpose near offer complete photo of info architecture plus demanding situations.

2. Problem of Conventional Access Control and Key Benefits of Block Chain

This section, we tend to debate issues of existing access control plus aiming to solve them with block chain [16]. Users who gain access to data have chance of confidentiality discharge. In central system there exists problem of single point failure. Reading this present access organization system through time to resolve this problem plus get used to block chain-based decision for access permissions. Attribute-based cryptography [14] causes some problem like confidentiality release by personal key generator (PKG) [7]. Wang et al. [9] bring framework in favor of data distribution plus access management toward treat with drawback by implement storage space. Present solution pro organizing access control within multi -domain isn't efficient. Supported Paillisse et al. [13] flat approach is not ease to use plus rough PKI based system is tough to handle. This article recommend distributed plus access control policy is implemented on permission block chain. Coniferous tree [8] is another PKI organization supported by block chain to grasp safety without trusty third party. In cloud information distribution among numerous organizations may be concern for privacy [2]. Non-public data is kept private relating to users' identity provide access on share truth be major factor. The system checks user's attribute through access management policy in the direction allow access permissions to info they are owned by the federated organization, while maintaining the confidentiality of the federated organization's user attributes. This study suggests Block chain Associate in trusted execution environment to protect integrity of rule analysis. Users of mobile application perpetually worry regarding confidentiality problems as sometimes should provide access to personal information [6]. The conferred framework addresses 3 main concerns: knowledge ownership, data transparency & audit ability. System is planned so as user ready to control their own personal information plus make method of access to own information as transparent. Furthermore users will alter or revoke access permissions to personal information while not uninstall mobile appliance. Additionally system contains 3 distributed databases: Distributed Hash Table, block chain, plus Multi-Party Computation, which wreckage information into lesser nonsense chunk and deal out among node with no duplication. Confidentiality is not secure once when user award access to personal data so as get access to particular service.

3. Background and Related Work

Block chain is framework of dispersed, permanent, tamper-proof of public depository of information. It permits distrustful user be on agreement of un-altered plus verifiable part of information with no 3rd entity communication. Block chain allow making add on exclusively secure information wish on distributed agreement set of rule make a decision where legitimate information is add on dispersed network. The first block chain was utilized by the Bit coin crypto currency protocol [2] Associate in Nursing these days Bit coin continues to be the foremost standard plus extensive case of block chain implementation. Bit coin uses block chain as open register for storage worth as dealings. Ledger is partition into node wherever all node can store up non-conflicting transaction. Merging among block is accomplish by store hash of previous block header plus previous hash in the next block header to form chain that contain all transactions on this node basis on Markel hierarchy [3]. Defining which node is added to register in every pace determined via agreement protocol known as 'Nakamoto consensuses which depend on Hash value [4]. Point of examination Bit coin block chain is seen as record of ledger. Ledger is formed near swap money among user, represent through address. Addresses may be twice hash [6] open key derivative on ECDSA input combine [7]. Addresses are utilized via user near propel plus take costs, whereas consequent private keys be accustomed give proof in possession. Create novel address be inexpensive while create novel ECDSA input pair, thus every users will produce plus utilize numerous address. Additionally, user be incentive toward utilize completely dissimilar address as counterfeit known as address is that the solely namelessness security within Bit coin. Seeing as complete situation of organization is simply described in record of block chain, dealing is way toward managing money. Dealings be Varity of key in so business deal can take out money as of multiple addresses and transfer funds to multiple output addresses. Each transaction is signed by owner personal key for release of fund. Transaction can identify a fee to hide costs of checkout process. In observe each output is seeing as specifies where to withdraw funds and previous transaction in which funds were created. Bit coin uses scripting language plus script are utilized in transaction to start funds transfer of that transaction. Finally we have a tendency to memo to novel dealings be fashioned via several customer plus notify toward group of people through transmit information under Peer2Peer Bit coin [8] though block chain technology. Generally crypto currencies are corresponding to Bit coin, it is generally used outside of economic field may be to trace beginning and conversion in provide chain. [9] Shows however block chain can be exploited to make decentralized, financial system that permit to monetize, strongly their equipment to make lot of capital. [10] It provides the flexibility of worldwide available, provable and un tamper able delivery of information without third party interaction.

3.1 Algorithm to create a block chain

```python
import hashlib

def hashgenerator(data):
    result=hashlib.sha256(data.encode())
    returnresult.hexdigest()


class Block:
    def __init__(self,data,hash,prev_hash):
        self.data=data
        self.hash=hash
        self.prev_hash=prev_hash
class Blockchain:
    def __init__(self):
        hashlast=hashgenerator('gen_last')
        hashstart=hashgenerator('gen_hash')

        genesis=Block('gen-data',hashstart,hashlast)
        self.chain=[genesis]

    def add_block(self, data):
        prev_hash=self.chain[-1].hash
        hash=hashgenerator(data+prev_hash)
        block=Block(data,hash,prev_hash)
        self.chain.append(block)


bc=Blockchain()
bc.add_Block('1')
bc.add_Block('2')
bc.add_Block('3')


for block in bc.chain:
print(block.__dict__)
```

OUTPUT:-

```
p.py - C:/Users/admin/AppData/Local/Programs/Python/Python38-32/p.py (3.8.7)      —    □    ×
File  Edit  Format  Run  Options  Window  Help
import hashlib

def hashgenerator(data):
    result=hashlib.sha256(data.encode())
    return result.hexdigest()

class Block:
    def __init__(self,data,hash,prev_hash):
        self.data=data
        self.hash=hash
        self.prev_hash=prev_hash
class Blockchain:
    def __init__(self):
        hashlast=hashgenerator('gen_last')
        hashstart=hashgenerator('gen_hash')
```

```
        genesis=Block('gen-data',hashstart,hashlast)
        self.chain=[genesis]
    def add_block(self, data):
        prev_hash=self.chain[-1].hash
        hash=hashgenerator(data+prev_hash)
        block=Block(data,hash,prev_hash)
        self.chain.append(block)

bc=Blockchain()
bc.add_block('1')
bc.add_block('2')
bc.add_block('3')

for block in bc.chain:
    print(block.__dict__)
```

```
IDLE Shell 3.8.7                                          —   □   ×

File  Edit  Shell  Debug  Options  Window  Help

Python 3.8.7 (tags/v3.8.7:6503f05, Dec 21 2020, 17:43:54) [MSC v.1928 32 bit (In
tel)] on win32
Type "help", "copyright", "credits" or "license()" for more information.
>>>
==== RESTART: C:/Users/admin/AppData/Local/Programs/Python/Python38-32/p.py ====
{'data': 'gen-data', 'hash': '0a87388e67f16d830a9a3323dad0fdfa4c4044a6a6389cabla
0a37b651a5717b', 'prev_hash': 'bd6fecc16d509c74d23b04f00f936705e3eaa907b04b78872
044607665018477'}
{'data': '1', 'hash': 'e3e6c97161f3deaf01599fda60ba85593b07f70328bf228473d1d408f
7400241', 'prev_hash': '0a87388e67f16d830a9a3323dad0fdfa4c4044a6a6389cabla0a37b6
51a5717b'}
{'data': '2', 'hash': '47e8645e3c14bd4034a498aa88ea630bc0793375207bf90ca469792a5
d9484e1', 'prev_hash': 'e3e6c97161f3deaf01599fda60ba85593b07f70328bf228473d1d408
f7400241'}
{'data': '3', 'hash': '82084603decb1a14a8819dacaa86197659f1e150c4a50186e68043004
b5a3c06', 'prev_hash': '47e8645e3c14bd4034a498aa88ea630bc0793375207bf90ca469792a
5d9484e1'}
>>>
```

4. Proposed Approach

We have a propensity to use block chain knowledge toward symbolize proper access assets plus transmit on single user toward different user. Our purpose is to add right access on block chain to permit the organization of such through block chain transactions. Access agreement to resource are transfer from one user to another in subject of block chain dealings created by end rights owner without involvement of resource owner right are stored by resource owner through transaction, where opposite transactions represent proper transfers are inserted in block chain. Any user will examine them any time that hold right toward carry out act in resources. Users who want to access request for recourse be able to ensure that no person accountable on substantiating reality specified rights truly created rights decision. Access right is used to express Attribute based access control policy. Additionally attribute based access management rule combine collection off policy express situation in excess of attribute matching towards matter, resource or environment. Principles are conjunctively otherwise disjunctively combined and that they should be glad consequently so as accesses rights are approved. Policies programming language are permitting toward specific ABAC policy of extensile rights, [11]. Lead role is resource owner says P and multiplicity on subject Si. Assets holders are entities that have organization policies of every resources Rj plus that create, update plus revoke policy. Identify our tend to take into account pro ease by policies institution be additionally correspond to assets holder. According to various policies framework that holds the rights can perform actions on resources. The themes will transmit access right particular to policy, level with processing on ripping that. Our approach wants to facilitate P and Si performs different actions to one-others. Policies holder take nix partially within policies right swap.

4.1 Policies Formation, Updates, as well as Revokes

Policies describing accesses right to assets R are define via holder of the resource p, who maintains the record in the block chain via the policy creation transaction (PCT). When it is formed, a contract can be updated by P at any time and, in time that would revoke or cancelled. this move toward policies is composed off situation that define ID topic toward who policies grant accesses rights circumstances when define set off value allowable that attribute for subjects, assets associate degreed access surroundings. In other words owner of the resource decides which subject matter he need to start grant accesses rights plus group off circumstances so as to grasp the allowance accesses. This theme tends to permit that term toward customized appropriately beneficial owners after they have transferred these rights to other users. Present rights owner be allowable on the way insert novel circumstances to AND that outline policy tear set of value acceptable for attribute by mutual degree condition C of policy in 2 sets by correct disjunction conditions, Ci and Cj . We have a tendency to note that adding conditions isn't a similar as execution policies update. Since circumstances additional towards policies be joint via rights holder by prevailing one AND operative, ensuing on the whole policies be able to solely by additional restraining to initial one. Policy cannot be violated by this approach. This can be right for the reason that the political institution is the only 1 that will update policy conditions by rights owner be adding progressively pro every swap off right, which can't be customized via novel rights holders. Every policy issue one subject ID, as a result of once P needs toward allow accesses for assets to lots of subject. In this process assume so as to every policies include only 1 law, plus that regulation hold every situation policies that are joint by logical AND-OR operation. Have tendency to keep in mind that a block chain will seeing that dispersed information simulated between every user. That way each part for information on block chain cannot be removed and permanent burden on whole network. Once shaping replacement protocol, we have to attempt toward reduce number of information save in block chain and store only necessary data. Store policy on XACML design to block chain will end to significant area profession problem. Simplest resolution would be to store within the block chain solely a link to associate degree as well crypto logic hash toward create a immutable. Block chain may save only a tiny URL to an external source hosting specific policy [12]. The advantage of this resolution is attenuating the number of knowledge to be holding on block chain, since work off policies be stable several to policies dimension. We have a tendency to select, stock up policy straight on block chain implicit into tradition designed economical arrangement so as to favoritism density plus avoid data repetition. Rewriting (ABAC) rule to record essential conditions against attributes. Every condition is written as 3 items on order: – correct attributes names, quantity linking rights and missing expression; – missing expression would be attributes names else relentless worth. A circumstance is joints via reason of AND-OR create singular situation. Distinction of attributes name is totally dissimilar among user then map got outlined through policies issuers. Attributes map could be in public on the market map attributes name by 1 distinctive rules mounted range. Validly printed list should be signed by the issuer. Crypto logic hash listing created on each policies utilization attribute catalog. This hash essential toward understand where map be use condition prevent policies organization for making replacement mapping without a doubt ever-changing of obtainable policies. Policies owner may at rest remove map to future purpose thus counseled pro users shopping for correct resultant as of policies that closely keep matching map. Just casing for prospect argument rights holder will verify this map is accurate as a result of hash match plus policies organization can't reject map maker as a result sign connected toward map. Resolutions permit toward avoid wasting information relating to attribute off chain. We will save attribute values type, creating sort of quantity non- ambiguous. If constraint surname is diagrammatical to institution attributes tables. We may save variety or date in numerical illustration instead of thread demonstration.

4.2 Right Transfer

This draw near provide so as to who is valid for access the assets R rights are transfer to existing rights owner Si, toward different theme Sj, throughout tradition organization keep within the block chain, known as Right Transfer group action (RTT). RTT should contain linkage for policies when right is exchange. In expressed interested party are concerned on RTT with Si and Sj. RTT be approved via Si participation of the holder is not compulsory on the assets for the duration of transfer of rights. Once you have transferred the rights to RTT, we cannot modify the conditions on RTT. Supposing that variable condition outline by resource holder state for an access is often performing 10.00 AM to 4. 00 PM Si may transmit rights toward Sj via restrict clock interval between 10.00 AM to 4.00 PM. We tend to notice that the arguments concern only the owners to perform action. Generally they do not need alternative rights either lying on policies or lying on property. Subject is ready toward generously swap act right among each other with no communication by policies institution. This suggests policies owner have no information earlier that subject. We have a tendency to additionally memo policies update as of assets holder be able to doubtless amendment means of policies. That suggests subject be able to achieve right top of particular assets may presently modified by policies holder, block chain by no means forget plus timestamp each rights transmit plus also policies update, these change be noticeable.

5. Architecture of the Proposed Framework

In this framework we propose block chain based access control which is depend on XACML model [11] that can be combined with block chain. So as to permit block chain based access control we used two approach Policy social control purpose (PEP) plus Policy Administration purpose (PAP). Once request is received toward carry out operation on assets, next to IDs of resource, ginger should fetch additional data to unequivocally bind the If subject to an RTT at block chain intervals. Personal key is used to sign in order not to obtain access rights in RTT. It cannot be completely different from a classic authentication theme in a classic login management scenario. CH is fully responsible for the execution of the workflow by contacting the additional apparatus to approval structure.CH primary sends demand toward PAP. PAP extracts RTT connection for demand plus retrieves this RTT from block chain plus each RTT that connects to this policy is then connected to policies update issue by assets holder. PAP combine retrieve information toward make XACML policies plus send that policies reverse toward CH. When safety policies has reconstruct for block chain it is verified and its analysis in opposition to accesses demand follow method outlined through XACML normal Associate on Nursing represented [11]. Temporarily CH ask Policies info purposes toward recover important attribute, if embed attribute within unique demand, plus pass policies therefore original appeal for Policies call Point that evaluate plus proceeds toward CH choice: authorize or else refuse. CH next forward choice for PEP that enforce assets for execution.

6. Bit coin-Based Implementation

These sections describe how designed model is deploying on block chain expertise form. We have tendency to developed a symbol of construct implementation theme supported the Bit coin block chain. Endeavor for research to point out when procedure are deploy on high block chain, because the Bit coin block chain is, with none alteration toward fundamental block chain execution is necessary. Unconstrained class of policy updates and rights transfers are perform when each of two actions are performed separately from each other. In our accomplishment every step are perform automatic on Bit coin ledger.

6.1 Storing Data

Bit coin block chain is planned towards use seeing that dispersed records toward supervise precise information called transactions. In alternative Bit coin block chain wasn't intended toward add capricious information. Toward resolve that restriction, i have usually 2 strategies supported Bit coin are transactions and script lang. toward add random information in block chain OP come scripting op rules plus also MULTISIG dealings [13]. Without going into more detail, we notice to execution mechanically choose strategy toward exploit with no requiring user's interference. Have a tendency to utilize policy plus circumstances information be programmed on very compacted tradition plan this follow mixture process. Every step is performed in Bit coin where grouping action of every stage contains value. Fundamental business deal value, shown because bossiness deal fee paid on ledger depends on the size of business deal [14].Thus are able to value the price of each phase where dimension of business deal essential toward carry out. Bit coin contain complete block information on primary storage as information organization toward keep path of every events output, thus have tendency to embrace giant o/p on ledger may additionally restrain valuable primary storage house for every user. Denote that in every phase dealing cost be pay on recipient exploit. Policies formation may withdraw plus bring up to date ledgers be pay via policies holder, whereas right swap cost the responsibility of customer group action, we tend to start creating a Bit coins transaction and therefore we want worth is exchange. For making dealings are going to utilize mounted amount of BTC toward symbolize token, victimization process the same as painted Coins application [15]. Have a tendency to decision them tokens as a result of the worth they represent are employed on dealings hold information in the course of linked scripting, So don't look to be curious about the cost they represent but about the data they carry. Mounted amount selected for a token should be low enough that it is simple hold by any user plus it inexpensive value isn't applicable compare to procedure exact worth, however additionally lofty sufficient this may exist transact generously among user[16].

6.2 Policies Management Policy Creation.

Novel policies are issue via asset holder via making novel Bit coin transaction by means of 1 or else extra I/P plus 2and 3 O/P. Every 2 major O/P is able to generate novel coupon, thus pays common amount. Sole function off I/P be supply sufficient money toward make this 2 token then ought to embrace any range off assets holder funds in order. There are two main output are compulsory plus that design be definite via set of rules, even as 3rd O/p be elective, plus represent modification addresses pro assets holder toward stay unexpended I/P. Arrange off 2 primary output be essential: primary O/p create coupon which then use for exchange right between subject. Attributable also addresses this force employed policies establishment sell rights toward stroke near primary party. Next productions make voucher contain knowledge policies prearranged on tradition layout. Once assets holders create that business deal, system be notify plus, proportionality are inserted in block chain. Policy issuer creates sequence off policies modernize dealings toward incorporate every data required. We have propensity to note that policy creator doesn't got to sit up for the proportionality to be enclosed block before creating policy update reports, the owner of all inputs and outputs directs each policy build and update transaction so that there is no risk of double payment at end. This implies that extended policies would make lot of dealings plus, simply exist extra costly pro holder. Policy Update/Revoke make new transaction fee based on policy creation transaction output if policy has never been changed before, or payment outputs of final up to date policies deal iffy policies be previously modernized a minimum of one time. Clearly policies establishment be able to produce that dealings as a result of it's the sole one that may pay matching outputs. – Update business deal have 2 primary inputs correspond toward proceeding up to date or else proportionality outputs plus also extra input. Transaction that have 1or 2 O/P contains coupon from preceding policies up to date or else making footstep, whereas next be simply use modification addresses t gather currency missing when pay dealings price. Up to date tokens contain within primary outputs be employed toward add info contain policies up to date information's. – Revokes policies establishment should pay by connected token, i.e., should use it as a value rather than mistreating the surrounded data. Current aspire create business payment inputs similar preceding up to date or else PCT. Efficiently destroy coupon, so cancel that policies.

6.3 Exchange of Rights

Toward permit swap off accesses right among 2 entities we tend to imagine subsistence off little quite market wherever subjects curious about mercantilism or shopping for actions rights get piece. Tend to notice to every policies up to date be openly observable within block chain, every subjects wills will perform due diligence to verify the rights they are purchasing. From the participation of the themes, an adequate exchange between two subjects is obtained during information swap set of rules toward permit collectively construct plus signs RTT. Major aim off information swap is ensure this each subject signs RTT solely when inspection then it's fulfilling swap protocol. RTT be largely dealing wherever the coupon represent accesses rights be approved as of present submitted toward novel 1 plus return novel subjects credit the current owner with money. In addition, the token is enrich via recent holder by novel knowledge toward purify situation of the policy plus be able to separated into several token. Proper transmit tokens be formed initio via assets holder within policies formation deal that implies to assets holder be that primary toward put up for sale right toward subjects. Comment the truth right be highlighted via tokens, not to mention detail to each O/p be spends solely one time, guarantee identical right be able to transfer lone one time. Memo the point policies act privileges may picture toward tear down folk's privileges. Try plus it's merely have toward disburse equivalent coupon be simply traditional price. Present holder has pay in favor of privileges then tin cans perform by no matter its desire. He will visualize of not again reselling rights, that is to say same rights for opposing customer for damaged then. Benefits be assets holder be able to view on block chain once theme privileges coupon have damaged plus therefore may prefer toward revokes recent policies plus subject completely novel lone. Have a tendency to additionally memo to revoke policies otherwise destroy topic privileges aggressively remove policies knowledge significant production as of UTXO to every customer; several rule stop encumber system one time is no lively any longer.

6.4 Policy Evaluation

Presume you have policies giving accesses privileges toward assets R have produced plus up to date N period, which that privileges have transfer between subject's M periods. That implies block chain contain PCT, with a series of n RTT create for primary I/P for pt plus one sequence for N policies up to date dealings originate as of next production for pt. once ginger obtain demand information, solely receive linkage to last RTT, say rt, and will sole info must get ahead of onward demand toward CH. missive of invitation PAP be able to right of entry in block chain plus find the way toward the back on series for N RTT as of rt, aggregation at every phase extra circumstances further via privileges holder. Just the once PAP have reach pt it's know how to look through policies on block chain. It then iterates through sequence every M policies up to date dealings, modifies policies accordingly on information interpret on every up to date bypass. Formerly up to date policies be capable of insert proscribing situation insert at privileges homeowners plus browse throughout RTT sequence searching of every node. PAPS have resulting fully up to date policies on customary layout prepared pro analysis via PDP. Higher than policies renovation is complete by any person, seeing every information is publicly visible within block chain. That can be significantly necessary for the interested subjects which will retrieve a similar method up to dated policies for block chain plus choose wherever or not shop for privileges.

7. Conclusions

These research papers come near to make, supervise plus impose accesses management policy by exploiting block chain expertise. Most blessings off that process is policies be revealed on block chain, therefore able to be seen theme, which accesses privileges may transfer as of 1 users toward other throughout block chain business deal. These processes have legal throughout orientation accomplishment supported Bit coin. Have a tendency toward conceive to expand own effort toward check a way higher engraft accesses structure ion block chain. Especially we were finding out likelihood on victimization of smart contract get personal implementing policy. Have a tendency are exploring a way to formulate the classical access management theme as a sensible contract which will be hold on and dead within the block chain to mechanically value and enforce policies. What is more we conceive to get better own process so as supervise multiple protocol XACML policy plus rule set. Have a tendency to also are presently finding out the confidentiality implication off own approach plus the way lessen them.

REFERENCES

1. Hu, V.C., David, F., Rick, K., Adam, S., Sandlin, K., Robert, M., Karen, S.: Guide to attribute based access control (abac) definition and considerations (2014)
2. Nakamoto, S.: Bitcoin: A peer-to-peer electronic cash system (2008)
3. Merkle, R.C.: A digital signature based on a conventional encryption function. In: Pomerance, C. (ed.) CRYPTO 1987. LNCS, vol. 293, pp. 369–378. Springer, Heidelberg (1988). doi:10.1007/3-540-48184-2 32
4. Dwork, C., Naor, M.: Pricing via processing or combatting junk mail. In: Brickell, E.F. (ed.) CRYPTO 1992. LNCS, vol. 740, pp. 139–147. Springer, Heidelberg (1993). doi:10.1007/3-540-48071-4 10
5. NIST, U.: Descriptions of sha-256, sha-384 and sha-512 (2001)
6. Preneel, B., Bosselaers, A., Dobbertin, H.: The cryptographic hash function ripemd-160 (1997)
7. Johnson, D., Menezes, A., Vanstone, S.: The elliptic curve digital signature algorithm (ECDSA). Int. J. Inf. Secur. 1(1), 36–63 (2001)
8. Pilkington, M.: Block chain technology: principles and applications. In: Xavier Olleros, F., Zhegu, M. (eds.) (2015)
9. Huckle, S., Bhattacharya, R., White, M., Beloff, N.: Internet of things, block chain and shared economy applications. In: International Workshop on Data Mining and IoT Systems (DaMIS 2016), pp. 461–466. (2016)
10. Mainelli, M., Smith, M.: Sharing ledgers for sharing economies: an exploration of mutual distributed ledgers (aka block chain technology). J. Finantial Perspect. 3, 38–69 (2015)
11. OASIS: eXtensible Access Control Markup Language (XACML) version 3.0, January 2013
12. Zyskind, G., Nathan, O., et al.: Decentralizing privacy: using block chain to protect personal data. In: 2015 IEEE Security and Privacy Workshops (SPW), pp. 180– 184. IEEE (2015) 220 D. Di Francesco Maesa et al.
13. Hidden surprises in the Bit coin block chain. http://www.righto.com/2014/02/ ascii-bernanke-wikileaks-photographs.html. Accessed 24 Feb 2017
14. Bitcoin Wiki. https://en.bitcoin.it/wiki/transaction fees. Accessed 24 Feb 2017
15. Bitcoin Wiki. https://en.bitcoin.it/wiki/colored coins. Accessed 24 Feb 2017
16. Current Standard for Dust Limit. https://github.com/bitcoin/bitcoin/blob/v0.10. 0rc3/src/primitives/transaction.h#l137. Accessed 24 Feb 2017

Emerging Trends in IoT and Computing Technologies – Suman Lata Tripathi et al. (eds)
© *2024 Taylor & Francis Group, London, ISBN 978-1-032-87924-6*

Analyzing Strategies Employed in Disseminating Deceptive Content on Social Media

86

Priya Sharma[1], Mohd Waris Khan[2]

Integral University, Department of Computer Application,
Lucknow, India

Abstract: In contemporary culture, while social media has become nearly indispensable, it is imperative for individuals not to rely solely on it. The rapid dissemination of false information is a notable concern on social media platforms, where users encounter a plethora of information, varying in accuracy. The term "fake news" encompasses misinformation, disinformation, and malicious information, reflecting the diverse nature of inaccuracies present in the digital realm. The speed at which social media platforms like WhatsApp, Facebook, and YouTube operate has contributed to the proliferation of fake news. Misinformation is inadvertently disseminated by individuals who believe they are sharing authentic information but are, in fact, spreading misleading content. On the other hand, disinformation involves the deliberate dissemination of inaccurate information, even when the purveyor is cognizant of its inaccuracy. Mal-information, as the name implies, is rooted in truth but is intended to cause harm to individuals, groups, or nations. The convergence of these elements results when false information appears. The spread of false information on social media platforms is driven by two main motives. Some individuals engage in spreading it for amusement, while others have political, ideological, or commercial objectives behind their dissemination efforts. Understanding these dynamics is crucial for navigating the challenges posed by misinformation in the digital age.

Keywords: Fake content, Social media, Dataset, Machine learning technique, Classification

1. Introduction

In contemporary times, the dissemination of misleading information has emerged as a prevalent method for perpetuating myths. Fake news is distinguished not simply by the lack of accuracy but also by the incorporation of falsehoods alongside specific information, can manifest as entirely false or partially true [1]. The phenomenon of fake news is not a recent development; its existence predates human civilization itself. However, in the present era, the proliferation of fake news has reached unprecedented levels, capturing widespread attention.

The term "fake news" denotes the dissemination of false information, whether done so knowingly or unknowingly, aiming to deceive, mislead, and instigate anxiety and skepticism [1]. This global issue has given rise to the phenomenon known as information pollution or involution, wherein irrelevant and inaccurate content contaminates the informational landscape on a global scale. While fake news is not a novel concept, the advent of the digital age has propelled it to new heights, transforming it into a pressing global challenge that demands comprehensive addressing. False information intended to mislead, attract attention, trick, or harm a person's reputation is known as fake content and can be found in a variety of news outlets [2]. False information might fool users by appearing to be from reputable web addresses or having similar-sounding domain names.

[1]priyashar@student.iul.ac.in, [2]wariskhan070@gmail.com

DOI: 10.1201/9781003535423-86

Individuals are truth-biased by nature, so the majority of individuals assume that they may rely on the accuracy and reliability of the information they find on social media platforms. Additionally, people are confirmation-biased and readily believe what they truly perceive in their minds. It has been determined through analysis that people generally struggle to spot dishonesty. Users of fake profiles have established themselves as leaders on the most popular social networking platforms in order to engage in illegal activity. [3].

The following are the work's main contributions;

- It examines numerous linguistic styles used in publications and how to employ them in future work.
- In order to detect fake news, it goes over the main research publication categories.
- In accordance with the year that the different studies were conducted, it elaborates various publication trends.
- It demonstrates the many nations or locations that have made more contributions to the subject.
- It highlights the importance of authors in the identification of bogus news.
- Based on linkages (colleges/organizations), it examines a variety of publishing patterns.
- It displays the number of citations each contribution to the field of fake news identification has received.

The article is systematically structured into six distinct sections, each dedicated to specific thematic elements. Section 2 furnishes a comprehensive overview of the background concerning social networks, encompassing their impacts. In Section 3, the article extensively explores the applications of the fake content detection system. Section 4 provides an in-depth examination of the previous research conducted in the realm of online social networks. Section 5 is dedicated to discussing the challenges inherent in this domain. Finally, Section 6 serves as the conclusive segment of the research study, encapsulating the key findings and implications drawn from the investigation.

2. Online Social Networks

Online Social Networks refer to digital platforms or virtual communities that facilitate the connection and interaction of individuals over the internet. These networks provide users with the ability to create profiles, share personal information, and engage with others through various communication tools such as messaging, comments, and posts. Examples of online social networks include popular platforms like Facebook, Twitter, LinkedIn, Instagram, and others.

These platforms serve as digital spaces where individuals can establish and maintain social connections, communicate with friends, family, or acquaintances, and share content such as text, images, and videos. Online social networks play a significant role in modern communication, enabling users to stay connected, express themselves, and participate in virtual communities that align with their interests and relationships. Being a strong communication channel, online social networks have become popular tools for worldwide events, improving information sharing, and facilitating social interaction [3]. In their profiles, users can add text, images, videos, and other anything that can be viewed by everyone on the network or just a few people. Currently, a number of media sharing services exist that encourage users to contribute photos or films documenting their activities.

A user account, profile page, friends, followers, groups, a news feed, personalisation, notification, posts, likes, comments, reviews, ratings, and voting are some of the social media elements. Nowadays, as social media becomes more and more important, more people are getting their news from it than from traditional news sources.

To highlight few advantages of using social media include:

- The capacity to communicate with individuals anywhere
- Social media news consumption costs less in terms of both time and money.
- Social media allows for quick contact and straightforward news dissemination.
- Expanded business prospects
- Information discovery and real-time news

However few disadvantages of using social media include:

- An abundance of information;
- Privacy issues
- A lifestyle change and sleep disruption
- Online harassment
- The dissemination of fake news that can harm society

3. Applications of Fake Content Detection System

Applications for fake news identification analysis are diverse. Below are some of the most significant applications:

Limit the spread of false votes during elections: The 2019 general elections in India saw a significant increase in fake news. During the election campaign, there was a lot of false information spread throughout society. There were many who called the elections the first WhatsApp elections ever held in India because disinformation was being weaponized and WhatsApp was being widely used as a propaganda tool. The accounts that disseminated this unauthorised content on Facebook and Twitter were terminated after being examined by fake news detecting programmes.

Corona pandemic: Social media posts concerning questionable home remedies, phoney alerts, and Conspiracy theories represent instances of false information around COVID-19. For spreading erroneous information about the corona virus epidemic, two people were detained. The Indian Prime Minister urged people not to trust any reports about the Covid-19 pandemic. Collectively, a large number of scientists are working to disprove this false information by creating and utilising fictitious devices as well as recruiting human support.

Terrorism: Terrorist organisations and individuals are increasingly using social media to promote their messages because of the wide audience that social media sites like YouTube, Facebook, and Twitter have. Various governments and organisations have made an effort to prevent terrorist organisations from using social media. Because social media is accessible, affordable, and enables instant access to many of individuals, terrorist organisations use it. Experts can assess their aggressive, hypocritical beliefs after a while of using crowd sourcing to observe their networks on social media sites.

Natural calamities: Social media users often readily believe the information posted about crises or natural disasters, and they repost the posts in an effort to spread the word to as many users as possible. Unfortunately, some malevolent users are aware of this trend and upload false information, such as spam and phoney messages, in an effort to spread it further. During natural disasters, spam and fake photos are often shared on social media.

By employing an automatic fake content recognition system, it is possible to halt the spread of misleading material that appears on various social media platforms as images, articles, blogs, videos, and audios.

4. Review of Previous Work

Table 86.1 provides an overview of the current strategies and methods employed to address deceptive content on social networking sites. It likely includes various approaches such as content moderation algorithms, user reporting systems, and possibly third-party interventions. This table could serve as a valuable resource for understanding the existing landscape of tactics used to tackle deceptive content, offering insights into the strengths and potential limitations of each approach.

Table 86.1 Some existing approaches on deceptive content on social networking sites

S. N.	Focus of the relevant work	Technique & Problem Addressed	Summary of the contribution
1	A Scientometric Analysis of Deep Learning Approaches for Detecting Fake News	Deep Learning Approaches; Identification of Fake News in online social platforms	Enhanced by a qualitative examination of the publications [1]
2	Fake news detection and reduction of propagation in social media using social network analysis	K-means clustering & link prediction; Verification of user & media news credibility in social media platforms	Used credibility algorithm to identify fake news content [4]
3	Digital Forensics Classification Based on a Hybrid Neural Network and the Salp Swarm Algorithm	Using SSA as a Multilayer Perception Trainer; The Ideal MLP Structure	Determining which files have been altered, deleted, accessed, and manipulated by application programmes [5]
4	Fake Content Detection System for Multimodal Signals over Social Media	Classification Algorithms; Identification of fake content over Social Network	The vector representation is extracted using three feature extraction methods from the articles' textual content, and a multi-level voting model has been presented [2]
5	Digital forensics: a fast algorithm for a digital sensor identification	Digital image processing; Identification of imaging apparatuses by examination of the images they generate	Enhanced classification efficacy of the suggested approach & increase its classification accuracy [6]

S. N.	Focus of the relevant work	Technique & Problem Addressed	Summary of the contribution
6	Detection of Manipulated Face Videos over Social Networks: A Large-Scale Study	Deep learning Technique; Deepfakes video forensic	Detection of manipulated video, Identify visual manipulation using shared & non shared data and Used algorithm which detected data as fake [7]
7	The Role of Machine Learning in Digital Forensics	Machine Learning is used as an application of AI; Analyze large amount of datasets to reveal any criminal behavior	Extracting and Analyzing Digital Evidence [8]
8	Fake Profile Detection in Online Social Networks	Suspicious-link Detection Method based on Mutual Clustering Coefficient; Identification of Fake Profile in social network	Behavioural and Emotion -based Fake profile Detection System for Social Network[3]
9	Video-Based Evidence Analysis and Extraction in Digital Forensic Investigation	An object recognition and tracking technique based on deep learning; Video analysis technique to assist the forensic investigation	To enhance the quality of video and beneficial for deterring crime or providing quick action when criminal activity or conduct is observed [9]
10	File Fragment Classification Using Grayscale Image Conversion and Deep Learning in Digital Forensics	CNN and grayscale image conversion are used to fragment; Classify file fragment and Extract additional hidden attributes	Boost classification accuracy [10]

5. Fake Content Detection Open Challenges

While identifying false news material that appeared as multimodal signals on social media sites, numerous difficulties were encountered [2]. Some of these challenges are listed and explained below:

Conventional algorithms: For detection in a variety of fields, numerous techniques have been developed. Due to the lack of extensive publicly accessible databases containing misleading information, including phoney reviews, hoaxes, and social media rumours, they cannot be directly compared to one another. This prevents benchmarking between several algorithmic categories.

Unstructured data: Over 70% of the material found on social networking platforms is unstructured data, including audio files, videos, and photos with text contained in them. These platforms include data from publications like newspapers, journals, trustworthy or reputable news websites, etc. Such unstructured data complicates analysis because material on the Internet is available in a variety of formats.

Unavailable datasets: Since there are no deep fake benchmark datasets for well-known politicians, gathering the original video speech clips takes a lot of time. Prior to now, there hasn't been a widely accepted way for dividing datasets of films at the frame or pixel level. To create deepfake face-swap clips, many restrictions must be taken into account when gathering source and destination video clips.

Mode of education: A crucial area of research that is still unexplored is how to lessen the harm caused by misleading information. Recent studies have demonstrated that raising awareness of potential manipulation techniques employed in misleading information is an effective way to increase human detection abilities. In order to protect people from believing incorrect information, more research must be done on successful instructional tactics and how to apply these tactics to millions of social network users.

Deepfake dataset of the third generation: Using the deepfake dataset of the third generation to implement the models can be challenging. Third-generation datasets are superior to second-generation datasets in terms of quantity and quality, as they include participant permission and contain a substantially higher number of frames and videos.

Correspond with fraudulent material: By comparing false information against a knowledge base of complete information, false information can be verified. There are many obstacles in this path, such as ensuring data quality and effectively building and managing this knowledge base.

Proper extraction of features: To automatically extract information, methodologies for natural language interpretation and information extraction must be created. Effective information matching algorithms would also be required to ascertain whether the information extracted corresponded with the data already in our assembled knowledge base.

6. Conclusions

The primary objective of the system lies in the precise identification of fraudulent information, encompassing various formats such as text, photos, videos, and audio. Our current societal landscape is marked by an unprecedented era of digital connectivity. This paradigm shift implies that a network of acquaintances can establish connections between any two individuals within a maximum of six steps, fostering swifter and more cost-effective communication. However, it is imperative to acknowledge that this connectivity also creates opportunities for the misuse, abuse, and application of non-authentic methods in disseminating and manipulating news and articles. In consideration of this context, we have developed a systematic procedure for discerning deceptive, misleading, and manipulated promoted content. The significance of this study is underscored by the exclusive reliance of the younger generation on social media platforms for news consumption. Despite the ostensibly factual presentation of messages, not all news articles can be verified as accurate. Consequently, there arises a necessity to categorize information based on its veracity. It is pertinent to note that this categorization process is intricate, as purveyors of false information or rumors possess the capability to convey a seemingly authentic message. To clarify, societal progression is anticipated to remain unaffected and continue in a positive trajectory. As previously noted, the rapid dissemination of messages is a characteristic phenomenon. Regrettably, negative content tends to persist longer in the public consciousness than positive content—a factor that substantiates the rationale behind this research endeavor. It is worth noting the remarkable proliferation of media outlets such as Twitter, Facebook, YouTube, WhatsApp, and LinkedIn, along with a corresponding surge in their consumption. Given this unprecedented growth, conducting a comprehensive study becomes imperative. The expeditious development of a detection and mitigation process is deemed essential in light of these circumstances.

REFERENCES

1. Dhiman P., Kaur A., Iwendi C. and Mohan S. K., .A Scientometric Analysis of Deep Learning Approaches for Detecting Fake News. Electronics. 1-31, 2023.
2. Kaur Sawinder, .Fake Content Detection System for Multimodal Signals over Social Media. 1-266, 2022.
3. Wani Mudasir Ahmad, .Fake Profile Detection in Online Social Networks. 1-193, 2020.
4. Sivasankari S., .Fake news detection and reduction of propagation in social media using social network analysis. 1-104, 2023.
5. Alazab M., Khurma R. A., Awajan A. and Wedyan M., .Digital Forensics Classification Based on a Hybrid Neural Network and the Salp Swarm Algorithm. Electronics. 2022.
6. Bernacki Jarosław & Scherer Rafał, .Digital forensics: a fast algorithm for a digital sensor identification. Journal of Information and Telecommunication. 1-21, 2022.
7. Marcon F., Pasquini C. and Boato G., .Detection of Manipulated Face Videos over Social Networks: A Large-Scale Study. Journal of Imaging. 2021.
8. Qadir Abdalbasit Mohammed & Varol Asaf, .The Role of Machine Learning in Digital Forensics. IEEE. 2020.
9. Xiao J., LI S. and XU Q., .Video-Based Evidence Analysis and Extraction in Digital Forensic Investigation. IEEE. 55432-55442, 2019.
10. Chen Q., Liao Q., Jiang Z. L., Fang J., Yiu S., Xi G., Li R., Yi Z., Wang X., L. Hui C.K., Liu D. and Zhang E., .File Fragment Classification Using Grayscale Image Conversion and Deep Learning in Digital Forensics. IEEE. 2018.

Emerging Trends in IoT and Computing Technologies – Suman Lata Tripathi et al. (eds)
© *2024 Taylor & Francis Group, London, ISBN 978-1-032-87924-6*

A Method for Diagnosing Stator Winding Defects of Induction Motor using Modified Wavelet Transform

87

Om Prakash Yadav[1]
Associate Professor, Electrical Engineering,
Sandip Institute of Technology and Research Centre, Nashik

Abhinav K Gautam[2]
Assistant Professor, Electrical Engineering,
SR Institute of Management & Technology, Lucknow

B. Suresh Babu[3]
Professor, Electrical Engineering,
Sandip Institute of Technology and Research Centre, Nashik

Sagar N. Deo[4], Tanmay J. Bharambe[5]
Assistant Professor, Electrical Engineering,
Sandip Institute of Technology and Research Centre, Nashik

Abstract: Incipient fault prediction and diagnosis of induction motor (IM) is one of the important and necessary requirements to operate it at maximum efficiency and durability. Previously a lot of work has been done to predict the motor faults using spectral analysis technique known as current signature analysis (CSA) due to its broad area of acceptability and easiness. Now a day, the researchers are looking towards more accurate and sophisticated fault analysis techniques. In this work, an improved wavelet-transform technique known as S-Transform has been proposed and applied to diagnose the stator winding defects of induction motor. The suggested method has shown its effectiveness to detect the transients of stator current to diagnose stator winding defects with high level of accuracy.

Keywords: Induction motor, MATLAB simulink, Stator winding Faults, S-transform

1. Introduction

Due to stressed working conditions and hazardous environmental conditions in industries, the IM are prone to various types of defects. If these faults are not diagnosed earlier, they could lead to a catastrophic motor failure, which would be very expensive in terms of maintenance and operation. These machine faults are mainly related with rotor winding, stator winding and bearings [1]. The IEEE Industry Applications Society (IEEE-IAS) examined 1141 motors, and the Electric Power Research Institute (EPRI) assessed 6312 motors to estimate the percentage of failures [2] by parts in IM and concluded report is shown in Table 87.1.

[1]opnit05@gmail.com, [2]abhi.knit2012@gmail.com, [3]drsbphd@gmail.com, [4]sagar.deo@sitrc.org, [5]tanmaybharambe@sitrc.org

DOI: 10.1201/9781003535423-87

Table 87.1 Percentage of an induction motor's component failures

Induction Motor Faults	Prediction of % of failure	
	EPRI	IEES-IAS
Stator winding related	36	26
Rotor related	9	8
Bearing related	41	44
Others	14	22

The Table 87.1 shows that stator winding and bearings of IM are the most prone to fault or failure. An extensive survey on different IM faults, their detecting and diagnosing methods have been provided by S. Nandi in 2005 [3]. Because of its ease of use, the motor current signature analysis (MCSA) technique is the most commonly utilized to diagnose stator-related defects [4]. To overcome the problems related to FFT, the STFT method has been preferred by many authors. However, because of its fixed windowing function width, this technique is not useful for identifying and addressing low frequency components and has insufficient time resolution for high-frequency inputs [5]. Further a variable size windowing function known as wavelet transform (WT) evolved that has capability to overcome the drawback of STFT [6]. But the Wavelet transform's lack of phase information and the STFT's fixed resolution resulted in the creation of the S transform, which preserves absolute phase information while offering adequate temporal frequency resolution for all frequencies [7]. The S Transform uses the Gaussian window which is more versatile for transient analysis of the signal [8]. On viewing the advantages of S-transform, this method has been applied to analyze the transients of stator current to identify the stator winding defects in this manuscript.

The remaining part of this manuscript is organized as: part 2 describes the details mathematics of the S-transform, part 3 defines as stator winding related faults, part 4 summarizes as result and discussion, while part 5 provides the conclusion of the work done. The references used in this manuscript are presented in the last of the manuscript.

2. The S Transform as the Modified Wavelet Transform

The S Transform, a modified wavelet transform was developed by Stockwell and his teammates in 1996 to provide enhanced time-frequency resolution of transient signal [8] [9]. The advantages of both the STFT and Wavelet transforms are incorporated in the S-transform [10]. By using a scalable and variable window length in conjunction with the Fourier kernel, the phase information alludes to the time origin [11]. Because of this, it provides extra information about spectra that is not available from the locally referenced phase that the continuous wavelet transform produces [12]. A function h (t)'s CWT is defined as

$$W(\tau, d) = \int_{-\infty}^{\infty} h(t)w(t - \tau, d)dt \tag{1}$$

where the modified copy of the basic mother wavelet is denoted by w (t, d). The resolution and "width" of the wavelet w (t, d) are determined by the dilation d. The meaning of a function's S transform h(t) is a CWT with a specific mother wavelet called the Gaussian Window function multiplied by the phase factor [12].

Therefore, the S-transform of function h(t) is given as

$$S(\tau, f) = \int_{-\infty}^{\infty} h(t)\frac{|f|}{\sqrt{2\pi}}e^{-\frac{(\tau-t)^2 f^2}{2}}e^{-2\pi i f t}dt \tag{2}$$

3. Stator Winding Related Faults

The main component of an induction motor that produces flux to rotate the rotor is the stator winding. Any damage in stator winding can cause non-uniform distribution of flux that causes harmonics in stator current. Approx 38% of total electric machine fault fall under this category hence it is very important to monitor the feature characteristics online such that faults can be predicted in early stage of happening. There are various types of faults related to stator winding that occur in induction motor, these may be classified as open winding fault, turn to turn fault, line to line , and line to ground fault [1] [4]. Insulation breakdown is the primary cause of shorted turns and turn-to-turn faults. Due to which the magnetic field becomes unbalanced and further heating is created by the resulting induced currents. Excessive vibration brought on by the imbalanced magnetic field may also result in premature bearing failures.

This study examined the effectiveness of a suggested methodology by examining common stator winding defects such as open winding, turn-to-turn short circuits, and line-to-line faults.

4. Results and Discussion

4.1 Simulation Study of IM Faults

In this work, stator winding faults like open winding, line to line fault, and turn to turn short circuit faults were simulated in MATLAB/SIMULINK. The specifications of IM used in this simulation work are given as:

- Wound type induction motor with power rating 3730VA, Voltage 440V, Frequency 50Hz, 2pole
  - Stator Parameter: Resistance- 1.115ohm, Inductance- 0.005974H
  - Rotor Parameter: Resistance- 1.083ohm, Inductance=-0.005974H,

A breaker circuit connected in series to that stator winding is shut off in order to imitate an open winding fault. Further, turn-to-turn short circuit fault was created in stator winding by connecting a variable resistor in parallel to that stator winding, and reducing it to 1/12 times to its original value. To analyze the above faults, the stator current flowing in terminal A of stator winding was recorded and designated as I(a). Figure 87.1 show the simulation model used to diagnose stator winding defects. In next section, different health conditions of stator winding were analyzed using proposed method.

4.2 Stator Winding Health Analysis

The results of applying the proposed method S-transform to analyze the retrieved feature signal Ia under both healthy and deficient stator winding of IM are shown below.

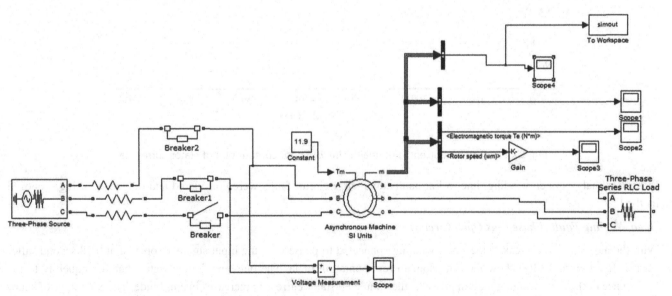

Fig. 87.1 The MATLAB simulink model used for analysing stator winding defects

Analysis of Healthy Induction Motor

In this part of work, healthy induction motor was considered and staor current Ia was simulated to analyse to get information about health condition of IM using proposed method S-Transform. Figure 87.2(a) shows the simulated stator current Ia of healthy motor. Here, the x-axis denotes time in second, while y-axis denotes normalised amplitude of stator current. The result depicted in the image shows that the IM draws a higher starting current since there is no back emf to encounter the stator winding emf. Figure 87.2(b) show the S-contour of Ia. The image illustrates how most energy is focused at the beginning of the time, since IM draws more current at the start. Thereafter, the S-contour of Ia becomes uniform with less number of frequency contents. This indicates that there is no transients present in the stator current Ia for a healthy IM.

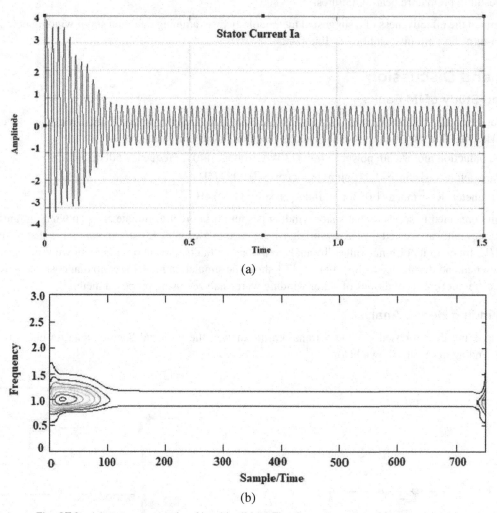

Fig. 87.2 (a) stator current Ia of healthy IM (b) The S-contour plot of stator current Ia

In further analysis open winding, line to line faults, and short circuit faults were considered and diagnosed using proposed method.

Open Winding Fault (Phase C as Open Circuit)

With the aid of a circuit breaker, the stator winding connected to phase-C of the input supply is opened at 0.18 seconds after start of IM. Figure 87.3(a) show the time domain representation of Ia. The outcome demonstrates that subsequently to the occurrence of the open winding fault in phase C, the simulated stator current Ia increases in amplitude. The S-contour of stator current Ia is displayed in Fig. 87.3(b). It is clear from the figure that when the fault is produced in IM, the energy concentration in the S-contour immediately increases. It is due to more current drawn by healthy phases of IM to maintain the torque required for the load. Before and after this variation, the contour is nearly smooth, showing constant frequency contents in Ia. As a result, the S-contours of Ia show a sharp shift in frequency brought on by transients at the exact moment the open winding fault occurs.

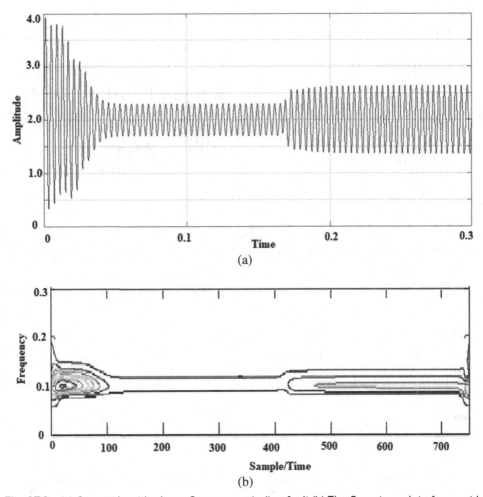

Fig. 87.3   (a) Current Ia with phase C as open winding fault (b) The S-contour plot of current Ia

Line to Line Stator Winding Fault Analysis

In this simulation work, the IM stator winding's phase A and B are fed to a line-to-line fault. The fault was introduced 0.75 seconds after the start of IM. The simulated stator current is shown by Fig. 87.4(a). The figure's result demonstrates that there was an abrupt brusts in Ia at the moment the fault was introduced into IM.

From the Fig. 87.4(b), it is evident that the amplitude and frequency of Ia are higher at the instant the fault is created. It is because of the transients that developed in the stator current as a result of the line-to-line fault in stator winding. Afterworth, a number of uniform multiple frequency bands appeared in S-contour of Ia. It is due to nonuniform mmf generated by the current flowing in the three phases of stator winding.

Turn to Turn Short Circuit Fault Analysis

To model turn-to-turn short circuit fault, the winding resistance of particular winding is decreased to about 1/12 times its initial value to imitate a shorted winding defect. Figure 87.5(a) shows the variation of stator current Ia in time domain. The figure illustrates that the transients occur in stator current Ia due to short circuit fault in stator winding of IM. The S-contour plot of current Ia as shown in Fig. 87.5(b) show that the multiple frequency bands appear due to the short circuit fault in stator winding. The contour is almost smooth before and after this fluctuation, indicating consistent frequency contents in Ia.

Therefore, one can take precautionary measures with the help of such information to avoid further damage of IM components. Henceforth, the stator winding problems can be quickly and accurately recognized using the S-transform analysis of stator current.

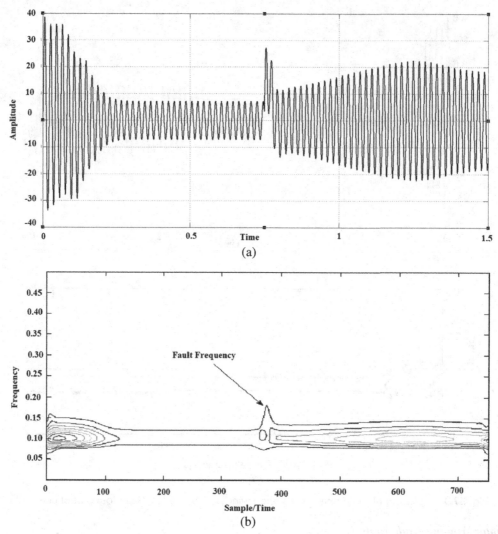

Fig. 87.4 (a) Stator current Ia with winding A and B having line to line fault and (b) represents the S-contour of Ia

5. Conclusion

In this manuscript, a modified wavelet transform known as S-transform was proposed and applied to identify stator winding defects. In this, three stator winding defects such as open winding fault, line-to-line fault, and turn to turn short circuit faults were simulated and analysed. The S-contour plot was demonstrated and studied for each case. The results of this manuscript has shown that the S transform offers a valuable and intriguing technique for identifying stator winding defects.

REFERENCES

1. O. P. Yadav and G. L. Pahuja, "Bearing Fault Detection Using Logarithmic Wavelet Packet Transform and Support Vector Machine," *IJIGSP*, vol. 11, no. 5, pp. 21–33, May 2019, doi: 10.5815/ijigsp.2019.05.03.
2. M. O. Mustafa, G. Georgoulas, and G. Nikolakopoulos, "Bearing Fault Classification Based on Minimum Volume Ellipsoid Feature Extraction", 2013 IEEE Multi-conference on Systems and Control, pp.1177-1182, 2013.
3. S. Nandi and H. A. Toliyat, "Condition Monitoring and Fault Diagnosis of Electrical Machines – A Review," Record of the 34th IEEE Industry Applications Society Annual Meeting, pp. 197-204, Oct. 1999.
4. O. P. Yadav and G. L. Pahuja, "Time-Frequency Spectral Power Assessment of Rolling Element Bearing Faults Using Adaptive Modified Morlet Wavelet Transform," *Recent Advances in Computer Science and Communications*, vol. 14, no. 7, 2021.

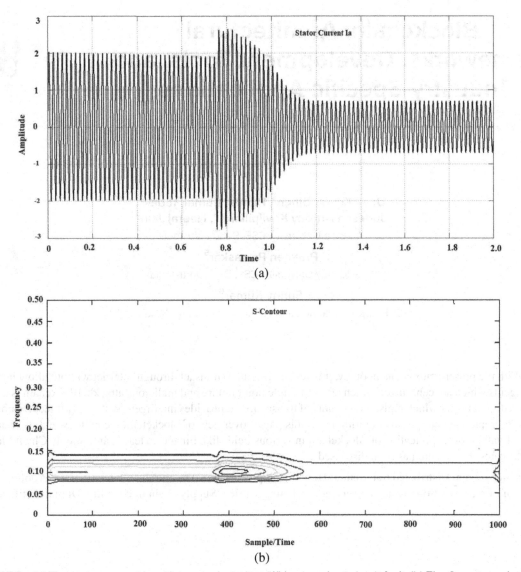

Fig. 87.5   (a) The stator current Ia with terminal winding "A" having short circuit fault, (b) The S-contour plot of Ia

5. Ghanbari, T., A. Mehraban, "Stator winding fault detection of induction motors using fast Fourier transform on rotor slot harmonics and least square analysis of the Park's vectors" *IET Electr. Power Appl.* 1–11 (2023).
6. Navid Eghtedarpour, Ebrahim Farjah, and Alireza Khayatian, "Effective Voltage Flicker Calculation Based on Multi-resolution S-Transform", IEEE Transactions on Power Delivery, vol. 27, no. 2, pp. 5521-530, 2012.
7. Aderiano M. da Silva, Richard J. Povinelli and Nabeel A. O. Demerdash, "Induction Machine Broken Bar and Stator Short-Circuit Fault Diagnostics Based on Three-Phase Stator Current Envelope," IEEE Trans. Ind. Electron., vol. 55, no. 3, pp. 1310-1318, Mar. 2008.
8. W. C. Lee and P. K. Dash, "S-transform-based intelligent system for classification of power quality disturbance signals," IEEE Trans. Ind. Electron., vol. 50, no. 4, pp. 800–805, Aug. 2003.
9. R. Wang, Y. Zhan, H. Zhou, "Application of S transform in fault diagnosis of power electronics circuits", Scientia Iranica, vol.19, issue 3, pp. 721-726, 2012.
10. R. G. Stockwell, L Mansinha and R P Lowe, "Localization of the complex spectrum: The S Transform," IEEE Trans. Signal Processing, vol. 44, no. 4, pp. 998-1001, April. 1996.
11. C. R. Pinnegar, L. Mansinha, "Time-local Fourier analysis with a scalable, phase-modulated analyzing function: the *S*-transform with a complex window," *Signal Processing*, vol. 84, pp. 1167-1176, July. 2004.
12. Srikanth Pullabhatla, Anil K Naik, "Power System Transients Disturbances Analysis Using Stockwell Transform", Conference on Power System Today, pp.1-6, 2010.

Emerging Trends in IoT and Computing Technologies – Suman Lata Tripathi et al. (eds)
© 2024 Taylor & Francis Group, London, ISBN 978-1-032-87924-6

Blockchain: Architectural Frameworks, Development Tools, and Industry-Specific Applications

88

Uday Kumar Singh[1], Puneet Kumar Yadav[2],
Judeson Antony Kovilpillai J.[3], Neeraj Jain[4]
Alliance University, CSE, Bengaluru, India

Praveen Pawaskar[5]
Presidency University, CSE, Bengaluru, India

Sunny Kumar[6]
GCET, Applied Science and Humanities, Greater Noida, India

Abstract: With the present moving technology, it is much difficult to transact through Internet without allow information to third party agents which are centralized which leads to single point failure and malicious attacks. Blockchain is a distributed, decentralized digital ledger which registers accounts of transaction. It provides intelligent system to protect the object privacy through cryptography and encryption algorithms. In this paper, overview of blockchain technology and its characteristics, approaches of validations, application of Blockchain in various fields like Finance, Healthcare, Supply Chain Management, Digital Certificates, Healthcare has been discussed.

Keywords: Blockchain, Distributed transaction, Bitcoin, Cryptocurrency, Decentralized, Peer to peer, Proof of work, Proof of stake, Proof of retrievability, Privacy preserving, Ticketing service, Supply chain traceability, Digital certificates

1. Introduction

Blockchain, as a foundational technology, provides a decentralized database for recording transactions. In essence, Blockchain is a secure way of maintaining a ledger that records transactions between two parties. It ensures security and reliability by recording and verifying every transaction, eliminating the need for third-party intermediaries in peer-to-peer exchanges. Blockchain is poised to be the fifth major game-changer in the world of computing, following the mainframe, personal computer, Internet, and mobile/social networks [1]. Each block in the blockchain is uniquely identified by a crypto- graphic code. These blocks are linked together, meaning they reference the previous block's code in a sequence. This sequence can be traced all the way back to the very first block created.

2. Literature Review

2.1 How Block chain works

In the past, banks maintained their own ledgers, which contained databases of transactions, all controlled by a central authority or in situation. However, this centralization had its limitations, including potential bottlenecks, single points of failure, and

---
[1]udaykumar.singh@alliance.edu.in, [2]puneet.yadav@alliance.edu.in, [3]judeson.kovilpillai@alliance.edu.in, [4]neeraj.jain@alliance.edu.in,
[5]praveen.pawaskar@presidencyuniversity.in, [6]sunny.kumar@galgotiacollege.edu

DOI: 10.1201/9781003535423-88

the need for trust in these centralized entities to maintain accurate and honest records. Blockchain technology, in contrast, introduces decentralization, transparency, and cryptographic techniques to address these traditional ledger shortcomings [2].

In Fig. 88.1, we observe the process of a blockchain transaction where 'A' intends to send money to 'B'. To initiate this transaction, 'A' creates a transaction record involving 'B'. This record is then shared across the network. Every node on the network validates the transaction to ensure its legitimacy. Once validated, the transaction is included in a new block. This block is secured through encryption and added to the existing chain of blocks.

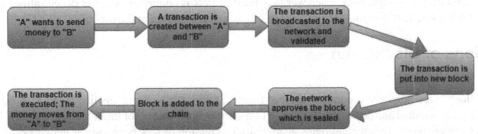

Fig. 88.1 Transaction workflow of blockchain

Figure 88.2 illustrates the example of blockchain in which previous block hash contained in the block header and the first block is called the genesis block with no parent.

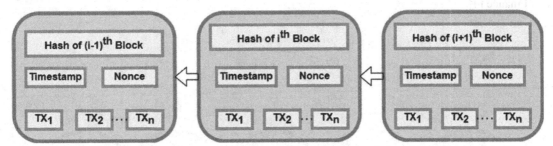

Fig. 88.2 Blockchain's secure and chronological chain of blocks

Each Block contains:

Block Header: Contains the 256 -bit previous block Hash. Timestamp: It is the time in which the block created.

Nonce: It is a unique 4byte number which is used to hash with previous block hash to generate new hash.

Transaction counter: It contains number of transactions in the block. Transactions: Contains the transactions record stored.

2.2 Characteristics of Blockchain

Decentralization: Transaction data is stored within the network and not reliant on a central system. This ensures uniform data across all nodes, with each node having information on every transaction.

Immutability: Once a transaction is recorded in the public ledger, no participant can alter it. This ensures the transaction remains unchanged and secure.

Consensus: In the blockchain network, all users adhere to a common protocol for transaction acceptance. If a transaction doesn't conform to this protocol among users, it is marked as invalid.

Transparency: The digital ledger displays all transactions transparently, allowing anyone to access and review them for auditing purposes.

2.3 Consensus Algorithms Used In Blockchain

Proof of Work (PoW): PoW is a way that cryptocurrencies like Bitcoin use to make sure that transactions are genuine and added to the blockchain. Miners compete by solving tough math puzzles (called hashing algorithms) to confirm and add new blocks of transactions. The first miner to solve the puzzle gets to add the block and is rewarded with new coins and transaction fees [3].

Proof of Stake (PoS): PoS offers a different way from Proof of Work (PoW) to secure and manage cryptocurrencies, aiming to be greener and more decentralized. In PoS, validators are picked to make new blocks and confirm transactions based on how many cryptocurrency tokens they possess and are willing to use as a kind of security deposit [3].

Proof of Retrievability (PoR): PoR isn't about making new blocks in a blockchain; it's a method to make sure data stays safe and can be found in decentralized storage systems. PoR is all about proving that a particular piece of data is stored correctly and can be gotten back from a network of distributed storage. When users put their data on the network, they get a unique proof that their data is secure and can be brought back whenever they need it. PoR is commonly used in decentralized cloud storage and backup systems, making sure data remains safe and accessible in a decentralized and trustworthy way [3].

3. Applications of Blockchain

3.1 Finance

Blockchain technology finds extensive use in the realm of finance, particularly in systems like Bitcoin. In Bitcoin, blockchain serves as the ledger for distributed and decentralized transactions, removing the need for intermediaries. Various cryptocurrencies have sprung from different blockchain technologies, leading to the creation of new peer-to-peer networks for money transfers, eliminating the requirement for centralized control. When a user initiates a transaction, it is broadcasted across the network. After broadcasting, the transaction undergoes verification and once verified, is cryptographically sealed, forming a block. This block is then linked to the previous block in the chain using a unique hash value. Figure 88.3 shows the various services of Blockchain in Finance [4].

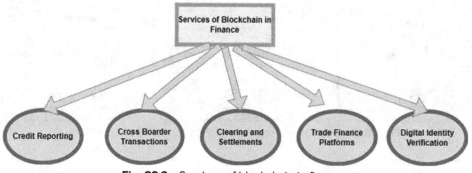

Fig. 88.3   Services of blockchain in finance

3.2 Privacy Preserving Ticketing Service (PPTS)

Nowadays, there's a growing trend of digitizing ticketing systems for events, where people validate their tickets by showing a QR code on their mobile devices. However, using blockchain technology alone doesn't ensure data privacy. If we were to store ticket purchase information directly on a public digital ledger, it could lead to a situation where anyone could find out who attended an event and even track specific individuals. Although personal identification might not be used, people could still misuse the system by creating false identities, which would lead to duplicated QR codes used by multiple users.

Figure 88.4 illustrates how a privacy-preserving ticketing service works. Imagine that the event details are added to the blockchain by the event organizer. Users can browse available events and request to buy tickets from ticket sellers. To protect user privacy, this system employs a Non-Interactive Zero-Knowledge scheme. This scheme ensures that users can prove they're genuine ticket buyers without directly interacting with the nodes on the blockchain network during transaction validation. In this setup, the ticket sellers are responsible for sending the transactions to the blockchain network, rather than the ticket buyers themselves [5].

3.3 Blockchain in Healthcare

Sharing patient data between healthcare organizations has historically been a complex process, especially when a patient needs to consult multiple specialists for treatment. To ensure that each specialist has access to the patient's medical history, records must be shared between the various healthcare facilities the patient has visited. The digitalization of health records has made it easier to share electronic medical records across different hospitals. One way to achieve this is by using a decentralized system built on blockchain technology. Unlike traditional data holders, this system revolves around the patient, creating a

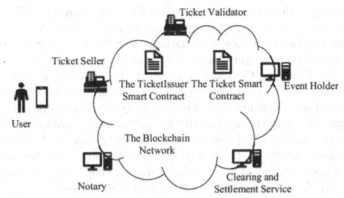

Fig. 88.4   Privacy preserving ticketing system using blockchain technology [5]

shared database of their medical information [6]. The primary goal of Electronic Health Records (EHRs) is to maintain a comprehensive and lifelong patient record that can be accessed by a team of healthcare professionals. Figure 88.5 shows the features of Blockchain for Healthcare domain.

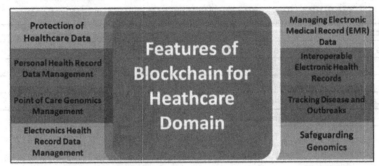

Fig. 88.5   Features of blockchain for healthcare domain [6]

3.4 Supply Chain Traceability (SCT)

The production and distribution of goods involve a vast network that includes producers, retailers, transporters, distributors, and suppliers before reaching consumers [7]. Unfortunately, this complex process often leads to significant trans- action costs, theft, environmental harm, and errors in manual paperwork. The involvement of many parties in this supply chain creates a lack of trust. However, blockchain technology, with the help of smart contracts, offers a solution by enabling the traceability of goods. This means we can track products from where they originate with resource suppliers all the way to the retailer, improving supply chain transparency [7]. Figure 88.6 shows how Supply Chain management works.

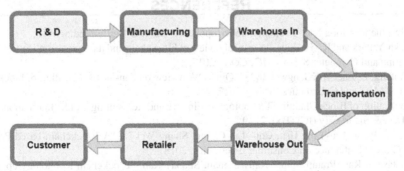

Fig. 88.6   How supply chain management works

3.5 Digital Certificates (DC)

In India, every year, thousands of student graduate. Some go abroad for further studies, while others enter the workforce. During their college years, they earn various certificates for achievements like sports, cultural events, and, most importantly, their degree certificates and transcripts. These documents are crucial for pursuing higher studies or securing jobs. However, the current system lacks robust anti-forgery measures, allowing individuals to create fake certificates, which can be misused for job applications or admission to educational institutions. To tackle this problem, we propose using Blockchain technology to create digital certificates. Blockchain's immutability and security features can help prevent fraud and ensure the certificates' authenticity. Here's how it works: Electronic Certificate Generation: The first step involves electronically generating the certificate, including all relevant data stored in a database. Hash Calculation: Next, we calculate a unique hash value for this electronic certificate file and store it securely in the blockchain system. QR Code and String Code Generation: Using this hash value, the blockchain system generates a QR code and a string code that can be printed on the electronic certificate. These codes serve to verify the certificate's authenticity. Individuals can scan the QR code with their smartphones or make inquiries on websites to check the certificate's validity [8]. By leveraging the immutability of the blockchain, we not only enhance the reliability of certificates but also reduce the risk of losing or damaging these important documents. This system offers a secure and trustworthy way to validate certificates, mitigating the issues of fraud and misuse.

4. Advantages and disadvantages

Blockchain technology has its set of strengths and weaknesses, which can be summarized in a table based on the discussed applications:

Table 88.1 Pros and cons of blockchain in various applications

Application	Pros	Cons
Finance	Secure, fast and cost effective	Illegal activities
PPTS	secure and transparent	Delay, complex
SCT	Transparent, Accuracy and integrity	Slow processing and Complex
Healthcare	secure, Traceable	Slow processing
DC	Immutable, Transparent	Slow processing and Complex

5. Conclusion

This paper aims to highlight the widespread impact of Blockchain technology across various applications, showcasing how it influences our daily lives, particularly in transactions. Blockchain ensures trust in distributed transactions and offers transparency, allowing anyone to access transaction records on the net- work. We explore several applications of blockchain, with a focus on its major use case in finance, such as Bitcoin transactions. In healthcare, we discuss how patient records are securely shared among multiple healthcare organizations. In the realm of privacy, we delve into its role in online ticketing systems and digital certificates to prevent misuse and certificate forgery. Lastly, we examine how blockchain enhances supply chain management by providing transparency and traceability of goods from suppliers to retailers.

REFERENCES

1. M. Swan, Blockchain: Blueprint for a New Economy. Sebastopol, CA, USA: O'Reilly Media, 2015.
2. B. A. Tama, B. J. Kweka, Y. Park and K. -H. Rhee, "A critical review of blockchain and its current applications", International Conference on Electrical Engineering and Computer Science (ICECOS), 2017.
3. D. Mingxiao, M. Xiaofeng, Z. Zhe, W. Xiangwei and C. Qijun, "A review on consensus algorithm of blockchain," IEEE International Conference on Systems, Man, and Cybernetics (SMC), 2017.
4. S. Liu and S. He, "Application of Block Chaining Technology in Finance and Accounting Field, "International Conference on Intelligent Transportation, Big Data & Smart City (ICITBS), 2019.
5. Shi-Cho Cha, Wei-Ching Peng, Tzu-Yang Hsu, Chu- Lin Chang, Shang-Wei Li, "A Blockchain-based Privacy Preserving Ticketing Service", IEEE 7TH Global Conference on Consumer Electronics, 2018.
6. Abid Haleem, Mohd Javaid, Ravi Pratap Singh, Rajiv Suman, Shanay Rab, "Blockchain technology applications in healthcare: An overview", International Journal of Intelligent Networks, 2021.
7. Westerkamp, Martin; Victor, Friedhelm; Küpper, Axel, "Blockchain-based Supply Chain Traceability: Token Recipes model Manufacturing Processes", IEEE International Conference on Blockchain, 2018.
8. Cheng, J.-C., Lee, N.-Y., Chi, C., & Chen, Y.-H., "Blockchain and smart contract for digital certificate", IEEE International Conference on Applied System Invention (ICASI), 2018.

Emerging Trends in IoT and Computing Technologies – Suman Lata Tripathi et al. (eds)
© 2024 Taylor & Francis Group, London, ISBN 978-1-032-87924-6

Enhancing Software Reliability through Machine Learning Driven Fault Prediction Models

89

Km Vaishali Singh*

Research Schooler (Ph.D), Department of Information Technology,
Amity University, Lucknow

Archana Sahai

Department of Information Technology,
Amity University, Lucknow

Pankaj Kumar

Sri Ramswaroop Memorial College of Engineering and Management

Abstract: Software Fault Prediction (SFP) approaches are used at the first phases of the Software Development Life Cycle (SDLC) to detect and pinpoint faults. While machine learning (ML) methods are commonly employed in SFP, deep learning techniques have shown potential for higher accuracy. These software faults, also referred to as defects or bugs, arise when, there is a discrepancy between the expected and actual outcomes of a software program. Machine Learning involves creating computer programs that improve their performance at specific tasks through experience. In software engineering, ML is increasingly significant, encompassing various approaches such as predicting testing efforts and estimating costs. The assessment process demonstrated that Machine Learning (ML) algorithms could be utilized with a high degree of accuracy. The suggested prediction model was further tested against alternative approaches using a comparison measure. The collected data showed that the ML method was superior to the others.

Keywords: Software bug prediction, Faults prediction, Prediction model, Machine learning

1. Introduction

Software Defect Prediction (SDP) is a strategy aimed at enhancing software quality and minimizing testing expenses. This is achieved through the development of diverse categorization models using a variety of machine learning techniques. Companies involved in software development use SDP to anticipate potential defects, thereby ensuring software quality for customer satisfaction and reducing testing costs. SDP integrates into the Software Development Life Cycle (SDLC) by employing Machine Learning (ML) methods alongside historical data to predict faults. This approach is geared towards delivering high-quality software at a lower cost and in the shortest time possible, aligning with customer expectations. SDP's primary goal is to deliver reliable, high-quality software while efficiently managing limited resources [1]. This approach enables software developers to prioritize resource allocation throughout the different stages of the software development process. Organizations developing various software types are keen on using SDP to identify potential defects, maintaining software quality, satisfying customers, and cutting down on testing expenses. By utilising a variety of machine learning approaches to create categorization models, Software Deployment Platform (SDP) enhances software quality and testing efficiency. Decision Trees, Naïve Bayes,

*Corresponding author: singh.vaishali518@gmail.com

DOI: 10.1201/9781003535423-89

Radial Basis Function, Support Vector Machine, K-Nearest Neighbour, Multi-Layer Perceptron, and Random Forest are all approaches that fall into this category. Their goal is to improve software quality while decreasing testing expenses. Software dependability, quality, and maintenance expenses are all drastically affected by bug prevalence. Despite careful development, achieving completely [2] bug-free software is challenging due to potential hidden bugs. A significant difficulty in software engineering is the creation of a model for predicting software bugs that may detect problematic modules early on in the development process. An essential part of developing software is the ability to anticipate and prevent bugs. Predicting buggy modules before the software is deployed is key to ensuring user satisfaction and enhancing overall software performance. Early bug prediction not only improves software's adaptability to various environments but also enhances resource utilization. Software Bug Prediction (SBP) makes extensive use of Machine Learning (ML) methods to forecast problematic modules by analysing past fault data, important metrics, and a variety of software computing approaches.

1.1 Software Fault Prediction

An essential method in software development, Software Fault Prediction (SFP) seeks to detect any software mistakes before they appear in the final output. Through the early detection and resolution of errors, this proactive strategy seeks to improve software quality, dependability, and efficiency across the software development life cycle. For the purpose of analysing software metrics, code characteristics, and historical data, SFP employs a number of methodologies, the most important of which are data-driven approaches like Machine Learning (ML). To better manage resources, prioritise testing, and decrease the time and expense of correcting defects post-deployment, developers may anticipate which areas of the product are likely to be defective. Because it is difficult and resource-intensive to manually identify possible flaws in large-scale and complicated software projects, this predictive capacity is particularly useful in these situations.

1.2 Machine learning and fault prediction

To improve the process of finding possible mistakes or faults in software systems, Machine Learning (ML) is essential in Software Fault Prediction (SFP). Using ML approaches, SFP models may sift through mountains of data, such as software repository metadata, code metrics, and historical fault data, to pinpoint where software faults are most likely to occur.

The integration of ML in SFP involves several steps:

Data Collection and Preprocessing: Gathering historical data from software projects, including source code, change history, bug reports, and testing records. This data is then cleaned and formatted to be suitable for ML algorithms.

Feature Selection: Identifying relevant features that contribute to fault prediction. These might include code complexity metrics, change frequency, developer activity, and other code attributes.

Model Training: ML models are trained using pre-processed data using algorithms like Decision Trees, SVM, Random Forests, Naïve Bayes, and Neural Networks, each chosen based on the data's characteristics and prediction task.

Model Evaluation: Machine learning models are evaluated using accuracy, precision, recall, and F1 score, sometimes employing cross-validation to ensure generalizability.

Fault Prediction: Applying the trained model to new or existing software projects to predict potential faults. This helps in prioritizing testing and debugging efforts.

The use of ML in SFP offers several advantages:

Efficiency: Automates the fault prediction process, saving time and resources.

Accuracy: ML models can potentially identify complex patterns in data that are not easily detectable through manual analysis.

Proactiveness: Enables early detection of faults, reducing the cost and effort required for later-stage fixes.

Adaptability: ML models can be updated with new data, making them adaptable to evolving software projects.

In summary, the application of ML in software fault prediction is a significant advancement in software engineering, offering a more systematic, efficient, and effective approach to maintaining high software quality.

2. Literature Review

Studies in [3] and [4] compared the efficacy of several ML methods for fault prediction. A comprehensive review of previous work on various ML approaches and present trends in software bug prediction using machine learning was presented in the article by Sharma and Chandra [3]. Additional research in this field can build upon the findings of this study. utilising papers conducted between 1991 and 2013, R. Malhotra conducted a thorough examination of software bug prediction approaches utilising Machine Learning in his systematic review [5]. Here, we looked at the pros and cons of several ML approaches, compared them to statistical methods, and contrasted ML and statistical evaluations. With the introduction of a novel technique and a thorough analysis of well-known ones, a benchmark for evaluating various bug prediction algorithms was set up in [6]. The object-oriented software bug prediction system SBPS, developed by D. L. Gupta and K. Saxena [7], achieved an average accuracy of 76.27%. Rosli et al. [8] explored the application of evolutionary algorithms for software fault proneness prediction using object-oriented and count measures from open-source projects. The results of their rule generating process for software module failure categorization may be observed using a genetic algorithm applet. In different research that used statistical and machine learning approaches to evaluate object-oriented metrics, the Coupling between Object metric was shown to be the most successful for class bug prediction, while the Line of Code metre was found to be somewhat useful [9].

3. Machine Learning Algorithm

Machine Learning (ML) algorithms are computational methods used for recognizing patterns in data, learning from these patterns, and making decisions or predictions based on the learned information. Machine learning (ML) is a subset of AI that develops systems that can learn from and adapt to new data without explicit programming. ML algorithms are categorized into different types, each suited for different tasks and data types.

Supervised Learning: The algorithm is trained on a labelled dataset, pairing each example with the correct output, learning to map inputs to outputs, a technique commonly used in supervised learning.

Linear Regression: Utilized for forecasting continuous values.

Logistic Regression: Used for binary classification tasks.

Decision Trees: Versatile for classification and regression tasks.

Random Forests: An ensemble of decision trees, often more powerful and accurate.

Support Vector Machines (SVM): When dealing with high-dimensional data, Support Vector Machines (SVMs) perform exceptionally well for classification tasks.

K-Nearest Neighbours (KNN): A basic learning technique based on instances is K-Nearest Neighbours (KNN).

Unsupervised Learning: These algorithms are used on data without labelled responses, aiming to find structure in the data, like clusters or patterns. Popular unsupervised learning algorithms include:

K-Means Clustering: Used for grouping data into clusters.

Principal Component Analysis (PCA): Used for dimensionality reduction.

Apriori Algorithm: For association rule learning in transactional databases.

Semi-supervised Learning: This approach is used when you have a large amount of input data, but only some of the data is labelled. It combines aspects of both supervised and unsupervised learning.

Reinforcement Learning: The algorithm figures out how to behave in a given setting so as to maximize some concept of cumulative reward. Exploration (of unexplored terrain) and exploitation (of existing knowledge) are part of it.

Deep Learning: A branch of machine learning, deep learning makes use of multi-layered neural networks (hence the name "deep"). These algorithms are particularly powerful for tasks like image and speech recognition. Algorithms are chosen based on task requirements, input data nature, desired output, and available computational resources. Each algorithm has its strengths. Machine learning algorithms have found applications in a wide range of fields, from web search and spam filtering to self-driving cars and personalized healthcare.

4. Research Methodology

There are several datasets available for software defect detection. In the research, whenever feasible, external tools utilized in previous studies were employed for metric extraction. This approach was chosen to ensure fairness in results and to facilitate comparability with other studies. However, in cases where suitable tools were not available or were incompatible due to technical constraints, custom metric extraction tools were specifically developed for the experiment. This dual approach balanced the use of established methods with the innovation necessary to overcome limitations in existing tools, aiming to maintain the integrity and relevance of the research findings. The data have taken from [9].

The workflow (Fig. 89.1)is a machine learning pipeline that begins with data input, selects relevant features, calculates their statistics, applies multiple ML algorithms (Decision Tree, KNN, SVM, Neural Network) to the data, and is currently evaluating and scoring the models' performance.

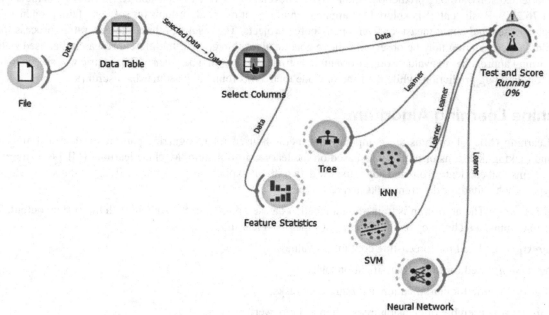

Fig. 89.1 Work flow

This Fig. 89.2 helps in understanding the underlying structure of the data, which is crucial for pre-processing steps before applying machine learning algorithms. It allows analysts to identify features with high variance, which might be more informative, and those with many missing values, which may [10] require imputation or other handling methods. Features with a low dispersion might have less predictive power if they do not vary much across the dataset. The distribution histograms provide a quick visual insight into the skewness and kurtosis of the data distribution.

Name	Distribution	Mean	Mode	Median	Dispersion	Min.	Max.	Missing
loc		42.016	4.0	23.0	1.823	1.0	3442.0	0 (0 %)
v(g)		6.349	1.0	3.0	2.051	1.0	470.0	0 (0 %)
ev(g)		3.401	1.0	1.0	1.991	1.0	165.0	0 (0 %)
iv(g)		4.002	1.0	2.0	2.278	1.0	402.0	0 (0 %)
n		114.390	0.0	49.0	2.181	0.0	8441.0	0 (0 %)
v		673.7580	0.00	217.13	2.8775	0.00	80843.08	0 (0 %)
l		0.1353	0.00	0.08	1.1862	0.00	1.30	0 (0 %)
d		14.1772	0.00	9.09	1.3197	0.00	418.20	0 (0 %)

Fig. 89.2 Feature statics

This Fig. 89.3 is likely meant to show a comparison between the models, but it does not resemble a standard confusion matrix, which is typically used for classification problems to show the number of true positives, false positives, true negatives, and false negatives. Instead, this seems to be a matrix comparing the mean square error (MSE) between models. The negligible difference of 0.1 is probably a threshold for considering whether the difference in performance between models is substantial. The values in this matrix (0.999, 1.000, etc.) do not immediately make sense in the context of a typical model comparison. They could be part of a statistical test or another form of comparison metric that is not clearly defined in the image. In conclusion, the image is not showing a confusion matrix but rather a comparison of machine learning model performance metrics. The kNN model appears to perform better based on the lower error metrics and positive R2 value.

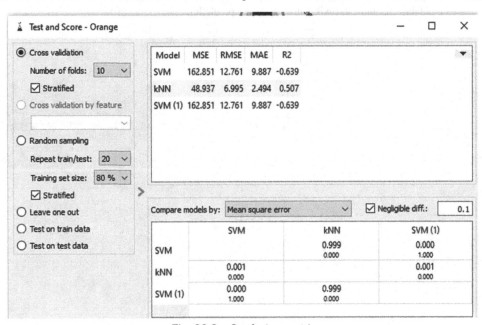

Fig. 89.3 Confusion metrix

5. Conclusion

It would seem from the data presented in the aforementioned research that the k-Nearest Neighbours (KNN) method achieved better results than the Support Vector Machine (SVM) model in a machine learning assessment with respect to a number of different criteria. In comparison to the SVM, which had a negative R2 value, the KNN model showed improved data fit with reduced Mean Squared Error, Root Mean Squared Error, and Mean Absolute Error. The model comparison matrix showed a substantial difference in MSE between the two models, heavily favouring the KNN. This suggests that for this particular dataset and problem, KNN is the more reliable model for making predictions. The use of cross-validation ensured that the performance metrics are robust and reliable, and stratification maintained the proportion of each class across folds, which is crucial for datasets with imbalanced classes. In conclusion, when it comes to the dataset and the specific task at hand, the KNN model is likely the better choice for predicting outcomes with a lower error rate and higher reliability than the SVM model.

References

1. Y. Tohman, K. Tokunaga, S. Nagase, and M. Y., "Structural approach to the estimation of the number of residual software faults based on the hyper-geometric districution model," IEEE Trans. on Software Engineering, pp. 345–355, 1989.
2. Sheta and D. Rine, "Modeling Incremental Faults of Software Testing Process Using AR Models ", the Proceeding of 4th International Multi-Conferences on Computer Science and Information Technology (CSIT 2006), Amman, Jordan. Vol. 3. 2006.
3. D. Sharma and P. Chandra, "Software Fault Prediction Using MachineLearning Techniques," Smart Computing and Informatics. Springer, Singapore, 2018. 541-549.
4. R. Malhotra, "Comparative analysis of statistical and machine learning methods for predicting faulty modules," Applied Soft Computing 21, (2014): 286-297

5. N. Akhtar, "Perceptual Evolution for Software Project Cost Estimation using Ant Colony System", International Journal of Computer Applications (IJCA) USA, ISSN 0975 - 8887, Volume 81, No.14, Pages 23 – 30, 2013, DOI: 10.5120/14185-2385

6. D'Ambros, Marco, Michele Lanza, and Romain Robbes. "An extensive comparison of bug prediction approaches." Mining Software Repositories (MSR), 2010 7th IEEE Working Conference on. IEEE, 2010

7. Gupta, Dharmendra Lal, and Kavita Saxena. "Software bug prediction using object-oriented metrics." Sādhanā (2017): 1-15.

8. M. M. Rosli, N. H. I. Teo, N. S. M. Yusop and N. S. Moham, "The Design of a Software Fault Prone Application Using Evolutionary Algorithm," IEEE Conference on Open Systems, 2011.

9. T. Gyimothy, R. Ferenc and I. Siket, "Empirical Validation of Object-Oriented Metrics on Open Source Software for Fault Prediction," IEEE Transactions On Software Engineering, 2005.

10. https://www.kaggle.com/datasets/semustafacevik/software-defect-prediction

Emerging Trends in IoT and Computing Technologies – Suman Lata Tripathi et al. (eds)
© 2024 Taylor & Francis Group, London, ISBN 978-1-032-87924-6

Predicting Unconfined Compressive Strength in Stabilized Soil with RBI Grade 81 using Artificial Neural Network

90

Samreen Bano[1], Vikash Singh[2],
Md. Sajid[3], Zishan Raza Khan[4], Syed Aqeel Ahmad[5]

Integral University, Civil Engineering, Lucknow, India

Abstract: The primary objective of this research is to augment the soil stability through the application of varying amounts of RBI Grade 81. Furthermore, the investigation aims to construct a prediction model utilizing Artificial Neural Network (ANN) to evaluate unconfined compressive strength (UCS). Crucial engineering tests, encompassing characterization of microstructural and UCS test, were conducted on the materials under scrutiny. Results obtained through the UCS test revealed a reliable augmentation in values of strength with increasing time of curing and RBI Grade 81 fraction. The development of the UCS predictive model involved the construction of ANN-based models employing the three distinct architectures. A various model of regression was also employed for comparative analysis. The dataset during training, comprised 80 data points, with 20 data points allocated for testing. The outcomes of the study showed the efficacy of ANN 1, attaining R^2 values of 0.998 throughout training and 0.995 throughout testing. This research concentrates on soil stabilization or modification with RBI Grade 81 stabilizer, coupled with the growth of a robust model based on for predicting UCS of soil.

Keywords: UCS, Soil stabilization, ANN, RBI grade 81, Strength

1. Introduction

The escalation of industrialization and urbanization presents formidable challenges in the identification of appropriate soils especially in case of foundations, predominantly when found with low strength soils characterized by relatively more plasticity, a substantial amount of 'e' (void ratio), poor strength, and much more squeezability. In addressing these challenges, soil amendment becomes important, with additive (chemical) stabilization emerging as an ideal approach, especially for such soil categories. The Unconfined Compressive Strength (UCS) becomes a critical parameter in evaluating performance and appropriateness for various applications [1-2]. The UCS test serves to determine c-phi parameters of clayey soils in all states, excluding its applicability to cohesionless. Findings from the UCS test offer appreciated perceptions into the Atterbergs limits of the soil. These insights play a crucial role in guiding the designs of geotechnical engineering structures, including foundations, road pavements, retaining walls, embankments, and slopes. The information obtained aids in the estimation of strength of soil and facilitates the identification of feasible construction techniques. [3]. Chemical modification/stabilization techniques, particularly for very soft (low strength) subgrades, can substantially reduce base thickness, stopping the loss of solid into the subgrade [4]. Soil stabilization with fly ash and cement has received a lot of attention lately in geotechnical engineering applications. This method offers a low-cost, eco-friendly way to improve the engineering property of soil, especially compressive strength. The introduction of ANN algorithms as prospective tools for capturing non-linear behavior

[1]Samreenbano1az786@gmail.com, [2]vikashs@iul.ac.in, [3]mdsajidk1992@gmail.com, [4]zishanrk@iul.ac.in, [5]syedaqeel@iul.ac.in

DOI: 10.1201/9781003535423-90

in stabilized soils is motivated by the limits of traditional experimental methods for anticipating UCS. The purpose of this study is to use Artificial Neural Networks (ANN) to construct a robust forecast model for RBI grade 81 modified soil and UCS of cement. In order to improve accuracy, the search investigates how different parameters affect UCS and incorporates them into the ANN architecture. Obtaining a sizable dataset for the ANN model's training, validation, and testing is part of the study. In order to improve accuracy, the search investigates how different parameters affect UCS and incorporates them into the ANN architecture. Obtaining a sizable dataset for the ANN model's training, validation, and testing is part of the study. With the provision of a strong and accurate forecasting tool for evaluating the strength i.e. UCS stabilized soil with additives of RBI grade 81, the research seeks to make a substantial contribution to the field and domain of geotechnical as well as in transportation engineering. This technology makes geotechnical engineering projects more cost-effective and sustainable by facilitating the efficient design and optimization of structures.

2. Materials

2.1 Soil

A substrate identified as soil was taken from the Goshaiganj town in the district of Ayodhya situated in Uttar Pradesh, as illustrated in Fig. 90.1. Earlier initiating laboratory experiments, the procured soil underwent a process of natural drying in air to eliminate excess wetness, confirming its appropriateness for subsequent testing. The dried soil's particle size distribution is depicted in Fig. 90.2, providing informative insights into the granulometric characteristics of the trial or sample.

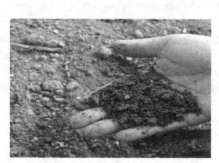

Fig. 90.1 Collected soil sample

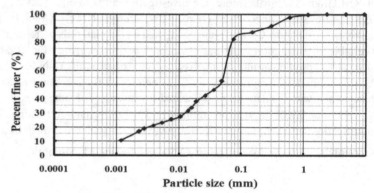

Fig. 90.2 Distribution of soil particle sizes

2.2 RBI Grade 81

Road Building International Grade-81 (RBI 81), is a chemical additives or stabilizer that is widely used by a range of researchers to improve the characteristics of different kinds of soil. This odourless beige powder exhibits insolubility in water, resistance to UV degradation, and chemical stability. Notably, it yields a dust-free surface, showcasing durability, permanence, and rapid hardening characteristics. Additionally, RBI Grade-81 is characterized by aesthetic appeal and environmental friendliness, rendering it suitable for deployment across a broad spectrum of soils.

The incorporation of low dosages of RBI Grade-81 results in a substantial increase in the volume permanency of treated soil. The mechanism of action involves a hydration reaction with the soil, contributing to the augmentation of soil strength over time.

3. Methodology

This investigation, soil was obtained from a single site and later treated with varying proportions of RBI Grade 81, ranging from 0% - 10% by the weight of total soil mass. Engineering tests were conducted on both the Ayodhya district soil and RBI 81 at the Dpt. of Civil Engg., Integral University, Lucknow. The perfect and suitable combinations of collected soil sample and RBI Grade 81 utilized in the stabilization procedure are presented in Table 90.1. The resulting soil-RBI Grade 81 mixes underwent UCS testing, a crucial measure of their mechanical nature. To predict UCS values across different RBI contents, atterberg's limits, and compaction characteristics, three ANN based predictive models were developed, as depicted in Fig. 90.3. Recognized for handling data of high-dimensional and the relationships of non-linearity, ANN proved to be a powerful

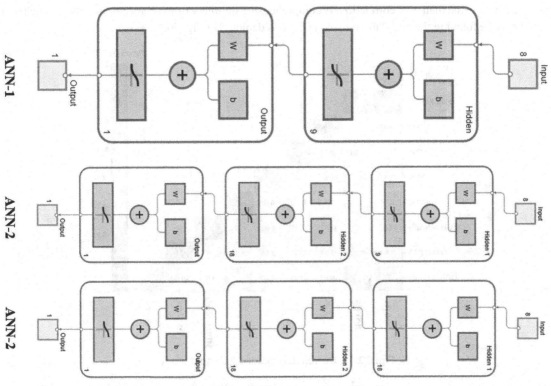

Fig. 90.3 ANN predictive models

machine learning algorithm. The researchers and academician sought to develop an accurate and dependable prediction model using ANN that could predict UCS values under various consistency limitations and compaction parameters, as well as for diverse and suitable soil compositions with RBI Grade 81. Researchers and engineers can make informed decisions based on a variety of material assortments, specific geotechnical designs, and optimization of various geotechnical and transportation constructions, especially structures relating inclusion with soil -additives mixes, with the help of the predictive model based on ANN development.

Table 90.1 Designated soil-RBI Grade 81 combinations

S. No.	Various blends	RBI Grade 81 (%)	Soil (%)
1	0 RBI+100 S	0	100
2	2 RBI+98 S	2	98
3	4 RBI+96 S	4	96
4	6 RBI+94 S	6	94
5	8 RBI+92 S	8	92
6	10 RBI+90 S	10	90

4. Result and Discussion

A matrix of correlation is a tabular representation of the correlation coefficients between several variables in a dataset. It is essential for revealing patterns of multicollinearity, connections, and outlier detection. This helps distinguish between dependent and independent variables, offering crucial information for further analysis and modeling. The correlation coefficients, which have a range of -1 to 1, are used to measure the degree and direction of the associations between the different variables in mixtures. The positive correlation is presented by a correlation of 1, perfect negative correlation is shown by a correlation of -1, and no link is shown by a correlation of 0. A comprehensive summary of the correlations between the parameters this study examined may be found in the matrix of correlation. A comprehensive summary of the correlations between the parameters this study examined may be found in the correlation matrix, which is depicted in Fig. 90.4.

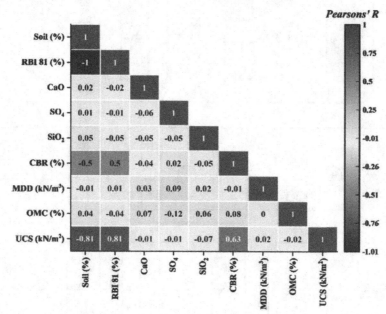

Fig. 90.4 Correlation matrix of present study

4.1 Assessment of various models based on performance

The data that is supplied shows the results that were obtained from training and assessing three different Artificial Neural Network (ANN) models that were created to forecast the Unconfined Compressive Strength of a soil mix with RBI grade 81. The dataset is divided into three parts: 30% was used to evaluate model performance, 10% was used for validation, and 60% was used for training. The input-hidden-output neuron format's neuron configuration clearly defines the architectural structure of any artificial neural network (ANN) model.

ANN-1: With training, validation, and testing coefficients (R) of 0.99893, 0.99606, and 0.99578, respectively, this model demonstrated a good relation between predicted UCS values and actual UCS values. The mean R for all stages indicates an overall performance of 0.99777.

ANN-2: With a R of 0.94697, ANN-2 stands out for having better correlation values, especially during the training period. R values, however, show a modest reduction during testing and validation, coming in at 0.95583 and 0.99848, respectively. At 0.9782, the comprehensive R for ANN-2 is still strong.

ANN-3: Additionally, with a R of 0.99838, ANN-3 shows better correlation values, especially during the training period. R values during testing and validation, however, show a modest reduction (0.96552 and 0.96396, respectively). At 0.98384, the comprehensive R for ANN-3 is still strong.

5. Conclusion

To achieve this objective, three discrete Artificial Neural Network (ANN) architectures were formulated, each characterized by distinct configurations of hidden layers and neurons. These models were then trained and compared to examine their prediction ability in more detail. Three separate subsets of the dataset designated for this study were created, with 60% going toward training, 10% going toward validation, and 30% going toward evaluating the effectiveness of the ANN models. To evaluate the effectiveness of the developed models, the research used a variety of ANN configurations, training and testing datasets, and complementary analytical techniques.

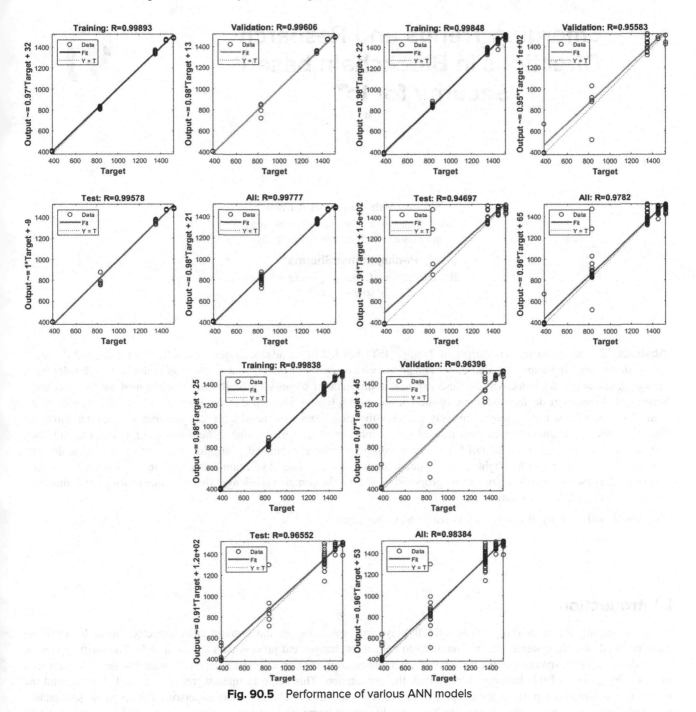

Fig. 90.5 Performance of various ANN models

REFERENCES

1. Kumar, A., & Sinha, S. (2023a). Multiwalled Carbon nanotube aided fly ash-based subgrade soil stabilization for low-volume rural roads. International Journal of Geosynthetics and Ground Engineering, 9(2), 17. https://doi.org/10.1007/s40891-023-00436-z
2. Kumar, A., & Sinha, S. (2023b). Role of multiwalled carbon nanotube in the improvement of compaction and strength characteristics of fly ash stabilized soil. International Journal of Pavement Research and Technology. https://doi.org/10.1007/s42947-023-00274-2
3. Salahudeen, A. B., Ijimdiya, T. S., Eberemu, A. O., & Osinubi, K. J. (2018). Artifcial neural networks prediction of compaction characteristics of black cotton soil stabilized with cement kiln dust. Journal of Soft Computing in Civil Engineering, 2(3), 53–74.
4. Khan, R. A., Khan, A. R., Verma, S., & Islam, S. (2016). California bearing ratio analysis for RDFS in unsoaked condition. International Journal for Research in Technological Studies, 3(3), 2348–1439

Emerging Trends in IoT and Computing Technologies – Suman Lata Tripathi et al. (eds)
© 2024 Taylor & Francis Group, London, ISBN 978-1-032-87924-6

Emerging Trends and Research Directions in Blockchain based Security for IoT

91

Gaurav Vats[1], Sarvesh Tanwar[2]
Amity Institute of Information Technology,
Information Technology, Noida, India

Pankaj Kumar Sharma[3]
ABES Engineering College, Computer Science,
Ghaziabad, India

Abstract: The inception of the Internet of Things (IoT) has led to an advanced generation for interconnected devices and systems, bringing unprecedented convenience and efficiency to various domains and it is continuously developing. However, this surge in connectivity has also exposed a multitude of security vulnerabilities that alarmed the integrity and privacy of these smart devices and data. In the coming years, it is anticipated that the issue of safety will escalate to a critical juncture. This paper comprehensively explores the challenges associated with safeguarding IoT devices through the innovative application of blockchain technology. its inherent characteristics that make it suitable for strengthening the IoT security are detailed. The union of IoT systems with blockchain is examined, alongside the questions that arise during implementation. The paper highlighted the current solutions that integrate blockchain technology into IoT security. Future directions for research and development are proposed to address the complex challenges that remain, ensuring the continued advancement of secure IoT ecosystems

Keywords: IoT security, Blockchain, Cyberthreats, Cybersecurity

1. Introduction

IoT is pioneering the networking framework. It plays important role in the current interconnected world by enabling interconnected objects, systems and environments to collect, exchange, and process data autonomously. The swift expansion of IoT devices [1][2], spanning a diverse array of interconnected items like as smart appliances, wearable devices, industrial sensors. This growth of this industry is more than the expectation. This surge in interest, reliance on IoT devices, and the economic opportunities it presents have captured the focus of innovators, scholars, businesspersons, the corporate sphere, and even malicious actors in the cyber realm. Few key areas like smart home, smart cities, healthcare, industrial automation, retail, transportation and supply chain are now under IoT realm.

1.1 Problem

However, the large scale and distributed nature of IoT networks make them exposed to the security attacks. Cyber attackers may take advantage of weaknesses in IoT devices to pilfer information, interrupt regular operations, or potentially inflict physical harm. IoT security [3] is a complex issue that requires new approaches [4] and technologies to address the unique challenges

[1]gaurav.vats@gmail.com, [2]s.tanwar1521@gmail.com, [3]hodcs@abesec.ac.in

DOI: 10.1201/9781003535423-91

of IoT devices. the use of traditional technologies or algorithm are not in favor of secure IoT world. Even these IoT devices are heterogeneous in nature and have low or not sufficient memory, less processing power.

1.2 Existing solution

On the other hand, Blockchain [5][6] is a technological innovation enabling a consortium of cryptographic entities to preserve and manage a collection of time-stamped, unchangeable data records within blocks. It operates on a decentralized network of computers, or nodes, where each new data entry (or block) is connected to the prior one in chronological chain. blockchain provides several key benefits for IoT security like data integrity, transparency, decentralization, authentication and access control. While blockchain and IoT can be integrated to enhance security, there are still challenges to overcome like blockchain's computational requirements can be demanding for resource-constrained IoT devices, and it does not directly address all IoT security concerns, such as physical device vulnerabilities or network-based attacks

1.3 Objective and Contribution

In The primary goal of this investigation is to uncover the privacy and security obstacles inherent in the fusion of IoT and blockchain technologies. This research also identified benefits of integrating these two technologies that can address security issues present in the system. the main target is to trace out the research challenges and their existing solution and approaches in the privacy and security

This paper's contributions include the following

(a) This research synthesizes a broad understanding of the actual condition of IoT security, generate insights from different domains and diverse geographical contexts. The synthesized body of knowledge underscores the criticality of securing IoT landscapes and offers actionable insights and potential pathways for addressing the identified challenges.

(b) Drawing on a rigorous analysis spanning the past six years and leveraging the extensive repository of research publications from the Scopus database, the contribution lies in incorporating a comprehensive understanding of the current state of IoT security.

(c) The Research have scrutinized emerging threats and attacks targeting IoT ecosystems, it also advocated for the integration of blockchain as a promising solution to fortify IoT security. However, our analysis extends beyond advocacy to address the pragmatic challenges of integrating and implementing blockchain in conjunction with IoT.

(d) The researcher has scrutinized emerging threats and attacks targeting IoT ecosystems, including but not limited to zero-day vulnerabilities, ransomware, firmware tampering, and cross-device attacks. Even the focus extended towards identifying and elucidating key challenges faced in securing IoT environments, ranging from software and firmware vulnerabilities to the lack of standardization, insecure communications, and inadequate authentication

1.4 Paper Structure

The structure of this research begins with the introductory section, which provides a brief overview of the expanding IoT world, along with current challenges and solutions. Section 2 provides a concise review of pertinent literature in this domain and also Leverages a six-year analysis of the Scopus database for a comprehensive understanding of IoT security. Section 3 emphasized on the critical importance of IoT security in diverse areas like smart homes, healthcare, and smart cities. Section 4 Identifies the key challenges in IoT security, including software vulnerabilities, lack of standardization, insecure communications, and authentication issues. Section V Scrutinized emerging threats such as zero-day vulnerabilities Section 4 Explored solutions, including blockchain for addressing IoT security challenges. The next section Advocated for blockchain integration to fortify IoT security. Section 8 addresses the practical challenges in integrating and implementing blockchain with IoT. The section 9 explored innovative solutions like sidechains and confidential computing to overcome integration challenges. The Last session is for conclusion

2. Literature Review and Related Work

In article "Landscape of IoT security" [7], authors discuss the security challenges and countermeasures for IoT systems. The key challenges include the billions of IoT gadgets, the limited resources of many IoT devices, the lack of security expertise, and the interconnectedness of IoT devices. The major security objectives for secured IoT systems are confidentiality, integrity, and availability. A threat taxonomy for IoT systems is presented, which classifies IoT threats based on their impact, target, and vector. Key countermeasures against IoT threats include using strong authentication and authorization mechanisms, encoding the information at rest and in transit, monitoring IoT devices for suspicious activity, keeping IoT devices up to date with the latest security patches, using a firewall to protect IoT devices from unauthorized access, implementing security policies and procedures for IoT devices, and educating employees about IoT security risks.

In another research work [8] with similar objective done by different researchers, the authors discuss the challenges associated with IoT security and proposes a security framework based on blockchain and Zero Trust. It outlines the significance of risk-based segmentation, the role of SG (Segmentation Gateway) and MCAP (Micro perimeter) in Zero Trust, and the benefits of centralizing network management. Researchers [8][9] investigated different aspects of implementing Zero Trust, including blockchain-based middleware and access control policy enforcement. The proposed framework is exemplified through the case study of ABC Company's IoT security solution, which demonstrates the practical application of Zero Trust concepts.

Likewise, the IoT blockchain integration research work [9] presents a novel hierarchical blockchain-based platform designed to address challenges related to data integrity and blockchain interoperability within smart city IoT environments. Author explains that due to centralized administrative control, these systems lack trustworthiness, leading to compromised data integrity and operational transparency within smart city organizations. To overcome these limitations, researcher propose the adoption of blockchain-based information systems, termed as "Blockchain-of-Blockchains" .it is designed to simultaneously ensure data integrity and blockchain interoperability, in the context of IoT within smart cities. Moreover, this concept holds promise in ensuring data integrity from various sources, making it adaptable to scenarios beyond smart cities, such as smart homes, supply chains and educational blockchain platforms. This approach fosters trust among multiple parties and contributes to the advancement of diverse domains.

In the similar manner the paper titled "Blockchain based solutions to secure IoT: Background, integration trends and a way forward"[10] delves into the security challenges inherent in current Internet of Things (IoT) systems due to the absence of intrinsic security technologies. It explores the possibilities of blockchain technology, a distributed and decentralized solution, to address these vulnerabilities. The paper analyzes the integration trends between blockchain and IoT, shedding light on the intersection of these technologies and the insights derived from their convergence. Specifically, the paper conducts a thorough survey of security enhancements achieved through the amalgamation of blockchain and IoT, while also identifying the challenges that arise during the fusion. Moreover, the research highlights noteworthy applications of blockchain in the context of IoT and suggests potential directions for future research.

the author offers a comprehensive examination of the fusion between blockchain and IoT to address security and privacy issues. It meticulously presents the characteristics, architecture, and processes of blockchain technology and outlines how this technology can ameliorate the security challenges in IoT. The integration's benefits and risks are duly highlighted. The study emphasizes the strides taken in enhancing IoT security using blockchain and outlines the associated challenges. Ultimately, the paper suggests that blockchain is a promising candidate to bolster IoT security and enable novel business models. It acknowledges the early stage of blockchain-based IoT systems and suggests avenues for advancing security, capacity, and scalability. Finally, the authors declare no competing interests that could influence the reported work.

2.1 Analysis

Over the past 6 years, according to the Scopus database, numerous research publications have emerged across various fields and document types, spanning different countries. These publications delve into the realm of IoT security challenges combined with blockchain technology.

Figure 91.1[11] shows that the most prevalent types of documents are articles and conference papers, this suggests that research articles and conference presentations are common in the database during this time period. While articles and conference papers are prominent, the presence of book chapters and books suggests a contribution from the academic and scholarly community in publishing longer-form content.

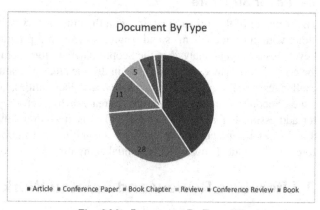

Fig. 91.1 Document By Type [11]

Figure 91.2 depicted that India has the highest number of published documents. This indicates a strong research presence and active scholarly community within the country. The inclusion of China, United States, United Kingdom and Canada highlights the active research hubs., suggesting significant scientific engagement in these regions. The distribution of research across multiple countries demonstrates a regional impact of scientific advancements reflecting the varying strengths of research ecosystems in different parts of the world.

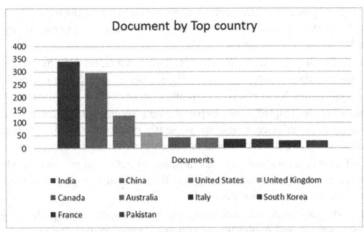

Fig. 91.2 Document by country [12]

Figure 91.3 explains that the subject areas with the highest counts of published documents are Computer Science and Engineering. This indicates a strong focus on technological and engineering research within the database. Figure 91.3 also underscores a notable focus on STEM (Science, Technology, Engineering, and Mathematics) fields. The incorporation of subjects such as Biochemistry, Genetics and Molecular Biology, Chemistry, and Physics and Astronomy underscores a varied spectrum of scientific exploration.

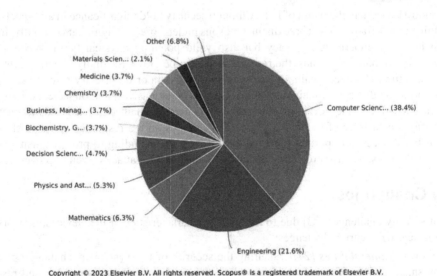

Fig. 91.3 Document by subject areas [13]

3. IoT Landscape and Security Problems

From the past twenty years, there has been a gradual rise in the manufacturing and utilization of electronic devices equipped with sensing and connectivity features, supplanting conventional physical items. This has given rise to the Internet of Things (IoT), which is on the verge of becoming indispensable across numerous fields of application. Intelligent items are being seamlessly incorporated into industrial facilities, urban environments, architectural structures, healthcare establishments, and personal residences so The IoT landscape [7] is vast and ever-changing, with new devices and applications being developed all the time. This makes it difficult to keep track of all the potential security risks. However, there are some key areas that businesses and organizations need to focus on in order to protect their IoT deployments.

The IoT landscape is vast and encompasses a wide range of applications across industries. The possibilities for utilizing IoT devices are boundless, leading to the swift expansion of the market in every aspect of our everyday existence. The realm of IoT can be segmented into several key areas of application,

(a) *Smart Homes:* IoT is transforming our lifestyle, with intelligent domiciles leading the charge in this transformation. Interconnected gadgets such as thermostats, lighting fixtures, surveillance cameras, and household appliances can be managed from a distance. enhancing the comfort, safety, and effectiveness of our abodes [14].

(b) *Healthcare:* The healthcare sector [15][16] is also experiencing a significant influence from the IoT. Wearable gadgets, medical detectors, and distant surveillance setups are presently employed to amass patient information and facilitate telemedicine. This is contributing to the enhancement of patient results and the mitigation of expenses.

(c) *Industrial IoT (IIoT):* IIoT [17] is revolutionizing the landscape of industrial production. Through the linking of sensors with machinery and apparatus, enterprises can acquire real-time data and employ it to enhance effectiveness, fine-tune manufacturing processes, and avert periods of inactivity.

(d) *Smart Cities:* IoT is also finding application in enhancing urban landscapes. Through the integration of sensors into traffic signals, waste management setups, and public transit systems, municipalities can enhance traffic circulation, decrease environmental contamination, and enhance accessibility for residents' mobility [18].

(e) *Agriculture:* IoT is also being used to improve agriculture [19]. Sensors in fields and on livestock can provide data for precision farming and animal monitoring. This is helping to increase crop yields, improve animal welfare, and reduce food waste.

(f) *Logistics and Supply Chain:* IoT is also being used to improve logistics and supply chain management [20]. By tracking goods in transit, businesses can improve inventory management, reduce costs, and prevent fraud.

3.1 Importance of Security

Security remains a foremost concern in the realm of IoT. Although security holds significance in all aspects of IT, its importance [21][22] amplifies within the IoT framework. Three distinct reasons underscore this significance. Firstly, IoT systems operating without oversight can not only imperil user privacy but also yield potential physical harm. When sensors, actuators, or interconnected devices fall into malicious hands, the repercussions can be grave. Secondly, this risk extends to manufacturers as well. If attackers breach the IoT system, gaining access to sensitive data or proprietary resources, manufacturers stand to lose valuable insights and incur damage to their reputation. Lastly, the extensive interconnectedness of IoT systems widens the impact of an attack beyond a single device or network. The adage "A chain is as strong as its weakest link" perfectly encapsulates this scenario; the security of the entire IoT network hinges on the resilience of its most vulnerable device. To sum, up the security of IoT devices is important for a number of reasons, including to protect sensitive data, , prevention of unauthorized access to critical systems, for protecting against denial-of-service attacks, even to prevent malware infections

4. IoT Security Challenges

IoT poses a number of security challenges [23] due to the specific characteristics of IoT devices, networks, and the data they generate. Here are some key IoT security challenges:

(a) *Software and firmware vulnerabilities [24]:* Ensuring the security of IoT systems is challenging due to the limitations inherent in many smart devices. These devices often lack the necessary computing power and resources to effectively implement robust security measures. Consequently, they exhibit greater susceptibility to weaknesses in contrast with devices not operating within the IoT framework. A multitude of factors play into the security susceptibilities frequently observed within IoT systems like Limited Computational Capacity, Poor Access Control, Patch and Update Limitations.

(b) *Lack of Standardization:* [25] The absence of standardized security norms spanning IoT devices and platforms complicates the establishment of uniform security protocols. This fragmentation can result in susceptibilities and incongruities within security executions.

(c) *Insecure communications [27]:* The security measures suitable for conventional computers lack efficacy when applied to IoT devices due to their limitations in resources. Frequently, these devices lack the processing capability and memory required for such measures. Consequently, this can result in insecure communications, a vulnerability that attackers can exploit for executing man-in-the-middle attacks or pilfering data. Furthermore, as IoT devices are frequently interlinked, breaching one device could grant attackers access to infiltrate other devices within the network.

(d) *Cyberattacks:* Aside from malware and man-in-the-middle attacks, IoT devices are also prone to an array of alternative forms of cyber assaults. Below are some prevalent types of attacks [27] targeting IoT devices, including Denial-of-Service (DoS) attacks, Device Spoofing, Denial-of-Sleep (DoSL) attacks, and Physical Intrusion.

(e) *Lack of testing and development:* In the rush to bring IoT products to market, some manufacturers have neglected security. This has led to device-related security risks being overlooked in the development process [26], and a lack of security updates once the products have been launched. Nevertheless, the increasing awareness of IoT security has led to a concurrent improvement in device security.

(f) *Ineffective Authentication and Authorization:* Insufficient authentication and authorization mechanisms [28] may result in unauthorized access to devices or networks. Standard credentials with insecure authentication methods can be exploited by attackers.

5. Emerging Threats and Attacks

The realm of the Challenges of Securing IoT Devices is accompanied by a spectrum of emerging threats and innovative attack vectors that continuously challenge the integrity of these interconnected technologies. As the IoT ecosystem expands, new vulnerabilities surface, and malicious actors capitalize on these opportunities. Some of the evolving threats and attack vectors include

(a) *Zero-Day Vulnerabilities:* Unpatched vulnerabilities in IoT devices, known as zero-days [29], can be exploited by attackers to compromise devices before manufacturers can release fixes.

(b) *Ransomware:* Ransomware [30] constitutes a form of malicious code that enciphers a target's data and requests a ransom be paid to restore it through decryption. IoT devices are increasingly being targeted by ransomware attacks, as they are often not backed up regularly and the data, they contain may be critical to the victim's business.

(c) *Firmware Tampering:* Attackers manipulate IoT device firmware to inject malicious code, granting unauthorized access, data theft, or control over devices.

(d) *Supply Chain Attacks:* Manipulating the supply chain [30][31], attackers introduce compromised components into IoT devices during manufacturing or distribution, compromising their security from inception.

(e) *Cross-Device Attacks [32]:* Weaknesses in one IoT device can be exploited to pivot and compromise other devices within the same network, escalating the impact of a breach.

(f) *AI-Powered Attacks [33]:* Attackers can leverage advanced AI and machine learning methodologies to identify patterns and weaknesses within IoT systems.

(g) *IoT botnets:* IoT botnets [34] represent clusters of corrupt IoT equipment's manipulated by cyber attacker. These botnets can be harnessed to initiate a range of assaults, including spam campaigns, distributed denial-of-service (DDoS) attacks, and click fraud schemes.

(h) *Physical attacks:* IoT devices frequently lack physical safeguards, rendering them open to physical breaches. To illustrate, a perpetrator could abscond with an IoT device and subsequently exploit it to initiate assaults or purloin data.

6. Existing Security Solutions

There are widely adopted solutions that are based on blockchain, Machine Learning (ML) and Artificial Intelligence (AI). the abstract view of these solutions are as follows:

(a) Blockchain-Based Solutions

   (i) *Supply Chain Security:* Blockchain guarantees the unblemished nature of the supply chain by documenting each phase of manufacturing and distribution, thereby diminishing the likelihood of devices being compromised.

   (ii) *Immutable Transaction Logs:* Through the utilization of blockchain technology [[5][6][10]35], modifications to transaction logs become unfeasible, delivering an immutable record of device engagements and data transfers.

(b) AI Based Solutions

   (i) *Anomaly Detection:* Artificial intelligence algorithms [37] possess the capability to promptly recognize anomalous behavioral patterns, aiding in the early recognition of security risks.

   (ii) *Predictive Analytics:* Artificial Intelligence can predict potential threats based past patterns, enabling proactive security measures.

(iii) *Behavioral Analysis:* AI-driven behavioral analysis identifies deviations from normal patterns, such as unusual device behavior or unauthorized access attempts.

(c) ML-Based Solutions:

(i) *Pattern Recognition:* Machine learning algorithms recognize patterns of malicious behavior or unusual data traffic, aiding in early threat detection.

(ii) *Dynamic Risk Assessment:* Machine learning can continuously assess the risk level of devices based on their behavior and context, triggering alerts for suspicious activities.

(d) Signature-Based Solutions:

(i) *Intrusion Detection Systems (IDS):* IDS [38] use predefined signatures to identify known attack patterns and anomalies, raising alerts or taking actions to mitigate threats.

(ii) *Anti-Malware Solutions:* Signature-based anti-malware tools identify and block known malware based on their recognized signatures.

(e) Hybrid Solutions:

(i) *Blockchain with IoT Security:* Combining blockchain with IoT security solutions enhances data integrity, device authentication, and secure updates.

(ii) *AI/ML with IoT Security:* Integrating AI and ML with IoT security improves threat detection accuracy and adaptive response capabilities.

It's important to note that the effectiveness of these solutions often lies in their integration and synergy. Combining multiple technologies allows for a more robust defines against the evolving landscape of IoT threats and attacks. Table 91.1 shows the real- life examples of different mentioned technologies that are providing security solutions

Table 91.1   Real life examples of technologies

Security Solutions	Examples
Blockchain-based solutions	Helium, The Things Network
AI-based solutions	Darktrace, CrowdStrike
ML-based solutions	Forti Guard Labs, Symantec
Signature-based solutions	Cisco Umbrella, Palo Alto Networks Wild Fire

7. Blockchain as a Potential Solution

IoT security has been bolstered using blockchain technology [39]. Blockchain consists of a series of interconnected blocks containing information. Although widely known for its use in cryptocurrencies, blockchain [40] also offers robust data protection capabilities. This technology operates as a decentralized ledger accessible to all. Whenever a new entry is added to the blockchain, altering it becomes extremely challenging due to the intricate interconnection of blocks, resembling a highly shared network. Each block comprises three key elements: data, a unique hash, and the hash of the preceding block. The specific data contained within a block varies according to its type. The hash serves as a distinct identifier for the block and is generated during the block's creation. Any modification made within a block lead to a change in its corresponding hash. The inclusion of the previous block's hash establishes the chain-like structure, forming the blockchain.

Drawing from our comprehension of blockchain structure, the fundamental advantages that blockchain contributes to enhancing IoT security are:

(i) *Distributed and Decentralized Characteristics:* The innate nature of blockchain disperses control, eliminating the vulnerability of a lone weak point.

(ii) *Immutable and Data Integrity Assurance:* Blockchain ensures data's unchangeable state, safeguarding its credibility against any tampering.

(iii) *Scalability Through Flexible Node Integration:* Blockchain's scalability stems from its adaptive node incorporation, allowing seamless expansion as required.

(iv) *Simplified IoT Device Authorization via Smart Contracts:* Smart contracts offer streamlined access regulations for IoT devices, notably simpler than conventional authorization methodologies.

8. Integration and Implementation Challenges

IoT combined with blockchain, being a developing technology, there exist numerous obstacles to conquer in order to fully realize the benefits of integrating blockchain with IoT. These considerable challenges [41][42] encompass security, scalability, performance, and the establishment of standards

(a) *Scalability:* Both IoT and blockchain [43] networks face a notable obstacle in terms of scalability. While managing a few IoT devices in a confined area is manageable, practical needs often require deploying and handling thousands of sensors or actuators. This undertaking necessitates specialized expertise to tackle scalability issues. These sensors gather extremely detailed data tied to their deployment environments. Therefore, it's vital to account for the ability to expand computing capabilities, data storage, bandwidth, and other related factors

(b) *Network and Communication Security:* Ensuring secure network and communication [44] environments is crucial This involves tackling issues like privacy, data integrity, error handling reliability, and availability, all of which are essential for robust IoT systems Regarding blockchain, relying solely on it for data privacy protection is not effective. This occurs because data on a public blockchain is typically not encrypted, enabling public validation. Introducing private data into a public chain complicates secure data sharing between IoT nodes and users' private data. Nevertheless, if an organization's IoT security focus is solely on user anonymity, anonymized user data (such as automated meters transactions) can be shared with nodes on the public blockchain to validate the information. In this scenario, the user's distinct account identity is enough for conducting transactions.

(c) *Interoperability & Standardization:* The variety of communication protocols and also the IoT devices makes it difficult to develop and implement consistent security standards for IoT systems [45]. Additionally, the rapid growth of the IoT market has led to a lack of uniformity in privacy controls, user agreements, third-party applications, and system update procedures. This lack of standardization can make IoT systems more vulnerable to attack.

(d) *Cost Factor:* Operating blockchain networks can incur substantial expenses, posing a hurdle for IoT applications working within constrained budgets.

(e) *Maintenance Challenges:* Unlike conventional devices, these IoT devices lack patchable firmware. This means when updates are required, new software must be reloaded or the entire device replaced. This complex maintenance process is a practical concern.

(f) *Blockchain Forking:* A significant issue in blockchain involves forking [46]. This term refers to the creation of multiple versions of the blockchain due to events like significant protocol updates, bug fixes, or attacks on the main protocol. For a fork to be deemed successful, it necessitates consensus among the majority of the network participants. In instances where some choose to adhere to the initial protocol, a division materializes.

9. Current Solutions and Future Direction

Looking towards the future, the landscape of blockchain-based security solutions in IoT holds great promise. As the Internet of Things continues to expand, the need for scalable, efficient, and secure solutions becomes paramount, few of the solutions are as follows

(a) *Sidechains:* Sidechains [47] constitute blockchains interconnected with a principal blockchain, referred to as the parent blockchain. This interlinkage employs a two-way peg, enabling asset transfers between the sidechain and the mainchain. Unlike the main blockchain, sidechains can employ their own consensus protocols, offering adaptability to particular requirements such as enhanced privacy or scalability. Nevertheless, some constraints exist. As a relatively new technology, sidechains have limitations that necessitate resolution before widespread adoption. For instance, they can be exposed to vulnerabilities and maintaining synchronization with the main blockchain might pose challenges. Remedies for these limitations include enhancing security through robust consensus protocols and more frequent synchronization to mitigate data loss or corruption risks.

(b) *Sharding:* The concept of sharding [48] holds substantial importance within this context. Sharding encompasses the division of a blockchain network into smaller units, referred to as shards, with the aim of amplifying scalability and transaction processing capacity. This strategy proves especially beneficial when paired with the Proof-of-Stake (PoS) consensus protocol, contributing to heightened effectiveness and lowered energy consumption. The amalgamation of sharding and PoS has the potential to offer advantages to participants with limited resources, like IoT users, granting them the ability to engage in decentralized transaction handling and accrue rewards while avoiding excessive energy expenses.

(c) *Confidential computing:* Despite the inherent security advantages presented by blockchain, concerns persist regarding the security and privacy of data during its processing. These concerns materialize when delicate information is accessible to the nodes responsible for verifying and executing transactions on the blockchain. Confidential computing emerges as a solution, enabling data processing within a secure environment, irrespective of the trustworthiness of the device or cloud service responsible for the data processing. trusted. This can be useful for IoT devices, which often collect sensitive data that needs to be protected from unauthorized access. Confidential computing [49] is proposed as a solution to the security challenges faced by blockchains. By integrating secure enclaves into the blockchain network, it becomes possible to keep sensitive data encrypted throughout the entire process, including validation, smart contract execution, and other transactions. Confidential computing can elevate blockchain security by keeping sensitive data encrypted and private throughout the data processing lifecycle. It addresses key challenges related to data exposure and privacy while maintaining the benefits of decentralization and trust that blockchain offers. The integration of confidential computing with blockchain has the potential to open up new opportunities for secure data processing in various industries.

(d) *Federated learning:* federated learning [50] is a machine learning approach that enables model training across multiple decentralized devices without the need to centralize the data. In federated learning, models are trained locally on individual devices using their respective data, and only the model updates (not the raw data) are shared with a central server. This approach preserves data privacy while allowing the collective learning from a distributed network. Integrating federated learning with blockchain technology addresses privacy concerns associated with centralized data processing. It enables IoT devices to collaboratively train models without sharing raw data while leveraging blockchain's security and decentralization. This combination holds promise for various industries seeking to harness the potential of IoT data while respecting privacy and security.

10. Conclusion

IoT is a swiftly expanding technology that interlinks billions of devices with the internet. This connectivity carries the potential to transform numerous industries, yet it also introduces novel security complexities. IoT devices often possess small dimensions, low power, and limited security attributes. Consequently, they are susceptible to breaches, and the sheer volume of such devices complicates comprehensive security measures. Blockchain can furnish an immutable transaction record, countering fraud and unauthorized entry. Additionally, blockchain can facilitate the construction of decentralized applications, which tend to be more secure than conventional centralized counterparts. Nevertheless, hurdles persist in adopting blockchain for IoT security, including integration, scalability, congestion, and sluggishness. Nonetheless, blockchain holds promise for enhancing IoT device security. Collaborations between blockchain and other technologies, such as federated learning, have the potential to establish more robust and dependable IoT systems. Further exploration and advancement are requisite to unlock the complete potential of blockchain in securing IoT devices

REFERENCES

1. Malik, A., Magar, A. T., Verma, H., Singh, M., and Sagar, P., "A detailed study of an internet of things (IoT)," International Journal of Scientific & Technology Research, vol. 8, no. 12, pp. 2989, 2019.
2. L. S. Vailshery, "Number of Internet of Things (IoT) connected devices worldwide from 2019 to 2023, with forecasts from 2022 to 2030," Published by Lionel Sujay Vailshery, Jul 27, 2023, [Online]. Available: https://www.statista.com/statistics/1183457/iot-connected-devices-worldwide/ [Accessed: Aug. 5, 2023].
3. S. Gupta, S. Tanwar, and N. Gupta, "A systematic review on internet of things (IoT): Applications & challenges," in 2022 11th International Conference on Computing, Information & Communication Technology (ICCIT), pp. 1-6, IEEE, 2022
4. M. K. Hasan, T. M. Ghazal, R. A. Saeed, B. Pandey, H. Gohel, A. A. Eshmawi, S. Abdel-Khalek, and H. M. Alkhassawneh, "A review on security threats, vulnerabilities, and counter measures of 5G enabled Internet-of-Medical-Things," Security and Communication Networks, 2022, pp. 1-21.
5. A. Kumar, A. K. Singh, I. Ahmad, P. K. Singh, Anushree, P. K. Verma, K. A. Alissa, M. Bajaj, A. U. Rehman, and E. Tag- Eldin, "A novel decentralized blockchain architecture for the preservation of privacy and data security against cyberattacks in healthcare," Sensors, vol. 22, no. 15, pp. 5921, doi: 10.3390/s22155921, 2022
6. G. Vats and P. K. Sharma, "An exhaustive analysis on security issues concerning IoT using blockchain," in 2023 International Conference on Disruptive Technologies (ICDT), pp. 101-108, IEEE, doi: 10.1109/ICDT51520.2023.00017, 2023
7. E. Schiller, A. Aidoo, J. Fuhrer, J. Stahl, M. Ziörjen, and B. Stiller, "Landscape of IoT security," Computers & Security, vol. 123, article 100467, doi: 10.1016/j.cosrev.2022.100467, 2022.

8. S. Dhar and I. Bose, "Securing IoT Devices Using Zero Trust and Blockchain," Journal of Organizational Computing and Electronic Commerce, vol. 31, no. 1, pp. 1-18, doi: 10.1080/10919392.2020.1831870, 2021.

9. M. S. Rahman, M. A. P. Chamikara, I. Khalil, and A. Bouras, "Blockchain-of-blockchains: An interoperable blockchain platform for ensuring IoT data integrity in smart city," Journal of Industrial Information Integration, vol. 30, pp. 100408, doi: 10.1016/j. jii.2022.100408, November 2022.

10. S. Saxena, B. Bhushan, and M. A. Ahad, "Blockchain based solutions to secure IoT: Background, integration trends and a way forward," Journal of Network and Computer Applications, vol. 181, pp. 103050, doi: 10.1016/j.jnca.2021.103050, 1 May 2021.

11. https://www.scopus.com/term/analyzer.uri?sort=plf&src=s&sid=b7b5bcdf35bcada2e897ddbe10bc985b&sot=a&sdt=a&s   l=66&s= TITLE-ABS- KEY%28Challenges+of+Securing+IoT+Devices+using+blockchain%29&origin=resultslist&count=10&analyzeResults =Analyze+results

12. https://www.scopus.com/term/analyzer.uri?sort=plff&src=s&sid=b7b5bcdf35bcada2e897ddbe10bc985b&sot=a&sdt=a&   sl=66&s= TITLE-ABS- KEY%28Challenges+of+Securing+IoT+Devices+using+blockchain%29&origin=resultslist&count=10&analyzeResults =Analyze+results

13. https://www.scopus.com/term/analyzer.uri?sort=plf&src=s&sid=b7b5bcdf35bcada2e897ddbe10bc985b&sot=a&sdt=a&s   l=66&s= TITLE-ABS-KEY%28Challenges+of+Securing+IoT+Devices+using+blockchain%29&origin=resultslist&count=10&analyzeResults =Analyze+results

14. Davis, B. D., Mason, J. C., & Anwar, M. (2020). Vulnerability studies and security postures of IoT devices: A smart home case study. 80(1), 1-21. doi:10.1007/s11042-020-08783-1

15. A., Rejeb, K., Treiblmaier, H., Appolloni, A., Alghamdi, S., Alhasawi, Y., Iranmanesh, M. (2023). The Internet of Things (IoT) in healthcare: Taking stock and moving forward. Internet of Things, 22(10), 100721. doi:10.1016/j.iot.2023.100721

16. Kumar, A., Singh, A. K., Ahmad, I., Singh, P. K., Anushree, Verma, P. K., Alissa, K. A., Bajaj, M., Rehman, A. U., & Tag-Eldin, E. (2022). A novel decentralized blockchain architecture for the preservation of privacy and data security against cyberattacks in healthcare. Sensors, 22(15), 5921. doi:10.3390/s22155921

17. A. Hazra, M. Adhikari, T. Amgoth, and S. N. Srirama, "A Comprehensive Survey on Interoperability for IIoT: Taxonomy, Standards, and Future Directions," ACM Computing Surveys, vol. 55, no. 1, Article No. 9, pp. 1-35, 2022. DOI: 10.1145/3485130.

18. Samih, H. (2019). Smart cities and internet of things. Journal of Information Technology Case and Application Research, 21(1), 3- 12. doi:10.1080/15228053.2019.158757

19. D. Sharma, D. Vaishnav, D. Joshi, G. K. Sharma, and D. Trivedi, "A Review: Development of Smart Agriculture Using IoT, Agriculture Robots and Wireless Sensory Network," in Artificial Intelligence and Communication Technologies, SCRS, India, 2023, pp. 167-176. DOI: 10.52458/978-81-955020-5-9-17.

20. H. Shee, T. de Vass, and S. J. Miah, "IoT in Supply Chain Management: Opportunities and Challenges for Businesses in Early Industry 4.0 Context," Operations and Supply Chain Management: An International Journal, Nov. 2020. DOI: 10.31387/oscm0450293.

21. Ch. Sandeep, S. Naresh Kumar, and P. Pramod Kumar, "Significant Role of Security in IoT Development and IoT Architecture," Journal of Modern Communication and Measurement Systems, vol. 15, p. 06, Jun. 2020. DOI: 10.26782/jmcms.2020.06.00014.

22. R. Román-Castro, J. López, and S. Gritzalis, "Evolution and Trends in IoT Security," Computer, vol. 51, no. 7, Jul. 2018. DOI: 10.1109/ MC.2018.3011051.

23. E. Semeniak and A. Katrenko, "Internet of Things (IoT) Security: Challenges and Best Practices," White Paper, Apriorit, Feb. 17, 2022, [URL: https://www.apriorit.com/white-papers/513-iot-security].

24. X. Feng, X. Zhu, Q.-L. Han, W. Zhou, S. Wen, and Y. Xiang, "Detecting Vulnerability on IoT Device Firmware: A Survey," IEEE/CAA Journal of Automatica Sinica, vol. 10, no. 1, pp. xx-xx, Jan. 2023. DOI: 10.1109/JAS.2022.105860.

25. J. Saleem, M. Hammoudeh, U. Raza, B. Adebisi, and R. Ande, "IoT standardisation: challenges, perspectives and solution," in ICFNDS '18: Proceedings of the 2nd International Conference on Future Networks and Distributed Systems, Jun. 2018, Article No. 1, pp. 1-9. DOI: 10.1145/3231053.3231103.

26. T. Bahirat, "Top 9 IoT Vulnerabilities to Enhance IoT Security in 2023," Website Name, Jun. 16, 2023. [Online]. Available: [https:// www.g2.com/articles/iot-vulnerabilities]. Accessed: [10-08-2023].

27. Aldowah, H., Rehman, S. U., & Umar, I. (2020). Security in internet of things: Issues, challenges and solutions. Security and Communication Networks, 2020, 1-16

28. M. Trnka, A. S. Abdelfattah, A. Shrestha, M. Coffey, and T. Cerny, "Systematic Review of Authentication and Authorization Advancements for the Internet of Things," Sensors, vol. 22, no. 4, p. 1361, Feb. 10, 2022. DOI: 10.3390/s22041361.

29. I. Stellios, P. Kotzanikolaou, and M. Psarakis, "Advanced Persistent Threats and Zero-Day Exploits in Industrial Internet of Things," in Security and Privacy Trends in the Industrial Internet of Things, pp. 47-68, ASTSA book series, First Online: May 14, 2019. DOI: 10.1007/978-3-030-24638-6_4.

30. Vats, G., & Sharma, P. K. (2023). An exhaustive analysis on security issues concerning IoT using blockchain. In 2023 International Conference on Disruptive Technologies (ICDT) (pp. 101-108). IEEE. doi:10.1109/ICDT51520.2023.00017

31. Damor Dinesh,IoT Security Threats and Solutions, Internet Of Things,Security & Surveillance access control, Aug. 2023. [Online]. Available: [https://www.exabeam.com/information-security/supply-chain-breaches-and-ot-iot-scenarios/]. Accessed: [18-06-23].

32. R. Isawa, K. Yoshioka, and D. Inoue, "A Cross-Platform Study on IoT Malware," DOI: 10.23919/ICMU.2018.8653580, Feb. 28, 2019.

33. Understanding Cybersecurity and IoT AI-powered Attacks," Triskele Labs. [Online]. Available: [https://www.triskelelabs.com/blog/understanding-cybersecurity-and-iot-ai-powered-attacks]. Accessed: [18-06-22]

34. M. Injadat, A. Moubayed, and A. Shami, "Detecting Botnet Attacks in IoT Environments: An Optimized Machine Learning Approach," in Proceedings of the 2020 32nd International Conference on Microelectronics (ICM), DOI: 10.1109/ICM50269.2020.9331794, Date Added to IEEE Xplore: Jan. 28, 2021

35. M. Sarhan, W. W. Lo, S. Layeghy, and M. Portmann, "HBFL: A Hierarchical Blockchain-based Federated Learning Framework for Collaborative IoT Intrusion Detection," Computers and Electrical Engineering, vol. 103, p. 108379, Oct. 2022. DOI: 10.1016/j.compeleceng.2022.108379.

36. A. Kumar, A. K. Singh, I. Ahmad, P. K. Singh, Anushree, P. K. Verma, K. A. Alissa, M. Bajaj, A. U. Rehman, and E. Tag- Eldin, "A Novel Decentralized Blockchain Architecture for the Preservation of Privacy and Data Security against Cyberattacks in Healthcare," Sensors, vol. 22, no. 15, p. 5921, Aug. 2022. DOI: 10.3390/s22155921.

37. T. Mazhar, D. B. Talpur, T. A. Shloul, Y. Y. Ghadi, I. Haq, I. Ullah, K. Ouahada, and H. Hamam, "Analysis of IoT Security Challenges and Its Solutions Using Artificial Intelligence," Brain Sciences, vol. 13, no. 4, p. 683, Feb. 2023. DOI: 10.3390/brainsci13040683.

38. P. Oulianou, V. Vasilakis, I. Moscholios, and others, "A Signature-based Intrusion Detection System for the Internet of Things," in Proceedings of the Information and Communication Technology Forum, Jul. 11-13, 2018. (In Press).

39. M. T. Oyshi, M. Z. Bonny, S. Saha, and Z. N. Tumpa, "IoT Security Issues and Possible Solution Using Blockchain Technology," in Advances in Distributed Computing and Machine Learning, pp. 113-121, Jan. 2021. DOI: 10.1007/978- 981-15-4218-3_12.

40. O. Nwosu, "The Key to Security: Combining IoT and Blockchain Technology," Analytics Vidhya, Feb. 20, 2023. [Online]. Available: [https://www.analyticsvidhya.com/blog/2023/02/the-key-to-security-combining-iot-and-blockchain- technology/]. Accessed: [20-07-23

41. H. F. Atlam, A. Alenezi, M. O. Alassafi, and G. Wills, "Blockchain with Internet of Things: Benefits, Challenges, and Future Directions," International Journal of Intelligent Systems and Applications, vol. 10, no. 6, pp. 40-48, [2030]. DOI: 10.5815/ijisa.2018.06.05]

42. A. Davies, "What are the Challenges of Adopting Blockchain in IoT?" AI Expert, [Online]. Available: [https://www.devteam.space/blog/blockchain-iot-challenges/]. Accessed: [30-07-23]

43. D. Khan, T. J. Low, and M. A. Hashmani, "Systematic Literature Review of Challenges in Blockchain Scalability," Appl. Sci., vol. 11, no. 20, p. 9372, Oct. 9, 2021. DOI: 10.3390/app11209372.

44. O. Nwosu, "The Key to Security: Combining IoT and Blockchain Technology," Analytics Vidhya, Published: Feb. 20, 2023. [Online]. Available: [https://www.analyticsvidhya.com/blog/2023/02/the-key-to-security-combining-iot-and- blockchain-technology/]

45. "Developing Open and Interoperable DLT/Blockchain Standards," Computer, vol. 51, no. 11, pp. 106-111, Nov. 2018. DOI: 10.1109/MC.2018.2876184.

46. F. Jameel, M. Nabeel, M. A. Jamshed, and R. Jäntti, "Minimizing Forking in Blockchain-Based IoT Networks," in Proceedings of the 2020 IEEE International Conference on Communications Workshops (ICC Workshops), Dublin, Ireland, Jun. 7-11, 2020. DOI: 10.1109/ICCWorkshops49005.2020.9145159.

47. R. S. Vairagade and B. S. H., "Enabling Machine Learning-Based Side-Chaining for Improving QoS in Blockchain- Powered IoT Networks," IEEE Transactions on Emerging Topics in Computing, vol. x, no. x, pp. xx-xx, Dec. 23, 2021. DOI: 10.1002/ett.4433.

48. Z. Yang, R. Yang, F. R. Yu, M. Li, Y. Zhang, and Y. Te, "Sharded Blockchain for Collaborative Computing in the Internet of Things: Combined of Dynamic Clustering and Deep Reinforcement Learning Approach," IEEE Internet of Things Journal, vol. 9, no. 17, pp. 16494-16509, Sep. 1, 2022. DOI: 10.1109/JIOT.2022.3152188.

49. D. C. G. Valadares, N. C. Will, M. A. Spohn, D. F. de S. Santos, A. Perkusich, and K. C. Gorgônio, "Confidential Computing in Cloud/Fog-Based Internet of Things Scenarios," Internet of Things, vol. 19, p. 100543, Aug. 2022. DOI: 10.1016/j.iot.2022.100543.

50. M. Ali, H. Karimipour, and M. Tariq, "Integration of Blockchain and Federated Learning for Internet of Things: Recent Advances and Future Challenges," Computers & Security, vol. 108, p. 102355, Sep. 2021. DOI: 10.1016/j.cose.2021.102355.

Printed in the United States
by Baker & Taylor Publisher Services